BREATHING

*Physiology, Environment
and Lung Disease*

BREATHING

Physiology, Environment and Lung Disease

AREND BOUHUYS, M.D.

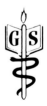

Grune & Stratton

A Subsidiary of Harcourt Brace Jovanovich, Publishers

New York   San Francisco   London

Library of Congress Cataloging in Publication Data
Bouhuys, Arend, 1925-
    Breathing; physiology, environment and lung disease.
    Includes bibliographies.
    1. Lungs—Diseases. 2. Environmentally induced
diseases. 3. Respiration. I. Title. [DNLM: 1. Air
pollution. 2. Lung diseases. 3. Respiration. WF102
B759b 1974]
RC732.B65   616.2'4   74-1283
ISBN 0-8089-0758-1

Grune & Stratton, Inc.
111 Fifth Avenue
New York, New York 10003

Library of Congress Catalog Card Number 74-1283
International Standard Book Number 0-8089-0758-1
Printed in the United States of America

To Henk, Margreet and Welmoed

Dum spiro, spero.

Contents

Preface

Respiratory physiologists have usually directed their research toward the solution of practical problems of human health. W. Einthoven studied mechanics of breathing in order to understand bronchial asthma. J. S. Haldane's interest in gas exchange was stimulated by his experience with people exposed to gas in mines. A. Krogh started a school of physiology aimed at improving human performance during exercise and sports. Today, many respiratory physiologists apply their knowledge to problems of air pollution, cigarette smoking, occupational exposures, and other environmental causes of lung disease.

If environmental lung disease is to be prevented and controlled, then systematic studies will be necessary in lung physiology and in lung function changes induced by environmental exposures. These studies must combine the tools of both physiology and epidemiology. Hence, this book has a dual focus. Its first part provides a framework of knowledge concerning respiratory physiology, emphasizing areas which are important in physiopathology. The second part deals with lung diseases induced by environmental exposures, with emphasis on the use of physiological, biochemical and other specialized techniques in epidemiological studies of environmental lung diseases.

The book is intended to provide physicians and medical students with basic concepts of respiratory physiology and environmental lung disease. However, I hope that many chapters will also be useful to others, including epidemiologists, environmental engineers, and public health professionals, who need information on respiratory function and its relevance to important public health problems. In addition, I hope this book may help to attract molecular biochemists and cellular biologists to research on environmental lung disease; their work is essential to increase our knowledge of cellular and subcellular systems in the lungs and airways.

Given the increasingly multidisciplinary nature of lung-disease research, I have tried to avoid medical jargon when possible. In addition, I have attempted to provide a guide through the maze of current literature in the areas covered by this book. As a result, many chapters resemble review articles on specific topics. The book grew out of lectures on respiratory physiology, inhaled pollutants, and lung diseases that I have presented during the past ten years to a variety of audiences. They included students, physicians and air pollution experts, public health specialists and textile mill managers, music teachers and union officials. What they had in common was an interest in breathing mechanisms, in how the lungs work, what harms them and what can be done to improve respiratory health. I hope this book will answer some of their questions and those of the many types of professionals whose work is needed to make progress against lung disease.

Arend Bouhuys, M.D., Dr. med. Sci.

Professor of Medicine and Epidemiology,
Director of Yale University Lung Research Center,
Fellow of the John B. Pierce Foundation,
Yale University School of Medicine,
New Haven, Connecticut

Acknowledgments

I am indebted to my colleagues and the staff of the Yale University Lung Research Center, who have contributed their work, thoughts, and criticism to this book, and who have relieved me from tasks both small and large while I wrote it.

I am also grateful to many sponsoring agencies and institutions which have supported my research and that of the Lung Research Center, including the National Heart and Lung Institute, the National Institute for Occupational Safety and Health, the National Air Pollution Control Agency, the Connecticut Lung Association, the John B. Pierce Foundation, and the estate of the late Beulah S. Hinds.

Each chapter has been reviewed by at least two colleagues; their comments have proved invaluable in preparing the final text. The reviewers are Drs. J. Brain, W. A. Burgess, J. Charpin, A. C. DeGraff, Jr., J. S. Douglas, L. E. Farhi, S. K. Friedlander, J. B. L. Gee, G. Giebisch, H. Heimann, J. Hildebrandt, R. E. Hyatt, M. J. Jaeger, D. E. Leith, P. Lieberman, P. T. Macklem, the late C. B. McKerrow, E. K. Motoyama, S. Permutt, D. F. Proctor, D. Rall, R. L. Riley, S. A. Rooney, R. S. F. Schilling, F. Speizer, R. S. Sikand, S. Weissman, J. B. West; R. Hosein, M.Sc., and J. B. Schoenberg, M.Phil., M.P.H. Special thanks are due to Dr. R. H. Kellogg for his detailed review of Chapter 10 and Dr. C. A. Mitchell for reviewing many chapters. Needless to say, any remaining errors, omissions and inaccuracies are my own.

The book would never have been completed without the meticulous and concerted hard work of Susan K. Hunsinger, M.S., who edited the manuscript in several stages, and greatly improved its organization and language. My thanks also to Dolores M. Piscitelli, who cheerfully took charge of the details associated with preparing a large number of illustrations, and to Salvatore Dattilo and my wife Fenna G. Bouhuys, who prepared them. Marion M. Bruch and other members of our secretarial staff typed and corrected many revisions of the manuscript. The assistance of Susan Hunsinger and of my wife in proofreading, reference checking and indexing was crucial in meeting a tight publishing schedule.

I am also indebted to the following authors, publishers and journals who gave their permission to use illustrations and tabular material for inclusion in the book:

Authors: O. Auerbach, R. Benesch, E. J. Caldwell, F. J. Clarke, S. W. Clarke, R. M. Cherniack, C. D. Cook, D. Crowley, P. Dejours, R. V. Ebert, J. Emery, L. E. Farhi, M. J. Fisher, R. E. Forster, D. L. Fry, J. George, J. C. Gilson, W. W. L. Glenn, R. B. Helgerson, W. W. Holland, D. Hourihane, R. E. Hyatt, R. H. Kellogg, R. Lefrançois, J. P. Lyons, J. Mead, J. Milic-Emili, E. K. Motoyama, J. T. Parer, H. Parker, J. B. Paton, E. P. Pendergrass, J. A. Pierce, D. F. Proctor, H. Rahn, P. E. Rauwerda, F. Ruff, P. W. Scherer, W. Schoedel, R. C. Schroter, H. Spencer, N. C. Staub, S. M. Tenney, E. R. Weibel, J. B. West, J. P. Wyatt, H. Yamabayashi.

Publishers and Journals: Academic Press, Inc.; Acta Medica Scandinavica; Acta Physiologica Scandinavica; American Journal of Medicine; The American Journal of Pathology; American Journal of Physiology; Annals of the New York Academy of Sciences; Annals of Surgery; American Physiological Society; Archives of Environmental Health; British Medical Journal; Clinical Science; Wm. Heinemann Medical Books, Ltd.; Journal of Applied Physiology; The Journal of Clinical Investigation; The Journal of Pharmacology and Experimental Therapeutics; S. Karger; The Lancet; Le Poumon et le Coeur; McGraw-Hill; Nature; Nederlands Tijdschrift voor Geneeskunde; Pergamon Press, Ltd.; Pflügers Archiv; Royal Dublin Society Scientific Proceedings; Science; Charles C Thomas, Publisher; Thorax.

The staff of Grune and Stratton, Inc., has given invaluable help in preparing the manuscript for publication. I remember with gratitude the initial stimulation I received from the late Siegmund F. Kurzer, Vice-President.

To all these persons, and many others, my sincere thanks.

PART I

Physiology

Unless we understand the function of an organ system, we cannot fully understand the diseases that affect it. The physiology of today remains the medicine of tomorrow—and in the years since E. H. Starling wrote these words the scope of both physiology and of medicine have greatly expanded and become more diversified. Part I of this book (Chaps. 1-11) is thus devoted to the physiology of breathing. In addition to presenting a framework of knowledge concerning lung development, lung and airway function, and the control of breathing, Part I also includes many clinical applications, both present and future. Since the second part of the book focuses on environmental exposures, the two parts together can be viewed as an attempt to apply one particular field of physiology to one particular area of medicine with prevention and control of environmental lung disease as the final goal.

To introduce the physiology section, Chapter 1 describes how the lungs develop from the first fetal months to the newborn infant's cry—and beyond. Chapters 2-3 focus on the airways which are more than passive conduits for inspired and expired gas. Chapter 2 describes airway morphology and structure, and discusses airway function in heat and water exchange and in protecting the lungs against entry and accumulation of foreign matter. Chapter 3 deals with gas transport mechanisms and the volume of conducting airways, the anatomical dead space.

Gas exchange (Chaps. 4-6) between inspired gas and tissues involves a complex chain of events. Chapter 4 describes an initial step in this process—the distribution of inspired gas to different regions of the lungs and its mixing with alveolar gas. Chapter 5 deals with the "dialogue" between air and blood in the alveoli, where O_2 and CO_2 exchange is chiefly determined by the ratio of alveolar ventilation and lung capillary blood flow. Chapter 6 traces oxygen transport from alveolar gas to the cells' mitochondria by diffusion through alveolocapillary and red cell membranes, binding to hemoglobin, and diffusion from capillary blood into the cells.

The section on lung mechanics (Chaps. 7-9) might be expected to focus on a simple pumping function: as the lungs and chest suck in atmospheric air and expel air containing less oxygen and more carbon dioxide, alveolar air is renewed. Although, for many purposes, such a simple model is sufficient, lung mechanics is more than the study of an ingenious pump system ventilating through a complex system of pipes. It also involves the basic physical properties of lung tissue and the details of lung structure which determine transmission of forces; lung mechanics can lead to study of airways and lungs as biological systems. Measurement of mechanical parameters, although an imperfect reflection of the physical system, helps assess changes in lungs and airways which result from disease, drugs, and other agents. In an attempt to treat lung mechanics in this broader sense, Chapter 7 describes the properties of the lungs and chest cage during volume displacements. The relations between driving pressures and airflow through airways are discussed in Chapter 8. Chapter 9 describes flow-volume curves and their applications.

The final chapters in the physiology section discuss the motor control of breathing. Chapter 10 describes breathing mainly as an involuntary motor act, controlled by a neuronal network in the brain stem which initiates rhythmic breathing and modifies its pattern guided by information concerning lung inflation, respiratory muscle tension and arterial blood gas composition received from different types of sensors. Chapter 11 focuses on breathing as a voluntary motor act in the service of interhuman communication via speech, singing, and wind-instrument playing. This function of the breathing apparatus emphasizes the integration of the control of breathing with the control of other motor acts.

Chapter 1

Development of the Breathing Apparatus

Growth and differentiation of tissues and organs are regulated by information contained in the genetic code. How this information is transcribed during the development of a fertilized egg into a full-grown organism remains a mystery. Gross morphological development is well understood in a descriptive sense, but we do not know the mechanisms that bring about the rapid and profound changes in a developing organism. How the biochemical machinery of the body and its capacity to respond to exogenous agents, such as drugs, develop is virtually unknown. The surfactant system of the lungs is a prime example of the difficulties remaining in this field. In this chapter, we will consider chiefly the lungs' morphological development, the maturation of the surfactant system, and the maturation of the neuromuscular system that controls chest motion and affects airway caliber. We will also review aspects of lung and chest growth that can be measured in vivo. Several other developmental aspects of breathing, such as fetal gas exchange and the initiation of breathing in newborn infants, have been discussed in recent monographs and reviews [3, 17, 21] (see also Chap. 10, p. 224).

MORPHOLOGICAL DEVELOPMENT

When the human fetus is about 3 mm long, the lungs begin to form. A groove develops from the foregut and ends in a small pouch. This pouch and a mass of tissue around it form the *primary lung bud*. The foregut grows rapidly and forms the esophagus and trachea. The primary lung bud splits into left and right buds, and these divide further to begin the bronchial tree. During the first 4 months of fetal life—the *glandular period*—the whole tissue mass grows rapidly. The primitive airways that are formed are open from the beginning: at no stage of lung development is the tissue solid.[21] The *canalicular period* follows, and the newly formed bronchi divide further and the amount of connective tissue between them decreases. Increased numbers of blood vessels now enter the lungs. Although the epithelium flattens out, there is still enough tissue between epithelium and blood

3

vessels to prevent effective gas exchange. At this stage, in a human fetus of about 30 weeks gestation, flattened epithelium was found in the terminal bronchioles and saccules, but no alveoli had as yet formed.[11] The airways terminated in relatively wide saccules from which, presumably, alveoli develop later on. Although there was a considerable amount of interstitial tissue between epithelium and blood vessels, the lung had some gas exchange capability; the infant survived 19 hours.

In the last 8 or 10 weeks of pregnancy, the *alveolar period* begins. The new alveoli are shallow and small, and they are formed only in the walls of the terminal saccules.[11] The epithelium flattens out further, and the amount of connective tissue between it and the blood vessels decreases. There is some dispute concerning the time of alveoli formation. Boyden [11] states that a few small and shallow alveoli are formed before birth, while Reid [42] believes that all alveoli are formed after birth. Part of the dispute may be a matter of semantics—are the superficial, thin-walled formations in the walls of the tubes shown in Figure 1-1 true alveoli or not? There is, however, agreement that most alveoli are formed after birth. According to Emery,[21] the development of an elastic tissue network is an essential part of new alveoli formation. At birth there are only a few elastic fibers around terminal airways; during postnatal growth collagen fibers are converted into elastic fibers, making this network more extensive and dense.

The elastic tissue network helps the lungs recoil to a smaller volume during expiration, and Emery [21] believes that it also promotes alveolar development. The elastic fibers curve around existing alveoli and indent their walls (Fig. 1-2). This is the first method of alveoli formation—*peripheral alveolar segmentation*. Similarly, the septa between the alveoli are indented; this is called *alveolar wall*

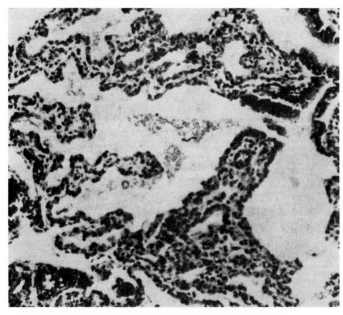

Fig. 1-1. Photograph ($\times$140) from the lung of a stillborn human fetus of 30 weeks gestation. The lumen is distended with liquor amnii. Note the formation of early alveolar ducts. Distinct connective tissue is obvious between the cavities. From Emery.[21]

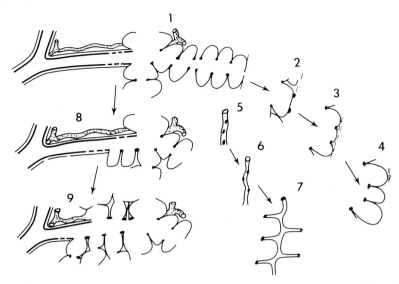

Fig. 1-2. Diagram showing methods of proliferation of alveoli as suggested by changes in the elastic tissue: (*1*) at birth; (*2, 3,* and *4*) peripheral alveolar segmentation; (*5, 6,* and *7*) alveolar wall compoundment; (*8* and *9*) fragmentation of terminal respiratory passage. From Emery.[21]

compoundment. Finally, there is a thick layer of elastic fibers in bronchiolar walls. Gaps develop in this network, and alveoli form by protrusion through holes in the elastic structure. Eventually, little of the bronchiolar wall remains but the ends of the septa (Fig. 1-3). This formation of alveoli by "eating away at the bronchioles" is called *fragmentation of terminal respiratory passages.*

In man, the total number of epithelialized airways increases slightly from birth up to age 1; from that age on the number declines. At the same time, the total number of alveoli increases rapidly. This is indirect evidence for conversion of conducting airways into alveolar ducts and alveoli. Boyden and Tompsett[12] observed in dog lung lobes that some airways disappeared in the process of alveolar formation. During the first 10 days after birth, conducting airways were rapidly altered into gas-exchanging units. Shortly before birth, airways lined with cuboid epithelium could be found at a distance less than 0.5 mm from the pleura. Ten days after birth, in another specimen, this distance was more than 3 mm. Boyden and Tompsett propose that the terminal nonrespiratory passages become "drawn out" during the rapid process of lung expansion after birth and that new alveoli develop from these as shown in Figure 1-2 (*8* and *9*). As many as six generations of airways, counting from the lobar stem bronchus, are transformed to respiratory units in this process. From these descriptions it appears that alveolar development is slower in man than in the dog. Schwieler and Skoglund[49] found considerable variability in the number of branches on the main stem bronchi of two lobes in 6- to 11-week-old cats. The anatomist is at a technical disadvantage when making the number of observations that satisfies statisticians!

From this theory of lung development one would expect that early damage to terminal conducting airways could permanently arrest alveolar formation.[21] Alveolar hypoplasia may, in fact, occur peripheral to obstructed airways,[43] but it

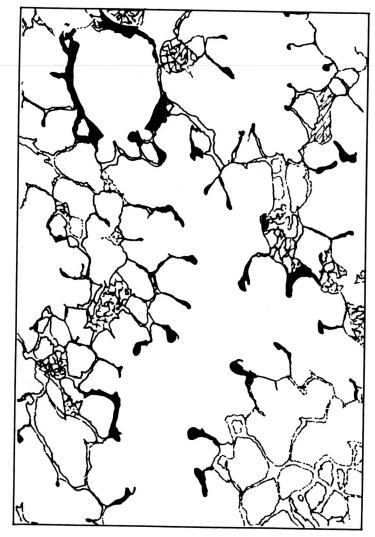

Fig. 1-3. Alveolar duct and alveoli, drawn after a preparation made by Staub.[52a] The rings of smooth muscle surrounding the entrance to the alveoli are seen as thickened endings of interalveolar septa.

is not certain whether, for instance, children who survive severe attacks of bronchiolitis sustain permanent damage to lung growth. Although controlled studies to answer this question are difficult to perform, it might help to know whether the total lung capacity remains small in children who have had severe bronchiolitis.

New alveoli are formed until at least age 7.[19] Data on a large number of lung samples have suggested that new alveoli might continue to form until early adulthood.[22] In any case, the increase in the number of alveoli during the teens is small. Large numbers of new alveoli are formed during the first decade of life, and at this age developmental arrest resulting from lung disease or even effects of pollutants on small airways might conceivably lead to permanent lung damage.

Cigarette smoke is perhaps the pollutant most worthy of concern in this context (Chap. 14).

Several aspects of morphological development have been traced in groups of small animals raised under controlled conditions. Rats treated with growth hormone become abnormally large, and their lung weight, lung volume, and alveolar surface area all grow in proportion to body weight.[7a] This is due to formation of new alveoli rather than to expansion of existing ones. If expansion were the main factor, alveolar surface would increase in proportion to the two-thirds power of lung volume; in fact, it increases more than that.

In newborn small animals, such as mice and rats, few alveoli are present at birth and these are similar in size to those of newborn infants and calves (diameter, 90–140 μm).[7b] Adult animals of these species have quite different alveolar diameters (about 20 μm in mice; 280 in men). Bartlett [7b] has pointed out that if newborn mice had more alveoli, their diameter would be very small and they would be highly susceptible to collapse.

Comparatively little is known about the development of specific tissue components of the lungs. A variety of *mucosal cells* occurs in small bronchioles of premature infants.[44b] In the rabbit, functional airway *smooth muscle* is present in the trachea at birth.[48] In smooth muscle cells (vas deferens of mice [57]), the Golgi apparatus and ribosomes appear at an early stage, while thin and thick myofilaments follow much later. There are apparently large differences between the development times of various kinds of smooth muscle. Bundles of *nerve fibers* are present around the trachea of a 35-mm long human fetus and begin to penetrate its wall to form an intrachondral plexus in the 100-mm fetus.[53] Nerve fibers to tracheal smooth muscle can be identified in the 100-mm fetus, and to mucous glands in the 140-mm long fetus. In the same study, nerve fibers to pulmonary arteries and veins were found in the 65-mm long fetus. The continued postnatal development of the *pulmonary arterial system* has been studied in human lung specimens.[16]

DEVELOPMENT OF THE ALVEOLAR LINING

Respiratory physiologists often picture the lungs as consisting of bubbles (alveoli) at the end of tubes (airways). Morphologists may scoff at such a naive idea, but this has been a productive model of the lungs. It led Von Neergaard [36] to realize that surface force could play an essential role in the lungs' recoil force. By comparing the recoil of air-filled lungs with that of liquid-filled lungs, he found that two-thirds to three-quarters of the total lung recoil force is caused by surface tension at the alveolar air-liquid interface. Recent measurements of stress relaxation [28] have suggested that surface tension accounts for 7/8 of the total viscoelastic force, and tissue proper for only 1/8, not far from Von Neergaard's estimate. Von Neergaard also realized that the newborn animal must overcome surface forces in the alveoli when inflating the lungs for the first time, and that this requires a large inspiratory force. But this force might be less if "the surface tension of the alveoli is decreased, in comparison with other physiological solutions, through enrichment by surface-active substances, according to Gibbs-

Thomson's law." This suggestion of Von Neergaard has been amply confirmed, although it took nearly 30 years.

The more recent history of lung surfactant is well known and has been ably reviewed.[33, 40, 45] Studies of fetal lambs have shown that surfactant material begins to develop at a well-defined moment during gestation (after about 128 days of a 147-day gestation).[38] After about 135 days gestation, enough surfactant has been formed to allow safe transition to air breathing after birth. When delivered before 135 days gestation, newborn lambs do not breathe well and their condition resembles the respiratory distress syndrome of human newborns.[44] This happens even when asphyxia is prevented, so that prematurity, and not asphyxia, appears to be the crucial event. In these studies the appearance of lung surfactant was usually deduced from measurements of the surface tension of lung extracts. More recently the anatomical substrate for surfactant formation has been clarified by electron microscope studies of the two main types of cells in the alveolar wall. Kikkawa et al.[31] compared the morphological appearance of alveolar type II epithelial cells (i.e., large cells with inclusion bodies) with the absence or presence of surface activity in lung extracts, at various stages of development in fetal and newborn lambs. Surface activity was first detected a few days after osmiophilic inclusion bodies appeared in type II cells (Fig. 1-4). These bodies first appear at about 121 days gestation, and they increase in number and size as the lungs mature. Large osmiophilic bodies are often found near the cell surface, where it is likely that they deposit their contents. Several investigators have now shown a lining layer of similar osmiophilic material on the surface of the alveolar epithelium. Although the layer's origin in the osmiophilic bodies of the type II cells

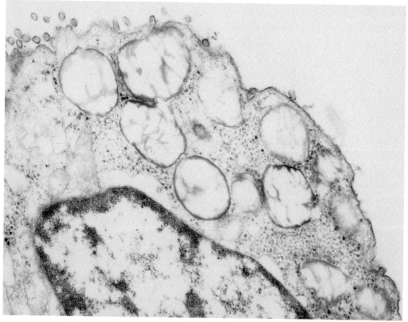

Fig. 1-4. Type II cell ($\times$10,000) in the lungs of a lamb fetus (135th day of gestation). There are clumped ribosomes and inclusion bodies in the cytoplasm. Surface activity is normal. From Kikkawa et al.[31]

is not fully established, it appears likely. The presence of the layer correlates with surface activity in lung extracts, and the layer is absent in immature animals whose lungs collapse after birth. The surface lining layer remains particularly well conserved when tissue is fixed by perfusing the pulmonary vessels rather than by filling the air spaces with liquid.[25]

The chemical nature of the surfactant material in vivo is not certain. Most likely it is a phospholipid compound. In particular, disaturated lecithin is probably an important component of surfactant; its presence correlates with alveolar surface area in 11 different vertebrate species, including man, and surfactant shows a similar correlation.[15] In vivo, the lipid component of surfactant may be bound to protein. Although tissue extractions may yield a protein-free lipid, this may result from lipoprotein breakdown during the preparative procedures.[46] King and Clements [32] have extracted four highly surface-active fractions, at least 40 times enriched, from dog lung. All consisted of lipid and protein, and all decreased surface tension and formed films on air-liquid interfaces. All four contained large amounts of lecithin.

Lung tissue can synthesize phospholipids from acetate in vitro; most of the acetate is incorporated in lecithin.[35] It is not certain which cells perform the synthesis, but type I cells are unlikely candidates since they possess few intracellular organelles. Type II cells, in contrast, appear to be highly active metabolically and thus more suitable for this role. Tombropoulos [54] concludes that microsomes, as well as mitochondria, can synthesize lecithin from its components; mitochondria are better in synthesizing long-chain fatty acids from acetate, while microsomes are more active in esterification. Recent work by Page-Roberts [39] shows that a purified lamellar body fraction from rat lung was surface-active and had a much higher phospholipid content than that of mitochondrial and microsomal fractions. Further studies [44a] show that the phospholipid content of the lamellar body fraction is similar to that of lung wash (which represents surfactant), and that its saturated fatty acid content is much higher than that in other fractions. These findings support the importance of the lamellar body in synthesizing surfactant.

In humans, prematurity and its accompanying lack of surfactant production are associated with a severe and often fatal condition known as the idiopathic respiratory distress syndrome (IRDS) of the newborn. As a result of insufficient surfactant, the lungs have a greatly increased recoil force and tend to collapse during each expiration, often resulting in atelectasis. Recently, clinical improvement has been obtained when such infants were ventilated with continuous positive airway pressure, to counteract the lung's increased recoil.[26] Another feature of the respiratory distress syndrome is the formation of curious hyaline membranes in the air spaces of the lungs. The membranes are probably formed from fibrin, derived from transudation of plasma into the air spaces.[25a] In the healthy fetal lamb, the alveolar epithelium is an effective barrier against passage of such large molecules as proteins, and thus normal alveolar fluid contains very little protein.[37] When immature lambs are ventilated, this barrier breaks and the alveolar epithelium then becomes permeable to proteins. Therefore, leakage of the alveolar epithelium appears to promote hyaline membrane formation in the lungs of infants with respiratory distress.

The respiratory distress syndrome is self-limiting—if the infant survives long enough, the lungs mature and sufficient surfactant will be formed. Clinically, most surviving infants appear to have no permanent pulmonary damage, although lung fibrosis occurs in some.[50] Thus, such symptomatic treatment as continuous positive pressure may be essential for survival. In addition, it may be possible to speed up surfactant formation with drugs. There is evidence that treating the unborn rabbit with corticosteroids may accelerate surfactant formation and increase survival chances after transition to air breathing.[32a, 34] However, the mechanism of action is as yet unclear. Direct injection of cortisol or thyroxine into the rabbit fetus (2–3 days before premature delivery) caused an earlier appearance of surfactant and maturation of type II cells (Fig. 1-4). Also, the lungs were better aerated after delivery than those of control litter mates.[34, 56a] Experiments with drugs that affect microsomal or mitochondrial metabolism or specific steps in the synthesis of lung lipids could help unravel the events in lung maturation and at the same time yield important therapeutic results. Along these lines, Kikkawa and Motoyama [30] have recently treated rabbits with an inhibitor of cholesterol synthesis (AY-9944) and found that this delayed lung tissue maturation while at the same time abnormally large numbers of type II cells appeared. Morphological development and surfactant maturation did not proceed at the same pace. It seems obvious that there are specific biochemical pathways for surfactant formation, and these appear to be, in part, independent of tissue growth and alveolar formation.

NEUROMUSCULAR MATURATION

Coordination of breathing requires a mature neuromuscular apparatus to move the chest bellows. To do this, all components of the system must function adequately—coordinating centers as well as peripheral nerve fibers, neuromuscular junctions, and muscle fibers. The newborn infant lacks coordinated control over many motor acts; there is also evidence that central as well as peripheral nerve fibers need to mature considerably after birth in many animals. But the steps that limit motor control development are not clear. Is it the learning process, or is it immaturity of one or other anatomical components of the system? With more insight into this basic question, we might eventually be able to correlate physiological events at the cellular level with behavioral aspects of development in infants and children. In respiration, this may improve understanding not only of the development of control over breathing itself (Chap. 10), but also of other motor acts, such as speech, that use the respiratory bellows (Chap. 11).

Here we describe some aspects of development of peripheral neuromuscular elements. Peripheral myelinated nerve fibers mature considerably after birth, increasing in both number and diameter.[52] When mature, the fibers are better able to transmit impulses continually and at high frequencies.[47] In part, their relative functional incompetence in the immature stage may be a consequence of their small size. In addition, metabolic factors may be important.[48] Autonomic nerve fibers, too, increase in number and size during postnatal development.[58] For instance, the hearts of 1–2-day-old rabbits contain few adrenergic fibers; they also contain little epinephrine.[23]

Physiological experiments also suggest that post-natal maturation occurs in peripheral nerve fibers. In our laboratory, Schwieler developed a technique that provides information on the functional competence of vagal and sympathetic nerve fibers to the trachea and the heart in rabbits.[48] Supramaximal stimulation at different rates was used in tracheotomized animals varying in age from less than 1 day to more than 6 months. The effects on the trachea were measured by recording the pressure inside a thin-walled balloon placed in a segment of the trachea above the tracheostomy. The response to vagal stimulation is shown in Figure 1-5. In older animals, contractions are well maintained at stimulation frequencies up to 200 impulses per second. In younger animals, however, they decrease before the end of the stimulation period at 30 and 50 impulses per second, and at 100 impulses per second the initial amplitude is also reduced. This decreasing response was not due to smooth muscle exhaustion, because less than 1 minute later a sustained maximum response could again be obtained by simply reducing the stimulation rate to 20 or 30 impulses per second. It also seemed unlikely that the neuromuscular junction limited the response to high-frequency stimulation. Other experiments showed that physostigmine can prevent the decrease of vagal responses at high stimulation frequencies. This made it clear that the end organ can follow repetitive stimuli at high frequencies, if only enough transmitter substance is available. Thus, these experiments suggested that the ability of immature vagal efferent fibers to conduct impulses at high rates is limited. In addition, these immature fibers are highly sensitive to effects of general anesthesia. For instance, in the results shown in Figure 1-6, sodium pentobarbital decreases the heart's response to vagal stimulation. The effect is seen in an adult as well as in an immature animal, but in the latter much less of the drug is required.

The response to stimulation of efferent sympathetic fibers often depends on the initial state of the tracheal muscle. For instance, in the experiment outlined in Figure 1-7, vagal stimulation contracted the tracheal muscle, while sympathetic stimulation alone had no effect. Only when the muscle tone was first increased by stimulating the vagus did sympathetic stimulation result in tracheal muscle relaxation. Like the vagal responses, sustained sympathetic responses in newborn animals occurred only at low stimulation frequencies.

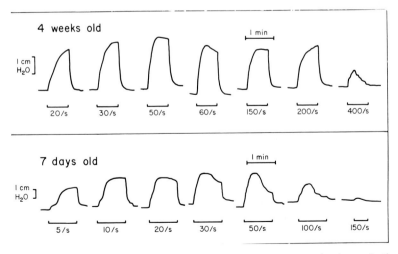

Fig. 1-5. Intratracheal pressure changes in response to supramaximal vagal stimulation in a 4-week-old and a 7-day-old rabbit. From Schwieler et al.[48]

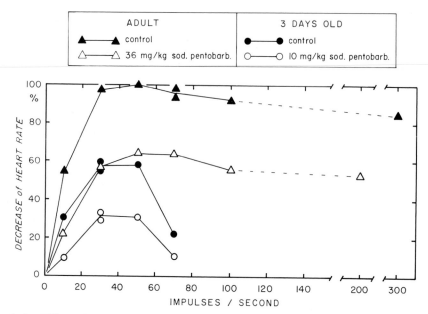

Fig. 1-6. Effect of sodium pentobarbital on heart rate response to supramaximal vagal stimulation in an adult and a 3-day-old rabbit. Control responses were obtained 1–2 hours after administering 1.5 gm/kg urethan and 20 mg/kg sodium pentobarbital to adult animal and 1 g/kg urethan and 10 mg/kg sodium pentobarbital to 3-day-old animal. Each dot represents decrease in mean heart rate (as a percentage of control value) produced by vagal stimulation for 20 sec. About 4 times more sodium pentobarbital is required in adult animal to produce a response decrease similar to that in 3-day-old animal. From Schwieler et al.[48]

From these results, as well as from other studies,[2, 18] it seems clear that the rabbit's trachea and heart have a functional efferent autonomic innervation at birth or very soon thereafter. But, apparently, important functional changes occur during the first 4–6 postnatal weeks, and these enable the nerve fibers to better conduct impulses at high stimulation rates for prolonged periods of time. Yet, the immature nerve fibers appear to participate effectively in reflex events. For instance, Downing[18] observed baroreceptor reflex activity on the heart in newborn rabbits. It seems likely, however, that the immature fibers can handle

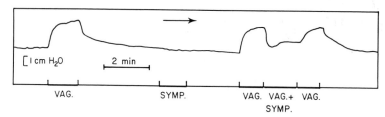

Fig. 1-7. Intratracheal pressure changes in response to supramaximal stimulation of right cervical vagal and sympathetic trunks at a stimulation frequency of 30 impulses per second in a 5-week-old rabbit. Tracheal smooth muscle relaxes in response to sympathetic stimulation only during simultaneous vagal stimulation. Upward deflection = pressure increase. From Schwieler et al.[48]

only short-lasting responses. During some of these evoked responses, vagal and sympathetic fibers fire at rates up to about 60 per second,[56] and immature fibers can transmit such impulse traffic only for short periods of time. In contrast with its competence during electrical stimulation and baroreceptor reflexes, the heart in newborn rabbits and other immature animals apparently does not respond to tonic vagal influences.[1, 2, 55] Vagotomy or atropine administration do not increase heart rate until a few weeks after birth. Perhaps even low-frequency stimuli (involved in maintaining vagal tone) are poorly conducted over long periods of time in immature autonomic fibers.

Impulse transmission decreases at high stimulation frequencies in immature pyramidal neurons in kittens,[29] as well as in preganglionic and postganglionic autonomic fibers. Since similar results have been obtained with somatic sensory nerve fibers, [20, 51] this may be a property of immature nerve fibers in general. It is hard to assess the physiological significance of nerve fiber immaturity in the development of such integrated responses as breathing and speech. If central [29] and peripheral [20, 48, 51, 52] neurons have common immature features, it is difficult to determine which component limits development of integrated motor acts and responses. Perhaps responses that require only low-frequency impulse traffic can develop earlier than those that require high rates of nerve-impulse conduction.

LUNG VOLUMES AND MECHANICS IN GROWING CHILDREN

Morphological data on lung development are difficult to obtain in sufficient quantity. On the other hand, measurements of lung volumes and other aspects of lung function are easily made, at least in older children, and these can clarify several aspects of growth. As children grow, their chest cages, lungs, and airways increase in size. This results in bigger lung volumes, larger maximum flow rates, and reduced resistance to airflow through airways. These changes correlate with height and age of the growing individual. Measurements of volumes and flow rates are useful to determine whether the lungs of a pediatric patient conform to normal limits,[41] but they can also increase understanding of lung growth in healthy children. The rationale and technical aspects of several of the tests are discussed in other chapters; here I discuss aspects that bear on lung and chest growth in older children, in whom accurate data can be obtained relatively simply.

Lung Volumes

Measurements of lung volumes are basic to most other lung function tests. The use of the body plethysmograph allows repeated and accurate studies of lung volumes, even in small children. Other methods, using gas dilution, require several minutes of quiet breathing through a mouthpiece, and errors due to leakage around the mouthpiece are a constant worry. With the plethysmograph, each volume measurement takes only a few seconds. Most children learn the maneuvers easily, and they like the space-age environment of the body box. The methods are also well suited for studying children with lung diseases.[60, 61]

Figure 1-8 shows data for total lung capacity (TLC), vital capacity (VC), and forced expiratory volume in 1 second ($FEV_{1.0}$) in boys and girls. (For defini-

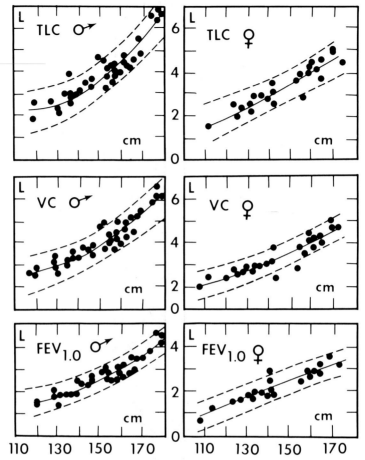

Fig. 1-8. TLC, VC, and FEV$_{1.0}$ versus body height (standing) in boys and girls. The drawn lines are regression equations; 95% confidence limits indicated by dashed lines. From Zapletal et al.[62]

tion of these variables, see p. 189.) In teen-agers, both TLC and VC increase with height much more in boys than in girls. Table 1-1 contains additional data on lung volume in the same group of children and adolescents. The relations between lung volume and body height clearly depend on the degree of lung inflation. At minimum volume (RV), lung volume is linearly related to height in both sexes (Table 1-1). At maximum inflation (TLC), lung volume increases progressively more (per unit height increase) as growth proceeds, particularly in boys. TLC and VC values for adolescents are similar to those of adults of the same height and sex,[8] but observations in the age group 16–24 years are limited, and hence the prediction of "normal" TLC and VC data in this age range is relatively uncertain.

Pleural Pressure

A recent study of Zapletal et al.[59] suggests that lung elastic recoil increases with height in children who are less than 150 cm tall. For instance, in a 120-cm

Table 1-1
Statistical Analysis of Lung Volumes (L) Versus Body Height (cm)

y	Sex	N	a *	b	c	130 cm	150 cm	170 cm
TLC	♂	37	+15.1397	−0.22713	+0.001002	2.55 ±0.51	3.62 ±0.46	5.49 ±0.47
	♀	24	+1.7592	−0.03394	+0.000300	2.41 ±0.40	3.41 ±0.40	4.66 ±0.42
VC	♂	39	+7.9942	−0.12509	+0.000605	1.96 ±0.40	2.85 ±0.35	4.21 ±0.43
	♀	26	+0.1694	−0.01217	+0.000189	1.78 ±0.27	2.60 ±0.25	3.56 ±0.27
FRC	♂	37	+9.3716	−0.14152	−0.000602	1.15 ±0.36	1.70 ±0.34	2.71 ±0.36
	♀	24	−2.1776	+0.02556	0	1.11 ±0.27	1.66 ±0.25	2.17 ±0.28
RV	♂	37	−1.0519	+0.01270	0	0.60 ±0.27	0.85 ±0.26	1.11 ±0.29
	♀	24	−0.8046	+0.01092	0	0.61 ±0.23	0.83 ±0.22	1.05 ±0.24
$FEV_{1.0}$	♂	33	+6.6314	−0.10261	+0.000499	1.73 ±0.31	2.47 ±0.29	3.61 ±0.32
	♀	21	−3.0378	+0.03640	0	1.69 ±0.30	2.42 ±0.29	3.15 ±0.30

* a, b, c=Coefficients in regression equations of the type $y=a+bx+cx^2$, where y is the measurement and x is height in cm. N=number of observations. Data for height 130, 150, and 170 cm are predicted values ± standard error for future individual measurements according to the regression analysis. Data from reference 62.

tall child, the average Pst(l) at 90 percent of TLC was 13.8 cm H_2O, compared with 19.2 cm H_2O in a child 160 cm tall, and 20.4 cm H_2O in a 180-cm tall person. Several factors may account for the increase of static lung recoil in small children. The increased density of the lung's elastic fiber network [21] may be important, as was confirmed by Hartung in the discussion of Zapletal's paper.[59] Another contributing factor may be unbalanced growth of the chest and lungs, with the chest growing slightly faster, leading to some added stretch of lung tissue. It is sometimes thought that much of lung growth after about age 8 is merely inflation of preexisting tissue. Chest cage growth may well be the primary factor, but without an increase in lung tissue mass, lung inflation would lead to much larger increases of lung recoil force than are actually found. In young children, increased lung elastic recoil, as well as more rapid chest cage growth, lead to increased static recoil pressures. In older children (over 150 cm tall), further growth of the chest and lungs appears to proceed in a balanced fashion, with increased lung tissue mass keeping pace with the increased chest volume. Thus, several quantitatively ill-described factors (chest cage recoil, muscle force), each of which is a function of development and growth, must affect lung size and TLC. In spite of this, TLC appears to be a useful guide to lung size in growing children and adolescents.

Maximum Expiratory Flow-Volume (MEFV) Curves

These curves [62] provide an impressive picture of lung growth (Fig. 1-9). They are obtained by recording flow rates during a maximally forced expiration, starting at TLC (i.e., after maximum inspiration), as a function of lung volume (see Chap. 9). Both vital capacity (on the abscissa) and maximum expiratory flow rates (on the ordinate) increase, and hence MEFV curves become much larger as children grow. Quantitative information on flow can be obtained by reading instantaneous maximum flow rates (MEF) at different volume points, e.g., 25 or 50 percent of VC, or 50 percent of TLC.

Such flow rates on MEFV curves correlate positively with body height (Fig. 1-10), but their relationship to lung volume is even more interesting. To compare flow rates among four subjects with widely differing lung volumes, lung volume is expressed as a percentage of TLC on the abscissa in Figure 1-9B. Concurrently, flow rates (in liters per second) of each individual are divided by his TLC and expressed as TLC per second.[9] This sizing adjustment is required because a maximum flow of, say, 2 liters/sec, is large for small lungs, but small for large lungs. The growth of the MEFV curve is almost solely related to TLC and not to sex; growth produces a geometrically similar enlargement of the MEFV curve. This is also shown in Figure 1-10B; maximum flow rates, at a fixed lung-volume level, become independent of height when expressed in units of TLC per second. This is, of course, just another way of stating that maximum flow is proportional to TLC in a group of subjects of widely varying body and lung sizes.

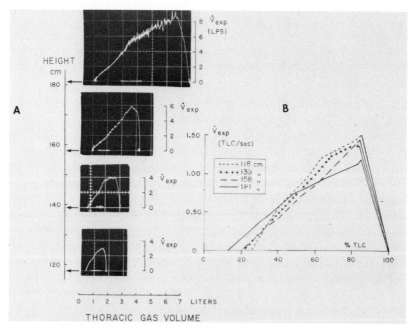

Fig. 1-9. *A*. MEFV curves of 4 boys; standing height indicated on scale at left. All curves have been lined up to fit the TGV scale at the bottom. TLC at right-hand side, RV at left-hand side on each curve. *B*. MEFV curves of *A* replotted with lung volume in percentage of TLC on abscissa and maximum flow rates in TLC per second on ordinate. From Zapletal et al.[62]

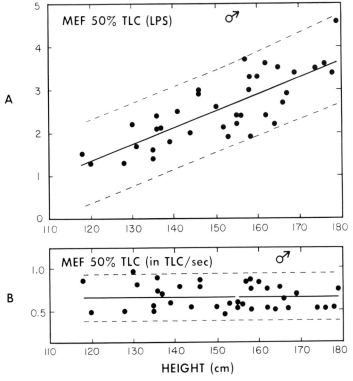

Fig. 1-10. *A*. Maximum expiratory flow rate at 50% TLC versus standing height in boys. Drawn line, regression equation; dashed lines, 95% confidence limits. *B*. Same data with flow rates in TLC per second. Drawn and dashed lines—average and 95% confidence limits, respectively. From Zapletal et al.[62]

The rule holds true at all volumes within the vital capacity range at which flow rates were measured; Tables 1-2 and 1-3 summarize these data.

Airway Conductance

Similar relations hold for airway conductance (Chap. 8). Measurements of conductance (Gaw) during panting need to be combined with determinations of lung volume (thoracic gas volume, TGV) measured with the body plethysmograph. Values for conductance at functional residual capacity (FRC) are shown in Figure 1-11. As with the maximum flow rates, division of Gaw by each individual's TLC yields a ratio that does not correlate with body height. Average values for these ratios at different lung volumes are given in Table 1-3.

Models of Lung Growth

As lung size increases, maximum expiratory flow rates and airway conductance increase in proportion to TLC. The simplest model that can explain this finding is a lung-airway system which grows isotropically, i.e., with equal relative increases of linear dimensions.[62] In such a model, airway volume grows in proportion to

Table 1-2
Statistical Analysis of MEF Versus Body Height

y	Sex	N	a *	b	r	130 cm	150 cm	170 cm
MEF 25% VC	♂	39	−2.3069	+0.02817	+0.76	1.36 ±0.41	1.92 ±0.40	2.48 ±0.43
	♀	26	−1.8576	+0.02483	+0.76	1.35 ±0.42	1.87 ±0.40	2.36 ±0.43
MEF 50% VC	♂	39	−4.5848	+0.05430	+0.87	2.48 ±0.50	3.35 ±0.47	4.65 ±0.53
	♀	26	−3.3655	+0.04477	+0.86	2.45 ±0.50	3.35 ±0.49	4.25 ±0.53
MEF 75% VC	♂	39	−6.8220	+0.07811	+0.86	3.32 ±0.75	4.89 ±0.73	6.46 ±0.80
	♀	26	−5.1934	+0.06367	+0.82	3.08 ±0.87	4.36 ±0.85	5.63 ±0.92
MEF 50% TLC	♂	37	−3.4163	+0.03946	+0.80	1.73 ±0.50	2.50 ±0.46	3.29 ±0.50
	♀	24	−2.3030	+0.03162	+0.80	1.81 ±0.42	2.44 ±0.41	3.07 ±0.44
MEF 60% TLC	♂	37	−5.1176	+0.05660	+0.87	2.24 ±0.53	3.37 ±0.52	4.50 ±0.55
	♀	24	−3.3956	+0.04413	+0.85	2.34 ±0.47	3.22 ±0.47	4.11 ±0.52
PEF	♂	39	−6.9865	+0.08060	+0.85	3.49 ±0.84	5.10 ±0.82	6.72 ±0.90
	♀	26	−5.3794	+0.06594	+0.82	3.19 ±0.87	4.51 ±0.84	5.83 ±0.92

* a, b=Coefficients in regression equations of the type $y=a+bx$, where y is the measurement and x is height in cm. N=number of observations. r=correlation coefficient of measured variable vs. height; all values are significant at $P < 0.001$. Data for height 130, 150, and 170 cm are predicted values ± standard error for future individual measurements according to the regression analysis. MEF is given in liters per second. Data from reference 62. Definition of MEF measurements: see Table 9-1, p. 187.

lung volume, and linear dimensions of alveoli and airways increase in proportion to the cube root of volume. If we represent airways by a single cylindrical tube in which airflow is laminar, Gaw will be proportional to TLC. The proportionality of maximum expiratory flow rates and TLC fits the same model. Other functional data, as well as anatomical measurements, support the hypothesis of isotropic growth. For instance, Hart et al.[27] have shown that anatomical dead space increases approximately in proportion to TLC (Table 1-4). For alveoli, Dunnill [19] concluded that between about 7 and 18 years of age alveolar diameter increases with the cube root of the change in lung volume. The same is true for frontal and sagittal bronchial diameters.[10, 62] Hislop et al.[27a] recently measured airway diameters in human lung specimens from the main bronchi to the terminal bronchioles and concluded that "the infant bronchial tree may be regarded as a miniature version of the adult pattern and . . . this . . . persists during postnatal growth." Thus, isotropic growth appears to be the rule throughout the bronchial tree.

Table 1-3
MEF in TLC per Second and Gaw in TLC per Second per cm H_2O
at Different Lung Volumes

Volume Level	MEF, TLC per Second		Gaw, TLC per Second per cm H_2O	
	Boys (N=37) *	Girls (N=24)	N	Boys and Girls
25% VC	0.50 ± 0.12	0.55 ± 0.12	21	0.071 ± 0.017
50% VC	0.93 ± 0.14	0.98 ± 0.16	21	0.105 ± 0.025
75% VC	1.27 ± 0.18	1.27 ± 0.24	21	0.141 ± 0.038
50% TLC	0.66 ± 0.14	0.72 ± 0.14	22	0.090 ± 0.020
60% TLC	0.88 ± 0.13	0.94 ± 0.15	21	0.106 ± 0.026
FRC			25	0.085 ± 0.015
PEF	1.33 ± 0.21	1.31 ± 0.24		

* N=number of observations. Values are means ± SD. Data from reference 62.

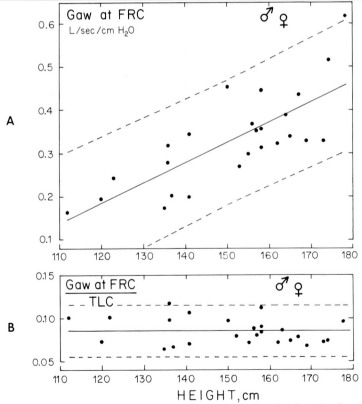

Fig. 1-11.   *A*. Airway conductance at FRC versus standing height. *B*. Same data with conductance in TLC per second per cm H_2O. Regression lines and 95% confidence limits as in Fig. 1–10; Gaw at FRC$=-0.3819+0.00472\times$height (cm). From Zapletal et al.[62]

Table 1-4
Anatomical Dead Space in Children

Body Height (cm)	V_D* (liters)	TLC (liters) †		$\dfrac{V_D}{TLC} \times 100$	
		M	F	M	F
125	0.068	2.4	2.2	2.83	3.09
150	0.105	3.6	3.4	2.92	3.09
175	0.150	6.0	5.0	2.50	3.00

* Average data of Hart et al.;[27] data for both sexes were pooled since they did not differ significantly.

† Average data of Zapletal et al.[62] for males and females.

Applications

The data in the preceding paragraphs simplify the interpretation of mechanical tests of lung function in children in the age range suitable for this type of measurement. Since airway conductance and maximum expiratory flow rates are proportional to TLC, one can distinguish between the effects of growth and of disease on lung mechanics. This should be especially helpful in longitudinal studies of children throughout their growth periods. TLC is an easily measured value related to overall growth of the lungs and chest cage. Therefore, it seems a better standard for comparison than body height, since the latter does not directly reflect chest and lung growth. These concepts have been applied in clinical studies of lung function in children with asthma and cystic fibrosis.[60]

Even a simple visual inspection of MEFV curves yields valuable information. The curves in Figure 1-9 are typical of those found in children and adolescents. In children with lung disease or in those who regularly smoke cigarettes, MEFV curves are shaped differently (Chap. 9). In healthy children, the MEFV curve can be used to predict certain performance limits during exercise and other activities. For instance, maximum flow rates required for playing wind instruments (Chap. 11) can be up to 2 liters/sec. A small boy (Fig. 1-9A, lowest curve) can achieve such a flow rate only over a volume range of about 0.8 liters. That is, he can maintain a tone on a horn that requires a flow of 2 liters/sec for only 0.4 seconds at the most. With such a physiological handicap, it is amazing that so many small children do well in compositions written for people with lungs like those that, in Figure 1-9, provided the top MEFV curve!

EXOGENOUS FACTORS IN LUNG DEVELOPMENT

Several recent studies suggest that environmental factors can influence lung growth. We already discussed the effect of corticosteroid hormone on surfactant development (p. 10). Bartlett[5] found that lung development was impaired in young rats kept in a hyperoxic environment (46.8 percent oxygen) for 2 weeks. This was probably due to a local effect of oxygen. In experiments with young rats kept for about 3 weeks at high altitude (inspired oxygen tension about 100 mm

Hg), morphometric data obtained independently by two groups of investigators [6, 14] showed a significant increase in alveolar surface area. Mean alveolar diameter remained unchanged,[6] and calculated diffusion capacity increased.[14] This apparently useful adaptation of lung growth to a hypoxic environment is not a result of hyperventilation; rats kept for 3 weeks in 5 percent CO_2 in air were unaffected.[6]

Exercise (for 20 days at sea level) did not influence lung growth of rats significantly,[4] and treatment with thiouracil or thyroxin to decrease or increase, respectively, metabolic rates also had no effect.[4]

In man, acromegaly leads to increased lung size,[13] and there have been suggestions that lung growth may be enhanced in natives of high-altitude areas. In one study,[24] data on children at high altitude were compared with similar data on children at sea level, but the two sets of data were collected by different investigators, with a time interval of more than 20 years. Thus, the comparison seems inadequate and confirmation is needed. The high-altitude children appeared to be shorter in stature, while their chest circumference and vital capacities, at similar ages, appeared to be larger than those of sea-level children.

SUMMARY

During intrauterine development, the lungs go through a glandular, a canalicular, and finally an alveolar period. Most alveoli are formed after birth, partly by segmentation of existing alveolar units, partly by fragmentation of terminal bronchioles. New alveoli continue to form at least until the age of about 8 years, and some alveolar formation may continue in the teens.

The newborn infant's lungs may collapse and he may develop the respiratory distress syndrome if birth occurs prematurely, before sufficient surfactant material is formed. Surfactant, which is mainly composed of surface-active phospholipids, may be synthesized by alveolar type II epithelial cells and is secreted to form an alveolar surface lining that decreases surface tension at the air-liquid interface. Surfactant begins to form during the alveolar period of lung development, and recent work indicates that corticosteroids and other drugs can accelerate this process.

Airway smooth muscle is well developed at birth and is supplied with functional vagal and sympathetic nerve fibers (in animals). During postnatal development, these fibers increase in size and become better able to conduct high-frequency impulses. Somatic nerve fibers undergo a similar postnatal development. Maturation of somatic fibers may be a prerequisite for the development of motor control of breathing; the functional importance of autonomic nerve fiber maturation is less clear.

As children grow, their chest cages and lungs become larger. Total lung capacity, vital capacity, and maximum expiratory flow rates increase, while airflow resistance in the bronchi decreases. During growth maximum flow rates and airway conductance increase in proportion to the total lung capacity, so that the ratios MEF/TLC and Gaw/TLC are constant at any relative lung volume (in percentage TLC). This facilitates the interpretation of lung-function tests in growing children. Static lung recoil pressure increases in young children. Lung-function data support the hypothesis that the lungs and airways as a whole grow isotropically, and morphological studies have confirmed this view. The lungs of rats kept at high altitudes grow faster and have a larger gas exchange surface area than those of rats kept at sea level, and this adaptive mechanism may also operate in children born and raised at high altitudes.

REFERENCES

1. Adolph EF: Ranges of heart rates and their regulations at various ages (rat). Am J Physiol 212:595–602, 1967
2. Anrep B von: Ueber die entwicklung hemmenden Funktionen bei Neugeborenen. Arch Ges Physiol 21:78–80, 1880
3. Avery ME, Wang NS, Taeusch HW Jr: The lung of the newborn infant. Sci Am 228: 74–85, 1973
4. Bartlett D Jr: Postnatal growth of the mammalian lung: influence of exercise and thyroid activity. Respir Physiol 9: 50–57, 1970
5. Bartlett D Jr: Postnatal growth of the mammalian lung: influence of low and high oxygen tensions. Respir Physiol 9: 58–64, 1970
6. Bartlett D Jr, Remmers JE: Effects of high altitude exposure on the lungs of young rats. Respir Physiol 13:116–125, 1971
7a. Bartlett D Jr: Postnatal growth of the mammalian lung: influence of excess growth hormone. Respir Physiol 12:297–304, 1971
7b. Bartlett D Jr: Postnatal development of the mammalian lung, in Goss RJ (ed): Regulation of Organ and Tissue Growth. New York, Academic Press, 1972, pp 197–209
8. Boren HG, Kory RC, Syner JC: The Veterans-Administration-Army cooperative study of pulmonary function. II. The lung volume and its subdivisions in normal men. Am J Med 41:96–114, 1966
9. Bouhuys A, Jonson B: Alveolar pressure, airflow rate, and lung inflation in man. J Appl Physiol 22:1086–1100, 1967
10. Boyd E: Outline of physical growth and development. Minneapolis, Burgess, 1942
11. Boyden EA: The pattern of the terminal air spaces in a premature infant of 30–32 weeks that lived nineteen and a quarter hours. Am J Anat 126:31–40, 1969
12. Boyden EA, Tompsett DH: The postnatal growth of the lung in the dog. Acta Anat (Basel) 47:185–215, 1961
13. Brody JS, Fisher AB, Gocmen A, DuBois AB: Acromegalic pneumonomegaly: lung growth in the adult. J Clin Invest 49:1051–1060, 1970
14. Burri PH, Weibel ER: Estimation de paramètres fonctionnels du poumon par morphométrie: Adaptation du poumon en croissance au taux d'oxygène dans l'air ambiant. Bull Physiopathol Respir (Nancy) 6:495–499, 1970
15. Clements JA: Comparative lipid chemistry of lungs. Arch Intern Med 127: 387–390, 1971
16. Davies G, Reid L: Growth of the alveoli and pulmonary arteries in childhood. Thorax 25:669–681, 1970
17. De Reuck AVS, Porter R (eds): Development of the Lung, Ciba Foundation Symposium. Boston, Little, Brown & Co, 1967
18. Downing SE: Baroreceptor reflexes in newborn rabbits. J Physiol (Lond) 150: 201–213, 1960
19. Dunnill MS: Postnatal growth of the lung. Thorax 17:329–333, 1962
20. Ekholm J: Postnatal changes in cutaneous reflexes and in the discharge pattern of cutaneous and articular sense organs. A morphological and physiological study in the cat. Acta Physiol Scand (Suppl) 297:1–130, 1967
21. Emery J (ed): The Anatomy of the Developing Lung. London, William Heineman Medical Books, 1969
22. Emery JL, Wilcock PF: The post-natal development of the lung. Acta Anat (Basel) 65:10–29, 1966
23. Friedman WF, Pool PE, Jacobowitz D,

Seagrens C, Braunwald E: Sympathetic innervation of the developing rabbit heart. Biochemical and histochemical comparisons of fetal, neonatal, and adult myocardium. Circ Res 23:25–32, 1968

24. Frisancho AR: Human growth and pulmonary function of a high altitude Peruvian Quechua population. Hum Biol 41:365–379, 1969

25. Gil J: Ultrastructure of lung fixed under physiologically defined conditions. Arch Intern Med 127:896–902, 1971

25a. Gitlin D, Craig JM: The nature of the hyaline membrane in asphyxia of the newborn. Pediatrics 17:64–71, 1956

26. Gregory GA, Kitterman JA, Phibbs RH, Tooley WH, Hamilton WK: Treatment of the idiopathic respiratory-distress syndrome with continuous positive airway pressure. N Engl J Med 284:1333–1340, 1971

27. Hart MC, Orzalesi MM, Cook CD: Relation between anatomic respiratory dead space and body size and lung volume. J Appl Physiol 18:519–522, 1963

27a. Hislop A, Muir DCF, Jacobsen M, Simon G, Reid L: Postnatal growth and function of the pre-acinar airways. Thorax 27:265–274, 1972

28. Horie T, Hildebrandt J: Dynamic compliance, limit cycles, and static equilibria of excised cat lung. J Appl Physiol 31:423–430, 1971

29. Huttenlocher PR: Functional properties of pyramidal neurons during development of cerebral cortex in the kitten. Fed Proc 28:825, 1969

30. Kikkawa Y, Motoyama EK: Effect of AY-9944, a cholesterol biosynthesis inhibitor, on fetal lung development and on the development of Type II alveolar epithelial cells. Lab Inves 28:48–54, 1973

31. Kikkawa Y, Motoyama EK, Cook CD: The ultrastructure of the lungs of lambs. Am J Pathol 47:877–903, 1965

32. King RJ, Clements JA: Surface active materials from dog lung. I. Method of isolation; II. Composition and physiological correlations; III. Thermal analysis. Am J Physiol 223:707–733, 1972

32a. Kotas RV, Avery ME: Accelerated appearance of pulmonary surfactant in the fetal rabbit. J Appl Physiol 30:358–361, 1971

33. Morgan TE: Pulmonary surfactant. N Engl J Med 284:1185–1193, 1971

34. Motoyama EK, Orzalesi MM, Kikkawa Y, Kaibara M, Wu B, Zigas CJ, Cook CD: Effect of cortisol on the maturation of fetal rabbit lungs. Pediatrics 48:547–555, 1971

35. Nasr K, Heinemann HO: Lipid synthesis by rabbit lung tissue in vitro. Am J Physiol 208:118–121, 1965

36. Neergaard K von: Neue Auffassungen ueber einen Grundbegriff der Atemmechanik. Z Ges Exper Med 66:373–394, 1929

37. Normand ICS, Reynolds EOR, Strang LB: Passage of macromolecules between alveolar and interstitial spaces in foetal and newly ventilated lungs of the lamb. J Physiol (Lond) 210:151–164, 1970

38. Orzalesi MM, Motoyama EK, Jacobson HN, Kikkawa Y, Reynolds EOR, Cook CD: The development of the lungs of lambs. Pediatrics 35:373–381, 1965

39. Page–Roberts BA: Preparation and partial characterization of a lamellar body fraction from rat lung. Biochim Biophys Acta 260:334–338, 1972

40. Pattle RE: Surface lining of lung alveoli. Physiol Rev 45:48–79, 1965

41. Polgar G, Promadhat V: Pulmonary Function Testing in Children: Techniques and Standards. Philadelphia, WB Saunders Co Inc, 1971

42. Reid L: Embryology of the lung, in De Reuck AVS, Porter R (eds): Development of the Lung, Ciba Foundation Symposium. London, Churchill J & A, 1967

43. Reid L, Simon G: The role of alveolar hypoplasia in some types of emphysema. Br J Dis Chest 58:158–168, 1964

44. Reynolds EOR, Jacobson HN, Motoyama EK, Kikkawa Y, Craig JM, Orzalesi MM, Cook CD: The effect of immaturity and prenatal asphyxia on the lungs and pulmonary function of newborn lambs: the experimental production of respiratory distress. Pediatrics 35:382–392, 1965

44a. Rooney SA, Page–Roberts BA, Motoyama EK: The phospholipid composition of the lamellar body fraction from the lung. (Submitted for publication)

44b. Rosan RC, Lauweryns JM: Mucosal cells of the small bronchioles of prematurely born human infants (600–1700 g). Beitr Pathol 147:145–174, 1972

45. Scarpelli EM: The Surfactant System of the Lung. Philadelphia, Lea & Febiger, 1968

46. Scarpelli EM, Colacicco G, Chang SJ: Significance of methods for isolation and characterization of pulmonary surfactants. Respir Physiol 12:179–198, 1971

47. Schwieler GH: Respiratory regulation during postnatal development in cats and rabbits, and some of its morphological substrate. Acta Physiol Scand (Suppl) 304:1–120, 1968

48. Schwieler GH, Douglas JS, Bouhuys A: Postnatal development of autonomic efferent innervation in the rabbit. Am J Physiol 219:391–397, 1970

49. Schwieler GH, Skoglund S: Individual variations in the bronchial tree in cats of different ages with special reference to the post-natal development. Acta Anat (Basel) 56:70–78, 1964

50. Shepard FM, Johnston RB Jr, Klatte EC, Burko H, Stahlman M: Residual pulmonary findings in clinical hyaline-membrane disease. N Engl J Med 279:1063–1071, 1968

51. Skoglund S: The activity of muscle receptors in the kitten. Acta Physiol Scand 50:203–221, 1960

52. Skoglund S, Romero C: Postnatal growth of spinal nerves and roots. A morphological study in the cat with physiological correlations. Acta Physiol Scand 66 (Suppl) 260:1–50, 1965

52a. Staub NC: The interdependence of pulmonary structure and function. Anesthesiology 24:831–854, 1963

53. Taylor IM, Smith RB: Intrinsic innervation of the human foetal lung between the 35 and 140 mm crown-rump length stages. Biol Neonate 18:193–202, 1971

54. Tombropoulos EG: Lipid synthesis by lung subcellular particles. Arch Intern Med 127:408–412, 1971

55. Wekstein DR: Heart rate of the pre-weanling rat and its autonomic control. Am J Physiol 208:1259–1262, 1965

56. Widdicombe JG: Action potentials in parasympathetic and sympathetic efferent fibres to the trachea and lungs of dogs and cats. J Physiol (Lond) 186:56–88, 1966

56a. Wu B, Kikkawa Y, Orzalesi MM, Motoyama EK, Kaibara M, Zigas CJ, Cook CD: The effect of thyroxine on the maturation of fetal rabbit lungs. Biol Neonate 22:161–168, 1973

57. Yamauchi A, Burnstock G: Development of smooth muscle. J Anat 104:1–15, 1969

58. Yamauchi A, Burnstock G: Post-natal development of the innervation of the mouse vas deferens. A fine structural study. J Anat 104:17–32, 1969

59. Zapletal A, Misur M, Samanek M: Static recoil pressure of the lungs in children. Bull Physiopathol Respir (Nancy) 7:139–143, 1971

60. Zapletal A, Motoyama EK, Gibson LE, Bouhuys A: Pulmonary mechanics in asthma and cystic fibrosis. Pediatrics 48:64–72, 1971

61. Zapletal A, Motoyama EK, van de Woestijne KP, Gibson LE, Bouhuys A: Use of the body plethysmography in children. Prog Respir Res 4:228–235, 1969

62. Zapletal A, Motoyama EK, van de Woestijne KP, Hunt VR, Bouhuys A: Maximum expiratory flow-volume curves and airway conductance in children and adolescents. J Appl Physiol 26:308–316, 1969

Chapter 2

Conducting Airways

The main purpose of the airways that lead from the atmosphere to the alveoli is to conduct inspired air to the gas-exchanging surfaces and to eliminate expired air. In addition, they have other important functions—warming and humidifying air, removing aerosol particles and soluble gases from inspired air, producing voice sounds, and chemically monitoring inspired air. The latter depends on special receptors for the sense of smell, while the air-conditioning functions depend on the mucosal surface area, the nature of airflow over it, and the properties of its mucus. The voice function makes more subtle demands on upper airway function to generate and to articulate speech sounds. This task, the essence of human communication, is associated with important changes in the shape and structure of the upper airways during man's evolution (Chap. 11).

UPPER AIRWAYS

Nose

During quiet breathing, a healthy person breathes through the nose. Although its volume is only about 20 ml, folds make the mucosal surface area large—about 160 cm² (Fig. 2-1)—rendering the nose an effective air-conditioning device. Unless it is first passed through the nose, dry air damages the mucosa of airways; for patients who must breathe through a tracheostomy tube, special air-conditioning devices prevent drying and crust formation in the trachea ("artificial nose").[27, 60] The effectiveness of air conditioning in the upper airways is apparent, for instance, in experiments with dogs exposed to inspired air at −40°C and at +40°C during normal breathing.[2] Just below the larynx, inspired air was fully saturated with water vapor and had reached body temperature (37°C), regardless of the inspired air temperature.

A man who inspires dry air at 0°C must evaporate about 420 gm water per 24 hours to saturate all inspired air with water vapor. Since this requires about

25

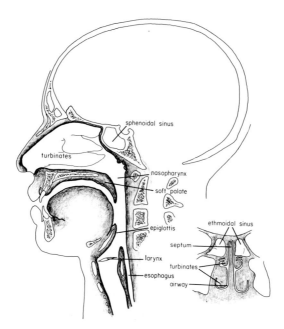

Fig. 2-1. Sagittal section through the human head to show anatomical relations in the upper airways. *Inset.* A transverse section through the nose shows how mucosal folds (turbinates) narrow the airway passage and provide a large surface area for heat and water exchange. From reference 42.

2200 calories/24 hr, he would use nearly all of his metabolic heat production merely to warm and humidify the air he inspired. Clearly, protective mechanisms prevent this—much of the added heat and water are recovered on expiration. Cold inspired air cools the nasal mucosa, and the expired air meets a cool mucosa on its return. Hence, expired air cools when it reaches the front portion of the nose, and water condenses on the mucosa. This water is available for evaporation during the next inspiration of cold air. Any excess water on the mucosal surface causes the "runny nose" when one is out in the cold. With this type of counter-current heat exchange mechanism,[54] the nose recovers water and calories from the expired air before they are lost to the atmosphere. In contrast, when the inspired air is warm, the mucosa remains warm during inspiration, and the expired air leaves the nose at a temperature of 37°C, saturated with water vapor. Thus, the upper airways contribute to heat loss when we are in a warm environment.

To facilitate air conditioning, then, it makes sense to breathe through the nose. But the anatomy that enables the nose to be effective for this purpose—narrow passages between well-vascularized mucosal folds—creates a high resistance to airflow. Just as in our houses, effective air conditioning requires energy. The nose's resistance to airflow is about twice that of the mouth (Chap. 8), and during quiet breathing, the nasal passages contribute nearly half the total flow resistance. We normally prefer to accept the extra work that breathing through the nose requires, only switching to mouth breathing during talking, sighing, and exercise. The control mechanisms that determine the choice of mouth or nose breathing are not clear. Opening the mouth is a part of the act of talking or sighing. I doubt whether it can be explained in terms of flow rate increases or some other local mechanical event, since it does not seem to follow but rather to anticipate these events. We may have learned mouth breathing during exercise simply because we discovered it was easier during hard work. Subjectively, the decreased effort during mouth breathing is obvious whenever we breathe at increased frequency and at high flow rates. Very little air passes through the nose when we breathe through the mouth, because of the nose's high resistance in contrast to the low resistance of the oral cavity. In newborn infants, the morphology of the nasal and oral passages suggests that the reverse is true; the obligate nose breathing of infants may be due to a lower nasal flow resistance.[36]

Linear air velocities in the nose are not uniform and may reach high values in certain areas even when total flow rates are moderate.[43] The highest velocities occur in the anterior part of the middle meatus. High velocities during inspiration lead to partial collapse of the alae nasi and may, along with accompanying sensations, trigger the switch to mouth breathing.

Pharynx

Well-known accidents can occur at this crossroad, with food, liquid, or air taking inappropriate directions (Fig. 2-1). Fenn[13] wondered about the possible advantages of this curious design. Why should we have a crossing of food and air passages at all? One answer may be structural economy—the tongue helps to process food, to speak, and to condition air somewhat during mouth breathing. In primates and other mammals, the pharynx is much less developed than in man,[29] and the epiglottis and larynx are much closer to the nasopharynx. Thus, the dangers of food and liquid running into the airway are much less in animals than they are in man. The pharynx is essential for articulated speech (Chap. 11), and perhaps the disadvantages of the human design are simply accidental to its advantages for communication.

The crossing of food and air allows interaction between the senses of taste and smell. Of the two, smell is more sensitive, and although some of its survival function has been lost during man's evolution, it retains great psychological importance. It leaves long-term memory imprints, as those immortalized by Proust's description of the smell of madeleines dipped in tea.[44] Proctor[43] has observed that the nasal sensors are placed outside the mainstream of the inspired air, so that they are not really in a good position to sample the air. This may be another design disadvantage that man incurred when his upper airways adapted to speech.

Swallowing

Bosma[4] has reviewed the pharyngeal stages of deglutition. Triggered by the arrival of a food bolus at the back of the mouth, a fixed sequence of movements, lasting 0.3–0.5 seconds, passes the bolus from the mouth to the esophagus. The tongue brings the bolus into the middle part of the pharynx (oropharynx), while the palate prevents it from entering the nasopharynx. While the bolus passes over the epiglottis, swallowing begins with a headward movement of the pharynx, accompanied by upward motion of the hyoid bone and its attachments, including the larynx. During this time, the epiglottis curves down over the airway, and breathing is momentarily interrupted. As the pharyngeal sphincter muscle propels the food bolus downward, the hypopharyngeal sphincter muscle at the entrance of the esophagus relaxes. This allows food to enter the esophagus; at all other times, the hypopharyngeal sphincter is tightly closed, preventing air from entering the esophagus, where—as elsewhere in the chest cage—pressure is normally less than atmospheric.

The nervous control of swallowing is closely linked with that of breathing. During a swallow, breathing is interrupted, and every swallow is followed by an expiration. In newborn infants, swallowing, suckling, and breathing follow in a fixed sequence.[4] Swallowing is a good example of a motor act in which an obligatory series of motor events can be triggered voluntarily or by reflex. It fits the concept of a programmed motor act (Chap. 11). Bosma[4] stresses its all-or-nothing character, independent of afferent modification. Much training, not always successful, is required to teach laryngectomized patients to use their hypopharyngeal sphincter in a quite different way, namely, as a substitute larynx (esophageal speech[11]).

Larynx

The larynx acts as a valve that prevents food or liquid from entering the trachea. It is also a major obstacle for the respiratory physiologist: since the larynx is a major site of flow resistance during breathing, it complicates the measurement of lower airway resistance. The use of the larynx during phonation and speech is discussed elsewhere (Chap. 11). One component of the larynx, the cricoid cartilage, located at the upper end of the trachea, has special importance during breathing. The only complete cartilaginous ring around the trachea, the cricoid cartilage alone can keep the trachea open during forced inspirations, when the pressures inside the trachea are less than atmospheric. Without the tethering function of the cricoid cartilage, the trachea would be much more subject to dynamic compression during forced inspirations.

The glottal opening is larger in men than in women, and, as a consequence, unilateral paralysis of a vocal fold causes more respiratory embarrassment in women than in men. Schiratzki[53] documented this with measurements of subglottic pressure and upper airway resistance. In patients with vocal fold paralysis, lung volume and forced expiratory volumes ($FEV_{1.0}$; Chap. 9) are often normal, while maximum voluntary ventilation (MVV) may be low.[53] This is one of the rather rare instances where the MVV test, which requires the subject to breathe in and out as deep as possible and at a high rate of breathing, detects an abnormal condition that may not be revealed by the $FEV_{1.0}$ and other tests based on single expirations. There appear to be no reports on visual observations of paralyzed vocal folds during maximum voluntary ventilation maneuvers. One suspects that the passive to-and-fro movements of the paralyzed fold, "in the wind" as it were, create much extra energy loss and increase laryngeal resistance.

THE BRONCHIAL TREE

Morphology of Branches

Table 2-1 gives names, numbers, and dimensions of the trachea and its branches. Figure 2-2 illustrates the main features of large conducting airways (*A*) and of the transition between conducting and gas-exchanging airways in terminal lung units (*B*). Illustrations of airway morphology are available elsewhere.[20, 56] To correlate form and function, quantitative morphological data are a prerequisite; this "morphometric" approach to the study of lung structure was introduced by Weibel and Gomez.[63] The quantitative data thus obtained can be used to develop concepts or models of lung morphology that clarify lung and airway physiology. The first of these is Weibel's model (Fig. 2-3).[62]

The first generations of the bronchi are named after easily recognized parts of the lungs with surface landmarks—lobes and segments. Subsequent generations decrease in size and gradually lose the cartilaginous support in their walls as they branch further. The last generation of "small bronchi" contains little cartilage. The next several generations are given a distinct name, bronchioles; they are distinguished from bronchi by the absence of cartilage. Yet further along, alveoli appear in the walls; because of their participation in gas exchange, these airways are called respiratory bronchioles. The walls of the airways become more and more studded with alveoli, until nothing remains of their walls but the septa between alveoli (Fig. 1-3); the bronchioles have then become alveolar ducts. These branch through a few more generations of decreasing length and terminate in the alveoli. The average total pathway length from the cricoid cartilage to the alveoli is about 24 cm, half of which is the length of the trachea; individual pathway lengths vary considerably. Ross documented this for the dog lung.[51]

In Weibel's model, each airway that branches is assumed to divide into two equivalent branches (*regular dichotomy.*) Weibel also described another model,[62] based on the assumption of *irregular dichotomy,* but this has not been as widely used. Parker et al.[40] found dichotomous branching in small but not in larger airways. The problem of defining the type of branching is illustrated in the diagrams of Figure 2-4, which express the same bronchial tree two different ways. One model (*B*) considers all branching points as Y junctions leading into two equivalent branches. The other (*A*) considers them as T junctions: the smaller branch is a minor sidebranch, the other continues as the main stem of the T. As models, these two concepts differ importantly. Which one is more realistic depends on precise measurements of branching angles at the junctions and of all branch diameters. Since lung volume affects airway diameters and branching angles, one's choice of model might differ depending on lung inflation.

Several quantitative observations confirm the general validity of the regular dichotomy model introduced by Weibel.[62] Parker et al.[40] counted alveoli and alveolar ducts in one lobule, about 0.34 ml of inflated human lung tissue, and found an average of 13 alveoli per alveolar duct or sac. Weibel estimated the total number of alveoli at 300×10^6; with the data of Parker et al., this gives a total of $300/13 = 23 \times 10^6$ alveolar sacs and ducts (16×10^6 in generations 19–23 of Weibel's model). Horsfield and Cumming[22] found 224×10^3 most distal respira-

Table 2-1
The Bronchial Tree

Generation	Name	Diameter† (cm)	Length† (cm)	Total Cross Section† (cm²)	Number per Generation†	Small Airway Counts
0	Trachea	1.8	12.0	2.54	1	
1	Main bronchi	1.22	4.76	2.33	2	
2	Lobar bronchi	0.83	1.90	2.13	4	
3	Segmental bronchi	0.56	0.76	2.00	8	
4	Subsegmental bronchi	0.45	1.27	2.48	16	
5		0.35	1.07	3.11	32	
thru	Small bronchi					
10		0.13	0.46	13.4	1.02×10^3	
11		0.109	0.39	19.6	2.05×10^3	
thru	Bronchioles					
13		0.082	0.27	44.5	8.19×10^3	7.6×10^3 §
14		0.074	0.23	69.4	16.38×10^3	13.4×10^3 §
&	Terminal bronchioles					
15		0.066	0.20	113.0	32.77×10^3	24.8×10^3 §
16		0.060	0.165	180.0	65.54×10^3	51.6×10^3 §
thru	Respiratory bronchioles					
18		0.050	0.117	534.0	262.14×10^3	224×10^3 §
19		0.047	0.099	944.0	524.29×10^3	23×10^6 §
thru	Alveolar ducts					
23 *		0.041	0.050	11800.0	8.39×10^6	
24	Alveoli	244 μm††	238 μm††	43–80 m² ‖		300×10^6 ††

Nomenclature according to Staub.[56]

* 23rd generation also named alveolar sacs.

† Data from Weibel;[62] regular dichotomy model based on lungs inflated to 4.8 liters = 75% of TLC.

†† Average data from 5 normal lungs. (see pp. 61, 66 in ref. 62).

§ Data of Parker et al.[40] for alveolar ducts and generation 18; others derived from their counts of small airways in human lung lobule.

‖ Total alveolar surface area. (see p. 67 in ref. 62).

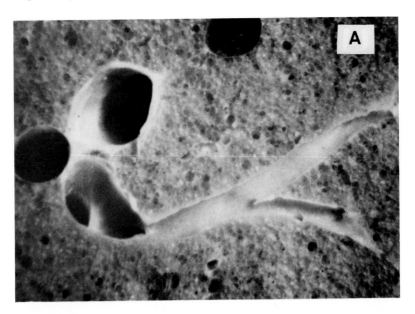

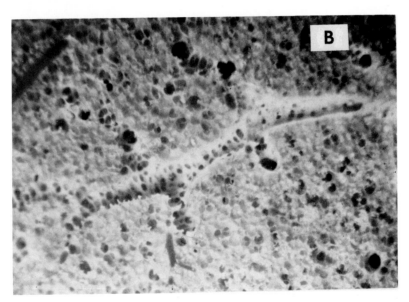

Fig. 2-2. Microscopic sections of rapidly frozen cat lungs, prepared by Staub. *A.* Segmental bronchus and branches. A small bronchus emerges from the lower branch and its longitudinal section shows another branching. The pulmonary artery is close to the airway (*left*); the pulmonary vein is at a distance from the airway (*top*). The airway branches are embedded in peripheral lung tissue. *B.* Transition of a terminal bronchiole with scattered alveoli in its wall (*upper right*) into more alveolated respiratory bronchioles and alveolar ducts, toward the left. The transition between conducting and gas-exchanging airways cannot be defined precisely. Reproduced with permission from teaching slides of Dr. Norman Staub (see also reference 56).

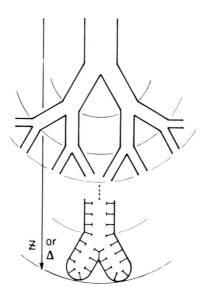

23 generations regular dichotomy

Fig. 2-3. Airway generations in the regular dichotomy model; z indicates length of pathway from entrance
to trachea. Modified from Weibel.[62]

tory bronchioles (262×10^3 in Weibel's model). Estimates for the larger bronchioles (Table 2-1; last column) also reasonably agree with the regular dichotomy
model.

Weibel's model has been criticized as "being based more on a mathematical
concept than on direct observation." [40] Such criticism ignores the basic requirements of a good model—it must be based on facts, and it must summarize and

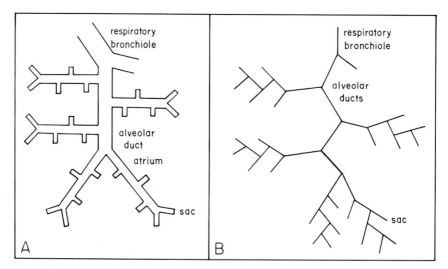

Fig. 2-4. The same branching pattern of the bronchial tree can be schematized in
different diagrammatic models. Discussion in text. From Parker et al.[40]

simplify them in a mathematical concept. Since Weibel's model fits this definition, it is a useful representation of airway dimensions. Few physiologists, for instance, were aware of the tremendous increase in total cross-sectional area of the airway as one approaches the alveoli until Weibel's data brought this fact home. Although more data have become available since Weibel's book was published in 1962, these have as yet not led to an equally elegant and useful concept of bronchial tree structure. Other models, such as those of Figure 2-4, are more complex than Weibel's and seem to be about equally far removed from anatomic reality. They will supersede Weibel's model only if it can be shown that they better predict or describe important features of lung mechanics or gas exchange.

Physiological events are often described as occurring in "small" or "large" airways. This distinction is arbitrary, considering the wide range of airway sizes; the definition depends on one's purposes. Small bronchi are small in relation to other bronchi (generations 1-4; Table 2-1), but large in relation to bronchioles. Hence, cartilage may be a more useful factor than size in distinguishing large from small airways. Airways without cartilage (approximately 11th generation and smaller) would then be small airways, while all cartilaginous airways would be considered large. Among small airways, the bronchiolar walls have well-developed smooth muscle layers and no protection from cartilage. This definition of small airways may be useful in discussions of smooth muscle function. (see Chap. 8, p. 156) Other ways of dividing the bronchial tree into small and large airways are: (1) location downstream (large) or upstream (small) from an equal-pressure point in the airways;[34] (2) blood supply via bronchial (large) or pulmonary (small) blood vessels;[37] (3) dynamic compression during forced expiration occurs only in large and not in small airways;[5] and (4) small airways are those smaller than the airway in which a pressure-measuring catheter is lodged.[31] Each definition is useful in the context for which it was proposed—confusion results when definitions are used inappropriately. Accurate anatomical information on the site of events in airways during life may clarify some of these problems. It is unrealistic, however, to expect that more elaborate morphological studies will necessarily lead to better understanding of function. Morphological data are easily visualized but difficult to quantitate, while functional data are by nature quantitative and conceptual, but often hard to translate into concrete structural form. Thus, one encounters basic difficulties in correlating structural and morphological detail with physiological measurements and concepts.

The Walls of the Airways

Airway walls consist of epithelium, smooth muscle, cartilage, and glands in a framework of connective tissue.[18, 20, 55] The epithelium of the airways is composed of ciliated and goblet cells, together with columnar epithelial and basal cells (Fig. 2-5). In the bronchioles this pseudostratified epithelium is replaced by a simpler cuboidal cell epithelium with fewer goblet cells. Situated between the basal membrane of the epithelium and the cartilage of larger airways are seromucinous glands, ducts of which open onto the epithelial surface; these glands are absent in bronchioles. The smooth muscle network, arranged to allow changes of width as well as of length, discovered by Reisseisen, 1808,[39, 50] consists of transverse and longitudinal fibers. Only transverse fibers are found in deflated lungs, but this

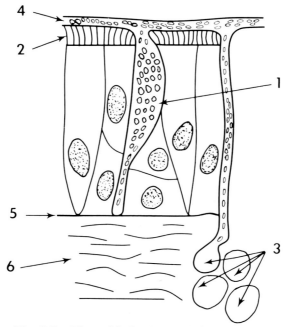

Fig. 2-5. The epithelial layer of the airways with a
goblet cell (*1*), cilia (*2*), and a submucous gland (*3*). The
cilia beat in the watery layer (sol phase) of the mucus; the
mucous layer (gel phase) lies on top of the cilia (*4*). The
epithelial layer is separated from the submucosal connective tissue (*6*) by the basement membrane (*5*). Schematic
drawing, not to scale.

is an artifact.[32] In small bronchi the amount of smooth muscle increases, occupying
the largest fraction of the wall thickness in the terminal bronchioles, where it becomes a conspicuous structure.[32] Nerve fibers, ganglia, and possible sensory elements in airway walls have been described.[28, 32] A dense network of adrenergic
nerve fibers, identified by fluorescence labeling of catecholamine stores, is present
in respiratory bronchioles of the cat.[7] Mast cells are found around airways and in
the pleura of the human lung.[21]

Glands and Goblet Cells

Both glands and goblet cells produce mucus, which coats the epithelial surface
of the airways. The number of these structures along the bronchial tree varies
greatly among different species and in the same animal. The rabbit, guinea pig,
mouse, and hamster are poorly endowed, while the cat has more than man.[24, 48]
The rat, which has more glands and goblet cells than most other small animals,
responds to irritant exposure with hypertrophy of the glands as well as with development of goblet cells in bronchioles where normally there are none; its mucus-
secreting system may be fairly similar to that of man.[48] In the epithelium of
trachea and large bronchi, there is about one goblet cell for every five ciliated
cells. The number of goblet cells decreases in smaller airways; bronchioles normally

contain few or none at all. Although glands and goblet cells are absent, a thin fluid layer can be identified on the mucosal surface in terminal bronchioles if the lungs are fixed by perfusion through the blood vessels.[16] The origin of this fluid is not known.

The seromucinous glands contain some cells that mainly produce serous liquid and others that produce mucus. The nasal mucosa contains similar glands, and the serous cell type appears to be more predominant than it is in lower airways.[6] Mucous glands are commonly hypertrophied in asthma [23] and in chronic bronchitis.[6, 47, 59] As an index of gland hypertrophy, Reid [47] proposed measuring the gland's thickness as a proportion of the total thickness of the bronchial wall in the same airway section. However, this "Reid index" can be determined accurately only in large airways.[59] A Reid index of more than about 0.50 is commonly associated with chronic bronchitis, in which the gland hypertrophy is limited to the bronchial tree and does not involve the nasal mucous glands.[6] Mucous gland hypertrophy correlates well with smoking habits and is more pronounced in airways of people who have smoked much.[35] Smoking does not seem to affect the nasal mucosal glands.[6]

High concentrations (300–400 parts per million) of sulfur dioxide in air induced hypersecretion of mucus and, after several weeks' exposure, extensive glandular hypertrophy as well as development of goblet cells in bronchioles.[48] These changes occurred without evidence of infection. Other authors [35] have concluded that, in man, smoking is more important than infection in the development of mucous gland hypertrophy. Thus, airway infections in chronic bronchitis may often be secondary to such factors as smoking, which not only cause mucous gland hypertrophy but probably also damage the lungs' cleansing mechanisms. The effects of cigarette smoking on human mucous gland hypertrophy may be largely reversible, as evidenced by the disappearance of sputum production in many young people who stop smoking. In Reid's SO$_2$-exposed rats,[48] however, the effects of 4–6 weeks' exposure did not disappear in a subsequent period of three months without exposure.

Mucus production by glands and goblet cells, and the physical and chemical composition of their secretions, pose interesting problems that have received far less attention than they deserve. Since it is difficult to collect human bronchial secretions without eliciting increased mucus production in the airway, most studies with human material use sputum—a pathological product, an inconstant and heterogeneous mix of abnormal lower airway secretions, saliva, and other extraneous material from the nose and mouth. In recent years, however, histochemical studies together with biochemical measurements of components of mucus have provided some basic information.[65]

Goblet cells have a prominent Golgi apparatus where vacuoles are formed. In the upper part of the cell, vacuoles are transformed into mucous granules and are then discharged on the epithelial surface. A similar process occurs in the seromucinous glands, although they produce a mixture of serous and mucous liquid which is perhaps less viscous than the product of goblet cells. Mucus has so-called viscoelastic properties because it contains long-chain mucoproteins (molecular weight >200,000), partly in a fibrillar structure. The peptide skeleton of these chains is combined with mucopolysaccharides containing sulfate and sialic acid radicles. With histochemical methods, these radicles can be marked, and at least six different types of intracellular mucus—occurring in different proportions in goblet and gland cells [49]—can be distinguished. Radioactive-labeled sulfate is incorporated in serous gland cells as well as in goblet cells.[19] According to Reid, proximal goblet cells form more sulfated mucopolysaccharides, while sialic acid appears to be the predominant radicle in smaller airways.[48] Serum albumin and γA-immunoglobulins are the main plasma proteins present in bronchitic sputum as well as in fluid aspirated from lower airways in man.[33] It is not clear whether these proteins are secreted by glandular elements, but at least one other protein, lactoferrin, is.[33] In addition, nonpurulent human airway secretions contain lysozyme.[33]

A baffling question is how the total production of secretion is regulated, using different production sites, so that just enough material is available to coat the airways with a layer of mucus sufficient for protection and for mucociliary transport. The amount of mucus a healthy man produces is not known. Toremalm [61] estimated mucus production to be about 15–20 ml/24 hr in laryngectomized patients with a tracheostomy. The number of secretory cells per unit airway wall surface area is perhaps roughly constant throughout the bronchial tree, so that the amount of mucus produced would be proportional to the surface area to be covered if all cells produced mucus at a constant rate. But it seems unlikely that production is indeed constant. Vagal stimulation in the cat increases mucus flow considerably, while atropine inhibits this effect.[14] Increased secretion could also be elicited by reflex and, more directly, by irritants, the latter unaffected by vagotomy or by atropine.[14] Injected intravenously, pilocarpine increased secretion in the cat.[14] In a different type of experiment, Formijne et al.[15] found that isoproterenol inhibits the incorporation of labeled glucosamine into mucin formed in rat tracheal tissue in vitro. Such data suggest that the secretion of mucous liquid, as well as the formation of one important ingredient of mucus, can be influenced by autonomic mediating substances. Thus, there are potential mechanisms for changes in the amount and composition of mucus produced in the airways, as a function of physiological conditions.

The physical properties of mucus are essential for its protective function as a relatively impermeable cover of the epithelium, for its ability to trap foreign materials, and for its mode of transport by the cilia. This topic is discussed together with other aspects of mucociliary transport later in this chapter.

Cilia

The ciliated epithelium of the airways is the motor organ for transport of mucus and the cells and particles imbedded in it to the pharynx, where it is swallowed. Ciliated epithelium covers the airway mucosa from the larynx down to the terminal bronchioles. There are about 200 cilia on each ciliated cell, with a length of 5–7 μm.[52] Cilia move to and fro with a rapid stroke in the direction of the airway opening and a slow return beat in the opposite direction. In airways with mucus-secretory elements, the cilia move in thin fluid and are covered with a mucous layer. This two-phase liquid system (Fig. 2-5) is essential for mucociliary transport.

Iravani [25] developed an ingenious method to observe ciliary motion in intact small airways in rat lungs in vivo. The ciliary beat is arrhythmic, stroboscopic images are never steady, and some coordination of the beat exists between several adjacent cells. The rate increases from the periphery to the main bronchus, as well as near branches, where the wall surface area is reduced by the opening of the branch.[25] In a 0.2-mm diameter rat airway, beat frequency was 13/sec at 35° C, and 2/sec at 20° C;[25] in the rabbit trachea, 20/sec at 37° C, and 7/sec at 20° C.[17] Species, site, and temperature are the important variables. In addition, the amount of material to be transported probably regulates beat frequency.[25]

The Mucociliary Ladder

The concept that most of the conducting airways are covered with a continuous and coherent sheet of mucus, which normally moves constantly toward the pharynx, has led to use of the term mucociliary ladder for this protective transport mechanism. Cell debris, inhaled particles, and any other matter that gets trapped in the mucus sheet will eventually be removed from the lungs. The rate of this transport is subject to a large number of ill-understood variables. The rate of displacement of a particle or droplet placed on the mucosa provides information only on overall transport. Such data need interpretation in terms of the biological mechanisms that affect the ciliary beat or the amount and the quality of mucus.

The mucociliary ladder eliminates material once it is subject to the impact of ciliary motion. But in the last 50 μm of the terminal bronchioles of the rat, no ciliary motion occurs.[25] Other protective mechanisms, including phagocytosis (Chap. 12), take over at this level. Presumably, live phagocytes can reach the first rung of the mucociliary ladder by their own motion.

The amount and the physical qualities of bronchial mucus are crucial for mucociliary transport. Several physical scientists have studied the rheological properties, or flow characteristics, of mucus, and the results do not provide easy answers.[9, 10, 30, 45, 57] Everybody who has ever had a cold knows that the secretions of the nasal mucosa vary with the stage of that disease, from thin serous liquid to a sticky and tenacious mucus. A similar difference exists between the sol and gel phases of the mucous layer in the lower airways (Fig. 2-5). Mucus viscosity is a complex concept, since mucus does not follow simple linear stress-shear relations, as do such homogeneous liquids as water and oil. Layers of mucus do not follow a regular laminar flow pattern. In conformance with a property of plastic materials, a certain minimum stress must be exerted before mucus moves at all. Because of its long-chain mucoproteins, mucus can store some of the energy spent on it, so that it can recoil from stretch. Thus, mucus has plastic and elastic, as well as viscous, properties. The same long molecules make mucus into a coherent layer, continuous with the filaments that emerge from the glandular ducts. In physiological conditions, the ciliary beat exerts enough force on the mucus blanket, on top of the cilia, to keep the material moving and to break the filaments that connect the sheet to the glands. Since the ciliary beat is so rapid, the mucus layer has no time to recoil between beats. Therefore it keeps moving as a relatively rigid sheet of material.

It might be useful to express the physical properties of mucus in numbers. Unfortunately, owing to the heterogeneity of the material and its complex properties, no physically meaningful numbers can be measured. Many attempts have been made to measure sputum viscosity. Puchelle and Benis[45] compiled data for human sputum viscosity varying from 0.017 poises to 61×10^5 poises, a difference of some eight orders of magnitude. These numbers include effects of viscosity as well as contributions of plasticity, elasticity, and heterogeneity. Sputum viscosity measurements have not yet been of great help to the clinician. In theory, a very watery mucus would require little energy for transport, but gravity might make it accumulate in the alveoli. Tenacious mucus, on the other hand, is difficult to set in motion but once started it is likely to keep moving because of its elasticity and coherence. On arriving in large airways, this kind of mucus often bypasses muco-ciliary transport altogether; it acts as a foreign body and elicits cough. During lavage of the lungs, large amounts of mucus can be removed,[58] probably by elimi-nating air-mucus interfaces rather than by altering the physical properties of mucus per se. Between the extremes of watery mucus and tenacious sputum may be some optimal set of physical properties that best serves the purposes of mucociliary transport. The tolerance for variations around such optimal properties may be rather large; this would decrease the requirements for controlling the quality and quantity of the secretion products.

The rate of particle transport by the mucociliary ladder has been measured in different species. Kilburn has reported transport rates in the lung of the bullfrog,[26] and Baetjer[3] developed a quantitative method for measuring transport rates in the conveniently long necks of chicks in vivo under nearly physiological conditions. She deposited 1 μl of a ^{131}I-labeled solution on the mucosa through a small hole at the lower end of the trachea and followed its progress with two detectors placed 3.2 cm apart over the upper part of the trachea. Transport rates so measured varied from 7.4 to 17.9 mm/min. In man, a labeled inert particle can be placed on the nasal mucosa and its rate of displacement followed with external detec-tors.[1,46] These methods produced variable results, even in the same subject during constant, controlled climatic conditions, with average rates from less than 0.10 to 23.6 mm/min in 58 subjects.[1] Often clearance was not continuous throughout the period of measurement, and, in localized areas on the mucosa, virtually no clearance was seen. Foreign materials might preferentially accumulate at such spots.

Mucociliary transport in the human bronchial tree can be studied only with indirect methods. The clearance of particles deposited on the mucosa by aerosol inhalation can be measured with external monitoring methods (Chap. 12). Quali-tative observations have been made from serial x-ray films after coating the airways with a contrast medium such as tantalum powder.[38] Parks et al.[41] concluded that exposure to mists, often used to treat patients with lung disease (water aerosolized by heated jet nebulizer or by ultrasonic nebulizer), caused no change in tantalum clearance rate in dogs. So far, there is no objective evidence that this treatment improves the removal of secretions from lower airways. It is sometimes believed that mist droplets, when inhaled into the airways, render mucus less viscous. However, adding water droplets to air already saturated with water vapor does not result in deposition of significant amounts of water.[64] Also, water and mucus do not mix to form a homogeneous liquid, and addition of water, therefore, does not liquify mucus. After auto- or allotransplantation of a lung in dogs,[12] tantalum clearance was delayed up to 120 days. Decreased glandular mucus secretion, as a consequence of denervation, may be one factor in this delay,[12] but it is difficult to exclude subtle local impediments at the suture site.

Transport measurements reflect an average value of rates that may vary con-siderably in time and place during the observations. With a method that detects arrival of a marker at some distance, the result depends on the first arrivals, i.e., the faster rates. Short-term changes in transport rates can be detected if they are large enough. Other methods (e.g., tantalum clearance) assess the amount of material that stays behind. This is a function of the slowest transport rates and is the relevant information if one wants to know how much of a toxic material remains in the lungs after a given period of time.

SUMMARY

The conducting airways have an important function in protecting the lungs' gas-exchanging parts from exposure to cold, dry, or contaminated air. The nose's functions of heat and water exchange and the prevention of food and liquid from entering the airways during swallowing are both essential protective mechanisms. The branching pattern of the bronchial tree can be described in different ways; Weibel's regular dichotomy model is adequate for many purposes. Small and large airways need to be defined in some context, and several criteria can be used for this purpose. The bronchial wall's structures—consisting of epithelium, glands, smooth muscle, connective tissue, and cartilage—vary with airway size. Glands, goblet cells, and ciliated epithelium are essential parts of the mucociliary clearance mechanism that helps eliminate foreign matter from the lungs.

REFERENCES

1. Andersen I, Lundquist GR, Proctor DF: Human nasal mucosal function in a controlled climate. Arch Environ Health 23:408–420, 1971

2. Armstrong HG, Burton AC, Hall GE: The physiological effects of breathing cold atmospheric air. J Aviat Med 29: 593–597, 1958

3. Baetjer AM: Effect of ambient temperature and vapor pressure on cilia-mucus clearance rate. J Appl Physiol 23:498–504, 1967

4. Bosma JF: Deglutition: Pharyngeal stage. Physiol Rev 37:275–300, 1957

5. Bouhuys A: Airway dynamics and bronchoactive agents in man, in Bouhuys A (ed): Airway Dynamics; Physiology and Pharmacology. Springfield, Charles C Thomas, 1970, pp 263–282

6. Burton PA, Dixon MF: A comparison of changes in the mucous glands and goblet cells of nasal, sinus, and bronchial mucosa. Thorax 24:180–185, 1969

7. Dahlström A, Fuxe K, Hökfelt T, Norberg KA: Adrenergic innervation of the bronchial muscle of the cat. Acta Physiol Scand 66:507–508, 1966

8. Dalhamn T: Mucous flow and ciliary activity in the trachea of healthy rats exposed to respiratory irritant gases (SO_2, H_3N, HCHO). Acta Physiol Scand 36 (suppl 123):1–161, 1956

9. Davis SS, Dippy JE: The rheological properties of sputum. Biorheology 6: 11–21, 1969

10. Denton R, Forsman W, Hwang SH, Litt M, Miller CE: Viscoelasticity of mucus. Its role in ciliary transport of pulmonary secretions. Am Rev Respir Dis 98:380–391, 1968

11. Diedrich WM: The mechanism of esophageal speech, in: Sound Production in Man. Ann NY Acad Sci 155, Article 1, 1968, pp 303–317

12. Edmunds LH Jr, Stallone RJ, Graf PD, Sagel SS, Greenspan RH: Mucus transport in transplanted lungs of dogs. Surgery 66:15–21, 1969

13. Fenn WO: Perspectives in phonation. In: Sound Production in Man. Ann NY Acad Sci 155, Article 1, 1968, pp 4–8

14. Florey H, Carleton HM, Wells AQ: Mucus secretion in the trachea. Br J Exp Pathol 13:269–284, 1932

15. Formijne P, van der Schoot JB, de Nie I: On the formation of mucin in tracheal mucosa of the rat. Biochim Biophys Acta 83:239–241, 1964

16. Gil J: Ultrastructure of lung fixed under physiologically defined conditions. Arch Intern Med 127:896–902, 1971

17. Hakansson CH, Toremalm NG: Studies on the physiology of the trachea. I. Ciliary activity indirectly recorded by a new "light beam reflex" method. Ann Otol Rhinol Laryngol 74:954–969, 1965

18. Hale FC, Olsen CR, Mickey MR Jr: The measurement of bronchial wall components. Am Rev Respir Dis 98:978–987, 1968

19. Havez R, Deminatti M, Roussel P, Degand P, Randoux A, Biserte G: Étude des glycoprotéines carboxyliques et sulfatées de la sécrétion bronchique humaine. Clin Chim Acta 17:463–477, 1967

20. Hayek H von: Die menschliche Lunge. Berlin, Springer, 1953. (Translation by Krahl VE: The Human Lung, New York, Hafner, 1960)

21. Holczabek W: Die Mastzellen der Lunge des Menschen. Deutsche Z gerichtl Med 54:175–177, 1963

22. Horsfield K, Cumming G: Morphology of the bronchial tree in man. J Appl Physiol 24:373–383,1968

23. Huber HL, Koessler KK: The pathology of bronchial asthma. Arch Intern Med 30:689–760, 1922

24. Hughes T: Microcirculation of the tracheobronchial tree. Nature 206:425–426, 1965

25. Iravani J: Flimmerbewegung in den intrapulmonalen Luftwegen der Ratte. Pfluegers Arch 297:221–237, 1967

26. Kilburn KH: Mucociliary clearance from bullfrog (Rana cantesbiana) lung. J Appl Physiol 23:804–810, 1967

27. Koch Hj, Allander C, Ingelstedt S, Toremalm NG: A method for humidifying inspired air in posttracheotomy care. Ann Otol Rhinol Laryngol 67:991–1004, 1958

28. Larsell O, Dow RS: The innervation of the human lung. Am J Anat 52, 125–146, 1933

29. Lieberman P, Crelin ES: On the speech of Neanderthal man. Linguistic Inquiry 2:203–222, 1971

30. Litt M: Mucus rheology. Relevance to mucociliary clearance. Arch Intern Med 126:417–423, 1970

31. Macklem PT, Mead J: Resistance of central and peripheral airways measured by a retrograde catheter. J Appl Physiol 22:395–401, 1967

32. Macklin CC: The musculature of the bronchi and lungs. Physiol Rev 9:1–60, 1929

33. Masson PL, Heremans JF, Prignot J: Studies on the proteins of human bronchial secretions. Biochim Biophys Acta 111:466–478, 1965

34. Mead J, Turner JM, Macklem PT, Little JB: Significance of the relationship between static recoil and maximum expiratory flow. J Appl Physiol 22:95–108, 1967

35. Megahed GE, Senna GA, Eissa MH, Saleh SZ, Eissa HA: Smoking versus infection as the aetiology of mucous gland hypertrophy in chronic bronchitis. Thorax 22:271–278, 1967

36. Moss ML: Veloepiglottic sphincter and obligate nose breathing in the neonate. J Pediatr 67:330–331, 1965

37. Nadel JA, Corn M, Zwi S, Flesch J, Graf P: Location and mechanism of airway constriction after inhalation of histamine aerosol and inorganic sulfate aerosol, in Davies CN (ed): Inhaled Particles and Vapours II. London, Pergamon, 1966, pp 55–67

38. Nadel JA: New technique for studying structural changes of airways in vivo using powdered tantalum, in Bouhuys A (ed): Airway Dynamics; Physiology and Pharmacology. Springfield, Charles C Thomas, 1970, pp 73–83

39. Oreckin-Duchemin H: Documents sur la vie et l'oeuvre de F.D. Reisseisen (1773–1828). Université de Strasbourg, Faculté de Médecine, 1971

40. Parker H, Horsfield K, Cumming G: Morphology of distal airways in the human lung. J Appl Physiol 31:386–391, 1971

41. Parks CR, Woodrum DE, Graham CB, Cheney FW, Hodson WA: Effect of water nebulization on normal canine pulmonary mucociliary clearance. Am Rev Respir Dis 104:99–106, 1971

42. Proctor DF: Physiology of the upper airway, in Fenn WO, Rahn H (eds): Handbook of Physiology, Section 3: Respiration, vol 1. Washington, D.C.,

American Physiological Society, 1964, pp 309–345

43. Proctor DF: Airborne disease and the upper respiratory tract. Bacteriol Rev 30:498–513, 1966

44. Proust, Marcel: A la recherche du temps perdu, I. Du Côté de chez Swann. Paris, Bibliothèque de la Pléiade, Edition Gallimard, pp 44–48, 1954

45. Puchelle E, Benis AM: Propriétés d'écoulement des secrétions bronchiques. Bull Physiopathol Respir (Nancy) 7:673–712, 1971

46. Quinlan MF, Salman SD, Swift DL, Wagner HN, Jr, Proctor DF: Measurement of mucociliary function in man. Am Rev Respir Dis 99:13–23, 1969

47. Reid L: Measurement of the bronchial mucous gland layer: A diagnostic yardstick in chronic bronchitis. Thorax 15:132–141, 1960

48. Reid L: An experimental study of hypersecretion of mucus in the bronchial tree. Br J Exp Pathol 44:437–445, 1963

49. Reid L: Histochemical and enzyme studies of bronchial mucus. Med Thorac 22:61–68, 1965

50. Reisseisen FD: Ueber den Bau der Lungen. Berlin, Rücker, 1822 (First published as thesis, Koenigliche Akademie der Wissenschaften, 1808)

51. Ross BB: Influence of bronchial tree structure on ventilation in the dog's lung as inferred from measurements of a plastic cast. J Appl Physiol 10:1–14, 1957

52. Satir P: Cilia. Sci Am 204:108–116, 1961

53. Schiratzki H: Upper airway resistance during mouth breathing in patients with unilateral and bilateral paralysis of the recurrent laryngeal nerve. Acta Otolaryngol (Stockh) 59:475–496, 1965

54. Schmidt-Nielsen K, Hainsworth FR, Murrish DE: Counter-current heat exchange in the respiratory passages: Effect on water and heat balance. Respir Physiol 9:263–276, 1970

55. Sorokin SP: Respiratory system, in: Greep RO (ed): Histology. New York, McGraw-Hill, 1966, p 573

56. Staub NC: The interdependence of pulmonary structure and function. Anesthesiology 24:831–854, 1963

57. Sturgess JM, Palfrey AJ, Reid L: The viscosity of bronchial secretion. Clin Sci 38:145–156, 1970

58. Thompson HT, Pryor WJ, Hill J: Bronchial lavage in the treatment of obstructive lung disease. Thorax 21:557–559, 1966

59. Thurlbeck WM, Angus GE: The variation of Reid index measurements within the major bronchial tree. Am Rev Respir Dis 95:551–555, 1967

60. Toremalm NG: A heat-and-moisture exchanger for post-tracheotomy care. Acta Otolaryngol (Stockh) 52:461–472, 1960

61. Toremalm NG: The daily amount of tracheo-bronchial secretions in man, a method for continuous tracheal aspiration in laryngectomized and tracheotomized patients. Acta Otolaryngol [Suppl] (Stockh) 158:43–53, 1960

62. Weibel ER: Morphometry of the Human Lung. Berlin, Springer-Verlag, 1963

63. Weibel ER, Gomez DM: Architecture of the human lung. Science 137:577–585, 1962

64. Wolfsdorf J, Swift DL, Avery ME: Mist therapy reconsidered; an evaluation of the respiratory deposition of labelled water aerosols produced by jet and ultrasonic nebulizers. Pediatrics 43:799–808, 1969

65. Yeager H Jr: Tracheobronchial secretions. Am J Med 50:493–509, 1971

Chapter 3

Anatomical Dead Space

In 1894, Loewy measured the volume of a plaster of paris cast of the human bronchi and found a value of 144 ml.[17] Nearly 80 years and many controversies later, the simplest answer to the question, "What is the volume of the conducting airways?" is still: about 150 ml. Because the conducting airways do not participate in gas exchange, this volume is called the anatomical dead space. Its size has important effects on gas exchange, and, if nothing else, it is a source of confusion for medical students and a delight for engineers who enjoy complex plumbing problems. The physiologist must neither oversimplify nor introduce needless complexities. Theoretical analyses that go far beyond what can be measured experimentally are unlikely to increase our understanding of gas exchange or lung disease. The Appendix (p. 55) summarizes several definitions of dead space. In this chapter, I discuss only anatomical dead space; physiological dead space is a concept closely linked with alveolar gas exchange (see Chap. 5).

MORPHOLOGICAL MEASUREMENTS

Loewy's estimate of 144 ml[17] was for the volume of the bronchial tree only. Rohrer[24, 25] did a more complete study, measuring the airway dimensions of a nearly collapsed right lung, down to bronchi of 1 mm in diameter (total volume for both lungs from the carina down—72 ml). He also estimated the volumes of the trachea (45 ml), pharynx (30 ml), and nose (15 ml). Thus, excluding airways less than 1 mm in diameter, he arrived at a value of 162 ml for the total dead space during nose breathing. A more recent estimate[19] is 138 ml for the total dead space, of which 72 ml is in the extrathoracic part of the airways. Thus, about 50 percent of the dead space is in the upper airways, and this volume depends greatly on the position of the jaw.[19]

Weibel's symmetrical model[37] (see also p. 30) is based on measurements made on a single lung specimen inflated to about 75 percent of total lung capacity

(4800 ml volume). This model has an anatomical dead space (from the glottis to the last, 16th generation of unalveolated bronchioles) of 175 ml. Thus, this would yield a total dead space of about 220 ml, assuming 45 ml for the pharynx and nose. In Weibel's model, the volume corresponding to Rohrer's 72 ml (carina to 1 mm bronchi) is less, about 60 ml, in spite of the larger lung volume. The volume of successive generations of airways in the bronchial tree (in Weibel's model) is indicated in Figure 3-4. The trachea and main bronchi contribute about 40 ml, the next 4 generations only 12 ml. Beyond the 10th generation, airway volume rapidly increases, owing to the large increase in total cross-sectional area of the smaller airways (Table 2-1, p. 30).

Loewy and Rohrer both knew that they had underestimated the volume of the small airways in their dead space values. The 17th generation, which carries the first few alveoli, has a volume of about 40 ml (Weibel's model, Fig. 3-4). It is difficult to determine which part of this generation should be assigned to the conducting and which part to gas-exchanging airways, since they gradually merge (Fig. 2-2B). Since the aggregate volume of these transition generations is large, morphological determinations of anatomical dead space volume have a large margin of uncertainty.

As a rule of thumb, anatomical dead space in man (in milliliters) is numerically equal to body weight in pounds, (i.e., 2.22 ml/kg body wt.).[22] Anatomical data in animals are few: 150 ml in inflated dog lungs,[26] 380 ml in the cow,[23] 1600 ml in the giraffe,[23] and 150 to 300 liters in fin whales.[30]

PHYSIOLOGICAL MEASUREMENTS

Physiological measurements depend on the fact that gas in the dead space retains the composition of inspired air, while gas in the alveoli contains less O_2 and much more CO_2 than inspired air.

Hence, dead space can be measured only for gases which are not absorbed or excreted in the upper airways and the bronchial tree. For instance, the dead space for water vapor is minimal since inspired gas is rapidly saturated with water vapor (Chap. 2, p. 25). Differences between O_2 and CO_2 dead space are discussed in Chap. 5 (p. 93).

During expiration, dead space gas emerges first, and alveolar gas later. Apparently, Wollaston (1766–1828) was the first to notice that the last portion of the expired air extinguishes a candle, and he concluded that this was because of its CO_2 content. In 1845, Vierordt[35] reported the first quantitative measurements: 3.72 percent CO_2 in the first half and 5.44 percent in the second half of the air expired during a deep expiration. Gréhant[13] concluded from an experiment with hydrogen inspiration that 170 ml of inspired gas was expired without change in composition.

In 1891, Christian Bohr[4] formalized these concepts in the following equation

$$V_E \cdot F_E = V_D \cdot F_D + V_A \cdot F_A, \tag{1}$$

where V_E, V_D, and V_A are the volume of expired gas, dead space gas, and alveolar gas, respectively, and F_E, F_D, and F_A are the average fractional concentrations of a reference gas in these volumes. The equation states that the amount of reference gas in the total breath equals the sum of the amounts contained in the first portion expired (the dead space) and the last portion expired (the alveolar gas). Since $V_E = V_D + V_A$, Eq. (1) can be rearranged to solve for V_D

$$V_D / V_E = (F_A - F_E) / (F_A - F_D) \tag{2}$$

Since no gas exchange takes place in the dead space, F_D equals the inspired gas concentration. The equation is usually solved with data for carbon dioxide (during air breathing) and nitrogen (after inspiration of 100% oxygen). In both cases F_D is close to zero and can be ignored, so that Eq. (2) simplifies to

$$\frac{V_D}{V_E} = \frac{F_A - F_E}{F_A} \tag{3}$$

V_E and F_E are measured by collecting the expired gas and determining its CO_2 or N_2 concentration. The remaining unknowns are V_D and F_A. Thus, one may use Eq. (3) to calculate V_D if F_A is known, or F_A if V_D is known or assumed. The controversy surrounding the Bohr equation and dead space has resulted from the difficulty in deciding acceptable values for F_A.

The Bohr equation treats expired air as if it consists of two distinct portions— dead space gas, with inspired gas concentration $F_I = F_D$, and alveolar air, with gas concentration F_A. The equation represents the situation at the end of inspiration as if the conducting airways were filled with inspired air, separated by a sharp gas front (i.e., a distinct boundary without intermixing of gas) from the alveolar gas 'in the respiratory zone. In this case, if one inspired 100 percent oxygen and analyzed the next expiration for nitrogen with a rapid analyzer, a recording like that of Figure 3-1A would be obtained. The first portion of expired air (OA) would contain no N_2 at all (pure oxygen from dead space), while the second portion (AD) would contain a constant N_2 concentration. The vertical line AB is recorded at the moment that the sharp front between dead space gas and alveolar gas passes the sampling site. In this graph, the rectangle $ABCD$ represents the amount of N_2 expired (surface area $AD \times AB = V_E \times F_E$).

Actually, no sharp front as implied in Figure 3-1A exists. Because of gas mixing (see below), a more gradual concentration change occurs. A test record from a rapid gas analyzer [9, 18] is shown schematically in Figure 3-1B. Some of the first recordings, made by Mundt et al.[18] with hydrogen as the test gas, are reproduced in Figure 3-2.

Only the first portion of the expired gas in Figure 3-1B contains no N_2 at all. In the next portion, N_2 concentration rises in an S-shaped pattern until a plateau value is reached. At C, a new oxygen inspiration begins, and the N_2 concentration seen by the analyzer drops to zero. Fowler[9] indicated a graphical technique to calculate dead space shown in Figure 3-1A and B. To determine the virtual volume of the anatomical dead space, we must find the virtual sharp front as it occurs in the idealized condition of A. Since the surface area under a concentration-volume curve represents an amount of gas, this can be done by finding the rectangle $ABCD$ of graph A that has the same surface area as the recording of graph B. To do this, a line AB is placed halfway up the S-shaped portion of B, so that the area of the two hatched triangles is equal.

To determine anatomical dead space as in Figure 3-1B, a graph of percentage of expired N_2 must be plotted against expired volume. This can be recorded

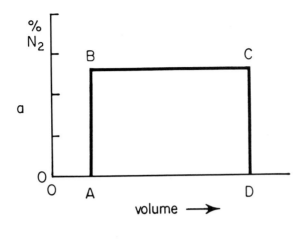

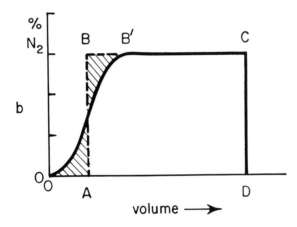

Fig. 3-1. (A). Idealized single-breath N_2 curve, assuming a square front of N_2 traveling through the airways. (B) Actual shape of single-breath curve (OB'CD).
Line AB represents the vertical N_2 front, placed so that the
surface area OB'CD equals surface area of ABCD. OA =
anatomical dead space; OD = total expired volume.

directly with electronic equipment (Fig. 3-3). The calculation of dead space in
Figure 3-1 can be used only if the plateau B'C is flat, or nearly so. The line B'C
represents alveolar N_2 concentrations, and if B'C slopes upward (as in many patients with lung disease), this means that alveolar gas is not homogeneous (Chap.
4). Under these conditions, the definition of average F_A becomes arbitrary, and
application of Bohr's equation is questionable. Modified dead space measurements
are feasible but do not fully solve the problem.[10]

When alveolar gas is not homogeneous, there are different methods for obtaining an average F_A value. One is to make a more or less educated guess from
alveolar gas concentration data; e.g., one could select the halfway point on line
B'C. Another method is to record the rate of mixing of lung gas with gas in a
spirometer.[3] The Bohr equation shows why these methods often yield V_D values

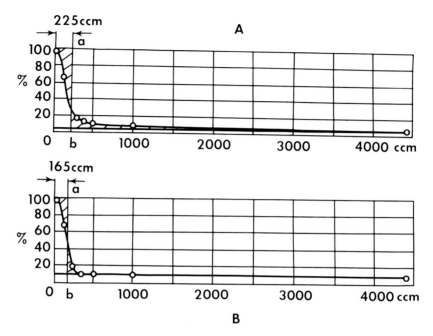

Fig. 3-2. Single-breath records of H_2 concentration in expired air (ordinate) versus expired volume (abscissa) after one inspiration of H_2. In both graphs, the vertical line ab represents the virtual front between dead space and alveolar gas. The hatched areas on either side of line ab have an equal surface area. *A.* If F_A is taken to equal the lowest H_2 concentration recorded in expired air, V_D is calculated by graphical analysis at 225 ml. *B.* If F_A is taken to equal the H_2 concentration at the transition point between the second and the third phase of the record, a V_D value of 165 ml is calculated. This value approximates the anatomical dead space; the larger value calculated from *A* includes an additional volume which reflects the slope of the alveolar plateau. From Mundt et al.[18]

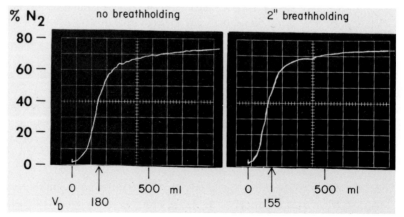

Fig. 3-3. Single-breath N_2 curves in a healthy subject. Two-second breath holding reduces dead space from 180 to 155 ml, end-inspiratory volume and other parameters being equal. Data from Chiang, Snyder, and Bouhuys (unpublished).

that include an increment resulting from nonuniform gas distribution. With 100% O_2 inspiration, Eq. (1) transforms to: $V_E \times F_E = V_A \times F_A$, or, the quantity of N_2 in expired gas equals the amount contributed by alveolar gas. $V_E \times F_E$ is determined experimentally. If one chooses an unduly high F_A value, e.g., at the end of the sloping plateau, V_A becomes too small and thus V_D too large (Fig. 3-2A). This effect of nonuniform ventilation was recognized by Mundt et al.[18] and is well illustrated in their curves (Fig. 3-2). Other methods of obtaining an average F_A use the pulmonary circulation as an averaging circuit. This leads to F_A values weighted in favor of lung regions with high perfusion rates. These methods give values for physiological dead space, discussed in Chapter 5.

In healthy subjects, a wide variety of methods [1, 3, 7, 9, 21, 27] gives values close to the anatomical volume of the conducting airways. In patients with nonuniform lung ventilation, no satisfactory method to arrive at such a value has as yet been devised.

THE INSPIRED GAS FRONT AND DIFFUSION
DURING INSPIRATION

Yandell Henderson et al.[15] noted in 1915 that some alveolar gas already emerged at the mouth when only 50 ml gas had been expired, an observation confirmed in more recent work.[6] They believed that this resulted from a laminar airflow pattern in the airways, with a peak linear velocity in the middle of the stream twice as large as the mean velocity (parabolic gas front). In this way, some alveolar gas, traveling at peak velocity, would reach the airway opening early during expiration. "The authors of this paper were obviously aware of the complications in mass transport by convection and diffusion during the unsteady flow of a non-uniform gas mixture in a pipe." [39]

A more detailed analysis of gas transport in conducting airways does not support the assumption of a parabolic gas front. Gas moves into the trachea and large airways by bulk transport in the direction of a pressure gradient (convective transport). The exact flow pattern is not clear; turbulent flow very likely prevails in the trachea and may even extend to segmental bronchi.[20] Branching also affects flow patterns,[31] and it is unlikely that fully developed laminar flow occurs at all in the airways. Wilson and Lin [39] estimated that the purely convective forms of transport dominate until the eighth generation. In these large airways, convection is so fast that no appreciable time is available for diffusion. When the tubes narrow and convection velocities slow down, radial diffusion, which smoothes out concentration differences along the radius of the tube, becomes an additional transport mode. This coupling of axial convection and radial diffusion as a combined mode of gas transport is called Taylor diffusion. Beyond the 12th generation, axial gas velocity becomes so slow that no radial concentration differences occur. Hence, transport occurs by convective block flow coupled with axial diffusion.[39]

A model of dead space proposed by Scherer [28, 29] lumps convective transport and radial (Taylor) diffusion since both result in net forward transport. This model illustrates several features of gas transport in the airways. An important feature of the bronchial tree is the increase of total cross-sectional area as a function of airway generation number (Table 2-1), or of distance into the airway (Fig. 3-4). No

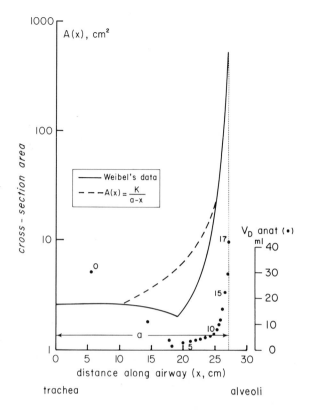

Fig. 3-4. Total cross-sectional area of all airways
[$A(x)$] as a function of distance into the bronchial tree;
0 is at the oral entrance of the trachea. The dashed line
is the hyperbola used in Scherer's model (see text). The
right-hand ordinate refers to the points which indicate the
anatomical dead space volume of airway generations 0-17
(0 = trachea). The point for each generation has been
placed at the mid-point of its length. Data from Weibel.[37]

accurate mathematical equation has as yet been fitted to this area function curve.
As a rough approximation, a hyperbola is suitable.[28]

How would a front of pure oxygen move into a lung represented by this
model? Near the entrance the cross-sectional area is small, hence velocities must
be high. As cross-sectional areas increase, velocities decrease, approaching zero in
the peripheral airways near the respiratory zone. To quantitate this movement of
the front, Scherer assumed a tidal volume of 500 ml and a sine-wave entrance
velocity. From the hyperbola, which describes the relationship between airway
cross-sectional area and distance along the airway, one can compute the position
and velocity of the oxygen front at any moment during the inspiration. Figure 3-5
shows the result. During the first 0.1 second, as the front begins to enter the
airways, the velocity of the air entering the trachea is almost equal to the velocity
of the front, which is then still in large airways with a cross section nearly equal to
that of the trachea. At about 0.3 seconds, front velocity begins to decrease, as the
front enters airways with an increasing cross-sectional area. At 1.0 second, velocity

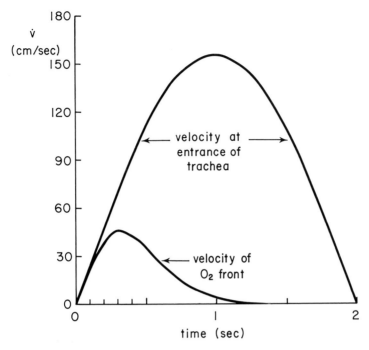

Fig. 3-5. Linear velocity of the gas front ($\dot{v}$) moving into the airways as represented by the hyperbolic function of Figure 3-4. The input velocity (at entrance of trachea) is a sinus function. When $\dot{v}$ at the trachea entrance is at its maximum, the O_2 front is already in small airways and has slowed down considerably. After Scherer.[28]

at the trachea entrance has reached its maximum, and half the tidal volume (250 ml) has entered the airways. The surface area under the area-function curve of Figure 3-4 has the dimensions of volume (abscissa in cm, ordinate in cm²); when 250 ml air has entered the airways, the front must be situated in very small airways, close to 27 cm from the trachea entrance. Hence, front velocity has decreased to nearly zero.

So far, the front has been treated as if it were a sharp gas concentration boundary throughout inspiration. But inspiration takes a certain time, and diffusion around the front will occur. Scherer[28] separated the effects of bulk flow and diffusion by changing coordinates. An apocryphal analog may illustrate this. Consider a group of people who start a train journey together at the bar of a commuter train out of Grand Central Station bound for Connecticut. Bulk flow begins when the train leaves and picks up speed. While this happens, the commuters pick up their drinks and disperse through the train. To measure their speed of dispersion, an observer must be on the train, not beside the track. To place an observer on the train means establishing the speed of the train as a reference velocity. The dispersion of the commuters is measured with respect to the position of the bar, which itself moves at the reference velocity. Similarly, Scherer used the position of the oxygen front at any time as his zero coordinate. He also assumed that radial diffusion is fast compared with axial diffusion; therefore, only axial diffusion along a single pathway into the lung was considered.

Figure 3-6 illustrates diffusion on both sides of the front. In the trachea, at

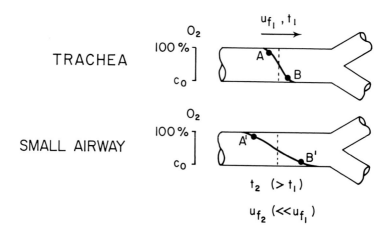

Fig. 3-6. Diffusion around the oxygen front which moves into the airways. In the trachea the diffusion zone is short; in a small airway it has increased in width. $c_0 =$ oxygen concentration in gas in airways before O_2 front moves in. Uf_1 and Uf_2 are the velocities of the front at times t_1 and t_2 respectively.

time t_1, there is a narrow zone around the front in which oxygen concentration changes from 100 percent to c_0. An instant later, at time t_2, the front is in a small airway and its velocity has decreased. In the interval $t_2 - t_1$, diffusion has enlarged the length of airway in which O_2 concentration decreases from 100% to c_0. The speed of individual molecules differs. For instance, a molecule moving from A to A' during t_2-t_1 has covered less distance than a molecule moving from B to B' in the same time interval. However, these differences are small, and for the analysis one may consider all molecules to move with the velocity of the front. In the new coordinate system one may solve the diffusion equation, assuming that there is an infinite oxygen reservoir at the mouth, and that at the alveolar end of the airway there is an infinite reservoir of well-mixed alveolar gas. With these boundary conditions, we ignore the complexities of alveolar mixing and consider only diffusion in pipes. We consider the alveoli as a source of gas with a constant nitrogen concentration. (Gas mixing in the alveolar units themselves is discussed in Chap. 4.) Assume that the lower diagram of Figure 3-6 represents the front and the diffusion zone around it at the end of inspiration. During expiration, the front and diffusion zone move back to the airway opening, now at increasing velocities since the front moves into larger airways, with a decreasing cross-sectional area. As soon as the front has left the small airways, diffusion becomes a minor transport mode because of the increased dimensions and gas velocities. An analyzer sampling gas expired at the mouth will therefore inscribe the S-shaped curve of Figure 3-1B, reflecting the blurring of the gas front caused by diffusion.

    The equations derived from this model [28] describe anatomical dead space (i.e., the volume down to the virtual square gas front) as a function of the constants K and a, which describe airway geometry (Fig. 3-4), and of breath-holding time. These equations fit dead space measurements reasonably well, using 0–5-second-periods of breath holding (see p. 52). Implications of the model for gas mixing in the lungs are discussed in Chapter 4.

UNEQUAL PATHWAY LENGTHS

The preceding section discussed one reason for the S shape of the expiratory N_2 curve after a breath of oxygen. This section deals with a morphological feature that can explain, at least in part, the same phenomenon. Study of human and dog lungs provides good evidence that pathway lengths from the trachea to the alveoli vary a great deal in different parts of the lungs. In the dog lung, Ross [26] found the shortest pathways (carina-alveoli) only about 2 cm long, and the longest about 14 cm. For the human lung, Weibel's data [37] on the distribution of airways of equal diameter also suggest a wide variability of pathway lengths. Most bronchi with an internal diameter of 2 mm belong to the 7th through 11th generations, with the total range varying from the 4th to the 13th. Pathway lengths for these, from the carina, vary from about 17 to 32 cm. The distribution of 0.5-mm diameter airways [37] suggests that total pathway lengths (carina-alveoli) may vary from roughly 22 to 40 cm (at 75% TLC). Since the volume of the common dead space (upper airway and trachea) is about 90 ml, and N_2 already begins to appear at the mouth after some 60 ml gas has been expired, unequal pathway lengths do not completely explain the S-shaped curves. To the extent that they account for part of it, airway models based solely on gas-transport mechanisms should underestimate the range of volumes over which the expired gas front is blurred when it arrives at the mouth during expiration.

STRATIFIED DEAD SPACE

The term stratified dead space has recently been proposed to designate that part of the conducting airways where diffusion is an important transport mode.[34] The delineation of this space is, unfortunately, not clear. The virtual boundary of the anatomical dead space is sharply defined by the position of the oxygen front in a model and by the Bohr equation in the experiment. The boundaries of stratified dead space are also virtual ones, and they can be defined only arbitrarily. Consider Figure 3-6: the stratified dead space might be the area between points A' and B', or one might choose points closer to or farther away from the 100 percent and c_0 limits. Strictly speaking, the limits are never reached but only approached asymptotically; so stratified dead space might be equal to total airway or even lung volume in this absolute sense. The concentration gradients in the diffusion zone around the front cannot be determined accurately. While the term stratified dead space implies a measurable volume with virtual but defined boundaries, such a space exists neither in theory nor in practice.

GAS TRANSPORT TIME

A bolus of CO injected into the trachea can be detected at the pleural surface by continuous monitoring for CO-hemoglobin with a photoelectric method. Wagner et al.[36] used this ingenious technique in anesthetized dogs to estimate the time it takes the CO bolus to travel from the trachea to the alveoli. The additional time needed for CO to diffuse across the alveolocapillary membrane and to bind to Hb is short compared to its transport time through the airways. During slow and fast inspirations, CO transport time was about 50 percent of the duration of inspiration. This corresponds well with Scherer's model (Fig. 3-5), in which the inspired gas front arrives in very small airways at about the midpoint of inspiration. However, the data obtained with Wagner et al.'s method do not allow firm conclusions concerning the modes of gas transport.[32]

FACTORS THAT MODIFY DEAD SPACE

Lung Volume

Airway caliber increases with lung distension,[16] and dead space volume therefore increases with lung volume. Since the increase is in the order of 2–3 ml per 100 ml increase in postexpiratory lung volume,[5] dead space should be measured as a function of lung volume.

Widdicombe [38] has pointed out that since about 50 percent of the dead space is in upper airways and trachea where little change in volume is expected, the intrapulmonary and particularly the small airways (bronchioles) may inflate much more in proportion with lung volume. For instance, his own data [38] indicate a total V_D of about 150 ml at a lung volume of 2 liters, and a V_D of about 250 ml at 5.5 liters—an overall increase of about 3 ml V_D per 100 ml increase in lung volume. If one assumes that x ml of dead space does not change with lung volume, and the remainder changes in proportion to lung volume, one has: $2000:5500=(150-x):(250-x)$, from which $x=93$ ml. This is close to Rohrer's value of 90 ml for the dead space of the extrathoracic airways and trachea.[24] The dead space of the bronchial tree increases from 57 to 157 ml with this lung volume increase, or 28.5 ml/liter.

Tidal Volume

The relation between dead space and tidal volume was the subject of the classical Haldane-Krogh controversy, reviewed elsewhere.[5] There is no evidence that tidal volume influences dead space in any way other than by increasing postinspiratory lung volume (see above).

Breath Holding

Even a few seconds' breath holding after inspiration of 100 percent O_2 lowers the dead space value [33] (Fig. 3-3). Breath holding for more than 5 seconds does not have much additional effect (Fig. 3-7). Scherer's model (see pp. 47–50) predicts the rapid decrease of V_D during the first few seconds, but after about 5 seconds the model and the data diverge. This results from the boundary conditions of the model; it assumes an infinite reservoir of alveolar gas. Therefore, diffusion in the model continues while in the lungs there is a finite amount of alveolar gas and hence a limit to the extent of diffusion. In intact man, the heartbeat may be an additional factor which promotes gas mixing during breath holding.[35a]

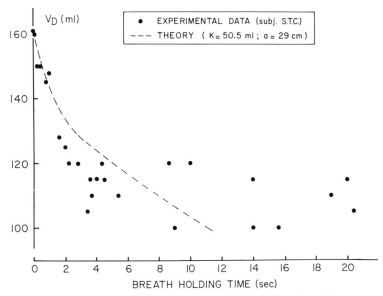

Fig. 3-7. Theoretical data for V_D as a function of breath-holding time are based on Scherer's model.[28, 29] Experimental data, on one subject, from Chiang, Snyder, and Bouhuys (unpublished).

Airflow Rates

Inspiratory flow rate has little effect on V_D if time and postinspiratory volume are kept constant (Chiang, Snyder, and Bouhuys, unpublished material). Also, expiratory flow rates varying from 1–5 liters/second had little influence on V_D in the same experiments (Fig. 3-8). This does not confirm an earlier report [2] of large decreases of dead space at high expiratory flow rates. By the time flow has reached

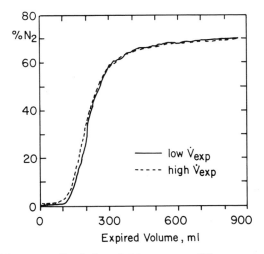

Fig. 3-8. Single-breath N_2 curve at different rates of expiratory flow (*drawn line:* $\dot{V} = 1.4$ liters/sec; *dashed line:* $\dot{V} = 5.7$ liters/sec) in healthy subject. Data from Chiang, Snyder, and Bouhuys (unpublished).

maximum values, the front has left small airways. Hence, differences in diffusion times due to the different duration of expiration should not affect dead space significantly. Decreasing dead space at high expiratory flows has been attributed to large airway compression,[2] but it is not clear how this would affect dead space.

Volume History

Froeb and Mead [11] demonstrated that in certain subjects anatomical dead space depends on volume history of the lungs. When dead space is measured after several expirations to residual volume, other parameters being equal, dead space is smaller than when the measurement is made after several inspirations to TLC. This phenomenon apparently varies individually. It was confirmed in some of the subjects of Chiang et al. (unpublished). The mechanisms of hysteresis of the dead space may be related to those which cause volume history dependence of airway resistance (Chap. 8). Temporary closure of airways at small lung volumes is probably an important factor.

Body Size

Hart et al.[14] determined dead space with the N_2 single-breath method in children, and Chiang et al. obtained similar data in children and adults. Their results are summarized in Figure 3-9. Dead space increases as a linear function of standing

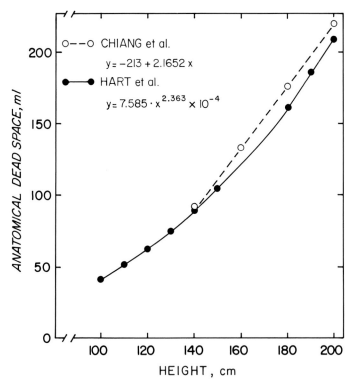

Fig. 3-9. Anatomical dead space as a function of standing height in two groups of subjects. The group of Hart et al.[14] included children; the group of Chiang et al. (unpublished) were healthy adults. Lines shown are regression lines fitted to experimental data.

body height, and also approximately in proportion to vital capacity and total lung capacity. In the 140-cm tall child, V_D is about 3.5% VC and 3% TLC, while in the 180-cm tall adult, these percentages are 3.4% VC and 2.4% TLC (see also Table 1-4, p. 20).

Effects of Drugs

In studies reviewed elsewhere,[5, 38] bronchodilator drugs increased dead space volume, while constrictor drugs decreased it. These responses have not been observed consistently.[8] In our laboratory, Chiang et al. (unpublished) found no consistent effect of isoproterenol inhalation, in doses known to decrease airway resistance, on dead space in healthy subjects (method as shown in Fig. 3-3). A large fraction of dead space is in upper airways and in the trachea, where major caliber changes induced by drugs are unlikely. In peripheral airways, more subject to caliber changes, other factors, such as airway closure and lung elastic recoil, also affect caliber. Thus, dead space measurements are not very suitable for the quantitative assessment of airway responses to drugs.

SUMMARY

The volume of conducting airways varies from about 150 to 300 ml, depending on the state of lung inflation. Although gas transport modes are complex and not completely defined, gas dilution methods (using an inert test gas) can measure this volume reasonably accurately in healthy men, using Bohr's equation. When lung ventilation is markedly nonhomogeneous, the definition of alveolar gas becomes arbitrary and the Bohr equation then does not measure dead space volume per se. Therefore, anatomical dead space is difficult to measure in many patients with lung disease.

Gas transport in the conducting airways can be studied with simplified mathematical models. Convection and diffusion are two important gas-transport modes. Unequal bronchial pathway lengths also influence the shape of the expiratory N_2 curve recorded at the mouth after oxygen inspiration. Gas-transport times from trachea to alveoli have been measured in animals but do not give insight into transport modes.

Dead space values measured in healthy persons are a function of body size, lung volume, the time course of the test maneuver, and, in some subjects, of lung volume history. Airflow rates have a minor effect, and changes induced by bronchoactive drugs are difficult to measure in the presence of the several other variables that influence anatomical dead space in vivo.

Appendix: Definitions of Dead Space

1. *Anatomical:*
    A. Morphological definition: the volume of the conducting airways, i.e., airways not lined with respiratory epithelium, measured from a cast of the bronchial tree. Most data exclude the supralaryngeal airways; the precise extent of the cast must be specified. This is a volume with "spatial boundaries identified by anatomical means."[12]

B. Functional definition: the volume of inspired gas that does not mix with alveolar gas, measured in vivo by gas-dilution methods as indicated by Fowler.[9] Synonymous term—series dead space.[8]

2. *Physiological:*

The volume of gas that is inspired and expired but takes no part in gas exchange in the alveoli, measured from V_{CO_2} and Pa_{CO_2} by assuming that PA_{CO_2} equals Pa_{CO_2} (Chap. 5).

3. *Alveolar:*

A volume of inspired gas that mixes with gas in alveolar spaces but takes no part in alveolar gas exchange, thus, a volume of gas in well-ventilated, non-perfused alveoli. Alveolar V_D = physiological V_D − anatomical V_D. Synonymous term—parallel dead space.[8]

4. *Instrumental or mechanical:*

The volume of mouthpiece, breathing valves, or other apparatus connected to the airways, in which inspired and expired gas are not separated. It is customary to subtract this volume from calculated dead-space volumes, but a more complex correction method is needed for calculation of physiological dead space.[33a]

5. *Personal:*

A term used to indicate the calculated dead-space volume, either physiological or anatomical V_D, minus instrumental dead-space volume.

6. *Respiratory:*

This general term needs qualification; the definitions 1–3 are more specific and, therefore, preferable.

REFERENCES

1. Bartels J, Severinghaus JW, Forster RE, Briscoe WA, Bates DV: The respiratory dead space measured by single breath analysis of oxygen, carbon dioxide, nitrogen or helium. J Clin Invest 33:41–48, 1954

2. Bashoff MA, Ingram RH Jr, Schilder DP: Effect of expiratory flow rate on the nitrogen concentration vs. volume relationship. J Appl Physiol 23:895–901, 1967

3. Birath G: Lung volume and ventilation efficiency. Change in collapse-treated and non-collapse-treated pulmonary tuberculosis and in pulmonectomy and lobectomy. Acta Med Scand 120 (suppl 154):1–168, 1944

4. Bohr C: Ueber die Lungenathmung. Skand Arch Physiol 2:236–268, 1891

5. Bouhuys A: Respiratory dead space, in Fenn WO, Rahn H (eds): Handbook of Physiology, Section 3: Respiration, vol. I. Washington, D.C., American Physiological Society, 1964, pp 699–714

6. Briscoe WA, Forster RE, Comroe JH Jr: Alveolar ventilation at very low tidal volumes. J Appl Physiol 7:27–30, 1954

7. Enghoff H: Volumen Inefficax. Bemerkungen zur Frage des schädlichen Raumes. Upsala Laekaref Foerh 44:191–218, 1938

8. Folkow B, Pappenheimer JR: Components of the respiratory dead space and their variation with pressure breathing and with bronchoactive drugs. J Appl Physiol 8:102–110, 1955

9. Fowler WS: Lung function studies. II. The respiratory dead space. Am J Physiol 154:405–416, 1948

10. Fowler WS: Lung function studies. V. Respiratory dead space in old age and in pulmonary emphysema. J Clin Invest 29:1439–1444, 1950

11. Froeb HF, Mead J: Relative hysteresis of the dead space and lung in vivo. J Appl Physiol 25:244–248, 1968

12. Gray JS, Grodins FS, Carter ET: Alveolar and total ventilation and the dead space problem. J Appl Physiol 9:307–320, 1956

13. Gréhant N: Recherches physiques sur la respiration de l'homme. J Anat Physiol Homme Anim 1:523–55, 1864

14. Hart MC, Orzalesi MM, Cook CD: Relation between anatomic respiratory dead space and body size and lung volume. J Appl Physiol 18:519–522, 1963

15. Henderson Y, Chillingworth FP, Whitney JL: The respiratory dead space. Am J Physiol 38:1–19, 1915

16. Huizinga E: Ueber die Physiologie des Bronchialbaumes. Pflueger's Arch 238:767–779, 1937

17. Loewy A: Ueber die Bestimmung der Grösse des "Schädlichen Luftraumes" im Thorax und der alveolaren Sauerstoffspannung. Arch Ges Physiol 58:416–427, 1894

18. Mundt E, Schoedel W, Schwarz H: Ueber den effektiven schädlichen Raum der Atmung. Pflueger's Arch 244:107–119, 1940

19. Nunn JF, Campbell EJM, Peckett BW: Anatomical subdivisions of the volume of respiratory dead space and effect of position of the jaw. J Appl Physiol 14:174–176, 1959

20. Owen PR: Turbulent flow and particle deposition in the trachea, in Wolstenholme GEW, Knight J (eds): Circulatory and Respiratory Mass Transport. Boston, Little, Brown & Company, 1969, pp 236–252

21. Pappenheimer JR, Fishman AP, Borrero LM: New experimental methods for determination of effective alveolar gas composition and respiratory dead space, in the anesthetized dog and in man. J Appl Physiol 4:855–867, 1952

22. Radford E Jr: Ventilation standards for use in artificial respiration. J Appl Physiol 7:451–460, 1955

23. Robin ED, Corson JM, Dammin GJ: The respiratory dead space of the giraffe. Nature 186:24–26, 1960

24. Rohrer F: Der Strömungswiderstand in den menschlichen Atemwegen und der Einfluss der unregelmässigen Verzweigung des Bronchialsystems auf den Atmungsverlauf in verschiedenen Lungenbezirken. Pflueger's Arch 162:225–299, 1915

25. Rohrer F: Die Grösse des schädlichen Raumes der Atemwege. Pflueger's Arch 164:295–302, 1916

26. Ross BB: Influence of bronchial tree structure on ventilation in the dog's lung as inferred from measurements of a plastic cast. J Appl Physiol 10:1–14, 1957

27. Rossier PH, Bühlmann A: The respiratory dead space. Physiol Rev 35:860–876, 1955

28. Scherer PW: Modeling of the dispersion of gases in the human bronchial tree. PhD Thesis, Yale University, 1971

29. Scherer PW, Chiang ST, Bouhuys A: A quantitative model of anatomical dead space. Fed Proc 29:396, 1970

30. Scholander PF: Experimental investigations on the respiration in diving mammals and birds. Hvalraadets Skr Nr 22, Norske Vid Akad 1–131, 1940

31. Schroter RC, Sudlow MF: Flow patterns in models of the human bronchial airways. Respir Physiol 7:341–355, 1969

32. Shair FH: Pulmonary gas transport time. Science 165:823, 1969

33. Shepard RH, Campbell EJM, Martin HB, Enns T: Factors affecting the pulmonary dead space as determined by single breath analysis. J Appl Physiol 11:241–244, 1957

33a. Singleton GJ, Olsen CR, Smith RL: Correction for mechanical dead space in the calculation of physiological dead space. J Clin Invest 51:2768–2772, 1972

34. Strieder DJ, Barnes BA, Levine BW, Kazemi H: Stratified dead space in excised perfused lungs. J Appl Physiol 29:486–492, 1970

35. Vierordt K: Physiologie des Athmens, mit besonderer Rücksicht auf die Ausscheidung der Kohlensäure. Karlsruhe, Groos, 1845, pp 130–133

35a. Wagner PD, Gaines RA, Mazzone RW, West JB: Mechanism of intrapulmonary gas mixing during breathholding in man. Physiologist 15:295, 1972

36. Wagner WW Jr, Latham LP, Brinkman PD, Filley GF: Pulmonary gas transport time: Larynx to alveolus. Science 163:1210–1211, 1969

37. Weibel ER: Morphometry of the Human Lung. Berlin, Springer–Verlag, 1963

38. Widdicombe JG: The regulation of bronchial calibre, in Caro CG (ed): Advances in Respiratory Physiology. Baltimore, Williams & Wilkins, 1966, pp 48–82

39. Wilson TA, Lin K–H: Convection and diffusion in the airways and the design of the bronchial tree, in Bouhuys A (ed): Airway Dynamics; Physiology and Pharmacology. Springfield, Ill, Charles C Thomas, 1970, pp 5–19

Chapter 4

Distribution of Inspired Gas

Effective ventilation of the alveoli requires mixing of inspired gas with alveolar gas. First, an adequate amount of inspired gas must reach the terminal lung units; this depends on bulk flow as the main transport mode. The amount of gas distributed to each unit is determined by gravity and structural factors (such as length of the airway, stiffness of the terminal unit). However, once inside terminal bronchioles and alveolar units where forward velocities of gas are nearly zero, gas travels primarily by diffusion rather than by bulk flow. The effectiveness of diffusion within the terminal units depends largely on their dimensions, which determine how far gas molecules must travel.

After inspiration, alveolar gas is not of equal composition throughout the lungs. This is because of (1) variations in dilution of alveolar gas with inspired gas, and (2) uneven lung blood flow and, hence, unequal exchange of O_2 and CO_2 in different lung parts. This chapter discusses only the first of these factors, non-uniform distribution of inspired gas, as a process independent of gas exchange. Chapters 5 and 6 deal with the second mechanism and with gas exchange itself.

MECHANISMS OF UNEVEN DISTRIBUTION

Several mechanisms contribute to uneven inspired gas distribution, but there is no comprehensive lung model that takes all of them into account. Hence, it is difficult to assess how much each mechanism contributes to the overall non-uniform distribution of inspired gas. The principal mechanisms are: (1) *regional* or *parallel ventilation differences,* which are related to unequal bronchial pathway lengths, unequal stress, and unequal compliance of lung tissue, and, under some conditions, to local airway resistance, especially at low lung volumes (airway closure); and (2) *series ventilation,* including stratification within terminal units, although this is probably not of practical significance in normal lungs. The first principal mechanism relates to the amount of inspired air delivered to each terminal unit, the second to the effectiveness of gas mixing in alveolar lung units.

Regional or Parallel Ventilation

The pathologist Tendeloo,[74] noting that tuberculosis and emphysema do not affect all parts of the lungs equally, thought this was due to unequal expansion of different lung regions. He attributed unequal ventilation to differences in tissue compliance (e.g., hilar versus peripheral parts) and uneven distribution of respiratory forces through the lungs. Physiological evidence for regional ventilation differences came much later when Martin and Young [53] measured the rate of N_2 washout (p. 71) in the right upper and lower lobes of human subjects. They concluded that the lower lobe is better ventilated (i.e., receives more ventilation per unit volume) than the upper lobe, a conclusion confirmed by radioactive gas techniques. For instance, when a small amount of radioactive xenon (^{133}Xe) is injected into the inspired airstream directly after a maximum expiration, most of the xenon is inspired into the lung tops (in the subject sitting upright; Fig. 4-1). When xenon is injected later during inspiration, most of it goes to lower lung zones and less to the lung tops. Thus, there are marked regional ventilation differences in healthy lungs, and these depend on lung volume.

EFFECT OF GRAVITY

The anatomical substrate for regional ventilation differences remained rather obscure until Glazier et al.[34] showed that when fixed in situ, alveoli in the top of the vertical dog lung are much larger than alveoli near the base of the lung. The difference in alveolar size suggested that lungs behave like a spring suspended at the top, with the upper coils distended much more than the lower ones, owing to the weight of the spring.[57] Other experiments have suggested that the distribution of pleural pressure around the lungs may be crucial. In isolated, perfused dog lungs, suspended vertically, inspired xenon is distributed uniformly, but when the same lungs are suspended in a foam which creates a hydrostatic pressure gradient around them, the nonuniform distribution pattern typical of vertical lungs in situ becomes apparent.[79]

With the radioactive gas methods, counting radioactivity externally over relatively large areas of the chest, one can estimate regional volume, as well as regional

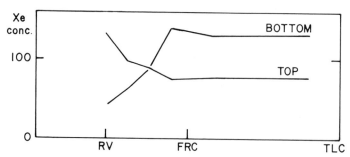

Fig. 4-1. Regional ventilation distribution determined with xenon. *Abscissa.* Lung volume at which Xe boli were injected into inspired airstream. *Ordinate.* Xe concentration as recorded with external counters over lung top and bottom, in percentage of value predicted if distribution were uniform. When inspired near RV, most Xe goes to the lung top; when inspired at or above FRC, most Xe goes to the bottom of the lungs. Average results in 5 young healthy subjects. Modified from reference 29.

expansion, relative to the volume of each counting zone at maximum inspiration.[17, 44, 57] The latter is called regional TLC (TLC$_r$), and regional volumes at lesser degrees of lung expansion are expressed as percentages of TLC$_r$.[57] Figure 4-2 is a diagram based on these measurements. Near the lung tops, regional FRC (FRC$_r$) is large, about two-thirds of TLC. In contrast, in the lower zones of the lungs of a seated person, FRC is only about one-third of TLC. Thus, these functional data in vivo in man agree with the data on alveolar size in dog lungs.[34]

Figure 4-3 is a different diagram based on similar data. If all lung regions expanded equally, regional volume everywhere would equal the same percentage of TLC, as indicated by the dotted lines in Figure 4-3. For instance, at residual volume (RV), regional volume would be about 25 percent of TLC$_r$ for all lung zones. In fact, regional volume in the lung tops is always larger than the dotted line shows, and in bottom zones it is less. The difference is most marked near RV. Although Figure 4-3 is based on data obtained during conditions of zero airflow, it shows approximately how a tidal breath is distributed. A tidal breath inspired from FRC (VT$_1$) goes predominantly to the lower lung zones. Between FRC and TLC, the relations between regional and total lung volumes are linear (Fig. 4-3), and the distribution pattern is comparable with the effects of gravity discussed above—lower zones are better ventilated than lung tops. This is because the lung tops are more expanded than the lower zones and hence operate on a flatter portion of the static recoil curve (see Fig. 7-1, p. 122). Experiments on the human centrifuge [17] confirm the importance of gravity in determining regional expansion: increased acceleration leads to divergence of the regional expansion lines in Figure 4-3B. Above FRC, the uppermost lung areas are ventilated less than the dependent zones, irre-

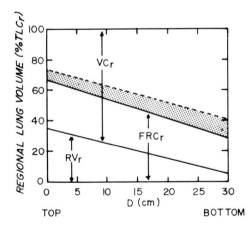

Fig. 4-2. *Ordinate.* Regional lung volume, as a percentage of regional TLC (TLC$_r$). *Abscissa.* Vertical distance, D, from lung top to lung bottom. At maximum inspiration, all lung regions are maximally expanded (100% on ordinate). At maximum expiration and at FRC, top regions are more expanded than lower ones. Regional VC is larger in lower zones than in the lung tops. *Shaded area.* Regional tidal volume, which is larger at the bottom than at the top. Modified from reference 57.

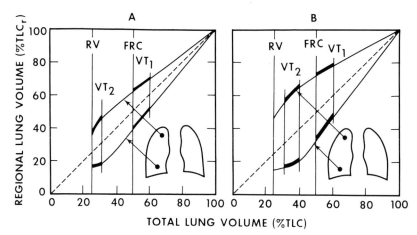

Fig. 4-3. *Ordinate.* Regional lung volume, in percentage of regional TLC_r. *Abscissa.* Total lung volume (% TLC). The dashed line of equality indicates regions which expand in proportion to total lung volume. The drawn line above the dashed line represents the expansion of an area in the top of a vertical lung, from RV to TLC; the lower drawn line represents the expansion of an area near the bottom of the lung. *A.* Control data; *B.* Data obtained during increased acceleration of gravity on human centrifuge. Heavy bars on lines indicate distribution of tidal volume above FRC (VT_1) and below FRC (VT_2). The slope of these bars indicates relative tidal volumes to each region. Particularly when gravity is increased, bottom zones receive little ventilation during tidals below FRC (bar nearly horizontal). Above FRC a larger fraction of VT goes to the bottom of the lungs (dependent region). Modified from reference 17.

spective of posture.[44] The difference is associated with the lungs' orientation in the gravity field and not with inherent properties of certain parts of the lungs.

Near RV, the lower lung zones are maximally deflated, because they are compressed by the lungs' own weight.[57, 77a, 79] Since this also impedes air entry into these zones, they receive little inspired air near RV (VT_2 in Fig. 4-3). Air entry into these dependent zones could be limited by alveolar collapse, closing of small airways, or closing of large airways. The exact mechanism is unclear, but since gas distribution near RV behaves as if airways in dependent zones were closed, the term airway closure is used to describe this mechanism. When gravity is increased (Fig. 4-3B), airway closure extends to a larger total lung volume. Posture also affects airway closure. If the alinear portions of the regional ventilation lines in Figure 4-3 are close to FRC, small postural changes can markedly influence gas distribution. For example, in the supine position FRC is moderately reduced, and the pattern of VT_1 might change into that of VT_2.

NONUNIFORMITY WITHIN LUNG LOBES

The external counters used to obtain the graphs of Figures 4-1–4-3 "see" radioactivity in large lung areas and do not detect ventilation differences within each area. These ventilation differences can be studied by passing catheters into large and small airways of one lobe to measure local N_2 clearance (p. 71). With this method, Suda et al.[73] found that inspired gas distribution within lobes and segments was markedly nonuniform. In fact, the differences within units as small as 20 ml were much greater than the ventilation differences between similar small units in the lung top and bottom. Since gravity effects must be negligible, they cannot explain nonuniform ventilation within such small lung segments. At least part of the ventilation inequalities in a 20-ml unit of lung must be due to unequal stress-strain relations or to unequal force distribution.[73] In such a unit, diffusion times (as calculated by Rauwerda, Table 4-1; p. 65) are too long to allow diffusion equilibration within the time span of a normal breath.

STRESS–STRAIN RELATIONS

Tendeloo [74] attributed unequal ventilation primarily to unequal distribution of the respiratory forces (stress) through lung tissue and unequal compliance of different lung parts. Later, physiologists proposed, by analogy with the theory of parallel electrical circuits, that the product of air flow resistance (R) and lung compliance (C) determines the rate of air entry into each lung region.[61] Regions where this product, the RC or time constant, is low should fill and empty faster than regions with a high RC constant. However, since peripheral airways have a very low resistance and hence a low time constant, RC constants in healthy lungs are probably too small to affect gas distribution.[56] Thus, bulk flow may largely be determined by elastic tissue properties and by stress distribution, rather than by airway resistance. Lung emptying patterns are influenced by expiratory flow rate,[43, 58] but this can be explained by local compliance variation as well as by the time constant theory.[78]

At small lung volumes, and also in older people or in patients with airway disease, regional airway-resistance differences are probably important in determining inspired gas distribution.[23, 29, 49] Increased airway muscle tone, as in asthma, increases nonuniform gas distribution (Chap. 18); again, changes in local airway resistance are the most likely determinant. At the end of the scale, airway closure (p. 62) in dependent lung zones and at low lung volumes implies infinitely high airway resistance to these zones and no air entry.

The difference between the top and bottom of a vertical lung is a good example of the importance of stress-strain relations. Since lung tissue in the top is stressed more, it is less distensible than lung tissue in the bottom zone. West has pointed out the consequences for lung pathology—emphysema is more common in the lung tops, and spontaneous pneumothorax due to rupture of lung tissue at the top occurs commonly in tall people.[77] These vulnerable regions, which may include the apical segment of the right lower lobe, may be under increased stress when lung volume decreases to near RV, as during shouting, laughter, or singing.

UNEQUAL PATHWAY LENGTHS

The varying length of bronchial pathways (p. 51) results in a sixfold range of transit times from the carina to the alveoli in the human lung.[40] The inspired gas front reaches the most proximal alveoli after 22 ml gas has passed the carina; 170 ml more must be inspired before the most distal alveoli are reached. This can account for a considerable degree of nonuniform gas distribution in normal lungs.[28, 40]

SEQUENTIAL FILLING AND EMPTYING

Fowler's sequential ventilation theory [31] continues to receive support.[75] It proposes that certain lung areas fill early in inspiration and expire late during expiration. For instance, when inspiring from RV (Fig. 4-3), the lung tops inspire first; the bottom zone receives a larger part of the inspired breath at higher volumes. During expiration, the bottom zones empty preferentially until airway closure occurs; the lung tops then contribute most of the remaining expired tidal volume. Thus, the area which fills first empties last. In contrast, the time-constant theory suggested a "first-in, first-out" sequence.[8] Both mechanisms may operate in the same lungs under different conditions. The first-in, first-out mechanism may predominate when time constants are increased, e.g., by airway obstruction. The "first-in, last-out" sequence may operate at low lung volumes and in other conditions when tidal volume overlaps with airway closing volume.

Series Ventilation

The mechanisms described above cause regional ventilation differences, or parallel nonuniformity, since the separate lobes, segments, and lobules are analogous to parallel elements in an electrical circuit. Alveoli, alveolar ducts, and larger airways are 'in series' elements, and if more inspired gas reaches terminal bronchioles than alveoli, there is series nonuniformity of ventilation. Parallel and series nonuniformity [64] are not mutually exclusive. The principal mechanisms of series ventilation are stratification in terminal units, collateral ventilation, redistribution of dead space gas, and pendelluft. None of these is quantitatively important in normal lungs, but each plays a role under abnormal conditions.

STRATIFICATION

According to Krogh and Lindhard: [46] ". . . the air in the airsacs (as well as in the atria) is not at the end of inspiration of the same composition throughout, because the inspired air is incompletely mixed with the air previously contained. The mixing takes place chiefly by diffusion and requires a certain time." This statement suggests a layering or stratified inhomogeneity of alveolar gas. Near the entrance to terminal units, gas composition would approach that of inspired gas; near the blood-air barrier, gas composition would be in equilibrium with blood. The opposite view is that diffusion within terminal lung spaces is fast enough for complete equilibration within the breathing cycle. Hence, any uneven composition of alveolar gas must be due to differences in regional ventilation.

Gas diffusion is no doubt an essential mode of transport in terminal airways and alveoli. The question is whether diffusion is a rate-limiting factor in gas-exchanging units. Since there is no precise anatomical delineation between conducting and gas-exchanging airways (see Fig. 2-2B), the debate on stratification is to some extent a matter of semantics. Two lines of evidence, from lung models and from gas exchange experiments, suggest that diffusional mixing in terminal lung units is rapid and that stratified inhomogeneity is minimal in normal lungs.

Rauwerda [63] used a 7-mm long cylindrical lung model to represent the diffusion path within a primary lobule. This distance is realistic in anatomical terms; according to Weibel's data (Table 2-1, p. 30), the average pathway length from the terminal respiratory bronchioles to the alveoli is less than 5 mm. In a 7-mm long cylinder, diffusion alone would decrease gas concentration differences to 16 percent of their initial value after 0.38 second.[63] Thus, diffusion appeared to be highly effective within the primary lobules. In larger units (lobules and lobes), diffusion times increase as the anatomical pathway lengths increase (Table 4-1). In his experiments, Rauwerda found that after an inspiration of oxygen, the early expired gas always contained more O_2 and less N_2 than gas expired later [63] (Fig. 4-4). When the breath was held before expiring, the difference between early and late samples decreased but did not disappear. Even after 60 seconds of breath holding, the early and late samples differed by about 2 percent O_2 and N_2. The first 30 seconds of breath holding appear to establish equilibrium in small lung units, where diffusion distances are short. However, even prolonged breath holding could not abolish concentration differences between lung regions that communicate via long pathways. Comparing these data to his model calculations (Table 4-1), Rauwerda concluded that (1) diffusion equilibrium would be reached in normal primary lobules within the duration of a normal inspiration, and (2) any concentration differences remaining after more than 30 seconds of breath holding should be attributed to regional ventilation differences between large units such as lung lobes. The dimensions Rauwerda chose for his lung model were anatomically realistic, but the model's cylindrical shape has been criticized.[24] However, more recent model computations largely confirm Rauwerda's conclusions.[48] A recent model of Cumming et al.,[27] which analyzes bulk flow and diffusion in alternating steps, yields little support for stratified inhomogeneity.

The present discussion may appear to contradict several studies with aerosols [59] and with heavy and light gases [25, 33, 62] which have confirmed that molecular weight and hence gas diffusivity markedly influence mixing of inspired gas in normal lungs. Heavy gases diffuse less and are expired first; lighter, more readily diffusible gases appear at the mouth only late during expiration [33] (*dashed line,* Fig. 4-5). Clearly, diffusion equilibrium is incomplete after a normal inspiration. However, these results show only that incomplete diffusion equilibrium occurs somewhere in the airways or in the alveoli; they offer no clues to the site of occurrence. Since stratified inhomogeneity is unlikely on the grounds discussed above, this site is

Table 4–1
Rauwerda's Diffusion Time Calculations

Part of the Lung	Diffusion Path (cm)	Diffusion Time § (sec)
Alveolar duct	0.05	0.002
Primary lobule	0.70	0.380
Lobule (small)	0.80 *	0.490
Lobule (large)	3.00 *	6.900
Lobe (small)	8.80 †	60.000
Lobe (large)	17.00 †	222.000
Lobe (small)	22.80 ‡	400.000
Lobe (large)	31.00 ‡	739.000

* From entrance of lobular bronchus to alveoli.
† Distance from carina to alveoli.
‡ Distance from trachea entrance to alveoli.
§ $t = (\alpha^2/D) \times 0.2$, where α = diffusion path length, and D = diffusion coefficient (0.260 cm^2/sec for O_2 into N_2 at 37° C). Data from Rauwerda.[63]

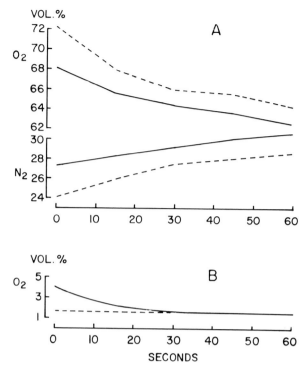

Fig. 4-4. Analysis of expired gas after inspiration of O_2 in a healthy subject. *A*. Lines drawn through points obtained in separate experiments with 0, 15, 30, 45, and 60 seconds' breath-holding. *Dashed lines.* Samples after 1-liter expiration. *Solid lines.* Samples after 2.5-liter expiration. The gas expired later contains less O_2 and more N_2. This difference decreases with breath holding, as indicated in *B* for O_2. *Abscissa.* Breath holding time. Modified from reference 63.

probably in conducting airways rather than in terminal lung units. This conclusion is in agreement with calculations based on a model in which bulk flow and diffusion operate simultaneously and continuously (Chap. 3, p. 50), calculations which suggest that diffusion in conducting airways can account for the effects of breath holding on dead space.

Another argument against stratified inhomogeneity is derived from experiments on gas exchange. If diffusional gas mixing influences gas concentrations adjacent to the alveolocapillary membrane, one would expect gases of high density to impede gas exchange. But even large increases in gas density do not impede gas exchange in man[68] or in dogs.[55] Only when dogs breathe hyperoxygenated liquid (with the density of water) does gas exchange become limited by diffusion in what used to be air spaces.[47]

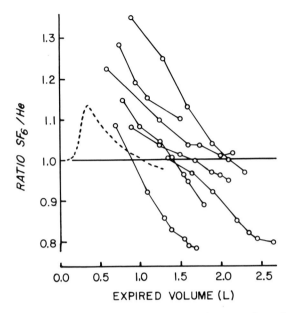

Fig. 4-5. Analysis of six successive samples of expired gas after inspiration of a gas mixture containing about 10% SF_6 and 30% He. *Dashed line.* Average data in 7 healthy subjects. *Solid lines.* Individual data in 7 patients with emphysema. Ratio SF_6/He $= 1.0$ when ratio in expired gas equals that in inspired mixture, i.e., 10/30. Early in expiration, the expired air is relatively rich in SF_6; later on, in He. Reproduced from reference 33.

COLLATERAL VENTILATION

Gas can pass through alveolar pores and through connections between respiratory bronchioles.[51] Polystyrene spheres less than 60 μm in diameter can pass between adjacent segments in human lungs.[38] Serial sectioning of small airways has demonstrated bronchiolar connections.[54] Collateral pathways normally do not contribute to uniform regional ventilation, since their flow resistance in human lungs is high.[39] In disease, collateral ventilation helps prevent collapse of lung regions behind occluded airways; these are then ventilated in series with lung units with open bronchi.[38] Since these areas are ventilated through other alveolar regions, they become, in West's terminology, a parasitic space, which seriously affects gas exchange.[76] Histamine and histamine-releasing drugs (curare, 48/80) reduce collateral ventilation in dogs,[18] perhaps because smooth muscle contraction occludes connections between respiratory bronchioles. If bronchial pathways become occluded, lungs without collateral ventilation pathways are vulnerable to atelectasis. Local tissue damage as well as drugs used in anesthesia can release histamine, and this may promote postoperative atelectasis in surgical patients.

DISTRIBUTION OF DEAD SPACE GAS

A large part of the anatomical dead space—the trachea and upper airways—is common to all parts of the lungs. At the end of expiration, this space is filled with a mixture of alveolar gas from all lung regions. During inspiration, this gas is distributed throughout the lungs. Thus, the common dead space, acting as a mixing chamber in series with the alveoli, tends to equalize alveolar gas concentrations throughout the lungs.[11] If one breathes through a long tube, this mixing is sufficient to turn N_2 washout curves into single exponential functions (Fig. 4-6).

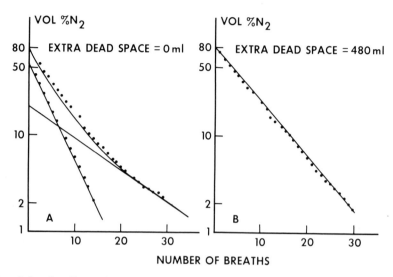

Fig. 4-6. Semilogarithmic plots of end-tidal N_2 concentration (log scale) versus number of breaths (linear scale) during O_2 breathing in a healthy subject. *A.* Control curve, analyzed as the sum of two exponential functions, each represented by a straight line. *B.* Washout curve from the same subject breathing through an extra dead space of 480 ml. Reproduced from reference 11.

PENDELLUFT

When different lung regions have grossly unequal time constants, one region may still inspire air while another region already expires. Thus, when ventilation is markedly asynchronous, alveolar gas may be shuttled back and forth (German: pendeln=to shuttle) between different lung regions, via the dead space. Pendelluft often contributes to ventilatory failure after severe chest injuries.[76]

MEASUREMENT OF NONUNIFORM DISTRIBUTION

Since inspired gas distribution is markedly uneven in obstructive lung disease, measurements of distribution are useful in diagnosing these conditions and in assessing treatment. Simple clinical tests (auscultation, percussion, and observation of chest movements) sometimes indicate regional lack of air entry, gross asynchrony or asymmetry of ventilatory movements, or decreased local air content. The chest x-ray film often provides similar qualitative information, and a more complex x-ray method (lung scanning after ^{133}Xe inhalation) can detect lung areas with poor or absent ventilation. However, the amount of ^{133}Xe seen on a scan cannot be related to the volume of each lung region. Thus, as usually applied, lung scanning provides qualitative, rather than quantitative, information.[57]

Here I shall discuss only quantitative methods, usually divided into single-breath and multiple-breath methods.[8, 14] Both use the principle of tracing a gaseous marker that undergoes little or no exchange with blood, i.e., a physiologically inert gas. Nitrogen is always available for this purpose; helium and radioactive xenon are also used. The marker can be traced by serial or continuous analysis of expired gas and, in the case of ^{133}Xe, by external counting as well.

Single-Breath Washout Curve

After 100 percent O_2 has been inspired, the N_2 concentration in expired gas increases rapidly as dead space gas is cleared (phases 1 and 2; Figs. 4-7 and 4-8). The concentration continues to rise slightly in phase 3 after dead space gas has been washed out, indicating nonuniform composition of alveolar gas. Several gas distribution tests use recordings of this type.[2, 22, 45] In healthy people, the slight slope of phase 3 may reflect a distribution of transit times [28] and some degree of sequential emptying.[75] Unequal $\dot{V}_A/\dot{Q}$ ratios (Chap. 5) contributes since all test gases are slightly soluble in blood; this can be eliminated by using two inert gases that are similarly affected by unequal perfusion.[30, 71]

In disease, several mechanisms may contribute to increased slopes of phase 3 (Fig. 4-7B). Stratified inhomogeneity may contribute when the lungs contain pathological spaces with large diffusion distances, as in emphysema. Time constant differences may be at fault when small airway narrowing is widespread, but unequally distributed, as in bronchitis or asthma. For clinical purposes, the percentage of N_2 difference between 750 and 1250 ml expired volume is used to quantitate phase 3 slopes.[22] The slopes are markedly influenced by lung volume,[42] flow

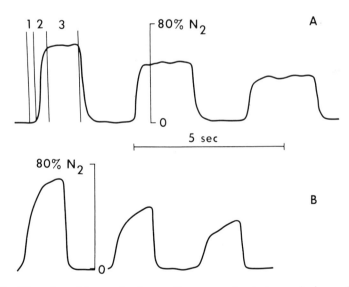

Fig. 4-7. Three breathing cycles from nitrogen washout curves during quiet breathing in a normal subject (A) and in a patient with emphysema (B). Washout of dead space gas ($1, 2$) followed by alveolar plateau (3). Phases 2 and 3 cannot be distinguished in emphysema, in which alveolar N_2% continues to increase throughout expiration.

rates,[43, 58] and posture.[3, 20] Therefore, standardized procedures are required for their use as a quantitative test. Gross abnormalities (e.g., the curves of Fig. 4-7B) are easily detected with any version of the test, but more subtle changes require careful assessment. Third phase slopes are more pronounced in healthy young adults than in healthy children, but do not increase beyond age 20.[2]

Expired gas and regional alveolar gas can be monitored simultaneously with the ^{133}Xe method. When inspired as a bolus at a volume close to RV, most Xe goes to the lung tops (Fig. 4-1). Figure 4-8 shows Xe concentration versus time

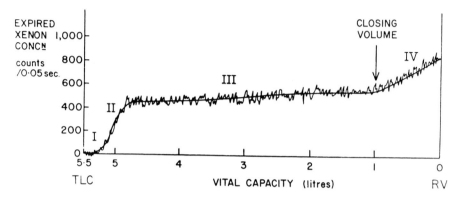

Fig. 4-8. Expired ^{133}Xe concentration (ordinate) as a function of lung volume, during a full VC expiration from TLC to RV. During the preceding inspiration, a bolus of ^{133}Xe was injected near RV. Phase 3 (alveolar plateau) and phase 4 (terminal rise) are indicated. Closing volume is about 1 liter above RV. Reproduced from reference 49.

in the next expiration. After phase 3, the curve shows a final rise (phase 4) at a volume close to RV. Dollfuss et al.[29] proposed that the high Xe levels in phase 4 show a large contribution of apical, Xe-rich zones to expired air. Lower zones appear to contribute progressively less to expired air, in phase 4, which agrees with the concept of airway closure in dependent lung zones (p. 62). The lung volume at which phase 4 begins is called airway closing volume (ACV).[2, 23, 49] In young adults, ACV is less than FRC, but in older persons with increased ACV some airways in dependent lung zones may be closed during quiet breathing.[49] Phase 4 can also be shown in N_2 single-breath curves if the subject expires to RV, then inspires O_2 to TLC, and holds his breath for 15–30 seconds before expiring to RV.[2] With the N_2 method, ACV was 10% of VC or less in children and young adults, and about 20 percent of VC in 40- to 50-year-old subjects.[2] The terminal rise (phase 4) in N_2 concentration was also increased in older persons.

Airway closing volume appears to rise with increasing expiratory flow.[43] Hyatt et al[41, 41a] reported that phase 4 begins when expiratory flow becomes limited by dynamic compression of intrathoracic airways (Fig. 4-9). These data suggest that airway closure in dependent lung zones is determined by dynamic compression of larger airways, rather than by alveolar collapse or closing of small airways. Thus, determination of ACV may have the same significance as measurement of flow rates at low lung volumes on MEFV curves (Chap. 9). That is, large closing volumes would correspond to low maximum flows. Several observations

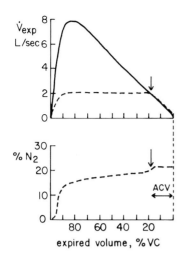

expired volume, % VC

Fig. 4-9. *Top.* MEFV curve of a healthy person (*drawn line*). (See Chap. 9 for discussion of these curves.) *Dashed line.* Expired flow rates during N_2 single-breath curve recording. *Bottom.* N_2 single-breath curve. 100% O_2 inspired from RV during previous inspiration. At the arrow, expiration becomes flow-limited; i.e., flow reaches the maximum value indicated by the MEFV curve (*top graph*). At the same moment, N_2% rises to a phase 4 (*bottom graph*). Airway closing volume (ACV) is indicated; its value depends on expiratory flow during the single-breath curve and increases with increasing flow.[11, 43] Modified from reference 41a.

support this interpretation. For instance, increasing age and cigarette smoking are both associated with large ACV's [2, 49] and with decreased flow rates on MEFV curves (Chap. 9).

Multiple-Breath Inert Gas Washout

If a tidal volume of oxygen is distributed to all parts of the lungs in proportion to their volumes, alveolar N_2 concentrations decrease by the same factor everywhere. This dilution factor depends on lung volume, tidal volume, and dead space. If the dilution factor is constant from breath to breath, alveolar N_2 concentrations ($F_{A_{N_2}}$) decrease exponentially after successive breaths of O_2. Hence, a graph of log $F_{A_{N_2}}$ versus the number of breaths then yields a straight line. In healthy persons these graphs are sometimes linear (Fig. 4-10A), but frequently they are not (Fig. 4-6A). This indicates nonuniform inspired gas distribution, which might be due to regional ventilation differences, or stratified inhomogeneity, or both. Since the curve does not provide information on mechanisms, it requires interpretation in conjunction with other data. The graph of Figure 4-6A changed into that of Figure 4-6B when the subject breathed through a long tube at the mouth—an example of the effect of redistribution of dead space gas (p. 68). The graph of Figure 4-10A changed into that of Figure 4-10B after inhalation of an airway-constricting drug—this probably reflects a variable increase of time constants in different lung regions, which changed the ventilation from a uniform pattern (*A*) to a nonuniform distribution (*B*).

Alinear N_2 clearance curves can be analyzed by a curve-stripping procedure (Figs. 4-6 and 4-10) into a sum of two or three exponential functions. Computer methods can eliminate observer bias from this procedure.[36] To quantitate nonuniform ventilation, several numerical indices, reviewed earlier,[8] are derived from clearance curves.[32, 64] New indices have been published more recently.[36, 60, 67] The accuracy of these procedures is limited by the accuracy of the experimental data, which may show considerable breath-to-breath variations (e.g., in Fig. 4-10B).

A simpler way of expressing N_2 washout data, independent of the shape of the clearance curve, is to calculate the lung clearance index [5]:

$$LCI = nV_T/V_L \tag{1}$$

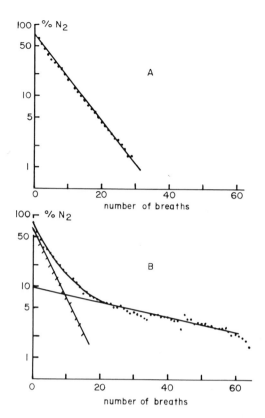

Fig. 4-10. Expired $N_2\%$ (log scale) versus number of breaths during N_2 washout. The points are end-tidal N_2 concentrations in successive expirations; the line through the points has been drawn freehand. The curve of *B* has been analyzed into two exponential components by curve-stripping. *A*. Control curve in healthy subject (LCI=7.5). *B*. Directly after inhalation of histamine aerosol (LCI=16.1). Histamine aerosol induces marked nonuniformity of ventilation. Reproduced from reference 10.

where LCI= lung clearance index, n=the total number of breaths during N_2 washout, V_T=tidal volume, and V_L=the lung volume that is being washed out. V_L=FRC when the washout is begun at the end of a normal expiration. Thus, LCI simply indicates the amount of ventilation required to eliminate N_2 during a clearance test, to a predetermined end-point, commonly $F_{A_{N_2}}=0.02$; this value ranges from 6–10 in healthy persons. LCI is related to the exponential functions which describe N_2 clearance, and this enables one to predict values for LCI as a function of tidal volume, at a fixed end-expiratory lung volume.[13] With tidal volumes greater than 600 ml, LCI is relatively independent of tidal volume. However, its experimental values are always higher than those predicted, even when N_2 clearance curves show a single exponential function.[13, 67] The actual values of LCI may reflect residual nonuniformity not detected by the analysis of exponential components. With tidal volumes less than about 600 ml, N_2 clearance is delayed because dead space is a large fraction of tidal volume, and LCI is increased.[13] This also happens when extra dead space is added at the mouth.[11] LCI increases because added ventilation is needed to clear the extra dead space volume. At the same time, N_2 clearance curves become linear (Fig. 4-6), because the dead space act as a mixing chamber (p. 68). Thus, LCI and clearance curves do not always change in the same direction.

N_2 clearance tests provide objective information about lung ventilation during quiet breathing, but their clinical potential (p. 74) has not been widely utilized because of technical complexity and the labor required for data analysis. Improved N_2 meters and electronic data processing may now increase their use. Some programs for curve analysis are already available.[66] New electronic circuits allow direct plotting of $F_{A_{N_2}}$ versus accumulated expired volume on semilogarithmic coordinates.[70] On-line computation of the amount of N_2 expired during each breath of the clearance test is feasible and allows rapid data analysis using the method of Fowler et al.[32]

PHYSIOLOGICAL FACTORS INFLUENCING DISTRIBUTION

Breathing Pattern and Lung Volume

Increases in tidal volume and in breathing rate have little effect on N_2 clearance.[13, 69] At small tidal volumes (<600 ml), N_2 clearance is delayed (see above). Lung volume may affect distribution if airway closing volume is close to FRC (p. 62). Incomplete mixing because of shortened diffusion times occurs at unphysiological breathing rates (>100/min).[65]

Age

Few data are available in newborns.[6] Older children (<12 yrs) nearly always have single exponential clearance curves; adolescents and adults have increasingly nonuniform distributions.[8, 19] Single-breath curves also vary with age (p. 70). The effects of age on regional ventilation differences have not been described in detail. Closing volume increases with age.[2, 49]

Posture

Regional ventilation patterns shift with posture, according to the direction of gravity.[44] Since closing volume is larger in the supine than in the upright position,[49] there is an overall increase in nonuniformity when supine.[15, 20]

Tissue N_2 Elimination

During O_2 breathing, N_2 is eliminated from tissue stores in the body. Unless a correction is made, this leads to overestimation of FRC, underestimation of LCI, and errors in N_2 clearance analysis.[7] Data on tissue N_2 elimination in man[50] and in dogs[35] can be used for approximate corrections.

Airway Smooth Muscle Tone

Histamine and other smooth-muscle-contracting substances increase nonuniform distribution[10] (Fig. 4-10). N_2 clearance is also prolonged after inhalation of textile dust or allergens (Chap. 17, 18). Epinephrine increases LCI in healthy subjects[9, 15] and relaxes airway smooth muscle. Since distribution becomes less uniform when airway tone is decreased, normal muscle tone may help minimize nonuniform distribution. The mechanisms controlling this adjustment of tone are unknown. The effect of constrictor drugs or dust on N_2 single-breath curves varies.[4, 21, 72] Severe airway obstruction is compatible with a normal phase 3 slope.[4, 72] The initial slope and its underlying mechanisms (e.g., sequential emptying or increased time constants) may affect the results and explain the variability.

INSPIRED GAS DISTRIBUTION IN DISEASE

N_2 clearance is often grossly delayed in asthma and chronic bronchitis. Clearance curves are markedly alinear, and LCI is increased. Slopes of phase 3 in single-breath curves are usually increased as well (Fig. 4-7B); in such instances it may be difficult to distinguish phase 3 and 4 and to determine airway closing volume (ACV).

Measurement of ACV has been suggested for early detection of *airway obstruction*.[49] An increase in ACV may be related to the decrease in maximum flow rates, which is also a sensitive test for airway obstruction (Chap. 9). When a patient with asthma is undergoing treatment, N_2 clearance may remain abnormal even though other tests ($FEV_{1.0}$, airway resistance) are normal.[52] Regional xenon distribution in asthma may be normal even when other indices (e.g., maximum midexpiratory flow) are low.[37] Nonuniformity in asthma is probably related to obstruction in intralobar or intralobular airways, and collateral ventilation (p. 67) may contribute to prolongation of N_2 washout.

In *emphysema*, gas distribution is highly nonuniform.[12, 16] Stratified inhomogeneity and collateral ventilation, as well as widespread airway obstruction, may contribute. The large concentration gradients which occur in these lungs when a SF_6-He mixture is inspired (Fig. 4-5)[33] suggest that diffusion distances are increased. Since infused xenon is not as effectively cleared from alveolar air as inhaled xenon,[1] the layers of gas close to blood vessels may have a slower turnover than layers closer to airways in connection with the atmosphere. Cumming et al.[26] have demonstrated dilated airway structures in different types of emphysema, and these provide an anatomical substrate for increased diffusion distances. Stratified inhomogeneity within such abnormal spaces can contribute considerably to the overall inefficiency of ventilation and to sloping third phases of single-breath curves.[14, 63]

The lungs are a nonuniform structure in which respiratory and gravity stresses are distributed unequally. Physiological tests of gas distribution can detect the consequences of these nonuniformities, especially when the tests maximize the effect of particular mechanisms of uneven distribution. Yet, many young and healthy adults have linear N_2 clearance graphs (Fig. 4-10A) and minimal phase 3 slopes (Fig. 4-7A). This indicates that their inspired tidal volume is distributed uniformly, or nearly so. Yet, such subjects do have regional ventilation inequalities as shown by radioactive gas methods. Although N_2 clearance may lack the sensitivity to show this inequality, it seems remarkable that gross regional ventilation differences might occur in persons with linear N_2 clearance graphs like the one of Figure 4-10A. Unfortunately, no comparison of regional studies with N_2 clearance graphs in the same subjects appears to have been made. It seems possible, however, that the effects of different factors leading to nonuniform distribution might cancel one another, or that there may be regulation processes which maintain uniform gas distribution. In any case, markedly nonuniform distribution of inspired gas, as defined by N_2 single- or multiple-breath tests, is found only in older persons and in patients with lung disease.

SUMMARY

Inspired air is distributed unequally to different regions in *normal lungs* because of regional or parallel ventilation differences, which include effects of unequal bronchial pathway lengths, unequal stress distribution, unequal lung compliance, and effects of the lungs' orientation in a gravity field. The latter leads to distortion of the lungs because of their weight, with relative overexpansion of alveoli in the lung top, while the lower zones are compressed and do not receive inspired gas near RV (airway closure).

In *diseased lungs,* increased airway resistance in obstructed airways, stratification of gas in enlarged alveolar spaces, collateral ventilation of lung regions behind occluded bronchi, and pendelluft cause increased nonuniform distribution of inspired gas.

Methods to quantitate unequal gas distribution in disease include single-and multiple-breath inert gas clearance tests. Single-breath curves (N_2 or ^{133}Xe) have phase 3 slopes that reflect unequal distribution, while their phase 4 reflects airway closure. Multiple-breath N_2 clearance is prolonged by unequal distribution; this can be quantitated by an analysis of exponential functions or by the lung clearance index.

Breathing patterns, age, posture, and airway smooth muscle tone are the principal physiological variables affecting inspired gas distribution. Gas distribution is often markedly unequal in asthma, bronchitis, and emphysema, or after severe chest injuries.

REFERENCES

1. Anthonisen NR, Bass H, Oriol A, Place REG, Bates DV: Regional lung function in patients with chronic bronchitis. Clin Sci 35:495–511, 1968
2. Anthonisen NR, Danson J, Robertson PC, Ross WRD: Airway closure as a function of age. Respir Physiol 8:58–65, 1969/1970
3. Anthonisen NR, Robertson PC, Ross WRD: Gravity-dependent sequential emptying of lung regions. J Appl Physiol 28:589–595, 1970
4. Arnoldsson H, Bouhuys A, Lindell SE: Byssinosis: Differential diagnosis from bronchial asthma and chronic bronchitis. Acta Med Scand 173:761–768, 1963

5. Becklake MR: A new index of the intrapulmonary mixture of inspired air. Thorax 7:111–116, 1952

6. Bolton DPG, Cross KW: Lung volume and mixing efficiency in the new-born infant. J Physiol (Lond) 208:25–26P, 1970

7. Bouhuys A: Influence of tissue nitrogen elimination on analysis of pulmonary nitrogen clearance curves. Acta Physiol Pharmacol Neerl 8:431–436, 1959

8. Bouhuys A: Distribution of inspired gas in the lungs, in Fenn WO, Rahn H (eds): Handbook of Physiology, Section 3: Respiration, vol I. Washington, D.C., American Physiological Society, 1964, pp 715–733

9. Bouhuys A, Jönsson R, Lichtneckert S, Lindell SE, Lundgren C, Lundin G: The effect of epinephrine and hexamethonium bromide on the pulmonary ventilation in man. Acta Physiol Pharmacol Neerl 8:437–446, 1959

10. Bouhuys A, Jönsson R, Lichtneckert S, Lindell SE, Lundgren C, Lundin G, Ringquist TR: Effects of histamine on pulmonary ventilation in man. Clin Sci 19:79–94, 1960

11. Bouhuys A, Jönsson R, Lundin G: Influence of added dead space on pulmonary ventilation. Acta Physiol Scand 39:105–120, 1957

12. Bouhuys A, Jönsson R, Lundin G: Non-uniformity of pulmonary ventilation in chronic diffuse obstructive emphysema. Acta Med Scand 162:29–46, 1958

13. Bouhuys A, Lichtneckert S, Lundgren C, Lundin G: Voluntary changes in breathing pattern and N_2 clearance from lungs. J Appl Physiol 16:1039–1042, 1961

14. Bouhuys A, Lundin G: Distribution of inspired gas in lungs. Physiol Rev 39:731–750, 1959

15. Bouhuys A, van Lennep HJ: Effect of body posture on gas distribution in the lungs. J Appl Physiol 17:38–42, 1962

16. Briscoe WA, Cournand A: Uneven ventilation of normal and diseased lungs studied by an open-circuit method. J Appl Physiol 14:284–290, 1959

17. Bryan AC, Milic-Emili J, Pengelly D: Effect of gravity on the distribution of pulmonary ventilation. J Appl Physiol 21:778–784, 1966

18. Call EP Jr, Lindskog GE, Liebow AA: Some physiologic and pharmacologic aspects of collateral ventilation. J Thorac Cardiovasc Surg 49:1015–1025, 1965

19. Chiang ST, Wang BC, Chi YL, Hsieh YC: Ventilatory components of lungs in relation to sex and age. Am Rev Respir Dis 104:175–181, 1971

20. Clarke SW, Jones JG, Glaister DH: Change in pulmonary ventilation in different postures. Clin Sci 37:357–369, 1969

21. Colldahl H, Pegelow KO, Pokorny J: The single-breath nitrogen-elimination test for the registration of provocation tests in allergy diagnosis. Acta Allergol (Kbh) 22 (suppl 8):79–97, 1967

22. Comroe JH Jr, Fowler WS: Lung function studies. VI. Detection of uneven alveolar ventilation during a single breath of oxygen. Am J Med 10:408–413, 1951

23. Craig DB, Wahba WM, Don HF, Couture JG, Becklake MR: "Closing volume" and its relationship to gas exchange in seated and supine positions. J Appl Physiol 31:717–721, 1971

24. Cumming G, Crank J, Horsfield K, Parker I: Gaseous diffusion in the airways of the human lung. Respir Physiol 1:58–74, 1966

25. Cumming G, Horsfield K, Jones JG, Muir DCF: The influence of gaseous diffusion on the alveolar plateau at different lung volumes. Respir Physiol 2:386–398, 1967

26. Cumming G, Horsfield K, Jones JG, Muir DCF: Inhomogeneity of ventilation in normal and abnormal lungs, in Cumming G, Hunt LB (eds): Form and Function in the Human Lung. Baltimore, Williams & Wilkins, 1968, pp 56–65

27. Cumming G, Horsfield K, Preston SB: Diffusion equilibrium in the lungs examined by nodal analysis. Respir Physiol 12:329–345, 1971

28. Davies AS: Gas transit times in the porcine lung. J Physiol (Lond) 222:76p–77p, 1972

29. Dollfuss RE, Milic-Emili J, Bates DV: Regional ventilation of the lung, studied with boluses of ^{133}Xenon. Respir Physiol 2:234–246, 1967

30. Farhi LE: Diffusive and convective movement of gas in the lung, in Wolstenholme GEW, Knight J (eds): Ciba Foundation Symposium on Circulatory and Respiratory Mass Transport. Lon-

don, J & A Churchill Ltd, 1969, pp 277–293

31. Fowler WS: Intrapulmonary distribution of inspired gas. Physiol Rev 32: 1–20, 1952

32. Fowler WS, Cornish ER, Kety SS: Lung function studies. VIII. Analysis of alveolar ventilation by pulmonary N_2 clearance curves. J Clin Invest 31:40–50, 1952

33. Georg J, Lassen NA, Mellemgaard K, Vinther A: Diffusion in the gas phase of the lungs in normal and emphysematous subjects. Clin Sci 29:525–532, 1965

34. Glazier JB, Hughes JMB, Maloney JE, West JB: Vertical gradient of alveolar size in lungs of dogs frozen intact. J Appl Physiol 23:694–705, 1967

35. Groom AC, Morin R, Farhi LE: Determination of dissolved N_2 in blood and investigation of N_2 washout from the body. J Appl Physiol 23:706–712, 1967

36. Hashimoto T, Young AC, Martin CJ: Compartmental analysis of the distribution of gas in the lungs. J Appl Physiol 23:203–209, 1967

37. Heckscher T, Bass H, Oriol A, Rose B, Anthonisen NR, Bates DV: Regional lung function in patients with bronchial asthma. J Clin Invest 47:1063–1070, 1968

38. Henderson R, Horsfield K, Cumming G: Intersegmental collateral ventilation in the human lung. Respir Physiol 6:128–134, 1968–69

39. Hogg JC, Macklem PT, Thurlbeck WM: The resistance of collateral channels in excised human lungs. J Clin Invest 48: 421–431, 1969

40. Horsfield K, Cumming G: Functional consequences of airway morphology. J Appl Physiol 24:384–390, 1968

41. Hyatt RE, Okeson GC: Expiratory flow limitation, the cause of so-called "airway closure" or "closing volume." Physiologist 14:166, 1971

41a. Hyatt RE, Okeson GC, Rodarte JR: Influence of expiratory flow limitation on the pattern of lung emptying in normal man. J Appl Physiol 35:411–419, 1973

42. Jones JG: The effect of preinspiratory lung volume on the result of the single breath O_2 test. Respir Physiol 2:375–385, 1967

43. Jones JG, Clarke SW: The effect of expiratory flow rate on regional lung emptying. Clin Sci 37:343–356, 1969

44. Kaneko K, Milic-Emili J, Dolovich MB, Dawson A, Bates DV: Regional distribution of ventilation and perfusion as a function of body position. J Appl Physiol 21:767–777, 1966

45. Kjellmer I, Sandquist L, Berglund E: "Alveolar plateau" of the single breath nitrogen elimination curve in normal subjects. J Appl Physiol 14:105–108, 1959

46. Krogh A, Lindhard J: The volume of the dead space in breathing and the mixing of gases in the lungs of man. J Physiol 51:59–90, 1917

47. Kylstra JA, Paganelli CV, Lanphier EH: Pulmonary gas exchange in dogs ventilated with hyperbarically oxygenated liquid. J Appl Physiol 21:177–184, 1966

48. LaForce RC, Lewis BM: Diffusional transport in the human lung. J Appl Physiol 28:291–298, 1970

49. LeBlanc P, Ruff F, Milic-Emili J: Effects of age and body position on "airway closure" in man. J Appl Physiol 28:448–451, 1970

50. Lundin G: Nitrogen elimination during oxygen breathing. Acta Physiol Scand 30 (suppl 111):130–143, 1953

51. Macklem PT: Airway obstruction and collateral ventilation. Physiol Rev 51: 368–436, 1971

52. McFadden ER Jr, Lyons HA: Airway resistance and uneven ventilation in bronchial asthma. J Appl Physiol 25: 365–370, 1968

53. Martin CJ, Young AC: Lobar ventilation in man. Am Rev Tuberc Pulm Dis 73:330–337, 1956

54. Martin HB: Respiratory bronchioles as the pathway for collateral ventilation. J Appl Physiol 21:1443–1447, 1966

55. Martin RR, Anthonisen NR, Zutter M: Effect of increased gas density on respiratory gas exchange in the anesthetized dog. Physiologist 13:256,1970

56. Mead J: The distribution of gas flow in lungs, in Wolstenholme GEW, Knight J (eds): Ciba Foundation Symposium on Circulatory and Respiratory Mass Transport. London, J & A Churchill, Ltd, 1969, pp 204–209

57. Milic-Emili J, Henderson JAM, Dolovich MB, Trop D, Kaneko K: Regional distribution of inspired gas in the lung. J Appl Physiol 21:749–759, 1966

58. Millette B, Robertson PC, Ross WRD, Anthonisen NR: Effect of expiratory flow rate on emptying of lung regions. J Appl Physiol 27:587–591, 1969

59. Muir DCF: Distribution of aerosol particles in exhaled air. J Appl Physiol 23:210–214, 1967

60. Okubo T, Lenfant C: Distribution function of lung volume and ventilation determined by lung N_2 washout. J Appl Physiol 24:658–667, 1968

61. Otis AB, McKerrow CB, Bartlett RA, Mead J, McIlroy MB, Selverstone NJ, Radford EP Jr: Mechanical factors in distribution of pulmonary ventilation. J Appl Physiol 8:427–443, 1956

62. Power GG: Gaseous diffusion between airways and alveoli in the human lung. J Appl Physiol 27:701–709, 1969

63. Rauwerda PE: Unequal ventilation of different parts of the lung and the determination of cardiac output (Thesis). Groningen, The Netherlands, University of Groningen, 1946

64. Robertson JS, Siri WE, Jones HB: Lung ventilation patterns determined by analysis of nitrogen elimination rates; use of the mass spectrometer as a continuous gas analyzer. J Clin Invest 29:577–590, 1950

65. Roos A, Dahlstrom H, Murphy JP: Distribution of inspired air in the lungs. J Appl Physiol 7:645–659, 1955

66. Rossing RG: Evaluation of a computer solution of exponential decay or washout curves. J Appl Physiol 21:1907–1910, 1966

67. Rusher JL, Stoll PJ, Lenfant C: Exercise-induced hyperpnea and uniformity and efficiency of pulmonary ventilation. J Appl Physiol 28:63–69, 1970

68. Saltzman HA, Salzano JV, Blenkarn GD, Kylstra JA: Effects of pressure on ventilation and gas exchange in man. J Appl Physiol 30:443–449, 1971

69. Scheid P, Piiper J: Analysis of test gas washout from lungs with varying tidal volume: theory. J Appl Physiol 31:292–295, 1971

70. Shinozaki T, Abajian JC Jr, Tabakin BS, Hanson JS: Theory and clinical application of a digital nitrogen washout computer. J Appl Physiol 21:202–208, 1966

71. Sikand R, Cerretelli P, Farhi LE: Effects of VA and VA/Q distribution and of time on the alveolar plateau. J Appl Physiol 21:1331–1337, 1966

72. Stanescu DC, Teculescu DB, Pacuraru R, Popa V: Effect of bronchoconstrictor aerosols on the alveolar plateau of the single breath O_2 test. Thorax 23:628–633, 1968

73. Suda Y, Martin CJ, Young AC: Regional dispersion of volume-to-ventilation ratios in the lung of man. J Appl Physiol 29:480–485, 1970

74. Tendeloo N Ph: Studien ueber die Ursachen der Lungenkrankheiten. Erster (Physiologischer) Teil. Wiesbaden, JF Bergmann, 1901

75. Tsunoda S, Young AC, Martin CJ: Emptying pattern of lung compartments in normal man. J Appl Physiol 32:644–649, 1972

76. West JB: Gas exchange when one lung region inspires from another. J Appl Physiol 30:479–487, 1971

77. West JB: Distribution of mechanical stress in the lung, a possible factor in localisation of pulmonary disease. Lancet 1:839–841, 1971

77a. West JB, Matthews FL: Stresses, strains, and surface pressures in the lung caused by its weight. J Appl Physiol 32:332–345, 1972

78. Young AC, Martin CJ, Pace WR: Effect of expiratory flow patterns on lung emptying. J Appl Physiol 18:47–50, 1963

79. Zardini P, West JB: Topographical distribution of ventilation in isolated lung. J Appl Physiol 21:794–802, 1966

Chapter 5

Distribution of Ventilation and Perfusion

Exchange of oxygen and carbon dioxide between alveolar air and the blood in pulmonary capillaries is the essential function of the lungs. The ultimate energy-exchanging reactions between oxygen and metabolic substrates take place in the mitochondrial membranes in cells.[11] To maintain these processes, the circulating blood transports oxygen and carbon dioxide, and gas exchange in the lungs maintains O_2 and CO_2 partial pressures at constant levels, adequate for tissue gas exchange. The amounts of gases exchanged in the lungs depend on the amount of ventilation reaching the alveoli per unit time ($\dot{V}_A$), and the amount of blood circulating through lung capillaries per unit time (perfusion of the lungs, $\dot{Q}$). Gas and blood do not reach individual alveolar units at equal rates. Hence, the ratio of ventilation to perfusion ($\dot{V}_A/\dot{Q}$ ratio) differs locally. Since the alveoli are ventilated only during inspiration, the $\dot{V}_A/\dot{Q}$ ratio also changes during the breathing cycle. The variations in $\dot{V}_A/\dot{Q}$ ratios give rise to differences in partial pressures of O_2, CO_2, and N_2 between alveolar gas and blood in the lung capillaries. The net effect of the distribution of $\dot{V}_A/\dot{Q}$ ratios throughout the lungs is that a fraction of inspired gas does not participate in gas exchange (physiological dead space), while a fraction of blood perfusing the lung does not alter its composition (venous admixture).

EXCHANGE OF INERT GASES

The exchange of O_2 and CO_2 is complicated by chemical reactions in the blood (Chap. 6). Hence, to focus on events in the lungs, we will first consider inert gases, i.e., those which do not react chemically with blood components. Their exchange depends on (1) alveolar ventilation, (2) perfusion of the lung capillaries with blood, (3) diffusivity through the pulmonary capillary membrane, and (4) solubility in blood. Diffusivity will be considered later; for present purposes we may assume that diffusion through the membrane does not limit gas exchange. The diagrams developed by Farhi[6] show the relationships between ventilation, perfusion, and solubility (Fig. 5-1*A, B*). The relative importance of ventilation

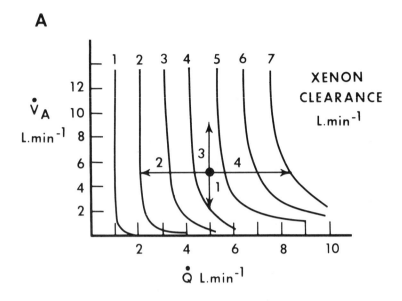

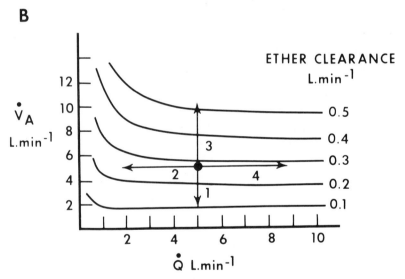

Fig. 5-1. Clearance of inert gases in the lungs. ● indicates clearance rates at normal average ventilation and perfusion rates ($\dot{V}_A = 5$ liters/min^{-1}; $\dot{Q} = 5$ liters/min^{-1}). Lines are isopleths of equal clearance rates for an insoluble (*A*, xenon) and a soluble (*B*, ether) gas. *A*. Xe clearance is largely determined by perfusion rate (*arrows* 2 and 4), and only slightly by ventilation rate (*arrows* 1 and 3). *B*. Ether clearance is largely determined by ventilation rate (*arrows* 1 and 3) and only slightly by perfusion rate (*arrows* 2 and 4). Modified from reference 6.

and perfusion in gas clearance depends on the solubility of the gas. Consider first xenon, a comparatively insoluble gas (Fig. 5-1A). At normal ventilation and perfusion rates (5 liters/min), dissolved xenon is cleared from blood at a rate of about 4.5 liters/min. This rate depends almost exclusively on perfusion of the lung capillaries; ventilation has little effect. Increasing or decreasing the rate of alveolar ventilation ($\dot{V}_A$), at constant perfusion rate, $\dot{Q}$, does not significantly alter xenon clearance (see arrows *1* and *3* in Fig. 5-1A). In contrast, decreasing perfusion ($\dot{Q}$) from 5 to 2 liters/min leads to a nearly equally large drop in xenon clearance, and an increase in $\dot{Q}$ from 5 to 8 liters/min leads to a proportionate increase in xenon clearance. Thus, the clearance of a relatively insoluble gas from blood depends mostly on how much of it reaches the gas-exchanging capillaries.

With a soluble gas, ethylether, the relations between ventilation and perfusion are different (Fig. 5-1B). Increasing $\dot{Q}$ fourfold from 2 to 8 liters/min at constant $\dot{V}_A$ (*2* and *4*) has only minimal effect on clearance, while a comparable increase in alveolar ventilation at constant $\dot{Q}$ (*1* and *3*) increases clearance about fivefold. These relations change when ventilation or blood flow are very low. With minimal alveolar ventilation (less than 0.5 liters/min), even large increases of perfusion cannot significantly increase xenon clearance; when perfusion is equally minimal, even large increases of ventilation cannot extract much more ether from blood.

Both alveolar ventilation and pulmonary blood flow are unevenly distributed throughout the lung.[19, 24] For instance, in the vertical lung, ventilation increases threefold from the lung top to the bottom (Chap. 4), and blood flow is even more dependent on gravity. According to West's calculations, blood flow increases from 0.07 liters/min in the top 7 percent of the lung volume to 1.29 liters/min in the bottom 13 percent.[24] Hence, the ratio of ventilation to perfusion ($\dot{V}_A/\dot{Q}$ ratio) decreases from 3.3 to 0.63 from the top to the bottom of the vertical lung. Although they receive little inspired air, the top alveoli are still overventilated in relation to blood flow since they receive almost no blood, and the bottom zones are relatively underventilated even though they receive a larger share of the inspired air.

The ratio between ventilation and perfusion has a pronounced effect on gas exchange. For inert gases, the partial pressures in alveolar gas depend solely on three variables: mixed venous partial pressure, solubility, and the $\dot{V}_A/\dot{Q}$ ratio. Figure 5-2 indicates the ratio between alveolar and mixed venous gas pressures as a function of solubility and the $\dot{V}_A/\dot{Q}$ ratio.[7] Relatively soluble gases (*1* and *3*) have alveolar pressures that nearly equal those in mixed venous blood at $\dot{V}_A/\dot{Q}$ ratios <1.0. The less soluble gas (*2*) always has an alveolar pressure much less than that in mixed venous blood, even when $\dot{V}_A/\dot{Q}$ is very low.

Figure 5-3 compares the behavior of an insoluble and a more soluble gas (i.e., gases *1* and *2* in Figure 5-2) by plotting their relative alveolar pressures against one another at different values of $\dot{V}_A/\dot{Q}$. At each value of $\dot{V}_A/\dot{Q}$, the insoluble gas (*2*) has a lower alveolar pressure, relative to mixed venous pressure, than the more soluble gas (*1*). Farhi and Yokoyama[7] have pointed out that the drawn curve in Figure 5-3 is a $\dot{V}_A/\dot{Q}$ line: the locus of all possible combinations of alveolar pressures of the two gases at given values of $\dot{V}_A/\dot{Q}$ ratios. The diagram considers the two gases in terms of their elimination from blood passing through the lungs. However, the basic relationships are similar whether one deals with

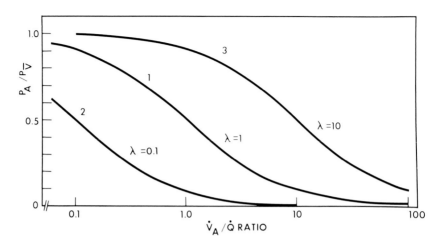

Fig. 5-2. Alveolar pressure (as a fraction of mixed venous pressure; $P_A/P_{\bar{V}}$ ratio) as a function of $\dot{V}_A/\dot{Q}$ ratio, for gases of increasing solubility (partition coefficient, $\lambda=$ 0.1, 1, and 10). At all values of $\dot{V}_A/\dot{Q}$, the relative alveolar pressure is higher for soluble than for insoluble gases. O_2 behaves approximately as gas *2*, CO_2 as gas *1* (See Fig. 5-3). After reference 6.

elimination or uptake, as Farhi and Yokoyama emphasized by constructing appropriate coordinates for CO_2 and O_2 partial pressures in the diagram of Figure 5-3. Thus, the physiological exchange of oxygen and carbon dioxide appears to follow rules similar to those for inert gases. Oxygen behaves as a relatively insoluble gas, and CO_2 as a soluble gas, with a ratio of partition coefficients of about 1:10.

EXCHANGE OF O_2 AND CO_2 IN ALVEOLI

The uptake of O_2 and the production of CO_2 are determined by the body's metabolic needs. Ventilation and blood flow adapt, through complex control systems, to restore altered O_2 and CO_2 pressures to normal. This results in adequate transfer of O_2 and CO_2 between the tissues and atmospheric air. Because of the chemical nature of the metabolic substrates, more O_2 is consumed than CO_2 is produced in the tissues. Thus, the respiratory quotient ($R=\dot{V}_{CO_2}/\dot{V}_{O_2}$) is usually less than 1. This means that less CO_2 is exchanged in the lungs than O_2, per unit time, unless the tissues release or store these gases. The total amount of O_2 and CO_2 exchanged by the body can be determined by measuring the amounts added or removed from inspired air. Thus, O_2 uptake and CO_2 production are measured from the amount of air ventilated and the concentrations, or partial pressures, of O_2 and CO_2 in the inspired and expired air. Since ventilation is the same for O_2 and CO_2, this cancels out when $\dot{V}_{O_2}$ is divided into $\dot{V}_{CO_2}$; therefore, R can be determined solely from the gas tensions. The equations relating R to the inspired and alveolar partial pressures of O_2 and CO_2 are described by Rahn and Fenn.[18] Figure 5-4 shows them graphically in an O_2 versus CO_2 diagram. If $R=1$, equal amounts of O_2 and CO_2 are exchanged, and the decrease in partial pressure of O_2 in alveolar gas equals the increase in the partial pressure of CO_2.

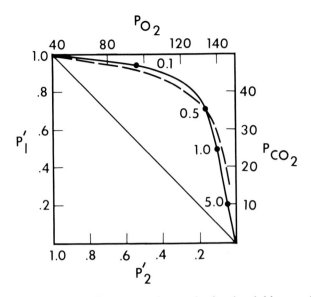

Fig. 5-3. *Abscissa. $P_A/P_{\bar{V}}$ ratio for insoluble gas 2 from Figure 5-2 (P'_2). Ordinate. $P_A/P_{\bar{V}}$ ratio for soluble gas 1 (P'_1).* The higher relative alveolar pressure of the more soluble gas *1* appears from the fact that all points that relate the two $P_A/P_{\bar{V}}$ ratios to one another are situated to the right of the diagonal line of equality, on the curved drawn line. Values for the $\dot{V}_A/\dot{Q}$ ratio can be placed on this line by reading $\dot{V}_A/\dot{Q}$ values from Figure 5-2. For instance, at $\dot{V}_A/\dot{Q} = 1.0$; $P'_2 = 0.1$, and $P'_1 = 0.5$. Points for $\dot{V}_A/\dot{Q} = 0.1, 0.5, 1.0$, and 5.0 are indicated on the curve. The dashed curve is the $\dot{V}_A/\dot{Q}$ line for O_2-CO_2 exchange (see text). Modified from reference 7.

In Figure 5-4, *I* represents the composition of inspired air: $P_{O_2}=150$ mm Hg; $P_{CO_2}=0$. A_1 is one possible composition of alveolar gas when $R=1$. At that point, oxygen tension has decreased 40 mm Hg (from 150 to 110) and P_{O_2} has increased from 0 to 40 mm Hg. When R is less than 1, the influx of CO_2 into the alveolar gas is less than the efflux of O_2 into the blood; hence, the sum of P_{O_2} and P_{CO_2} decreases. The total pressure of alveolar gas, of course, remains the same; the balance is made up by N_2. The solid line for $R=0.8$ shows that, at any point, the sum of P_{O_2} and P_{CO_2} is less than their sum in inspired air (150 mm). For example, at *A*, which represents one possible composition of alveolar gas, this sum is $102+40=142$ mm Hg. Thus, the composition of inspired gas changes into that of alveolar air along the pathway IA_1 or IA, depending on the value of *R*. The solid and dashed lines in Figure 5-4 represent all possible compositions of alveolar gas when $R=0.8$ or $R=1$, respectively. Lines for $R<0.8$ lie to the left of the drawn line; lines for $R>1$ lie to the right of the dashed line.

Where is the alveolar point located on the *R* line? This depends on the supply of inspired air (alveolar ventilation) and the uptake of O_2 (or output of CO_2) in or from blood. The equations developed by Rahn and Fenn [18] show that the ratios $\dot{V}_A/\dot{V}_{O_2}$ and $\dot{V}_A/\dot{V}_{CO_2}$ are the determining factors. Two values of the $\dot{V}_A/\dot{V}_{O_2}$

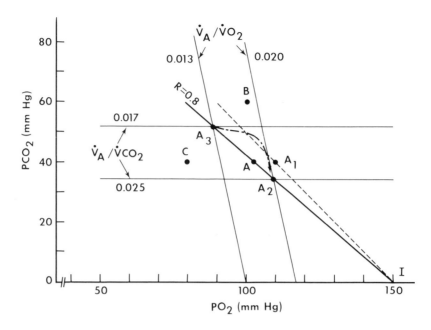

Fig. 5-4. O_2-CO_2 diagram.[17] Dashed line at 45° indicates $R=1$ ($P_{O_2}+P_{CO_2}$ $=150$ mm Hg$=PI_{O_2}$). Heavy drawn line for $R=0.8$. $\dot{V}_A/\dot{V}_{CO_2}$ and $\dot{V}_A/\dot{V}_{O_2}$ lines and individual data points are discussed in text. $I=$ inspired gas point. Alveolar point A is identical to point A in Figure 5-5. Units ($\dot{V}_A$ in liters/min; $\dot{V}_{O_2}$ in ml/min) are those used by Rahn and Fenn.[18] See also text footnote.

ratio are shown in Figure 5-4. The line marked .020 is the locus of all alveolar points consistent with a $\dot{V}_A/\dot{V}_{O_2}$ ratio$=0.020$. For instance, $\dot{V}_A$ might be 6 liters/ min BTPS* and $\dot{V}_{O_2}$ might be 300 ml/min STPD. Alveolar point A_2 lies on this line and also on the $R=0.8$ line; it is the only point consistent with both condi-tions. If, during light exercise, $\dot{V}_{O_2}$ increases from 300 to 460 ml/min while $\dot{V}_A$ remains constant at 6 liters/min, $\dot{V}_A/\dot{V}_{O_2}$ decreases to $6/460=0.013$. If R remains at 0.8, the only alveolar point consistent with the exercise conditions is A_3, the intersection of the $R=0.8$ line with a $\dot{V}_A/\dot{V}_{O_2}=0.013$ line. Thus, a small increase in O_2 uptake substantially changes the composition of alveolar gas if ventilation does not change. At A_3, P_{O_2} is 18 mm Hg higher, and P_{CO_2} is 20 mm Hg lower, than at A_2. Obviously, alveolar ventilation must be precisely controlled if the composition of alveolar air is to remain constant (Chap. 10). To maintain the alveolar point at A_2, $\dot{V}_A$ must increase in proportion to $\dot{V}_{O_2}$, i.e., from 6 to 9.2 liters/min, so that the $\dot{V}_A/\dot{V}_{O_2}$ ratio remains at 0.020.

Since R is the ratio of CO_2 production and O_2 uptake, each alveolar point must correspond to a level of CO_2 production consistent with R and $\dot{V}_A/\dot{V}_{O_2}$. For instance, if $\dot{V}_{O_2}=300$ ml/min and $R=0.8$, $\dot{V}_{CO_2}$ must be 240 ml/min. Thus, if

---

* This choice of units is convenient since ventilation is commonly expressed in terms of the physical condition of alveolar air (BTPS $=$ body temperature, ambient pressure, saturated with water vapor), while O_2 uptake and CO_2 output are measured in STPD conditions (0°C, 760 mm Hg, dry).

at A_2, $\dot{V}_A = 6$ liters/min and $\dot{V}_{O_2} = 300$ ml/min, $\dot{V}_A/\dot{V}_{CO_2}$ must be $6/240 = 0.025$. In the absence of CO_2 in inspired air, the ratio $\dot{V}_A/\dot{V}_{CO_2}$ is independent of P_{O_2}, and hence the lines for this ratio run parallel with the abscissa in Figure 5-4. The values for the ratio $\dot{V}_A/\dot{V}_{CO_2}$ decrease as P_{CO_2} increases. Thus, if $\dot{V}_A$ remains constant, the amount of CO_2 excreted can only increase if alveolar P_{CO_2} increases concomitantly. Each unit of expired alveolar gas then contains more CO_2 and total excretion increases. Similarly, if oxygen uptake increases while $\dot{V}_A$ is constant, alveolar O_2 tension decreases; more O_2 is extracted from each volume unit inspired gas.

The terms *hypoventilation* and *hyperventilation* indicate ventilation levels that result in abnormal alveolar gas tensions. They do not refer to set levels of 'normal' minute volumes of ventilation. Hypoventilation results in elevated P_{CO_2} and decreased P_{O_2} values (e.g., point A_3 in Fig. 5-4); hyperventilation decreases P_{CO_2} and raises P_{O_2}. During changes in ventilation levels, alveolar gas composition does not change as predicted by the R line between A_2 and A_3. For instance, during recovery from hypoventilation (A_3), extra CO_2 must be eliminated and extra O_2 taken up to reestablish equilibrium at the new alveolar gas composition, A_2. In steady-state conditions, alveolar gas tensions correspond to certain levels of CO_2 and O_2 which are stored in blood and in body tissues. The stores for CO_2 are considerably greater than those for O_2. Therefore, when a change in $\dot{V}_A$ leads to a change in alveolar gas composition, the oxygen stores assume the new level quicker than the CO_2 stores. As a consequence, alveolar P_{O_2} reaches its new steady-state value more rapidly than P_{CO_2}, and the pathway followed by alveolar gas describes a half loop (dashed arrow in Fig. 5-4).[18] Thus R does not remain constant but is temporarily elevated during the transition. A half loop in the reverse direction is followed when $\dot{V}_A$ decreases.

The management of patients with respiratory insufficiency, a condition which leads to hypoventilation and often severe hypoxia (low P_{O_2}) and hypercapnia (high P_{CO_2}), is often based on arterial blood gas data (p. 113). Determinations of R require expired gas collections, which is usually not feasible at the bedside. However, in a steady state, R should be less than 1 and therefore the sum of alveolar P_{O_2} and P_{CO_2} should be less than the inspired P_{O_2} (p. 83). This should also be true for arterial P_{O_2} and P_{CO_2}, since arterial P_{O_2} is usually at least several mm Hg lower than alveolar P_{O_2}, and arterial P_{CO_2} is close to alveolar P_{CO_2}. Hence, if arterial P_{O_2} plus arterial P_{CO_2} exceeds inspired P_{O_2}, one must suspect a technical error or a markedly unsteady state. The two can be distinguished if ventilation data are obtained at the time of blood sampling. To calculate $\dot{V}_A$ from total ventilation rate, one may assume an average value for anatomical dead space (Chap. 3), and with approximate data for $\dot{V}_{O_2}$ (from metabolic tables) one can estimate the $\dot{V}_A/\dot{V}_{O_2}$ ratio. This can be used to test the validity of arterial blood gas data. For instance, a $\dot{V}_A/\dot{V}_{O_2}$ ratio of 0.013 would be incompatible with an arterial $P_{O_2} = 100$ mm Hg and a $P_{CO_2} = 60$ mm Hg (Fig. 5-4B). However, because of the alveolar-arterial P_{O_2} difference, it would be compatible with an arterial blood point C ($P_{O_2} = 80$ mm Hg; $P_{CO_2} = 40$ mm Hg). Since alveolar gas can be sampled directly with rapid gas analyzers, it is possible to define alveolar points in persons in whom alveolar gas composition is fairly homogeneous. This is unfortunately not the case in most patients with respiratory insufficiency.

COMPOSITION OF ALVEOLAR GAS

Alveolar gas composition is not uniform throughout the lungs (Chap. 4); Figure 5-4 presents an idealized perspective. Additional elements of uncertainty concerning alveolar gas composition, not yet discussed in Chapter 4, include (1) variations during the breathing cycle, and (2) variations resulting from nonuniform perfusion of lung capillaries. The latter are discussed in relation to ventilation rates, i.e., as one determinant of $\dot{V}_A/\dot{Q}$ ratios.

Variations During the Breathing Cycle

Expiration is breath holding with a decreasing lung volume; CO_2 production continues into the contracting lung and hence alveolar P_{CO_2} increases. O_2 extraction also continues, with a resulting decrease in P_{O_2}. At the beginning of inspiration, dead space gas with a high CO_2 content is inspired into the alveoli; hence P_{CO_2} increases further in the first moment of inspiration, whereas P_{O_2} drops to a minimum. Then, fresh inspired air dilutes the alveolar gas; P_{O_2} rises and P_{CO_2} decreases until expiration starts again. The composition of alveolar air during a breathing cycle describes a loop on an O_2 versus CO_2 diagram;[4] the loop's excursions are normally small—some 2 mm Hg for P_{CO_2} and 3 mm Hg for P_{O_2}. Yet, even this slight deviation has implications for gas exchange.[16] Normally, peak flow rates occur early in expiration, after about one-third of its total duration.[2] If peak flow occurred later, the air would contain more CO_2, and more CO_2 would be transported in the same expired volume. With a late peak flow, the same gas exchange rate could be maintained with 6 percent less alveolar ventilation.[16] Thus, gas can be exchanged with less ventilation by delaying expiration and also by hastening inspiration. In Nye's model analysis the two together resulted in further economy of breathing. The combination is a gasping type of breathing called apneustic breathing (Chap. 10). Experiments in dogs have confirmed that this pattern can increase breathing efficiency. Arterial P_{O_2} increased within 30 seconds after altering the breathing pattern, while total ventilation, breathing rate, and tidal volume were unchanged.[12] This finding should be taken into account in selecting an optimal airflow pattern for artificial ventilation.

Ventilation-Perfusion Ratio

The $\dot{V}_A/\dot{Q}$ ratio has been discussed for inert gases (p. 82), and the concept of a $\dot{V}_A/\dot{Q}$ line was presented in Figure 5-3. In order to apply the ratio to O_2 and CO_2, perfusion must be introduced into the O_2 versus CO_2 diagram. This complicates matters because the relations between partial pressures and contents of O_2 and CO_2 in blood are not linear. In a steady state, gas exchange between tissues, blood, and lung air proceeds at the same average rate; that is, R must be the same for all exchanges. Obviously, the R for blood ($\dot{V}_{CO_2}/\dot{V}_{O_2}$) is determined by the contents of O_2 and CO_2 in arterial and venous blood. These contents can be related to corresponding partial pressures by referring to dissociation curves for O_2 and CO_2.[18] This enables one to plot combinations of P_{O_2} and P_{CO_2} that are consistent with given values of R. Figure 5–5 includes four such "blood R lines," all of which originate at the mixed venous point $\overline{V}$ and intersect the R lines for

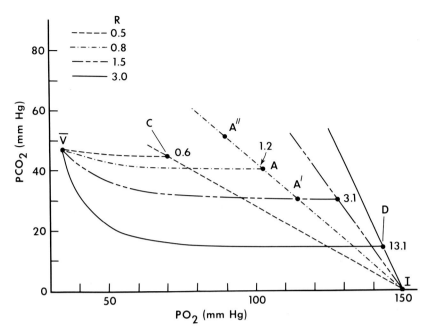

Fig. 5-5. R lines for blood and gas in an O_2-CO_2 diagram. $I=$inspired gas point; $\overline{V}=$mixed venous blood point. Gas R lines originate at I, blood R lines at $\overline{V}$. Alveolar point A is identical to A in Figure 5-4. Alveolar points A, A', and A'' are all situated on the $R=0.8$ line for gas; only A is situated on the $R=0.8$ line for blood. Hence, A represents the only composition of alveolar gas at which blood and gas can exchange O_2 and CO_2 at $R=0.8$, for the chosen values of I and $\overline{V}$. Points C and D explained in text. Values of $\dot{V}_A/\dot{Q}$ ratios indicated at each intersection of blood and gas R lines (0.6, 1.2, 3.1, and 13.1).

The O_2 and CO_2 pressures of mixed venous blood ($\overline{V}$) correspond to gas contents of about 129 ml/liter O_2 and 540 ml/liter CO_2, according to standard dissociation curves.[18] Arterialization of this blood at $R=0.8$ might add 40 ml/liter O_2 and eliminate $0.8 \times 40 = 32$ ml/liter CO_2. The gas contents of the arterialized blood would then be $129 + 40 = 169$ ml/liter O_2 and $540 - 32 = 508$ ml/liter CO_2. Referring again to standard dissociation curves, these contents correspond to a P_{O_2} of 52 mm Hg and a P_{CO_2} of 43 mm Hg. This is a point on the $R=0.8$ line for blood. Other points on the same line are obtained by assuming different values for O_2 uptake and CO_2 elimination. Points on other blood R lines are obtained by performing similar calculations with the appropriate R value, always starting with the composition of mixed venous blood. For details see reference 18.

alveolar gas. For instance, point A indicates the only possible composition of alveolar air compatible with steady-state gas exchange at $R=0.8$ for given values of points I and $\overline{V}$, the compositions of inspired air and of mixed venous blood. Point A also corresponds to a fixed value of the $\dot{V}_A/\dot{Q}$ ratio, just as the points on the curve of Figure 5–3 indicate $\dot{V}_A/\dot{Q}$ values derived from the exchange ratios of inert gases. For point A, $\dot{V}_A/\dot{Q}=1.2$ (Eq. 21 in reference 18).

Each of the intersections of blood and gas R lines in Figure 5–5 indicates blood and gas exchanging CO_2 and O_2 at a particular value of $\dot{V}_A/\dot{Q}$ (0.6, 1.2, 3.1, and 13.1). If a line is drawn through the mixed venous and inspired points as well as through the intersections of blood and gas R lines, the $\dot{V}_A/\dot{Q}$ line results (Fig. 5–6). Since $\overline{V}$ represents blood as it arrives in the lungs, unchanged by gas exchange, its $\dot{V}_A$ is zero, and its $\dot{V}_A/\dot{Q}=0$. In contrast, I represents inspired air unchanged by gas exchange; its $\dot{Q}$ is zero, and hence it stands for $\dot{V}_A/\dot{Q}=\infty$. Thus, $\dot{V}_A/\dot{Q}$ increases from zero to infinity along the $\dot{V}_A/\dot{Q}$ line, from $\overline{V}$ to I.

If ventilation and perfusion were uniformly distributed throughout the lungs, their ratio would be the same everywhere, and the composition of alveolar air would be constant at values consistent with one particular $\dot{V}_A/\dot{Q}$ ratio. In fact, neither ventilation nor $\dot{Q}$ is uniformly distributed and hence $\dot{V}_A/\dot{Q}$ varies locally and in time. In a vertical human lung, $\dot{V}_A/\dot{Q}$ varies from about 0.6 at the bottom to more than 3 in the lung top.[23, 24] That is, alveolar O_2 tensions vary from about 70 to 130 mm Hg, and P_{CO_2} from 45 to less than 30 mm Hg (see Fig. 5–6 and its legend). Since ventilation distribution is nonuniform even in small portions of the lungs (p. 62), some degree of $\dot{V}_A/\dot{Q}$ nonuniformity probably exists within subsegments and lobules. In addition, ventilation and blood flow in a single alveolar unit may be nonuniform. Thus, it is very unlikely that alveolar air ever has an ideally uniform composition. Yet, in healthy lungs the expired O_2 and CO_2 concentrations vary much less than one would expect from the wide range of alveolar tensions consistent with $\dot{V}_A/\dot{Q}$ ratios between 0.6 and 3 in the vertical lung. This is partly because areas with a low $\dot{V}_A/\dot{Q}$ contribute little to the expired

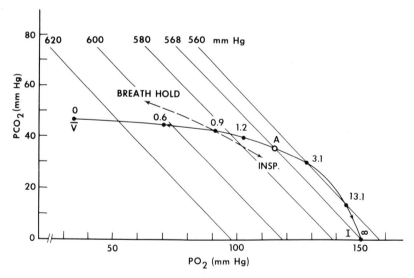

Fig. 5-6. $\dot{V}_A/\dot{Q}$ line in an O_2-CO_2 diagram. Inspired gas point, I; mixed venous blood point, $\overline{V}$. Numbers indicate $\dot{V}_A/\dot{Q}$ ratio at different points (from 0 at $\overline{V}$ to ∞ at I). In a vertical lung, $\dot{V}_A/\dot{Q}$ ratio varies from about 0.6 at the top to over 3.0 at the bottom. The graph indicates the wide range of alveolar O_2 and CO_2 tensions consistent with this range of $\dot{V}_A/\dot{Q}$ values. Dashed arrows indicate changes of alveolar gas composition during breath holding and during rapid inspiration, both starting at an alveolar point were $\dot{V}_A/\dot{Q}=0.9$. A decrease of $\dot{V}_A/\dot{Q}$ from 0.9 to 0.6 (*arrow*) leads to a lower PA_{O_2} but little change in PA_{CO_2}. At high $\dot{V}_A/\dot{Q}$ ratios, a further increase in ventilation (*arrow near I*) decreases PA_{CO_2} while PA_{O_2} increases little. Dashed diagonal lines are isopleths of alveolar P_{N_2} (see text). At A, $PA_{N_2}=PI_{N_2}$ (see also Fig. 5-7).

air; also, the dead space functions as a mixing chamber, which tends to equalize alveolar gas tensions (p. 68). Expired air, therefore, is a mixed gas weighted toward the composition of gas in high $\dot{V}_A/\dot{Q}$ areas. In contrast, the composition of arterial blood is determined largely by contributions from areas with a large blood flow, i.e., a low $\dot{V}_A/\dot{Q}$ ratio.

During breath holding alveolar P_{O_2} decreases much more than P_{CO_2} increases. This is partly because CO_2 is much more soluble in blood and tissues (including lung tissue [5]) than O_2 and partly because of the shape of the $\dot{V}_A/\dot{Q}$ line. During breath holding, alveolar ventilation stops, and hence gas exchange proceeds at a rapidly decreasing $\dot{V}_A/\dot{Q}$ ratio. On the other hand, after a rapid and deep inspiration, alveolar gas composition changes toward higher $\dot{V}_A/\dot{Q}$ values.[4] The dashed arrows in Figure 5-6 indicate the direction of these changes; these arrows deviate from the $\dot{V}_A/\dot{Q}$ line. Shifts of the mixed venous point are one reason for the deviation. Even within one circulation time, systemic circuits with short circulation times contribute blood with higher P_{CO_2} and lower P_{O_2} to mixed venous blood during breath holding. Also, cardiac output changes during breath holding, and this, too, affects the mixed venous point, since the arteriovenous O_2 and CO_2 differences are inversely related to cardiac output. The direction of alveolar gas changes during inspiration is also uncertain. As a result of dead space gas distribution, the composition of inspired air is not uniform in all lung areas (p. 63).[22] Thus, alveolar gas composition varies with inspiration and expiration, with time during breath holding, and with location in the lungs according to the $\dot{V}_A/\dot{Q}$ ratio. In addition, its exact value at any time is influenced by the position of the mixed venous point and of the inspired point for a given lung area. Because of these inherent uncertainties, it is difficult to reproduce a $\dot{V}_A/\dot{Q}$ line experimentally. However, in principle, this concept is well established and provides many important insights that can be confirmed by experimental data. Normally, $\dot{V}_A/\dot{Q}$ is between 0.8 and 1.0 in large parts of the lung. Increased perfusion leads to lower $\dot{V}_A/\dot{Q}$ ratios and decreases the alveolar P_{O_2}; increased ventilation leads to decreased P_{CO_2} tensions but has less effect on P_{O_2} (see Fig. 5-6 and its legend). Hence, in terms of total blood and gas flow, gas exchange is optimal when $\dot{V}_A/\dot{Q}$ ratios are about 0.8–1.0.

A-a PARTIAL-PRESSURE DIFFERENCES

Alveolar and arterial gas pressures would be equal if gas exchange in the lungs led to complete equilibration and if all arterial blood passed through the lungs. Neither is true. Arterial blood receives small contributions of venous blood through connections in the heart and from bronchial veins; a small amount of pulmonary blood flow may pass through unventilated zones ($\dot{V}_A/\dot{Q}=0$) or through arteriovenous anastomoses in the lung circulation. These result in a venous admixture in arterial blood, which reduces its P_{O_2} and slightly raises its P_{CO_2}. In addition, diffusion limits alveolocapillary equilibration for O_2 (Chap. 6); thus, even if all parts of the lungs exchanged gas at the same $\dot{V}_A/\dot{Q}$ ratio, alveolar and arterial gas tensions would differ. This alveolar-arterial difference is not the same for O_2, CO_2, and N_2. The (A-a)DO_2, or alveolar-arterial P_{O_2} difference, is determined partly by diffusion limitation, but mostly by the distribution of

$\dot{V}_A/\dot{Q}$ ratios. The P_{O_2} of arterial blood is weighted in favor of high perfusion, low $\dot{V}_A/\dot{Q}$ areas, while the P_{O_2} of mixed alveolar air is weighted in favor of well-ventilated alveoli, i.e., gas from high $\dot{V}_A/\dot{Q}$ areas. Figure 5-6 shows that, if alveolar gas tensions are close to the point where $\dot{V}_A/\dot{Q}=1.2$, and arterial gas tensions close to that for $\dot{V}_A/\dot{Q}=0.9$, this alone accounts for an (A-a)DO_2 of 12.5 mm Hg. The alinearity of the HbO_2 dissociation curve contributes to the (A-a)DO_2 in particular when O_2 tensions lie on the curved portion of that curve. The (A-a)DCO_2 has long been believed to equal zero. There is indeed no diffusion limitation for CO_2, but a distribution of $\dot{V}_A/\dot{Q}$ ratios can cause an (a-A) DCO_2 even though it is usually minimal. In particular, when there are substantial areas with a high $\dot{V}_A/\dot{Q}$ ratio, the P_{CO_2} of expired alveolar gas may be much lower than the P_{CO_2} of arterial blood. In contrast, areas with low $\dot{V}_A/\dot{Q}$ ratios do little to increase arterial blood P_{CO_2}; e.g., when $\dot{V}_A/\dot{Q}$ decreases from 0.9 to 0.6 (Fig. 5-6), P_{CO_2} increases only 2.5 mm. Changes in P_{CO_2} are much greater at the right-hand side of the $\dot{V}_A/\dot{Q}$ line where the ratios are high. Thus, a measurable (a-A)DCO_2 usually indicates the presence of lung areas with a high $\dot{V}_A/\dot{Q}$ ratio. This is the basis for its use as a diagnostic tool in pulmonary embolism, in which regional vascular occlusion causes part of the lungs to have a high $\dot{V}_A/\dot{Q}$ ratio. However, the difficulty in defining an acceptable value for alveolar P_{CO_2} limits its practical use. Temporary hyperventilation may decrease alveolar P_{CO_2} before blood P_{CO_2} follows, and the variations of P_{CO_2} in the normal breathing cycle (p. 86) are a substantial fraction of the venoarterial P_{CO_2} difference. In clinical settings, arterial blood is seldom collected under conditions approaching a steady state, and this alone makes refined interpretations of arterial and alveolar CO_2 tensions hazardous.

The A-a Nitrogen Difference

Blood leaving the alveoli contains N_2 in direct proportion to the alveolar P_{N_2}. The latter depends on the O_2-CO_2 exchange ratio, R. For instance, in Figure 5-5, the sum of O_2 and CO_2 tensions at point C ($R=0.5$) is 115 mm Hg, and at point D ($R=13.1$) 158 mm Hg. At both points, the sum of all partial pressures is atmospheric (disregarding alveolar pressures needed for airflow; Chap. 8). Thus, alveolar N_2 tension is $765-47-115=603$ mm Hg at point C and $765-47-158=560$ mm Hg at D. Blood leaving alveoli corresponding to C and D has a P_{N_2} of 603 and of 560 mm Hg, respectively. Isopleths for P_{N_2}, included in the $\dot{V}_A/\dot{Q}$ diagram of Figure 5-6, show that there is only one point (A) on the $\dot{V}_A/\dot{Q}$ line where $PA_{N_2}=PI_{N_2}$. At higher $\dot{V}_A/\dot{Q}$ values, PA_{N_2} is less; as the $\dot{V}_A/\dot{Q}$ ratio decreases, PA_{N_2} increases.[8, 19]

The arterial blood P_{N_2} reflects a mixture of blood with P_{N_2} values which vary as a function of $\dot{V}_A/\dot{Q}$. The average is weighted in favor of low $\dot{V}_A/\dot{Q}$ areas, since these contribute more to arterial blood than areas where $\dot{V}_A$ is high and $\dot{Q}$ is low. Also, as Figure 5-7 shows, alveolar P_{N_2} increases greatly in low $\dot{V}_A/\dot{Q}$ areas (*arrow* 2), while it decreases only slightly in high $\dot{V}_A/\dot{Q}$ areas (*arrow* 1). The point where $PA_{N_2}=PI_{N_2}$ is indicated by A (identical with A in Fig. 5-6). Hence, when significant areas in the lungs have low $\dot{V}_A/\dot{Q}$ ratios, arterial P_{N_2} will be relatively high. At the same time, expired alveolar gas reflects areas with higher $\dot{V}_A/\dot{Q}$ ratios and therefore has a P_{N_2} much closer to that of inspired gas.

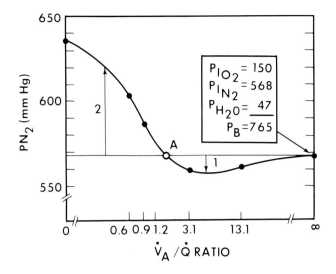

Fig. 5-7. Alveolar P_{N_2} (*ordinate*) as a function of $\dot{V}_A/\dot{Q}$ ratio (*abscissa*). At A, $PA_{N_2} = PI_{N_2}$ (see Fig. 5-6). Composition of inspired air in box. Arrows explained in text. Adapted from reference 19.

Hence, there will be an (a-A) P_{N_2} difference, which indicates the presence of areas with low $\dot{V}_A/\dot{Q}$ ratios in the lungs.[8]

Although alveolar P_{N_2} varies as a function of the $\dot{V}_A/\dot{Q}$ ratio throughout the lungs, no net exchange of N_2 between gas and blood takes place because the body tissues are saturated with N_2 during breathing of atmospheric air. In areas where PA_{N_2} is high, N_2 passes from alveolar air to blood; where it is lower, N_2 passes from blood to air. The amounts exchanged in either direction are equal and no net exchange occurs. Since the (a-A) P_{N_2} difference depends on these local exchanges of N_2 in areas with different $\dot{V}_A/\dot{Q}$ ratios, it is not influenced by shunts; in these, blood bypasses the alveoli and its P_{N_2} cannot be altered by gas exchange.

Many clinical conditions lead to hypoventilation of certain portions of the lung, for instance, prolonged bedrest, accumulation of secretions after general anesthesia, and inadequate aeration of the newborn's lungs. Thus, a method for detecting the presence of lung areas with low $\dot{V}_A/\dot{Q}$ ratios is clinically important. Since all body fluids are in equilibrium with arterial blood, as far as N_2 exchange is concerned, it is not even necessary to determine the arterial P_{N_2}; analysis of a urine sample (collected anaerobically) is sufficient. With this method, Abernethy et al.[1] found that recumbency at night, in healthy persons, increases the urinary-alveolar $(U-A)_{N_2}$ pressure difference; it was much lower during the day. The average P_{N_2} difference, 3.7 mm Hg before lying down, increased significantly, to 8.7 mm Hg 1 hour after lying down.[1] Therefore, recumbency increased non-uniform $\dot{V}_A/\dot{Q}$ distribution with a preponderance of low $\dot{V}_A/\dot{Q}$ areas. Healthy newborns have a normal $(U-A)P_{N_2}$ difference less than 10 mm Hg, but gradients up to 39 mm Hg were measured in infants with pneumonia.[13] The principal difficulty with the method is technical: it is extremely difficult to measure small variations in N_2 partial pressures. When the $(a\text{-}A)_{N_2}$ difference is 30 mm Hg (a highly abnormal value), arterial or urinary P_{N_2} is about 600 mm Hg, and the alveolar P_{N_2} about 570 mm Hg. A 1 percent error in the P_{N_2} measurement introduces an uncertainty of 6 mm Hg, 20 percent of the a-A difference. The analytical requirements have so far limited this method to small-scale research studies. As collection and analytical methods improve, this potentially important technique may be applied routinely.

In summary, A-a partial pressure differences can be measured for O_2, CO_2, and N_2. The presence of an abnormally high $(A\text{-}a)P_{O_2}$ difference indicates an abnormally wide range of $\dot{V}_A/\dot{Q}$ ratios in the lungs, including contributions of diffusion limitation and venous admixture. An $(a\text{-}A)P_{CO_2}$ difference indicates the presence of areas with high $\dot{V}_A/\dot{Q}$ ratios (hyperventilated, underperfused areas), while an abnormally large $(a\text{-}A)P_{N_2}$ difference suggests the presence of areas with low $\dot{V}_A/\dot{Q}$ ratios (hypoventilated, overperfused areas).

PHYSIOLOGICAL DEAD SPACE

Chapter 3 discussed the anatomical dead space, the volume of the airways without gas exchange function. Another definition of dead space is the ventilated airway and lung volume which does not participate in gas exchange (p. 56), the physiological dead space. It includes the anatomical dead space and any alveolar spaces that are not perfused via the pulmonary circulation. Physiological dead space is determined from the Bohr equation (p. 43) by substituting measurements of O_2 or CO_2 for those of the inert gases discussed in Chapter 3. Rahn [17] gave a graphical solution for the Bohr equation which illustrates several of its problems (Fig. 5-8). For CO_2, Eq. (3) on p. 44 can be rewritten by substituting partial pressures, which are proportional to gas concentrations, and by introducing measurements from Figure 5-8 (for the alveolar gas point A and expired air point E)

$$\frac{V_D}{V_E} = \frac{F_A - F_E}{F_A} = \frac{P_A - P_E}{P_A} = \frac{AB - DB}{AB} = \frac{AD}{AB} \tag{1}$$

A similar solution for O_2 yields

$$\frac{V_D}{V_E} = \frac{AF}{AC} \tag{2}$$

Since $AF/AC = AD/AB$, the dead space for O_2 equals that for CO_2. This graphical solution of the Bohr equation is feasible because the composition of expired air, a mixture of alveolar air with inspired air retained in the dead space, must be somewhere between points A and I on the diagram (Fig. 5-8). The smaller the dead space, the more the expired air point, E, approaches A. The larger the dead space, the more inspired air is mixed with the alveolar air, and the closer E will be to the inspired point, I. Eqs. (1) and (2) reflect these relations quantitatively.

As with anatomical dead space, the crux of the problem is the validity of alveolar air samples. The classical method is to collect the air last expired, at

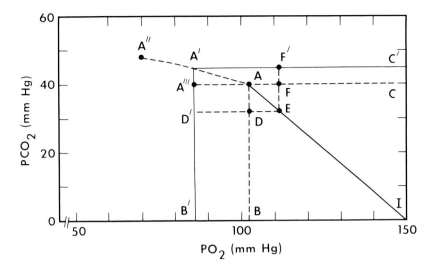

Fig. 5-8. Graphical solution of the Bohr equation in the O_2-CO_2 diagram (after Rahn[17]). See equations (1) and (2) in text. The true dead space for CO_2 is obtained from: $V_D/V_E = AD/AB = A''' D'/A''' B'$. The dead space for CO_2 obtained with the Haldane-Priestley method is given by: $V_D/V_E = A' D'/A' B'$, which is larger than $A'''D'/A'''B'$. Similarly, the dead space for O_2 is obtained from AF/AC which equals AD/AB. The Haldane-Priestley method yields a much larger value, indicated by $A'F'/A'C'$. See also text.

the end of a forced expiration (Haldane-Priestley method). However, no ventilation occurs during this forced expiration and hence alveolar gas composition changes as predicted from the breath-hold line in Figure 5-6. Depending on the depth and duration of expiration, the measured alveolar air composition might be that of point A' or A'' in Figure 5-8. Expired air, on the other hand, is collected independently during quiet breathing. Thus, with the Haldane-Priestley procedure one may find alveolar air at A' and expired air at E. Applying Eq. (1), one finds a dead space for CO_2 which equals $A'D'/A'B'$, and for O_2, $A'F'/A'C'$. This results in a larger dead space than would be obtained if the true alveolar gas composition during quiet breathing (point A) could be measured. $A'F'/A'C'$ is larger than $A'D'/A'B'$; hence one measures a larger dead space for O_2 than for CO_2, because A' deviates from the line AI, a consequence of the shape of the $\dot{V}_A/\dot{Q}$ line. Figure 5-8 can explain why Haldane's method gave large values for dead space. During exercise, the increased O_2 consumption would lead to a more rapid movement of point A along the breath-hold line, so that the error in determining alveolar gas composition increases. Thus, Haldane found that dead space increased greatly during exercise.[9] However, anatomical dead space only increases in proportion to end-tidal inspiratory volume, and Haldane's results during exercise do not allow conclusions about the size of the anatomical dead space (see also review of Haldane-Krogh controversy in reference 3). Early studies [10] suggested that the difference between O_2 and CO_2 dead space resulted from excretion of CO_2 in airways as well as in alveoli, while O_2 is taken up only in alveoli. There is no evidence for this; the difference between O_2 and CO_2

dead space with the Haldane method can be fully explained by changes in alveolar gas during prolonged expirations.

There is no satisfactory solution for the alveolar gas sampling problem. End-tidal samples eliminate the breath-holding effect of Figure 5-8 but include uncertainties related to timing and unequal distribution of $\dot{V}_A/\dot{Q}$ ratios; they are weighted in favor of relatively well-ventilated areas. Another weighting procedure is introduced if one collects arterial blood and uses its P_{CO_2} to represent alveolar P_{CO_2}. The assumption that there is no $(a-A)P_{CO_2}$ difference is not always valid (p. 90). Moreover, using the circulatory system as an averaging circuit means that the P_{CO_2} value is weighted in favor of lung areas with high perfusion rates. If blood flow is not uniform, high flow areas (such as the bases of the vertical lungs) contribute more to the arterial P_{CO_2} than low flow areas, such as the lung tops.

In healthy persons, anatomical and physiological dead space are nearly equal; that is, there are no ventilated, unperfused areas that can be measured with these methods. In lung disease, physiological dead space is often much larger than anatomical dead space, which suggests the presence of large ventilated but unperfused areas in the lungs. Some studies have shown that man's physiological V_D increases when he goes from the supine to the standing position; this is consistent with the development of underperfusion in the lung tops. The difference between physiological and anatomical dead space is called the alveolar dead space. This is the volume of a virtual space with a $\dot{V}_A/\dot{Q} = \infty$, which represents the effect of all gas-exchanging areas with a higher than average $\dot{V}_A/\dot{Q}$ ratio. The term indicates a non-gas-exchanging alveolar space. Like other dead space volumes, alveolar dead space is a virtual volume, since no sharp gas fronts separate inspired and alveolar gas (p. 49). In addition, even unperfused alveoli receive some CO_2 by inspiring gas from the common dead space. Calculations of alveolar dead space can be corrected for this rebreathing effect.[22] In practice, the importance of alveolar dead space is that it indicates an abnormally large degree of nonuniformity in $\dot{V}_A/\dot{Q}$ ratios throughout the lungs.

Physiological dead space [using arterial P_{CO_2} in Eq. (1)] increases with end-tidal inspiratory lung volume to an extent comparable to anatomical V_D. It also increases with tidal volume and breathing rate and is largest when both are high. In older persons, physiological dead space may range up to 350 ml at normal tidal volumes and breathing rates.[14]

VENOUS ADMIXTURE

The concepts of venous admixture and physiological dead space are used in a comprehensive model of alveolar gas exchange developed by Riley.[20, 21] Rather than describing gas exchange in terms of a continuous distribution of $\dot{V}_A/\dot{Q}$ ratios, it treats alveolar gas and arterial blood composition as the net result of (1) gas exchange in alveoli with a normal or ideal alveolar air composition; (2) dead space ventilation; and (3) venous admixture. The latter is the virtual amount of venous blood that, if admixed with blood oxygenated to complete equilibrium with ideal alveolar air, would account for the actual gas pressures in arterial blood. Thus, venous admixture is a concept similar to that of dead space. Apart from the venous blood contributed by direct shunts to the arterial side of the systemic circulation, and by venoarterial shunts in the pulmonary circulation, venous admixture reflects the distribution of $\dot{V}_A/\dot{Q}$ ratios. It is as if arterial blood were a mixture of blood in equilibrium with alveolar air at the average $\dot{V}_A/\dot{Q}$ ratio, and blood coming from shunts or lung areas where $\dot{V}_A/\dot{Q}$ is zero. For clinical applications, therefore, nonuniform distribution of $\dot{V}_A$ and $\dot{Q}$ can be expressed in two simple numbers—dead space and venous admixture.

CLINICAL APPLICATIONS

Many lung diseases lead to nonuniform distribution of $\dot{V}_A/\dot{Q}$ ratios in the lungs. Areas with obstructed airways have diminished alveolar ventilation but may still have a normal pulmonary blood flow; their $\dot{V}_A/\dot{Q}$ ratio is low. Areas with obstructed blood vessels have diminished perfusion but their alveolar ventilation may be normal; their $\dot{V}_A/\dot{Q}$ ratio is high. Whenever one lung area has a $\dot{V}_A/\dot{Q}$ higher than the average, another area must have a lower than average $\dot{V}_A/\dot{Q}$ ratio. Hence, areas with high and low $\dot{V}_A/\dot{Q}$ ratios coexist in the same diseased lung, as well as in the healthy vertical lung (p. 88). The resulting wide dispersion of $\dot{V}_A/\dot{Q}$ ratios can be recognized by measuring A-a partial-pressure differences, physiological dead space, and venous admixture. Many clinical studies using these methods have shown that nonuniform distribution of ventilation and perfusion is the main cause of arterial hypoxia and hypercapnia in lung diseases. In obstructive lung disease, nonuniform $\dot{V}_A/\dot{Q}$ ratios may increase even when ventilatory tests show relatively little abnormality. For instance, a recent study of hemp workers with byssinosis showed a marked decrease in arterial P_{O_2} during dust exposure that caused only a small decrease in $FEV_{1.0}$[15] (see also Chap. 17). Theoretical and technical problems associated with measuring alveolar gas tensions in steady-state conditions limit the clinical use of A-a partial pressure differences. Furthermore, little specific diagnostic information is derived from knowing the distribution of $\dot{V}_A/\dot{Q}$ ratios. Since arterial puncture is needed, the methods are not suitable for routine use in the early detection of functional abnormalities in lung disease. For the clinical management of patients with ventilatory failure, it is essential to know the causes (e.g., airway obstruction) and effects (hypoxemia, hypercapnia) of gas exchange disturbances. Although detailed studies of $\dot{V}_A/\dot{Q}$ distribution increase understanding of the disease process, they are usually not required for decisions on treatment.

SUMMARY

The exchange of O_2 and CO_2 in the lungs is determined by the ratio between alveolar ventilation $(\dot{V}_A)$ and pulmonary blood flow $(\dot{Q})$, by the gas tensions in inspired air and in mixed venous blood, and by chemical binding processes in blood. Since the latter do not occur with inert gases, their exchange illustrates the fundamental relations between $\dot{V}_A/\dot{Q}$ ratios and lung gas exchange without the complexities introduced by chemical binding of O_2 and CO_2.

The composition of alveolar gas varies throughout the lungs and during the breathing cycle and is markedly altered during breath holding and forced-breathing maneuvers. These variations occur as a function of the $\dot{V}_A/\dot{Q}$ ratio and can be illustrated graphically with gas and blood R lines, isoventilation ($\dot{V}_A/\dot{V}_{O_2}$ and $\dot{V}_A/\dot{V}_{CO_2}$) lines, and the $\dot{V}_A/\dot{Q}$ line in O_2-CO_2 diagrams.

The O_2 and CO_2 partial pressures in arterial blood are largely determined by the distribution of $\dot{V}_A/\dot{Q}$ ratios in the lungs, which can be assessed by measuring alveolar-arterial partial-pressure differences, physiological dead space, and venous admixture. An alveolar dead space and an (a-A)P_{CO_2} difference indicate areas with abnormally high $\dot{V}_A/\dot{Q}$ ratios. An abnormally large (a-A) or (U-A) (urinary-alveolar) P_{N_2} difference suggests the presence of areas with low $\dot{V}_A/\dot{Q}$ areas. Venous admixture includes the effects of low $\dot{V}_A/\dot{Q}$ areas and of lung blood flow shunts. The concepts and measurements discussed in this chapter have clinical applications in disorders of gas exchange (hypoventilation, hyperventilation, airway obstruction, pulmonary embolism) and in the interpretation of arterial blood gas data.

REFERENCES

1. Abernethy JD, Maurizi JJ, Farhi LE: Diurnal variations in urinary-alveolar N_2 difference and effects of recumbency. J Appl Physiol 23:875–879, 1967
2. Bouhuys A: Pneumotachography. Thesis, University of Amsterdam, (Assen, The Netherlands, Van Gorcum & Co.), 1956
3. Bouhuys A: Respiratory dead space, in Fenn WO, Rahn H (eds): Handbook of Physiology, Section 3: Respiration, vol I. Washington, D.C., American Physiological Society, 1964, pp 699–714
4. DuBois AB: Alveolar CO_2 and O_2 during breath holding, expiration, and inspiration. J Appl Physiol 5:1–12, 1952
5. DuBois AB, Fenn WO, Britt AG: CO_2 dissociation curve of lung tissue. J Appl Physiol 5:13–16, 1952
6. Farhi LE: Elimination of inert gas by the lung. Respir Physiol 3:1–11, 1967
7. Farhi LE, Yokoyama T: Effects of ventilation-perfusion inequality on elimination of inert gases. Respir Physiol 3:12–20, 1967
8. Farhi LE: Ventilation-perfusion relationship and its role in alveolar gas exchange, in Caro CG (ed): Advances in Respiratory Physiology. Baltimore, Williams & Wilkins, 1966, pp 148–197
9. Haldane JS: The variations in the effective dead space in breathing. Am J Physiol 38:20–28, 1915
10. Henderson Y, Chillingworth FP, Whit-ney JL: The respiratory dead space. Am J Physiol 38:1–19, 1915
11. Jöbsis FF: Basic processes in cellular respiration, in Fenn WO, Rahn H (eds): Handbook of Physiology, Section 3: Respiration, vol I. Washington D.C., American Physiological Society, 1964, pp 63–124
12. Knelson JH, Howatt WF, DeMuth GR: Effect of respiratory pattern on alveolar gas exchange. J Appl Physiol 29:328–331, 1970
13. Krauss AN, Soodalter JA, Auld PAM: Adjustment of ventilation and perfusion in the full-term normal and distressed neonate as determined by urinary alveolar nitrogen gradients. Pediatrics 47:865–869, 1971
14. Lifshay A, Fast CW, Glazier JB: Effects of changes in respiratory pattern on physiological dead space. J Appl Physiol 31:478–483, 1971
15. Lopez Merino V, Llopis Lombart R, Flores Marco R, Barbero Carnicero A, Gomez Guillen F, Bouhuys A: Arterial blood gas tensions and lung function during acute responses to hemp dust. Am Rev Respir Dis 107:809–815, 1973
16. Nye RE: Influence of the cyclical pattern of ventilatory flow on pulmonary gas exchange. Respir Physiol 10:321–337, 1970
17. Rahn H: A concept of mean alveolar

air and the ventilation-bloodflow relationships during pulmonary gas exchange. Am J Physiol 158:21–30, 1949

18. Rahn H, Fenn WO: A graphical analysis of the respiratory gas exchange; the O_2–CO_2 diagram. Washington D.C. American Physiological Society, 1955

19. Rahn H, Farhi LE: Ventilation, perfusion, and gas exchange—the $\dot{V}_A/\dot{Q}$ concept, in Fenn WO, Rahn H (eds): Handbook of Physiology, Section 3: Respiration, vol I. Washington, D.C., American Physiological Society, 1964, pp 735–766

20. Riley RL, Cournand A: "Ideal" alveolar air and the analysis of ventilation-perfusion relationships in the lungs. J Appl Physiol 1:825–847, 1949

21. Riley RL: Pulmonary gas exchange. Am J Med 10:210–220, 1951

22. Ross BB, Farhi LE: Dead-space ventilation as a determinant in the ventilation-perfusion concept. J Appl Physiol 15: 363–371, 1960

23. West JB: Regional differences in gas exchange in the lung of erect man. J Appl Physiol 17:893–898, 1962

24. West JB: Ventilation, Blood Flow and Gas Exchange, ed 2. Philadelphia, FA Davis Co, 1970

Chapter 6

Oxygen Transport Mechanisms

Oxygen is transported from points of higher to points of lower partial pressure. Figure 6-1 indicates its pathways from inspired to alveolar air, via the alveolocapillary membrane to arterial blood, and on to tissues and venous blood. From the atmosphere to the alveoli, and again from the lung capillaries to the tissue capillaries, O_2 is transported largely by bulk flow. Transport by diffusion occurs within the alveolar gas (p. 64), between alveolar gas and lung capillaries, and from peripheral capillaries into the tissues and the cells. Transport between air, blood, and tissue occurs via membranes, and therefore diffusivity (a constant depending on molecular weight) and solubility in membrane media determine the transport rates. O_2 never moves against the direction of partial-pressure gradients, and no active transport mechanisms are involved. Thus, O_2 exchange is governed by physical laws of diffusion and gas solubility. The application of these laws, however, is complicated by the thickness and heterogeneity of the membranes, the varying lengths of the diffusion pathways, and the nonlinear characteristics of the chemical binding process of O_2 in red blood cells.

The transport of CO_2 in blood involves physical solution and chemical binding as bicarbonate and to hemoglobin (carbamino reaction).[27, 55] CO_2 transport is closely linked with the processes that maintain the body's acid-base balance. The lungs are the major organ of CO_2 excretion, the rate of which is largely determined by the rate of alveolar ventilation. Passage from mixed venous blood to alveolar air decreases P_{CO_2} by only about 6 mm Hg; the major pressure drop is from alveolar to inspired air (Fig. 6-1). The relation between $\dot{V}_A$ and PA_{CO_2} has been discussed in Chapter 5. Deficient CO_2 elimination is nearly always a consequence of inadequate alveolar ventilation or of nonuniform $\dot{V}_A/\dot{Q}$ ratios, in particular of series ventilation [60] (p. 67). Alveolocapillary diffusion does not limit CO_2 transport. In contrast, O_2 transport can be impeded at several sites in the transport pathways and by diverse mechanisms. These factors are discussed in this chapter.

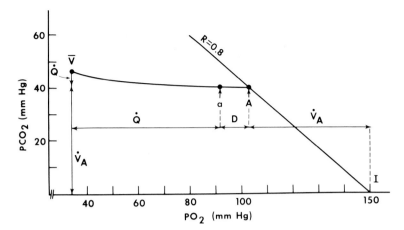

Fig. 6-1. The O_2-CO_2 diagram illustrates the relative importance of alveolar ventilation and lung blood flow for the transport of O_2 and CO_2. From the inspired point *I*, P_{O_2} decreases to its value at *A* by mixing of inspired and alveolar gas and further to a, owing to the (A-a) P_{O_2} difference. The largest P_{O_2} drop is from *a* to $\overline{V}$. Thus blood flow, $\dot{Q}$, accounts for the largest part of the decrease of P_{O_2} from *I* to $\overline{V}$. In contrast, P_{CO_2} drops only a few millimeters from $\overline{V}$ to *A*; CO_2 elimination is largely effected by alveolar ventilation $\dot{V}_A$. The relative importance of alveolar ventilation, diffusion, and cardiac output for gas transport is indicated by the relative lengths of the horizontal arrows labeled $\dot{V}_A$, *D*, and $\dot{Q}$ for O_2, and of the vertical arrows $\dot{V}_A$ and $\dot{Q}$ for CO_2.

GAS DIFFUSION IN THE LUNGS

The Alveolocapillary Diffusion Barrier

Oxygen must pass several layers of heterogeneous material on its path from alveolar gas to the interior of the red blood cell (Fig. 6-2). The length of this diffusion path varies from less than 0.5 μm to more than 2 μm. The membrane

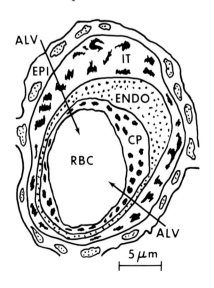

Fig. 6-2. Schematic drawing of diffusion pathway from alveolar air (ALV) to interior of red cells (RBC), via alveolar epithelium (EPI), interstitial tissue (IT), capillary endothelium (ENDO), and plasma in capillary (CP). Modified from reference 24.

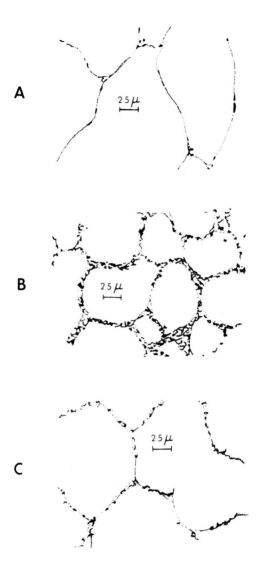

Fig. 6-3. 2-μm thick lung sections from greyhound dogs, prepared after freezing isolated lungs under different conditions. *A*. Top of a lung frozen in vertical position. Only a fraction of the alveolocapillary membrane is active in gas exchange because capillary blood flow is minimal (inflation pressure = 10 cm H_2O). *B*. Lower down in a lung prepared similarly. More capillaries are perfused, and most of the membrane is in contact with red blood cells (inflation pressure = 10 cm H_2O). *C*. Same preparation and location as in *B*, but with inflation pressure raised to 25 cm H_2O. This decreases blood flow and therefore the membrane surface area available for gas exchange. Drawn from micrographs of Glazier et al.[28]

surface area available for diffusion is limited by the total epithelial surface of the alveoli. However, often only a portion of the membrane functions in gas exchange (Fig. 6-3). When perfusion pressure is low, as in the top of the vertical lung (Fig. 6-3A), or when lung capillary blood volume is decreased by high inflation pressures (Fig. 6-3C), only a small fraction of the membrane is in contact with red blood cells in the capillaries.[28] With higher perfusion pressure, lower inflation pressure, or both, more capillaries are filled with red cells and most of the membrane surface area can then be active in gas exchange (Fig. 6-3B).

Diffusion Coefficient and Diffusion Capacity

The partial-pressure difference between points on either side of the interface between alveolar gas and capillary blood can be measured indirectly. However, the length of the diffusion pathway and the surface area of the diffusion membrane cannot be measured in the intact lung. Hence, the *diffusion coefficient* (a physical constant—the amount of gas transported per unit time, per unit surface area, per unit partial-pressure gradient along the diffusion pathway) cannot be determined. Since the diffusion characteristics of individual wall components (membranes, cytoplasm, cell nuclei) vary considerably, no useful assumptions can be made about the average diffusion properties of the total pathway.

Nevertheless, the overall diffusion characteristics of the interface can be assessed from the *diffusion capacity* of the lungs (D_L). In a small fraction, i, of the interface, the amount of gas transferred, $\dot{V}$, equals

$$\dot{V} = \frac{d_i \times s_i}{l_i} \tag{1}$$

where d_i is the diffusion coefficient of the interface, s_i is its surface area, and l_i is its length. $\dot{V}$ is the rate of gas transfer per unit time and per unit A-a partial-pressure difference. By adding transfer rates in all parts of the interface, one obtains the overall transfer rate, or diffusion capacity

$$D_L = \sum \frac{d_i \times s_i}{l_i} \tag{2}$$

where i has values from 1 to n, the total number of diffusion pathways. D_L can be calculated from the total rate of transfer, V, of CO or O_2 and its A-a partial-pressure difference

$$D_L = \frac{\dot{V}_{(CO,O_2)}}{PA_{(CO,O_2)} - P\bar{c}_{(CO,O_2)}} \tag{3}$$

where PA and P$\bar{c}$ are the alveolar and the mean capillary partial pressures of O_2 or CO. As an expression of overall gas transfer, D_L is determined by several unknowns including the diffusion coefficient, the membrane's surface area, the length of the diffusion pathway, and gas solubility in the membrane substance. D_L is expressed in units of ml gas STPD/min/mm Hg (see footnote, p. 84).

D_L and $\dot{V}_A/\dot{Q}$ Distribution

Figure 6-3 suggests that $D_{L_{O_2}}$ may depend more on the extent of contact between alveolar gas and red blood cells than on the inherent properties of the alveolocapillary membrane. Obviously, no gas transfer takes place in areas where either $\dot{V}_A$ or $\dot{Q}$ is zero. The discussion in Chapter 5 showed that gas transfer is optimal in terms of total gas and blood flow when local $\dot{V}_A/\dot{Q}$ ratios do not differ much from the average value for the lungs as a whole (p. 89). In high $\dot{V}_A/\dot{Q}$ areas, ventilation is wasted; in low $\dot{V}_A/\dot{Q}$ areas, perfusion is wasted and little or no O_2 is transferred in spite of an intact transfer surface. These areas are, in effect, lost in the calculation of D_L, with a resultant decrease in D_L for the lungs as a whole.

The effect of nonuniform $\dot{V}_A/\dot{Q}$ ratios on D_L depends on whether O_2 or CO is used for its measurement. When blood flows slowly in a lung region, little O_2 is taken up since its transfer is negligible once all hemoglobin is saturated. Hence, high $\dot{V}_A/\dot{Q}$ areas decrease $D_{L_{O_2}}$. This effect is minimal with the CO breath-holding method, since CO is used in small quantities and capillary Hb is not saturated even when blood flow stagnates. Both $D_{L_{O_2}}$ and $D_{L_{CO}}$ are affected by uneven distribution of inspired gas; in poorly ventilated units, gas transfer is limited by ventilation and not diffusion. When D_L is measured during tidal breathing (steady-state method), uneven distribution of inspired gas affects the result; in poorly ventilated units gas transfer is limited by ventilation and not by diffusion. This effect is less with the single-breath or rebreathing techniques (see below), which can be used for approximate prediction of diffusion limitations during exercise.[31, 43]

Thus, a low value of D_L does not necessarily indicate a defect in the alveolocapillary diffusion of gases. With complex graphical techniques, one can distinguish some patients in whom diffusion disturbances are more important than $\dot{V}_A/\dot{Q}$ ratio nonuniformity,[1] but in many instances a low D_L indicates primarily that gas and blood do not meet efficiently.[21, 29]

Rationale for D_L Measurements

The validity of D_L as a lung function test has been questioned.[8] If diffusion capacity does not measure diffusion, why measure it at all? However, D_L is valuable as a measure of overall transport between inspired gas and arterial blood, a fact better reflected by the term transfer factor T_L[13] than by diffusion capacity. A low D_L value often indicates lung disease, and D_L may be decreased in conditions where other test results are normal. For instance, a low D_L is often an early sign of asbestosis (Chap. 15) when lung volumes still remain normal. In patients treated with bleomycin (an anticancer agent), D_L may decrease before lung volumes change.[48] In other cases, slight degrees of interstitial lung edema may decrease diffusion capacity while leaving other function tests unchanged.[1] Therefore, decreased D_L values frequently have clinical significance. Convenient and reproducible test techniques, in particular the single-breath method for $D_{L_{CO}}$, provide objective data about gas transfer without arterial puncture.

Measurement of D_L

To solve Eq. (3), one needs to measure (1) the uptake of a gas from inspired gas into blood, and, simultaneously, (2) the partial-pressure difference between alveolar gas and capillary blood for the same gas. This is feasible for only two gases—O_2 and CO; in practice, the latter is now used almost exclusively.

DIFFUSION CAPACITY FOR O_2

Measurement of D_L for O_2 is too complex to be practical. O_2 uptake can be measured by collecting and analyzing expired gas, and the alveolar P_{O_2} can be determined, subject to the uncertainties discussed in Chapter 5. However, the mean capillary partial pressure of O_2 is difficult to measure. In normal persons, a measurable alveolocapillary gradient at the end of the capillary exists only when the subject breathes a hypoxic gas mixture. The arterial P_{O_2} does not equal $P\bar{c}_{O_2}$ in Eq. (3) because of contribution of venoarterial shunts. In addition, the P_{O_2} of blood passing through pulmonary capillaries does not increase in proportion to the distance along the path of contact with alveolar gas. The mean capillary O_2 tension ($P\bar{c}_{O_2}$) must be calculated by a complex integration procedure. The interpretation of D_L values is complex regardless of the gas used. For these reasons, simpler techniques such as the CO method are preferable.

DIFFUSION CAPACITY FOR CO

This measurement is based on the high affinity of hemoglobin for binding with carbon monoxide. When one briefly breathes a gas with small amounts of CO, all CO taken up in blood is mopped up by Hb. The value of $P\bar{c}_{O_2}$ [Eq. (3)] remains so near zero that it can be neglected for practical purposes, and only alveolar CO pressure must be measured. The amount of CO inhaled during a single test is insignificant in terms of CO toxicity. D_L for CO can be measured with different procedures.[24, 25] The single-breath or breath-holding method ($D_{L_{CO}}$ SB) is most practical for measurements at rest; either the breath-holding or the steady-state method ($D_{L_{CO}}$ SS) may be used for exercise studies.

Single-breath method ($D_{L_{CO}}$ SB). The test gas for this method commonly consists of 0.2%–0.3% CO, 21% O_2, and a suitable amount of helium (He) or neon (Ne), with N_2 as the balance. After a single inspiration of this gas mixture, from residual volume to TLC, the subject holds his breath for approximately 10 seconds. Then he expires rapidly, and a sample of expired air collected after at least 1000 ml of expiration is analyzed. This sample contains less CO and less He or Ne than the inspired mixture. The inert gas concentration drops because the inspirate is diluted with alveolar gas. If CO were not taken up in blood, its concentration would decrease by the same factor as the inert gas concentration. In fact, PA_{CO} is lower than that; the excess CO which disappeared is the amount taken up in blood. The inspired gas mixture may not be distributed evenly in the lungs, and this affects CO concentrations to the same degree as the He or Ne concentrations one measures By calculating the alveolar CO pressure from the dilution of He or Ne, one corrects PA_{CO} for nonuniform gas distribution. Since the breath-holding time is much longer than the duration of a quiet inspiration, the inspired gas has time to mix, by diffusion, even into spaces where it would barely penetrate during quiet breathing. Consequently, the value for $D_{L_{CO}}$ SB may overestimate gas transfer during quiet breathing. Another factor that works in this direction is that the breath is held at close to maximum inspiratory lung volume. Hence, $D_{L_{CO}}$ SB reflects the surface area of the gas-exchanging membrane available at that volume; the surface area at lung volumes near FRC may be considerably smaller.[43] Both factors may explain, in part, why the single-breath methods yield higher values in healthy people than the steady-state method (which uses the spontaneous breathing pattern at lung volumes near FRC).

$D_{L_{CO}}$ depends on the inspired O_2 concentration. O_2 and CO compete for binding with hemoglobin, with the odds increasingly favorable to O_2 the higher its partial pressure. Hence, the higher the PA_{O_2}, the less CO is taken up and the lower the $D_{L_{CO}}$. This relation is used in partitioning D_L (see below).

Rebreathing method.[35, 42]   This method is similar to the previous one but eliminates the need for breath holding and is technically more complex. In one version, the subject rebreathes a mixture containing CO, neon, acetylene, and O_2.[38] Successive expired gas samples are collected automatically.[37] The expirates are analyzed in a gas chromatograph (Fig. 6-4) and reflect (1) dilution of inspired gas in alveolar gas, measured from the dilution of Ne; (2) diffusion of CO; (3) disappearance of a soluble gas, acetylene, which is used to measure cardiac output. Disappearance curves during rebreathing are plotted for each of the three tracer gases, and this allows calculation of $D_{L_{CO}}$ and cardiac output.

Steady-state method ($D_{L_{CO}}$ SS).   With this method, CO uptake is measured during spontaneous breathing, at rest, or during exercise. The subject breathes a CO-air mixture (e.g., 0.1 percent CO) during several minutes.* When a steady state has been reached, expired gas is collected for CO uptake measurement, and PA_{CO} is determined simultaneously. End-tidal sampling gives satisfactory PA_{CO} data in healthy persons, but not in patients with nonuniform gas distribution or in patients who breathe rapidly with small tidal volumes. In these patients PA_{CO} can be estimated with the Bohr equation (p. 43), using arterial P_{CO_2} values to calculate the physiological dead space. This method [19] can be applied in most patients but does not solve the distribution problem. Physiological dead space is large when distribution is nonuniform (p. 94); the Bohr equation thus leads to a spuriously high PA_{CO} value and a too low D_L [Eq. (1)]. Regardless of the methods, therefore, $D_{L_{CO}}$ SS is low whenever the lungs are ventilated nonuniformly. Small degrees of nonuniformity, as after administering small doses of histamine aerosol to healthy subjects,[10] are enough to decrease $D_{L_{CO}}$ SS. Since the single-breath or rebreathing methods are less influenced by nonuniform distribution of inspired gas, they are preferred. The steady-state method requires corrections for back pressure of CO in blood, because the subject takes up much more CO than with the single-breath method. This correction is always necessary in smokers (Chap. 14).

---

* A protocol recommended for exercise studies includes the sequence: 0–2 min— exercise while breathing room air; 2–4 min—continue exercise; switch to 0.1 percent CO in inspired air; 4–7 min—collect expired gas; 5–6 min—collect arterial blood. (Unpublished committee report on standards of common measurements of lung function in interstitial lung disease for use in SCOR grant programs, National Heart and Lung Institute, 1972.)

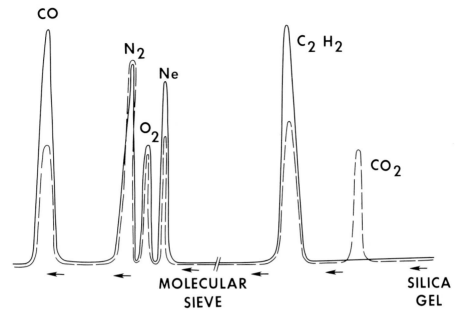

Fig. 6-4. Gas chromatographic analysis of inspired gas (*solid line*) and expired alveolar gas (*dashed line*) for determination of $D_{L_{CO}}$, lung volume, and $\dot{Q}$ with rebreathing method (see text). Composition of inspired gas = 0.5% CO, 0.5% C_2H_2, 0.5% Ne, balance air. The gas passes through a silica gel and a molecular sieve column. The decrease in C_2H_2 concentration in expired gas reflects its absorption into blood and is used for calculation of Q. The decrease in Ne % in expired gas reflects dilution of alveolar with inspired gas and is used to calculate lung volume and alveolar P_{CO} [for use in Eq. (3)]. The relative decrease of alveolar CO concentration is much larger than that of the Ne concentration, reflecting CO uptake in blood. The inspired and expired P_{CO} values are used to calculate CO uptake [$\dot{V}_{CO}$ in (Eq. 3)]. Curves recorded by A.C. DeGraff and P. Snyder, Yale University Lung Research Center.

PARTITIONING OF D_L

Diffusion is a gas flow per unit pressure difference; hence, D_L is a conductance and its reciprocal, $1/D_L$, is a resistance. Using electric circuit theory, one might say there are several resistance elements in series which together make up the total resistance, $1/D_L$, of the diffusion barrier between gas and the red cell interior (alveolar gas; alveolar and capillary endothelial cells and their basement membranes and interstitial spaces; blood plasma in the capillaries; and red cells). Of these elements, the resistance of the red cell can be measured separately, with red cells in a well-stirred fluid. The resistance depends largely on the time required for O_2 or CO to bind with Hb. The total conductance of the red cells in lung capillaries equals θ, the rate of gas uptake per milliliter of blood, measured in vitro, times the blood volume in gas-exchanging capillaries, Vc. The resistance of this part of the diffusion pathway is $1/\theta Vc$. The sum of all resistances equals $1/D_L$. Thus, D_L can be partitioned into two conductances [56] according to

$$1/D_L = 1/D_M + 1/\theta Vc \qquad (2)$$

where D_M is the diffusion capacity of all parts of the pathway between the alveolar gas and the wall of the red cell. Since it includes diffusion through the plasma layer, the term membrane diffusion capacity for D_M should not be taken literally.

Eq. (2) contains three unknowns. θ can be measured in vitro, which leaves two unknowns. A solution is feasible because the higher the PA_{O_2}, the lower the $D_{L_{CO}}$ (p. 104). Determination of $D_{L_{CO}}$ at a normal and at a high inspired P_{O_2} yields two values for D_L that can be substituted in Eq. (2). If one knows θ at the same alveolar P_{O_2} values, D_M and Vc can be calculated. Normal values for D_M average about 57 ml/min/mm Hg; Vc is about 90 to 110 ml. In disease, D_M and Vc usually change in the same direction, and therefore partitioning of D_L does not yield much additional clinical information. Also, it is not certain that values for θ measured in vitro apply in vivo: gas exchange conditions for red cells in narrow capillaries may differ from those for red cells suspended in dilute solutions in vitro.

Physiological Variables That Affect D_L

In healthy persons, D_L increases with height, decreases with age, and is larger in men than in women. A comprehensive review of normal values in healthy men and women is available.[14] D_L SB increases with lung volume. Posture also affects D_L, probably chiefly because it changes regional perfusion. For instance, D_L is smaller in the sitting position (in which the lung tops receive little perfusion) than in the supine. During exercise, many factors increase D_L—increased cardiac output, increased capillary volume, and flow redistribution with opening of previously unperfused capillaries. Athletes commonly have a large D_L, probably because of a combination of age, physique, selection, and training. A high D_L seems to be one determinant of athletic prowess.

Newcomers to high-altitude areas do not experience increases in D_L;[34] even a 6-week stay at 3100 meters (Leadville, Col.) did not induce increases of D_L in sea-level residents.[15] However, highlanders (natives and long-term residents at high altitudes) have significantly higher values for D_L, D_M, and Vc than sea-level residents.[15, 54] Their TLC is also larger than expected. Increased lung size and increased D_L may be adaptive responses under the stress of long-term altitude hypoxia. Yet, these findings may also be explained by selection—persons with small lungs or low diffusion capacities, or both, may not tolerate high-altitude residence and move away. The older Leadville natives had well-preserved D_L values, which again may represent adaptation or merely selection of the fittest.

Clinical Significance of D_L Measurements [26]

A low D_L value indicates a decreased gas transport capacity of the lungs. This may be a consequence of (1) small lungs or lesions that decrease the amount of functioning lung tissue, e.g., pneumonectomy; (2) obstructive lung disease leading to nonuniform $\dot{V}_A/\dot{Q}$ distribution; (3) interstitial lung disease with decreased ventilation, perfusion, and diffusion in many areas; or (4) emphysema with a decrease of gas-exchanging surface area. The test result does not discriminate within this group of varied lung lesions. Lung disease affects different components of alveolar walls, e.g., by thickening of basement membranes, by accumulation of water or fibrous tissue in the interstitial space, or by hyperplasia of type II alveolar cells. All of these can contribute to low D_L values. A normal D_L value, on the other hand, is strong evidence against major degrees of alveolar destruction and hence practically rules out emphysema. However, obstructive airway disease and emphysema often coexist; thus a low D_L value often reflects obstruction (with nonuniform $\dot{V}_A/\dot{Q}$ ratio distribution) as well as emphysematous alveolar tissue destruction.

In interstitial lung disease, including sarcoidosis, asbestosis, silicosis, beryllium lung disease, and other forms of disseminated granulomatous or fibrous disease, D_L is a rough guide to the extent of parenchymal involvement. Decreased diffusion surface area, abnormal $\dot{V}_A/\dot{Q}$ distribution, and, perhaps to some degree, thickening of the alveolocapillary diffusion barrier, all contribute to a reduced D_L in these diseases. In some instances, D_L decreases while other tests remain normal (e.g., early asbestosis; p. 355). In the management of patients with interstitial lung disease, measurements of D_L at regular intervals can help assess the effectiveness of therapy.

OXYGEN TRANSPORT IN BLOOD

Oxygen is carried in blood and is dissolved in plasma as well as bound to hemoglobin (Hb). The amount dissolved is small but crucial for the transfer of O_2 between air and Hb and between Hb and tissues. The O_2 carried "in bulk" within the red cells is bound to the iron atom of Hb. The capacity of Hb to bind with oxygen and unload it depends on a minute change in the radius of its iron atom, which occurs when O_2 is bound or given off, and which leads to changes in the stereochemical structure of Hb.[50-52] The relation between the structure of Hb and its physiological function is now largely understood. However, the red cell is more than a simple package of Hb since other chemical processes within the red cell affect their oxygen-carrying function.

Oxygen-Binding Pigments

In the human body, only Hb and myoglobin (Mb) play a role. Each consists of an iron-porphyrin compound (heme) and a protein. Each Fe atom in heme binds one O_2 molecule. If the reaction were a simple one between two molecules, the law of mass action predicts that the relation between the O_2 pressure and the degree of oxygenation (the dissociation curve) would be a hyperbola. This is true for Mb but not for Hb (Fig. 6-5). The Mb molecule has one heme group; its reaction with O_2 is bimolecular. The dissociation curve for Hb is not as simple; its explanation has required many years of research, reviewed by Barcroft in 1928,[4] by Roughton in 1964,[55] and most recently by Perutz.[50-52]

Hb Oxygenation

The molecular weight of Hb is 64,500. Its protein (globin) consists of two α chains (with 141 amino acids) and two β chains (146 amino acids each). Portions of each chain are coiled up in α-helical forms. Together, the peptide chains

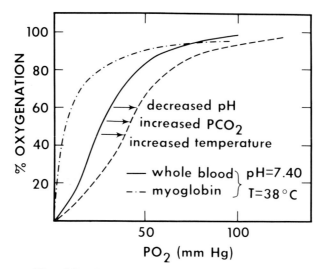

Fig. 6-5. O_2 dissociation curves for Hb and Mb. *Ordinate.* Percentage oxygenation (100% = full saturation of Hb or Mb with O_2). *Drawn line.* Typical curve for blood with normal Hb (HbA) under physiological conditions. Arrows indicate direction of change in position of curve as a function of pH, P_{CO_2}, and temperature. See also text. Modified from reference 55.

form a tetrahedral molecule (tetramer) in which the four subunits are held together by bonds between positive and negative ions (salt bridges, hydrogen bonds, and van der Waals forces). Each polypeptide chain is folded to form a pocket on the surface of Hb, in which the heme group fits, easily accessible to O_2 from outside. The position of the heme groups in such pockets explains why the volume of the Hb molecule does not increase when O_2 is bound to it.[18] The Fe atom is bound to a nearby site on the globin chain as well as to heme. When O_2 binds to the Fe atom, the small change in the radius of the Fe atom leads to a slight movement of the helical chains. These changes are associated with (1) changes in the position of peptide chains near the heme pocket and (2) disruption of the salt bridges between the chains and weakening of the bonding between the molecule's four subunits. Consequently, the quaternary structure of the molecule is changed considerably by slight displacements and rotations of amino acid groups near the heme pockets, because of oxygenation of one residue.

The four heme groups in Hb bind O_2 successively rather than simultaneously. Oxygenation of the first two or three heme groups of the tetramer leads to conformational changes about the heme pockets in the remaining chains and to disruption of the salt bridges between the molecule's four subunits. This increases the O_2 affinity of the chains with unoxygenated hemes. The shape of the dissociation curve reflects these successive binding reactions. O_2 binding to the first α chain is a bimolecular reaction.[57] After the first heme group is oxygenated, the O_2 affinity of the others increases and the dissociation curve slopes steeply upward. When three out of four heme groups have bound O_2, the rest of the binding process is again a bimolecular reaction. Therefore, the top parts of the dissociation curves of Mb and of Hb (if

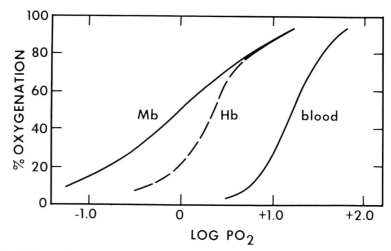

Fig. 6-6. Dissociation curves of myoglobin (Mb), stripped hemoglobin (Hb), and whole blood; P_{O_2} on log scale. After Benesch and Benesch.[6]

the effect of organic phosphate is removed; see below) coincide (Fig. 6-6).[6] The effect of oxygenation of one heme group on the O_2 affinity of the others, called *heme-heme interaction*,[52] ensures that, once the Hb molecule begins to unload O_2 in the tissues, the process proceeds rapidly because removing one O_2 molecule facilitates its unloading from the other three.

Bohr Effect

The Bohr effect also ensures adequate O_2 delivery to the tissues. Lowering the pH decreases the affinity of Hb for O_2, which promotes unloading of O_2 in the tissues, a consequence of binding of H^+ ions in the salt bridges that keep the Hb molecule in the deoxy strands.[52] At a lower pH, these do not split apart as easily, making O_2 binding more difficult. The binding of H^+ ions to the salt bridges also increases the capacity of Hb to bind CO_2. Hence, deoxygenated Hb binds more CO_2 than HbO_2 (Haldane effect). The Bohr and Haldane effects, which facilitate gas exchange in tissues, therefore depend on similar changes in the Hb molecule. In terms of the dissociation curve, a lower pH causes a shift to the right (Fig. 6-5). This is a graphical expression of the decreased O_2 affinity—at similar O_2 pressures, a smaller percentage of Hb is bound to oxygen.

2, 3-Diphosphoglycerate (2,3-DPG)

Although pH, P_{CO_2}, and temperature affect the affinity of Hb for O_2, these variables are close to constant in healthy persons. Therefore, a standard dissociation curve [16] has been widely used to study O_2 transport. But recent evidence suggests that metabolic mechanisms control O_2 binding. Changes in the O_2 affinity of Hb are important in several conditions, and standard Hb dissociation curves are not suitable to deal with these.

Organic phosphates in red cells, in particular 2,3-DPG, profoundly affect the Hb dissociation curve (Fig. 6-6). When all extraneous material is removed from the Hb molecule ("stripped Hb"), its O_2 affinity increases tenfold, and its dissociation curve approaches that of Mb. Addition of 2,3-DPG, which binds to the intact Hb molecule, moves the curve to the right and can return it to that of Hb in normal red cells. One molecule of 2,3-DPG may be bound per molecule of deoxyhemoglobin, probably to the β chains in the molecule's central cavity; under physiological conditions DPG is not significantly bound to oxyhemoglobin.[7, 52] The binding of DPG appears to stabilize the deoxy form of Hb. When the molecule is oxygenated, the central cavity becomes smaller and DPG is expelled. Adenosine triphosphate (ATP) acts similarly, but less effectively than 2,3-DPG.

2,3-DPG is formed by glycolysis in the red cell. Factors, such as increased intracellular pH, which stimulate glycolysis tend to elevate the levels of 2,3-DPG. This compound's formation is also subject to a feedback mechanism. Increased levels of 2,3-DPG in the red cell inhibit its further formation by inhibiting one of the glycolytic enzymes.[11] When 2,3-DPG is bound to Hb, the pool of free DPG diminishes and its formation is stimulated. This could explain why glycolysis increases when red cells are incubated under nitrogen—all Hb is in the deoxy form and binds DPG.[2] On the other hand, inhibiting glycolysis with chemical agents lowers red cell DPG content and increases the O_2 affinity of Hb. Thus, it is conceivable that DPG levels regulate O_2 binding by Hb under physiological conditions or in disease.[6, 11]

One instance where this regulatory role may be important is in adaptation to high altitude. The Hb dissociation curve of healthy humans shifts to the right within 24 to 36 hours after arrival at high altitudes (3000 or 4600 meters), an effect associated with an increased level of 2,3-DPG in the red cells.[39, 40] The process reverses on return to sea level. When long-term high-altitude residents are brought to sea level, their red cells and Hb also undergo the reverse change— DPG levels decrease and O_2 affinity of Hb increases. Hypoxia appears to induce DPG formation as part of an adaptive response to high altitude which promotes the unloading of oxygen from Hb and hence increases the oxygen availability to the body tissues. Recent work has also suggested that drugs may affect 2,3-DPG distribution in red cells.[46]

Oxygenation of Mb, Fetal Hb, and Hb Variants

Myoglobin. At partial pressures less than about 60 mm Hg, Mb binds more O_2 than Hb (Fig. 6-5). Thus, in muscle tissue, which contains Mb, hemoglobin can unload O_2 at a given P_{O_2} of, for example, 20 mm Hg, while Mb stores it. This oxygen-storage mechanism probably plays a role in increasing a man's total work output during intermittent exercise.[3]

Fetal hemoglobin (HbF). Small changes in the composition of the amino acid chains distinguish HbF from adult Hb (HbA). HbF has a higher O_2 affinity than HbA (Fig. 6-7).[49] "Stripped" HbF has a lower Hb affinity than HbA. Fetal blood is exposed to O_2 only after it has passed an additional diffusion barrier in the placenta, and hence the fetus has a lower arterial P_{O_2} than the mother. The high O_2 affinity of HbF insures adequate oxygenation of fetal blood despite lower partial pressures of O_2. That it also slightly inhibits unloading of O_2 in the tissues

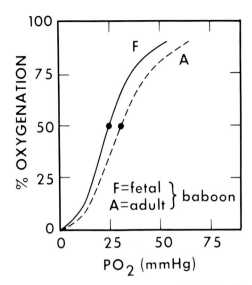

Fig. 6-7. Dissociation curves of Hb in blood of fetal and adult baboons. P50 indicated by dot on each curve. After Paton et al.[49]

apparently does not bother the fetus, whose intrauterine movements constitute only light exercise. The fetus' metabolic demands are much less subject to rapid and large changes than those of animals after birth.

Hb variants. There are many genetic variants of Hb in man—some lead to disease (sickle cell anemia, Cooley's anemia); others are rare traits discovered only by laboratory tests. They differ from HbA in the composition of the amino acid chains. In several variants, only a single amino acid residue is replaced by another. Yet, these changes are sufficient to alter the configuration of the Hb molecule, and especially the size and shape of the heme pocket. For many variants, the relation between stereochemical structure and physiological properties has been elucidated.[44] For example, Hb Zürich has an arginine group where HbA has a histidine group. The arginine residue is too large to fit in the heme pocket, and as a result, the heme pocket is wide open and O_2 is bound much easier than in HbA. Other Hb variants are less stable structures than HbA; they easily break apart into the four subunits. This, too, increases O_2 affinity.

Many Hb variants have a much higher or lower affinity to O_2 than HbA (Fig. 6-8).[58] Fortunately, there are compensatory changes in O_2 capacity: in general, the higher the O_2 affinity of the Hb variant, the larger the O_2 capacity. Hence, persons with a high O_2-affinity Hb variant, e.g., Hb Rainier, have a higher than normal O_2 capacity; persons with a low O_2-affinity variant, e.g., Hb Seattle, have a lower one.[47] Without this compensatory mechanism, persons with high O_2-affinity Hb variants where O_2 unloading is effective only at low O_2 tensions would suffer from O_2 deficiency in the tissues. Figure 6-8B shows how the changes in O_2 capacity normalize oxygen transport. With an arteriovenous O_2 difference of 4.5 vol%, mixed venous O_2 pressures vary only within a 10-mm Hg range in spite of the differences in O_2 affinity. The increased or decreased O_2 capacity allows O_2 trans-

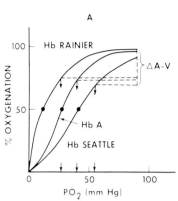

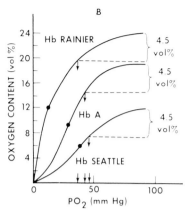

Fig. 6-8. A. Dissociation curves (% oxygenation scale) of blood with high affinity (Hb Rainier) and low affinity (Hb Seattle) hemoglobin variants, compared with blood with normal adult hemoglobin (HbA). ΔAV = Arteriovenous O_2 saturation difference (%). Arrows indicate mixed venous P_{O_2} of each blood for the same Pa_{O_2} and the same ΔAV. ● indicates P50. B. Dissociation curves for same bloods as in A, with O_2 content of blood on ordinate. Normal blood (HbA) has O_2 capacity (= 100% oxygenation) of 20 vol%; blood samples with Hb Rainier and Hb Seattle have a 20% higher and a 40% lower O_2 capacity, respectively. Because of the compensatory O_2 capacity changes, mixed venous P_{O_2} (*arrows*) is similar for blood with these variants when the arteriovenous O_2-content difference is the same (4.5 vol%). After Parer.[47]

port over portions of the dissociation curve where the slopes are similar.

These differences in O_2 capacity suggest that Hb production is controlled to meet the demands of oxygen transport. There is indeed evidence that venous O_2 tension influences the production of erythropoietin,[59] a hormone that regulates red cell production. When the number of red cells is drastically reduced by bloodletting, persons with Hb Rainier respond with a larger production of erythropoietin than persons with HbA. Because this compensatory mechanism involves production of new red cells, it takes time and is therefore useless under conditions involving acute changes in O_2 affinity of Hb.

OXYGEN TRANSPORT IN TISSUES

Oxygen molecules move along a gradient of decreasing partial pressure, from the red cell interior via blood plasma, through the capillary wall and the extracellular fluid, and through the cell membrane to the mitochondrial cristae. Electron transfers with the cytochrome chain of respiratory enzymes at the mitochondrial cristae are responsible for up to 90% of the cells' total O_2 consumption. Even within single cells, O_2 molecules are not distributed randomly. Also, there must be partial-pressure gradients, decreasing as one moves away from a capillary, in every tissue. For these reasons, the search for an average O_2 tension in tissues is not meaningful. But it is important to know what O_2 tensions must exist in capillary blood to insure adequate O_2 transfer to all cells.

With isolated mitochondria, a minimum O_2 tension of 0.5 mm Hg is required, and the critical intracellular P_{O_2} for intact cells is estimated at 3.5 mm Hg.[30] These are lower limits. Because of the partial-pressure gradients within a tissue, the capillary O_2 tension must be considerably higher to maintain these minimal values even in cells at a distance from the capillary or near its venous end where O_2 tension is low. The exact critical level is difficult to determine; one would need subtle indices of cell damage that could be related to capillary O_2 tensions.[61] Consciousness is lost when the internal jugular venous P_{O_2} falls below about 18 mm Hg (McDowell, quoted in ref. 32). A capillary oxygen tension of about 20 mm Hg is probably close to the lower limit that will prevent significant tissue hypoxia under most conditions and in most tissues.

Facilitation of Diffusion

Oxygen diffuses more rapidly in a layer of blood or Hb solution than in an equally thick layer of water. The presence of Hb or Mb in solutions appears to speed diffusion because the bound as well as the free O_2 can move by diffusion. For diffusion in red cells, experimental and theoretical results show that facilitation is not of great importance,[36] and Kreuzer[33] has concluded that the physiological importance of facilitated diffusion by Hb as well as Mb remains speculative. It is difficult to conceive how Hb could improve diffusion within the interior of red cells, where Hb molecules are tightly packed. In muscle tissue, facilitation of O_2 diffusion by myoglobin might make sense, but there is no evidence that it occurs.

OXYGEN TRANSPORT IN DISEASE

In disease, circulatory adaptations, blood viscosity, and many other factors outside the scope of this discussion are crucial for oxygen transport.[20] However, some clinical aspects of O_2 transport are particularly pertinent.

Although arterial O_2 and CO_2 tensions are often measured in patients with lung or heart diseases, they are rarely interpreted with accurate data on ventilation, cardiac output, and O_2 capacity of the blood. In extreme cases, a low arterial P_{O_2} clearly indicates inadequate O_2 transport. However, oxygen transport need not be normal when arterial P_{O_2} is within normal limits. The oxygen tensions in tissues are more nearly in equilibrium with venous than with arterial oxygen tensions. Low venous O_2 tensions can result from a large arteriovenous P_{O_2} difference, even if the arterial P_{O_2} is normal. This occurs when cardiac output is low and the tissues extract more O_2 from arterial blood to meet their metabolic demands. In patients with pulmonary edema, mixed venous O_2 tensions were lower than in bronchitic patients with ventilatory insufficiency, even though the latter had significantly lower arterial P_{O_2} tensions.[22] The bronchitics' larger cardiac output preserved tissue oxygenation in spite of a low arterial P_{O_2}. In the brain and the heart, where adequate oxygenation is particularly important, regional venous O_2 tensions are lower than the mixed venous value.[53] Thus, mixed venous O_2 tensions should always be well above critical levels to protect these hypoxia-sensitive tissues.

Improved interpretations of blood gas and associated data are feasible with computer programs that solve the alinear relations between ventilation, perfusion, and the characteristics of hemoglobin. Two groups of investigators have published their results from such programs in computer-produced tables [32] and nomograms [45] that allow calculations independent of any single standard dissociation curve and facilitate more complete interpretation of blood gas data. Kelman and Nunn's book [32] includes tables to calculate venous P_{O_2} if arterial P_{O_2}, arterial and venous O_2 content, temperature, and pH are known. Olszowska et al.[45] give examples to show the wide range of O_2 and CO_2 contents that may be associated with given values of P_{O_2} and P_{CO_2} in arterial blood, depending on O_2 capacity and the acid-base balance.

The principal causes of tissue hypoxia—inadequate arterial O_2 tension, anemia, and CO poisoning—indicate several important points for the clinical management of hypoxia.

ARTERIAL HYPOXEMIA

When arterial P_{O_2} decreases from 100 to 60 mm Hg, and the arteriovenous O_2 difference remains the same, the mixed venous P_{O_2} decreases only slightly (6 mm Hg; compare 1-1 and 2-2 in Fig. 6-9). This is because the mixed venous point is on the steep portion of the dissociation curve, where O_2 saturation changes

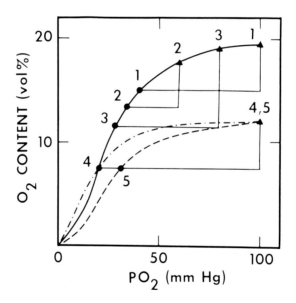

Fig. 6-9. Dissociation curves for blood with normal O_2 capacity (20 vol%, *solid line*) and low O_2 capacity (12 vol%, *dash-dot* and *dashed line*). Five different O_2 transport conditions (1-1 through 5-5) are shown. For each, the vertical line with arrow indicates the arteriovenous O_2-content difference (4.5 vol% for 1, 2, 4, and 5; 7.5 vol% for 3); the black circles on the dissociation curve indicate the corresponding mixed venous P_{O_2} values. Arterial $P_{O_2} = 100$ mm Hg (1, 4, and 5), 80 mm Hg (3), and 60 mm Hg (2). 4-4. O_2 transport in CO poisoning; 5-5. O_2 transport in anemia. See text for discussion. After reference 55.

considerably for each millimeter decrease of P_{O_2}. When the arterial point also reaches the steep portion of the curve, mixed venous P_{O_2} decreases almost as much as the arterial P_{O_2}, since both points are then on a nearly linear portion of the curve. However, this relationship holds only when the arteriovenous difference remains constant. If a slight arterial hypoxemia combines with a low cardiac output, the mixed venous point may drop to a dangerously low level. For instance, the person with an arterial P_{O_2} of 80 mm Hg and an arteriovenous difference of 7.5 vol% O_2 (corresponding to a 40 percent decrease in cardiac output) has a lower mixed venous O_2 tension than the person with an arterial P_{O_2} of 60 mm Hg and a normal cardiac output (compare 3-3 and 2-2 in Fig. 6-9).

Arterial hypoxemia in lung disease usually results from hypoventilation or nonuniform $\dot{V}_A/\dot{Q}$ ratios, or both. Since the relation between alveolar ventilation and alveolar P_{O_2} is nonlinear,[32] small changes in $\dot{V}_A$ can affect arterial P_{O_2} levels critically. For instance, under resting conditions a decrease of $\dot{V}_A$ from 5 to 4 liters/min may drop the alveolar P_{O_2} from 100 to 90 mm Hg, while a 1 liter/min decrease from 3 to 2 liters/min would decrease P_{O_2} from about 75 to 40 mm Hg.

Determination of mixed venous oxygen tensions may prove helpful in assessing tissue oxygenation in disease. Sampling via a pulmonary artery catheter is feasible but not always warranted;[22] a rebreathing method is also available.[12] Low values of mixed venous P_{O_2} indicate insufficient oxygenation, but normal values do not exclude oxygen deficiency in some tissues.

ANEMIA

Tissue hypoxia becomes a significant problem only when anemia is severe. In the example in Figure 6-9, a 40 percent loss of O_2 capacity is associated with a decrease of the mixed venous P_{O_2} from 40 to 32 mm Hg (compare 5-5 and 1-1 in Fig. 6-9). A compensatory increase in cardiac output often decreases the arteriovenous O_2 difference, so that the actual mixed venous P_{O_2} may remain normal.

CO POISONING

The shape of the O_2 dissociation curve in CO poisoning differs significantly from that in anemia.[55] It is placed to the left of the curve that corresponds to the same loss of O_2-binding capacity in anemia (compare 4-4 and 5-5 in Fig. 6-9). This displacement of the curve may be related to inhibition of 2,3-DPG synthesis [2] and results in low venous P_{O_2} values,[23] which contribute considerably to tissue hypoxia. Furthermore, the circulatory adaptations that follow when arterial P_{O_2} is low do not occur because P_{O_2} is normal (see also Chap. 10, p. 216).

Acute Changes of the Hb Dissociation Curve

The Hb dissociation curve changes as a function of blood loss, CO poisoning (see above), and physiological factors such as pH, P_{CO_2}, temperature (Fig. 6-5), and DPG metabolism. The position of the curve can be evaluated roughly if one knows (1) the O_2 capacity and (2) P50, the O_2 tension required to oxygenate 50% of the available O_2 capacity. A low value of P50 indicates high O_2 affinity of Hb and may signify decreased O_2 availability to the tissues. This measurement is particularly useful in conditions in which short-term changes in the dissociation curve's position are suspected. On the longer term, when compensatory changes in O_2 capacity may have occurred, P50 as well as O_2 capacity must be measured. The examples given for Hb variants (Fig. 6-8*B*) show that in that case O_2 transport may occur over a normal range of arterial and venous O_2 tensions, although the P50 varies from 12 mm Hg for Hb Rainier to 40.5 mm Hg for Hb Seattle.[47]

Acidosis and alkalosis. Blood pH variations can cause rapid changes in the position of the Hb dissociation curve. For instance, during treatment of diabetic acidosis, transient alkalosis may impair O_2 availability to the tissues.[5] When pH increases from 7.1 to 7.6, mixed venous P_{O_2} may decrease even though O_2 saturation at an arterial P_{O_2} of 100 mm Hg is slightly higher (Fig. 6-10). The acidotic patient can unload O_2 in the tissues at higher venous P_{O_2}'s. He can transport more oxygen for the same mixed venous P_{O_2} (cf. points at $P_{O_2}=40$ mm Hg in Fig. 6-10) and therefore requires a smaller cardiac output for the same O_2 uptake. In patients with heart disease, whose cardiac output can increase only within a small reserve, alkalosis can be especially dangerous while minor degrees of acidosis may be of some advantage in helping to oxygenate tissues.

DPG metabolism. Red cell DPG levels are altered in several clinical conditions, including lung disease with hypoxemia.[11, 41] During storage of blood, 2,3-DPG

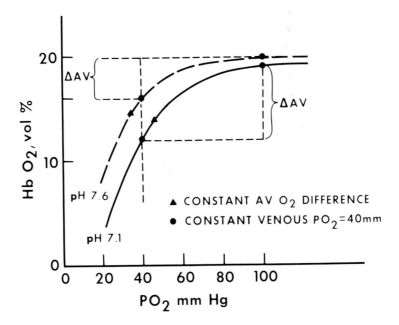

Fig. 6-10. Dissociation curves for alkalotic (pH = 7.6) and acidotic (pH = 7.1) blood. At the same mixed venous P_{O_2} (40 mm Hg; *black circles*), the person with acidosis transports more O_2 per 100 ml blood (i.e., has a larger arteriovenous O_2-content difference, ΔAV) than the person with alkalosis. At a constant ΔAV, the alkalotic person has a lower mixed venous P_{O_2} than the person with acidosis (compare *black triangles*).

disappears, and massive transfusions with stored blood can cause significant shifts to the left of the dissociation curve.[9] Patients who require large transfusions (after massive hemorrhage or surgical shock) usually have a decreased O_2 capacity. Therefore, to assess their O_2 transport, one needs to know the O_2 capacity and the P50, as well as the arterial P_{O_2}.

Treatment of Hypoxia

Although administration of supplementary oxygen is an obvious and seemingly simple mode of treating hypoxia, administration of gas with adequately monitored inspired O_2 concentrations requires accurate equipment and constant patient supervision. Monitoring of arterial P_{CO_2} tensions is also required, since patients with ventilatory insufficiency may retain CO_2 during oxygen treatment. Application of the principles of O_2 transport to medicine should include measuring parameters of the dissociation curve, in particular O_2 capacity and P50. Several methods to determine the dissociation curve [17, 17a, 58a] are now available which could improve evaluation and rational application of oxygen therapy.

As small computers and supporting software become more prevalent, computer-produced diagrams—based on quantitative relationships—will simplify the interpretation of blood gas data. The use of computer-produced tables and nomograms is a first step in this direction.[32, 45] Reliable hardware for measuring the primary data is already available (blood gas electrodes, mass spectrometer). Additional software and quality-controlled features must be developed to incorporate these techniques into user-oriented blood gas analysis systems that take blood samples as input and provide suitable diagrams and time charts as output. With the increasing need for intensive respiratory care in medical and surgical patients, such developments can lead to more effective, as well as more efficient, treatment of patients with ventilatory insufficiency and other conditions leading to tissue hypoxia.

SUMMARY

Oxygen diffuses from alveolar air, via the alveolocapillary diffusion barrier, to red cells in lung capillaries. In the red cells, oxygen is bound to hemoglobin and transported to tissues. The overall diffusion characteristics of the alveolocapillary interface can be assessed by measuring the diffusion capacity (D_L) using a single-breath, rebreathing, or steady-state method with CO in the inspired gas mixture. $D_{L_{CO}}$ depends on $\dot{V}_A/\dot{Q}$ distribution as well as on diffusion through the interface; a low $D_{L_{CO}}$ value often primarily reflects nonuniform ventilation-perfusion relations and is an early sign of certain lung diseases.

The binding of O_2 to hemoglobin involves successive binding of O_2 to Fe atoms in the four heme groups in Hb. Heme-heme interaction and the Bohr effect alter the affinity of Hb for O_2 during the binding process and promote O_2 unloading in the tissues. Organic phosphates in the red cell (primarily 2,3-DPG) also alter the O_2 affinity of Hb and may regulate O_2 binding. Myoglobin, fetal Hb, and Hb variants have O_2 affinities that differ from those of adult Hb (HbA). Through compensatory changes in O_2 capacity, O_2 transport may proceed normally in persons with high or low affinity Hb variants.

Significant tissue hypoxia probably occurs when the capillary P_{O_2} decreases below about 20 mm Hg. Facilitation of diffusion is of minor importance in vivo. In disease, the arterial as well as the venous P_{O_2} need to be taken into account when assessing tissue oxygenation. Moderate arterial hypoxemia can lead to tissue hypoxia when cardiac output is low and the arteriovenous oxygen content difference is large. Arterial hypoxemia in lung disease usually results from overall hypo-ventilation or nonuniform $\dot{V}_A/\dot{Q}$ ratios, or both. Alteration of O_2 transport in anemia, CO poisoning, alkalosis and acidosis, and following massive blood trans-fusion results in part from changes in the Hb-O_2 dissociation curve. These changes can be assessed by measuring P50 (the P_{O_2} required for 50 percent oxygenation of Hb) and the blood's O_2 capacity. To evaluate oxygen therapy and other modes of treatment in respiratory failure, one should consider all factors that result in tissue hypoxia rather than arterial P_{O_2} measurements alone.

REFERENCES

1. Arndt H, King TKC, Briscoe WA: Diffusing capacities and ventilation: perfusion ratios in patients with the clinical syndrome of alveolar capillary block. J Clin Invest 49:408–422, 1970
2. Asakura T, Sato Y, Minakami S, Yoshikawa H: Effect of deoxygenation of intracellular hemoglobin on red cell glycolysis. J Biochem (Tokyo) 59:524–526, 1966
3. Åstrand I, Åstrand P-O, Christensen EH, Hedman R: Myohemoglobin as an oxygen-store in man. Acta Physiol Scand 48:454–460, 1960
4. Barcroft J: The Respiratory Function of the Blood. Part II, Haemoglobin. London, Cambridge University Press, 1928
5. Bellingham AJ, Detter JC, Lenfant C: The role of hemoglobin affinity for oxygen and red cell 2,3-diphosphoglycerate in the management of diabetic ketoacidosis. Trans Assoc Am Physicians 83:113–120, 1970
6. Benesch R, Benesch RE: Intracellular organic phosphates as regulators of oxygen release by haemoglobin. Nature 221:618–622, 1969
7. Benesch RE, Benesch R, Renthal R, Gratzer WB: Cofactor binding and oxygen equilibria in haemoglobin. Nature [New Biol] 234:174–176, 1971
8. Bjure J, Söderholm B: "Pulmonary diffusing capacity"—a critical review of

its value as a lung function test. Scand J Clin Lab Invest 22:167–170, 1968.
9. Bordiuk JM, McKenna PJ, Giannelli S Jr, Ayres SM: Alterations in 2–3 diphosphoglycerate and O_2 hemoglobin affinity in patients undergoing open heart surgery. Circulation 43 (suppl 1): 141–146, 1971
10. Bouhuys A, Georg J, Jönsson R, Lundin G, Lindell S-E: The influence of histamine inhalation on the pulmonary diffusing capacity in man. J Physiol (Lond) 152:176–181, 1960
11. Brewer GJ, Eaton JW: Erythrocyte metabolism: interaction with oxygen transport. Science 171:1205–1211, 1971
12. Cerretelli P, Cruz JC, Farhi LE, Rahn H: Determination of mixed venous O_2 and CO_2 tensions and cardiac output by a rebreathing method. Respir Physiol 1:258–264, 1966
13. Cotes JE: Lung Function; Assessment and Application in Medicine, ed 2. Oxford and Edinburgh, Blackwell Scientific Publications, 1968
14. Cotes JE, Hall AM: The transfer factor for the lung; normal values in adults, in Arcangeli P (ed): Introduction to the Definition on Normal Values for Respiratory Function in Man. Alghero, Panminerva Medica, 1970, pp 327–343
15. DeGraff AC Jr, Grover RF, Johnson RL Jr, Hammond JW Jr, Miller JM: Diffusing capacity of the lung in Cau-

casians native to 3,100 m. J Appl Physiol 29:71–76, 1970

16. Dill DB, Edwards HT, Consolazio WV: Blood as a physicochemical system, XI. Man at rest. J Biol Chem 118:635–648, 1937

17. Duvelleroy MA, Buckles RG, Rosenkaimer S, Tung C, Laver MB: An oxyhemoglobin dissociation analyzer. J Appl Physiol 28:227–233, 1970

17a. Duc G, Engel K: A method for determination of oxyhemoglobin dissociation curves at constant temperature, pH, and pCO₂. Respir Physiol 8:118–126, 1969/70

18. Fenn WO: Partial molar volumes of oxygen and carbon monoxide in blood. Respir Physiol 13:129–140, 1971

19. Filley GF, MacIntosh DJ, Wright GW: CO uptake and pulmonary diffusing capacity in normal subjects at rest and during exercise. J Clin Invest 33:530–539, 1954

20. Finch CA, Lenfant C: Oxygen transport in man. N Engl J Med 286:407–415, 1972

21. Finley TN, Swenson EW, Comroe JH Jr: The cause of arterial hypoxemia at rest in patients with "alveolar-capillary block syndrome." J Clin Invest 41:618–622, 1962

22. Flenley DC, Miller HC, King AJ, Kirby BJ, Muir AL: Oxygen transport in acute pulmonary oedema and in acute exacerbations of chronic bronchitis. Br Med J 1:78–81, 1973

23. Forster RE: Carbon monoxide and the partial pressure of oxygen in tissue. Ann N Y Acad Sci 174:233–241, 1970

24. Forster RE: Diffusion of gases, in Fenn WO, Rahn H (eds): Handbook of Physiology, Section 3: Respiration, vol I. Washington, D.C., American Physiological Society, 1964, pp 839–872

25. Forster RE: Exchange of gases between alveolar air and pulmonary capillary blood: pulmonary diffusing capacity. Physiol Rev 37:391–452, 1957

26. Forster RE: Interpretation of measurements of pulmonary diffusing capacity, in Fenn WO, Rahn H (eds): Handbook of Physiology, Section 3: Respiration, vol II. Washington, D.C., American Physiological Society, 1965, pp 1453–1468

27. Forster RE, Edsall JT, Otis AB, Roughton FJW (eds): CO₂: Chemical, Bio-

chemical, and Physiological Aspects. Washington, D.C., National Aeronautics and Space Administration, 1969

28. Glazier JB, Hughes JMB, Maloney JE, West JB: Measurements of capillary dimensions and blood volume in rapidly frozen lungs. J Appl Physiol 26:65–76, 1969

29. Hatzfeld C, Wiener F, Briscoe WA: Effect of uneven ventilation-diffusion ratios on pulmonary diffusing capacity in disease. J Appl Physiol 23:1–10, 1967

30. Jöbsis FF: Basic processes in cellular respiration, in Fenn WO, Rahn H (eds): Handbook of Physiology, Section 3: Respiration, vol I. Washington, D.C., American Physiological Society, 1964, pp 63–124

31. Johnson RL Jr, Taylor HF, DeGraff AC Jr: Functional significance of a low pulmonary diffusing capacity for carbon monoxide. J Clin Invest 44:789–800, 1965

32. Kelman GR, Nunn JF: Computer Produced Physiological Tables, for Calculations Involving the Relationship Between Blood Oxygen Tension and Content. New York, Appleton-Century-Crofts, 1968

33. Kreuzer F: Facilitated diffusion of oxygen and its possible significance; A review. Respir Physiol 9:1–30, 1970

34. Kreuzer F, van Lookeren Campagne P: Resting pulmonary diffusing capacity for CO and O₂ at high altitude. J Appl Physiol 20:519–524, 1965

35. Kruhøffer P: Studies on the lung diffusion coefficient for carbon monoxide in normal human subjects by means of C¹⁴O. Acta Physiol Scand 32:106–123, 1954

36. Kutchai H: O₂ uptake by 100 mu layers of hemoglobin solution: theory vs. experiment. Respir Physiol 11:378–383, 1971

37. Lawson WH Jr: Rebreathing measurements of pulmonary diffusing capacity for CO during exercise. J Appl Physiol 29:896–900, 1970

38. Lawson WH Jr, Johnson RI Jr: Gas chromatography in measuring pulmonary blood flow and diffusing capacity. J Appl Physiol 17:143–147, 1962

39. Lenfant C, Sullivan K: Adaptation to high altitude. N Engl J Med 284:1298–1309, 1971

40. Lenfant C, Torrance J, English E, Finch CA, Reynafarje C, Ramos J, Faura J:

Effect of altitude on oxygen binding by hemoglobin and on organic phosphate levels. J Clin Invest 47:2652–2656, 1968

41. Lenfant C, Ways P, Aucutt C, Cruz J: Effect of chronic hypoxic hypoxia on the O_2-Hb dissociation curve and respiratory gas transport in man. Respir Physiol 7:7–29, 1969

42. Lewis BM, Lin T-H, Noe FE, Hayford-Welsing EJ: The measurement of pulmonary diffusing capacity for carbon monoxide by a rebreathing method. J Clin Invest 38:2073–2086, 1959

43. Miller JM, Johnson RL Jr: Effect of lung inflation on pulmonary diffusing capacity at rest and exercise. J Clin Invest 45:493–500, 1966

44. Morimoto H, Lehman H, Perutz MF: Molecular pathology of human haemoglobin: stereochemical interpretation of abnormal oxygen affinities. Nature 232:408–413, 1971

45. Olszowka AJ, Rahn H, Farhi LE: Blood Gases: Hemoglobin, Base Excess, and Maldistribution. Philadelphia, Lea & Febiger, 1973

46. Oski FA, Miller LD, Delivoria-Papadopoulos M, Manchester JH, Shelburne JC: Oxygen affinity in red cells: changes induced in vivo by propranolol. Science 175:1372–1373, 1972

47. Parer JT: Oxygen transport in human subjects with hemoglobin variants having altered oxygen affinity. Respir Physiol 9:43–49, 1970

48. Pascual RS, Mosher MB, Sikand RS, DeConti RC, Bouhuys A: Effect of bleomycin on pulmonary function in man. Am Rev Respir Dis 108:211–217, 1973.

49. Paton JB, Peterson E, Fisher DE, Behrmann RE: Oxygen dissociation curves of fetal and adult baboons. Respir Physiol 12:283–290, 1971

50. Perutz MF: Haemoglobin: The molecular lung. New Sci and Sci J 50:676–679, 1971

51. Perutz MF: Haemoglobin: Genetic abnormalities. New Sci and Sci J 50:762–765, 1971

52. Perutz MF: Stereochemistry of cooperative effects of hemoglobin. Nature 228:726–739, 1970

53. Rahn H, Fenn WO: A Graphical Analysis of the Respiratory Gas Exchange; the O_2-CO_2 Diagram. Washington, D.C., American Physiological Society, 1955

54. Remmers JE, Mithoeffer JC: The carbon monoxide diffusing capacity in permanent residents at high altitudes. Respir Physiol 6:233–244, 1969

55. Roughton FJW: Transport of oxygen and carbon dioxide, in Fenn WO, Rahn H (eds): Handbook of Physiology, Section 3: Respiration, vol I. Washington, D.C., American Physiological Society, 1964, pp 767–825

56. Roughton FJW, Forster RE: Relative importance of diffusion and chemical reaction rates in determining rate of exchange of gas in the human lung, with special reference to true diffusion capacity of pulmonary membrane and volume of blood in the lung capillaries. J Appl Physiol 11:290–302, 1957

57. St. Helen R, Roughton FJW, Fatt I: Polarographic studies of oxygen-hemoglobin equilibria at very low saturations. J Appl Physiol 30:575–579, 1971

58. Stamatoyannopoulos G, Bellingham AJ, Lenfant C, Finch CA: Abnormal hemoglobins with high and low oxygen affinity. Ann Rev Med 22:221–234, 1971

58a. Torrance JD, Lenfant C: Methods for determination of O_2 dissociation curves, including Bohr effect. Respir Physiol 8:127–136, 1969/70

59. Tribukait B: Experimentelle Untersuchungen zur Regulation der Erythropoiese unter besonderer Berücksichtigung der Bedeutung des Sauerstoffs. Acta Physiol Scand 58 (suppl 208): 1–47, 1963

60. West JB: Causes of carbon dioxide retention in lung disease. N Engl J Med 284:1232–1236, 1971

61. Zierler KL: Diffusion of gases in peripheral tissue, in: Physiology in the Space Environment, vol II, Respiration. Washington, D.C., National Academy of Sciences, National Research Council, 1967, pp. 79–86

Chapter 7

Pressure-Volume Relations

During breathing, the lungs inflate and deflate cyclically. The movements of the lungs and chest cage result from the force of respiratory muscles and the elastic properties of the structures themselves. In the chest cage, forces are generated actively by muscle contraction and passively by chest cage elastic recoil. The special properties of the pleural space allow transmission of these forces from the chest cage to the lungs. The forces applied by the chest cage are spent in overcoming opposing forces—chest and lung elastic recoil and airway resistance—in the lungs as well as in the chest cage. The interaction between applied and opposing forces causes pressures within the lungs and pleural space to deviate from atmospheric pressure. To understand lung and chest cage elastic recoil and the generation of pleural and alveolar pressures, pressure-volume diagrams of the lungs and chest are indispensable. The pressure-volume relations are also used to describe the maximum pressures that the respiratory muscles can generate, the work of breathing, and the factors that limit inspiratory and expiratory volume excursions. We shall consider first only conditions where airflow is zero or minimal, and, hence, where resistive and inertial forces are negligible. Airflow is introduced as an additional variable in Chapter 8; this chapter concentrates on the properties of the breathing pump, and Chapter 8 focuses on those of the airways, the complex plumbing system connected to the pump.

MOVEMENTS OF LUNGS AND CHEST

The lungs are enclosed by the rib cage, the soft tissues of the neck, and the diaphragm. These form the chest cage, which is expanded by the action of the diaphragm, the external intercostal muscles, and certain accessory muscles. The abdominal contents and wall are also displaced during breathing. Thus, the term chest wall, commonly used in lung mechanics, is an anatomical and physiological abstraction; the chest wall's properties are determined by all structures outside the lungs that move during breathing.

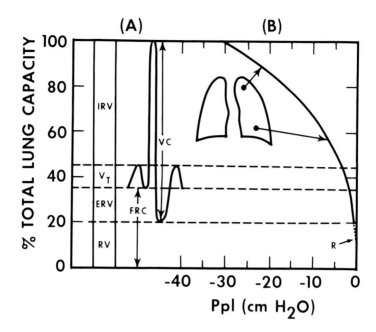

Fig. 7-1. *A.* Subdivisions of the total lung capacity (TLC). IRV = inspiratory reserve volume; V_T = tidal volume; ERV = expiratory reserve volume; RV = residual volume; FRC = functional residual capacity; VC = vital capacity. The spirographical curve shows two tidal breaths and a VC maneuver. *B.* Static pressure-volume or static recoil curve. *Abscissa.* Pleural pressure. R = resting position of the lungs (zero recoil force). Diagram of vertical lungs shows that areas in the lung top operate at higher volume than areas in bottom lung zones; the former have a lower compliance than the latter because of the curvature of the recoil curve (see also Chap. 4).

The lungs and chest always move together in healthy persons (see next section). During quiet breathing, the tidal volume (V_T) is a small fraction of the maximal volume excursion (the vital capacity, VC; Fig. 7-1). At the point of maximum expiration, the lungs still contain air (residual volume, RV), and further collapse can occur only when the chest is opened. The lungs then assume their resting volume (R in Fig. 7-1).

When excised lungs are inflated with air through the trachea, all linear dimensions increase by the same fraction; the lungs behave isotropically.[68] The lungs within the chest cage, however, can assume different shapes at the same volume. Thus, the configuration of lungs in situ depends not only on their volume, but also on the shape of the chest cage.[49] If lung volume is kept constant by closing the glottis, different configurations of chest and abdomen (and thus indirectly of the lungs) can be produced—first by expanding the chest and retracting the abdominal wall, and next by drawing in the chest and expanding the abdomen.

Role of the Pleural Space

The chest cage and the lungs are each covered with a pleural membrane that allows the lungs to move, to some extent, independently from the chest wall. Con-

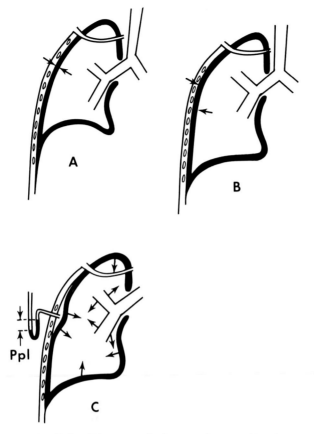

Fig. 7-2. Diagram of airways, lungs, pleural space (*black zone*), and rib cage. Points on the pleural membrane's two layers, which are in apposition (*arrows in A*), move apart when the lung expands in *B*. The retractile or recoil force (*arrows in C*) results in a distending force exerted on the airways and in subatmospheric (negative) pleural pressure.

sequently, when the lungs increase in volume, points that are in apposition near maximum expiration move apart (Fig. 7-2*A* and *B*). This enables the lungs to enlarge downward in response to contraction of the diaphragm. The pleural space contains no gas and only a minimal amount of liquid (about 2 ml) dispersed over a large surface area. Since the sum of the partial pressures of the gases in venous and even arterial blood is less than atmospheric,[27] any gas in the pleural space is absorbed into the blood. Also, any additional liquid is absorbed because capillary oncotic pressures in the pleura are low.[1] Therefore, the space between the pleural membrane is narrow (5–10 μm in cats[2]), and the lungs remain in close contact with the chest wall. This enables forces to be transmitted from the chest to the lungs and causes the lungs to follow all volume changes of the chest cage.

Viscoelastic Behavior of the Lungs

The lungs are elastic: they expand when stresses are applied and recoil passively when stresses are released. Lung tissue also has viscous properties: it responds to applied stress with some delay in deformation. Thus, the lungs are a viscoelastic, rather than a purely elastic, organ. The physical properties of such bodies are complex; [15, 68] a guide to terminology and definitions is available.[50]

Elastic recoil. The tensile strength of lung tissue is probably provided by strong, collagenic connective tissue fibers.[61] Although the extensibility of lung tissue is often attributed to the presence of elastic fibers, their close association with collagen fibers limits the extent to which the elastic fibers can be stretched. The recoil properties of the lungs as a whole relate less to the properties of the single fibers than to the arrangement of collagen and elastic fibers in a network (Fig. 7-3). When the lung tissue is stretched, the helical fiber network around alveoli and alveolar ducts uncoils.[65] Under the electron microscope, the alveolar surface is smooth and flat, regardless of lung volume.[32] The alveolar wall, therefore, distends and retracts without folding; it appears to have inherent elastic properties.[33, 72] The alveolar surface film (Chap. 1) also contributes considerably to the lung's elastic recoil, at higher lung volumes providing the major portion of the recoil force.[7]

Hysteresis. This term refers to "the failure of a system to follow identical paths of response upon application of and withdrawal of a forcing agent." [50] In air-filled excised lungs, pressure-volume curves during inflation and deflation differ markedly (Fig. 7-4). To a large extent, lung hysteresis is a function of the alveolar

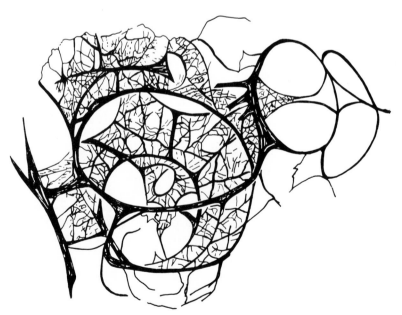

Fig. 7-3. Elastic fiber network arranged in a helical form around an alveolar duct and its alveoli. From reference 65.

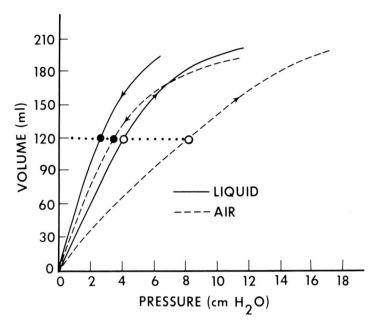

Fig. 7-4. Pressure-volume curves of cat lungs in situ inflated with liquid (Ringer-Locke solution) or air and subsequently deflated. The surface area between the inflation and deflation curves is greater for air than for liquid, reflecting the contribution of the air-liquid interface to hysteresis. Redrawn from reference 31.

surface film—hysteresis decreases when the lungs are filled with saline and the air-liquid interface is abolished. During quiet breathing, this may account for about 7/8 of the hysteresis of excised lungs.[39] How much the surface film contributes to hysteresis depends on lung volume and the direction of volume change. During inflation, the air-filled lung requires a much larger pressure than the liquid-filled lung; during deflation the difference is less (Fig. 7-4). The molecular mechanisms underlying hysteresis of film and of tissue may be similar.[39] Under some circumstances, smooth muscle contraction may also contribute to hysteresis.[17, 22] Lung tissues in man and in several mammals have similar hysteresis characteristics;[6] hence, basic mechanical properties of lung tissue appear to be independent of species variations. Another consequence of viscoelasticity is *stress relaxation*. When inflated lungs are held at constant volume, the distending pressure decreases with time, which may reflect realignment of tissue fibers and reorientation of the surface film.[39] Conversely, when pressure is constant, lung volume increases slightly with time (*creep of lung tissue*[75]). Opening of previously collapsed alveoli may contribute to stress relaxation and creep.

The difference between deflation and inflation pressure-volume curves in man is consistent with hysteresis-like behavior.[55] Similar characteristics of hysteresis have been found in tissue strips from persons with normal lungs and patients with lung diseases.[72] However, this study did not include tissue from lungs with extensive fibrosis.

Distribution of stress. Isolated strips of tissue, cut in different directions from a lung, are equally distensible.[33, 68, 72] In intact lungs, however, stress is not equally distributed and hence distension is not uniform.[77] In vertical lungs, stress increases downward and laterally, in part because of the force of gravity.[76] As a result, alveoli in the lung tops are more distended than alveoli in dependent zones (Fig. 7-1B; Chap. 4). Even during quiet breathing, alveoli near the lung tops may breathe near their maximum volumes. They are stressed considerably in normal conditions, which may explain the predilection of the lung tops for developing emphysema and large tuberculous cavities.[76]

If the lungs and all structures in it (airways, blood vessels) were homogeneous and the lungs were not distorted by the force of gravity, (1) all parts would expand isotropically (Chap. 1); (2) pleural surface pressure would be uniform; and (3) stress (force per unit area, or pressure) would be equal to pleural pressure at all boundaries within this ideal lung. Thus, airways and blood vessels would be subjected to exactly the same distending stresses that exist at the pleural surface. However, many structures within the lung have compliances that deviate from the mean. The dimensions of such structures change more or less than the average during distension, depending on whether they are more or less compliant than the lungs as a whole. Structures that stretch less than the lungs as a whole may be subject to stress magnification[57] since, for the same force at the boundary, they are proportionately more stressed the smaller their surface area. Hence, pressure variations in small lung blood vessels (in excised human lungs) are often greater than elastic recoil pressures.[66] The inverse relation between surface area and distending pressure, in the case of nonisotropic distension and recoil, promotes uniform lung expansion: if one unit is distended more than its neighbor, its surface area becomes larger and its distending pressure consequently decreases.[57]

STATIC PRESSURE-VOLUME CURVE

The lungs' elastic-recoil properties become clear only from a pressure-volume curve. To construct such a curve in man in vivo, one must measure lung volume with a spirometer or a body plethysmograph, which is easy, while simultaneously measuring pleural pressure, which is considerably more difficult.

Pleural Pressure (Ppl)

Because during life the lungs are always distended beyond their resting volume (R in Fig. 7-1B), they would collapse if not prevented by their apposition to the chest wall (Fig. 7-2). The collapsing tendency, or recoil force, of the lungs decreases the pressure in the pleural space below atmospheric (Fig. 7-2C). In lung mechanics, atmospheric pressure (Patm) is used as a zero reference pressure; the subatmospheric pressure in the pleural space is usually called a negative pressure, i.e., negative with respect to Patm $= 0$.

If measured by a fluid-filled catheter, the pressure within the intact pleural space is lower than the pressure measured in Figure 7-2C [1, 3]; the actual pressure includes an additional pleural liquid pressure created by the contact between the pleural membranes. As commonly measured by an air-filled catheter, Ppl is the pleural surface pressure, which is relevant to the elastic recoil of the lungs and chest wall. The interpretation of Ppl measurements is complicated by the fact that the pressure around the lungs is not uniform but increases, becoming less negative from the top to the bottom of vertical lungs. This reflects the distorted shape of the lungs in the thorax, resulting largely from gravity effects.[67] In a healthy, sitting man at FRC, pleural surface pressure is about -8 cm H_2O just below the apex and -2 cm H_2O near the bottom of the lungs; if the vertical height of the lungs is 25 cm, the gradient is about 0.3 cm H_2O/cm height. The effect of gravity on the chest wall and on the abdominal contents appears to contribute to the gradient.[21] The shape and height of the chest, the distribution of muscle force and of stress in the lungs, and the weight of lung tissue and blood are all relevant variables that contribute to the local variations of Ppl.[1]

Measurement of Ppl. The local variations of Ppl and the differences between pleural liquid and surface pressures make it difficult to interpret direct measurements of Ppl in terms of overall lung elastic recoil. Although indirect methods also suffer from limitations, they are at least more practical in man. One indirect method uses the fact that the intrathoracic esophagus is relaxed except during swallowing, and the pressure within its lumen reflects pleural pressure fairly well.[21] Esophageal pressures can be measured by inserting a balloon catheter, a method that depends on precise technical details.[59, 73] Another indirect method uses the retraction of the skin in the suprasternal notch as a measure of lung recoil force.[9]

Determination of Static Lung Recoil Pressure

The difference between pleural surface pressure (Ppl) and Patm equals the sum of two pressure differences: (1) that between the pleural surface and the alveoli (created by lung elastic recoil), and (2) that between alveoli and the atmosphere (the driving pressure for airflow). Thus

$$(Ppl - Patm) = (Ppl - Palv) + (Palv - Patm) \qquad (1)$$

and since $(Ppl - Palv) = -Pst(l)$, and Patm is the zero reference pressure

$$Ppl = -Pst(l) + Palv \qquad (2)$$

where $Pst(l)$ is the static recoil pressure of the lungs and Palv the pressure in the alveoli.

Increased pull of the lungs on the pleural surface [i.e., larger $Pst(l)$] reduces pleural pressure (makes it more negative), hence the negative sign for $Pst(l)$. $Pst(l)$ depends on lung volume (Figs. 7-1 and 7-5). If the relation between $Pst(l)$ and volume is known, Palv can be determined. Conversely, $Pst(l)$ can be determined from Ppl measurements if Palv is known. For instance, at A (Fig. 7-5), Ppl $= -20$ cm H_2O; $Pst(l) = +10$ cm H_2O. From Eq. (2): $-20 = -10 + $ Palv; hence Palv $= -10$ cm H_2O. Negative, i.e., subatmospheric, alveolar pressures lead to inspiration. Palv is negative at all points left of the curve in Figure 7-5; that area is associated with inspiration. For B in Figure 7-5, Palv $= +20$ cm H_2O.

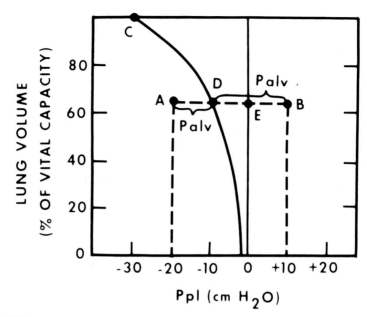

Fig. 7-5. Pressure-volume diagram of lungs in man. Curved line through C and D is the static recoil curve (see also Fig. 7-1). The diagram shows graphical solutions to Eq. (2). At point A, $Ppl = -AE$ and $Pst(l) = DE$. Substituting in Eq. (2), $-AE = -DE + Palv$; hence, $Palv = -AD = -10$ cm H_2O. Similarly, at B, $Palv = +BD = +20$ cm H_2O. $C =$ static recoil pressure at maximum lung inflation.

Palv is positive for points to the right of the curve; this area is associated with expiration.

When $Palv = 0$, $Ppl = -Pst(l)$ [from Eq. (2)]. The locus of all points where $Palv = 0$ is the elastic or static recoil curve of the lungs (Figs. 7-1 and 7-5). Palv can be made zero by holding the breath with all airways open; alveolar pressure then equals Patm. Thus, the static recoil curve can be determined experimentally if the subject inspires maximally (to point C, Fig. 7-5), and then exhales stepwise, holding the breath with glottis open at several intervals of about 0.5 liters. At each of these points, $Palv = 0$ and $Ppl = -Pst(l)$. The principle of the method can be shown clearly with an experiment on singing (Fig. 7-6). Here, the subject inspired maximally and sang a tone with periodic interruptions. The tone was constant in pitch and loudness and hence required a constant driving pressure (Chap. 11). To provide the pressure for phonation, Palv is elevated each time the note is struck. On the other hand, during each interruption (glottis open), Ppl decreases to the level of $Pst(l)$.

The lung static recoil curve is steep at low lung volumes: deflated lungs are highly distensible (Fig. 7-1B). As volume increases, the slope of the curve diminishes, indicating that the lungs increasingly resist further inflation. To measure $Pst(l)$ by breath holding may require training the subject. Easier methods for use in patients include very slow exhalations with open glottis to achieve nearly static conditions[11] and interruption of airflow at the mouth.[44] Measurement of thoracic gas volume with a body plethysmograph provides data for an absolute

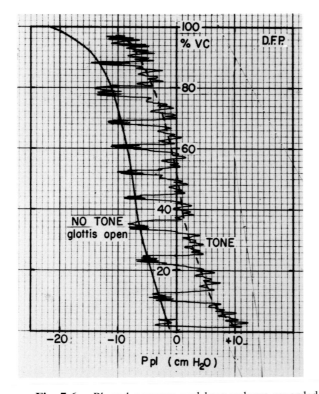

Fig. 7-6. Pleural pressure and lung volume recorded during singing of a tone at constant pitch and loudness. The subject initiated the tone at a lung volume close to 100% of VC and interrupted phonation 10 times. During the brief interruptions he held his breath with his glottis wide open. The noise in the Ppl recording is the result of fluctuations in esophageal pressure caused by the heart-beat. The course of Ppl during phonation is indicated by the dashed line. During the interruptions, Ppl decreases to the value of Pst(l) at the prevailing lung volume. *Solid line.* Static recoil curve of the lungs for this subject. Subglottic pressure $= 7.5$ cm H_2O at 50% of VC (horizontal distance between solid and dashed lines). From reference 13.

volume scale, as a percentage of TLC (Fig. 7-1). This is important in particular when short-term variations of Pst(l) occur, as in asthma (p. 140).

Lung Compliance

The slope of the Pst(l) versus volume curve reflects lung compliance, or the ease with which the lungs can be expanded. Since the curve is markedly alinear outside the tidal volume range, compliance depends on the breathing level. When lung stiffness increases as a pathological phenomenon, compliance is low; but increased stiffness is also a normal consequence of lung inflation to near TLC.

Only complete static recoil curves give a full picture of lung elastic recoil; compliance values are valid only for the tidal volume range over which they were measured and are generally difficult to interpret.

Dynamic Lung Compliance

In healthy persons who breathe quietly, Palv is zero throughout the lungs at the end-tidal points, i.e., the points of flow reversal between inspiration and expiration. These two points on the pressure-volume loop (Fig. 7-7C) therefore coincide with the static recoil curve. Measuring Ppl and volume at these points gives a compliance value, measured during breathing and called dynamic compliance (Cdyn), which is equal to the compliance measured from the static curve (static compliance, Cst). However, Cdyn does not always equal Cst. For instance, when airway obstruction causes some lung regions to fill slowly during inspiration, these areas receive less inspired air as breathing rate increases. The amount of air inspired for a given pleural pressure change thus depends on the duration of inspiration: the shorter the inspiration, the less air inspired. Under such conditions, Cdyn is frequency-dependent and decreases as breathing rate increases.[79] This phenomenon can be used to assess airway obstruction in disease. Its accurate recording requires control of lung volume levels, rapid response of the pressure-sensing device (for use with high breathing rates), and considerable cooperation and training of the subject. Frequency dependence of Cdyn is usually but not always associated with nonuniform inspired gas distribution (N_2 washout [25, 42]).

Variables Influencing Lung Static Recoil

At comparable lung volumes, as a percentage of VC or TLC, mammals with widely different lung sizes have similar static recoil pressures. The same holds true for growing children (Chap. 1). Since in healthy individuals, compliance in absolute units is a measure of lung size rather than of lung-tissue properties, young children and small animals have a small lung compliance. Advancing age is associated with decreased lung recoil,[74] although individual variability is considerable.[45] Whether the rate of aging of elastic structures in the lungs parallels that in other elastic tissues (e.g., the lens or skin) is not clear. Since the amount of elastic and collagen material does not change with age, loss of recoil force is perhaps best explained by degeneration of structure rather than by altered properties of individual elastic fibers.[65] Elastic recoil curves vary individually and are difficult to obtain in large groups of subjects. This limits their usefulness in detecting effects of environmental variables (smoking, air pollutant exposure) on lung recoil. Deep breaths and sighs increase dynamic compliance.[26] Regular deep breaths, perhaps elicited by chemoreceptor stimulation[8] and vagal afferent impulses,[34] may help prevent atelectasis, particularly in small animals that have small, easily collapsible alveoli (p. 7). The sighing mechanism is active in immature animals and may contribute to the events that initiate breathing after birth.[8] Stress distribution in the lungs affects local recoil forces (see p. 126).

STATIC PRESSURE-VOLUME CURVES
OF THE LUNGS AND CHEST

This section elaborates on the pressure-volume diagram by adding a curve that represents properties of the chest wall. This allows us to determine how the respiratory bellows generates pleural and alveolar pressures.

Generation of Pleural Pressure

Pleural pressure is actively altered by contraction of respiratory muscles.[19] The action of the muscles is reinforced or opposed by elastic recoil forces in the chest wall. The active and passive forces in the chest wall can be analyzed if one considers Ppl as the pressure difference between the atmosphere (zero reference) and the pleural space, separated by the chest wall

$$Ppl - Patm = Ppl = Pmus + Pst(w) \qquad (3)$$

where Pmus is the pressure developed by the muscles and Pst(w) the pressure developed by the recoil force of the chest cage. To solve Eq. (3) one measures Ppl at different lung volumes while the subject voluntarily relaxes all respiratory muscles. This maneuver makes Pmus = 0, and thus Ppl = Pst(w). During relaxation, lung volume normally returns to the resting breathing level (FRC). Thus, to measure Ppl during muscle relaxation at volumes other than FRC, one must keep volume at the desired level by closing the airways. To generate the curve of Figure 7-7A, the subject inspires maximally and holds the breath momentarily. This is the same maneuver used in Figure 7-5; during breath holding at TLC, Ppl is at point C in both figures. Next, a valve in the breathing tube is closed and the subject relaxes all muscles. At TLC, the chest cage tends to collapse through its own recoil and, since no air can escape, this creates a positive pressure in the pleural space. Hence, Ppl becomes positive and volume decreases slightly because of gas compression (point C'). At a small lung volume (e.g., at D) the chest cage tends to expand when the muscles are relaxed. Ppl then becomes more negative while lung volume increases slightly through decompression (to point D'). The reader can perform these maneuvers by closing his mouth and nose manually and relaxing at different lung volumes. If one relaxes near full inspiration, the positive pressure in the chest is transmitted to the mouth. It is more difficult to relax near full expiration; if the maneuver is successful, one notices that the chest tends to inspire air. Between these extremes is a volume where Pst(w) is zero (E; at about 60 percent of the VC). This is the resting position of the chest cage, i.e., the volume it would assume if no outside forces (muscle force and lung recoil) acted upon it. The resting volumes of the chest cage and the lungs differ considerably. During life, the properties of the pleural space lead to a resting volume of the lungs and chest that is less than the resting volume of the chest and more than that of the lungs. Since the lungs are more distensible than the chest, the combined resting volume lies closer to that of the chest than to that of the lungs.

Once the Pst(w) versus volume curve is known, Pmus can be determined from Eq. (3) for any value of Ppl. Examples are given in the legend of Figure 7-7B. When Ppl is greater than Pst(w), the muscles exert expiratory force and Pmus

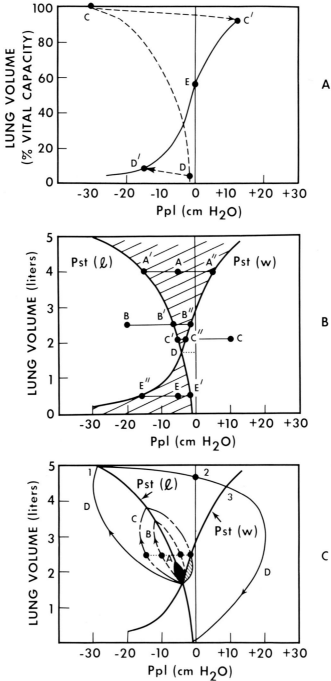

Fig. 7-7. Pressure-volume diagrams of lungs and chest in man. *A*. Dashed curve through *C* and *D* = static lung recoil curve. Drawn curve through *C'* and *D'* = static chest-wall recoil curve. *E* = resting position of the chest cage (volume at which the chest cage exerts no elastic forces on its contents). To obtain the chest wall curve, the subject inspires maximally (to *C*) and relaxes against a closed mouthpiece. The chest wall recoil then compresses the gas in the lungs, and Ppl becomes positive (dashed line

is positive. All points to the right of the Pst(w) curve are associated with expiratory muscle force. When Ppl is less than Pst(w), muscle force is inspiratory and Pmus is negative [all points to the left of the Pst(w) curve].

Any value of Pmus is the net result of contracting different muscles, including agonists and antagonists. Simultaneous contraction of inspiratory and expiratory muscles may result in a net muscle force which is small in comparison to muscular effort. Pmus is zero not only when all muscles are relaxed, but also when agonists and antagonists exert equal forces in opposite directions. The voluntary muscle relaxation used to produce the Pst(w) versus volume curve may not always be complete, and the numerical values of Pmus are then incorrect. Nevertheless, the curve indicates the mechanical behavior of the chest cage accurately, if not in precise quantitative terms.

Generation of Alveolar Pressure

Figure 7-7B includes the Pst(l) and Pst(w) curves. Five Ppl values are indicated (A-E); for each of these, equations (2) and (3) can be solved graphically by reading horizontal distances from the Ppl point to the Pst(l) and the Pst(w) curve (see legend to Fig. 7-7). At B, Palv and Pmus have a negative sign: muscle force is inspiratory, and the negative Palv would lead to inspiration. At C, both are positive: expiratory muscle force (with the glottis open) leads to expiration. At D, both Pmus and Palv are zero. Here, the elastic recoil of the lungs (pulling inward) and the recoil of the chest (pulling outward) just balance one another. This is the resting, end-expiratory breathing level to which lungs and chest return when all muscles are relaxed and the airways are open. Pmus and Palv have opposite signs at A and E. Point A is associated with expiration ($+$Palv) and inspiratory muscle force ($-$Pmus). Point A lies in the upper hatched area; points in this area reflect expiratory air movement braked by inspiratory muscle force. Without this brake, relaxing the chest cage would lead to higher pleural and alveolar pressures, e.g., up to $+20$ cm H_2O (A'') at the same volume as for A. Conversely, in the lower hatched area, the expiratory muscle force is not strong enough to prevent inspiration. To continue expiration at these small volumes, Pmus needs to be sufficient to increase Ppl to points to the right of the Pst(l) curve.

When Palv $\neq 0$ and the airways are open, air is inspired or expired and conditions are no longer static (Chap. 8). The development of Palv is, however,

---

CC'). When relaxing at low lung volume, starting at D, lung volume expands and Ppl decreases (dashed line DD'). B. Static lung [Pst(l)] and static chest wall [Pst(w)] recoil curves, to show graphical solution of Eqs. (2) and (3). At point A, Palv $= +AA'$ and Pmus $= -AA''$. At B, Palv $= -BB'$ and Pmus $= -BB''$. At C, Palv $= +CC'$ and Pmus $= +CC''$. At D, Palv $=$ Pmus $= 0$. At E, Palv $= -EE'$ and Pmus $= +EE''$. *Hatched areas.* See text for discussion. C. Pst(l) and Pst(w) curves with three pressure-volume loops with different tidal volumes (A, B, C) and a maximum inspiratory and expiratory maneuver (D). Hatched area indicates portion of breath C where positive expiratory muscle force is used. Dotted horizontal line and points indicate magnitude of resistive pressures on loops B and C. See text for further discussion.

best discussed on the basis of the pressure-volume diagram. During quiet breathing (loop A in Fig. 7-7C), inspiration is associated with inspiratory muscle force. During expiration, Palv is positive but the loop remains to the left of the Pst(w) curve. Expiration results from elastic recoil of the lungs, initially braked by inspiratory muscle force ($-$Pmus). During a deep and slow breath (loop B) the pattern is similar, but when flow rates are increased the loop widens because higher alveolar pressures are required (loop C). The expiratory portion of loop C crosses the Pst(w) curve, indicating that expiratory muscle force is applied during the last part of the expiration. Loop D represents a rapid inspiration to TLC, followed by a forced expiration to RV. During expiration Palv reaches values up to +30 cm H_2O. Initially, Palv increases because the inspiratory muscles relax (from *1* to *3*). At *2*, Ppl becomes positive; at *3*, Pmus=0. Beyond point *3*, expiratory muscles contract, further increasing Ppl and Palv. Throughout the expiration Pmus remains positive, while Palv gradually decreases and reaches zero when airflow stops at the residual volume level. Considerable expiratory muscle force is required to maintain lung volume at that level. At each point of all loops, Palv and Pmus can be determined as shown in Figure 7-7B. The relations between Palv and airflow rates are discussed in Chapter 8. Special breathing maneuvers (for singing, speech) can also be studied with pressure-volume diagrams (Chap. 11).

WORK OF BREATHING

The product of volume and pressure has the dimensions of work according to its physical definition. Since different muscle efforts may yield the same Pmus, the actual effort for a given amount of work performed on the lungs and chest may vary widely. When agonists and antagonists contract simultaneously, considerable effort is exerted but little work is accomplished. The product of volume and pressure, shown graphically as a surface area on a pressure-volume diagram, indicates only the amount of physical work performed in displacing air at the mouth. This work results partly from muscle force and partly from potential energy stored in the elastic structures of lungs and chest.

The part played by stored energy follows from the Pst(l) and Pst(w) curves. At A' (Fig. 7-7B), the lungs recoil with a pressure of +15 cm H_2O. At the same volume, the chest recoils inward with a pressure of +5 cm H_2O. Thus, the lungs and chest recoil together, in the direction of expiration, with a total pressure of +20 cm H_2O (A''' in Fig. 7-8). The different sign accorded to Pst(l) in Figures 7-7 and 7-8 may be confusing. In the former figure, pressure is measured outside the recoiling lungs; the lungs tend to pull away from the site of pressure measurement (Fig. 7-2C), and lung recoil is measured as a negative pressure. At the same time, lung recoil leads to pressure on the air in the lungs and to expiration. Thus, for the purpose of Figure 7-8, Pst(l) has a positive sign. A similar calculation for a point at a low lung volume (E''' in Fig. 7-8) shows a net recoil force of lungs and chest in the inspiratory direction—lung elastic recoil is small but the chest cage tends to expand with considerable force. The same calculation at other lung volumes yields the curve through A''' and E'''

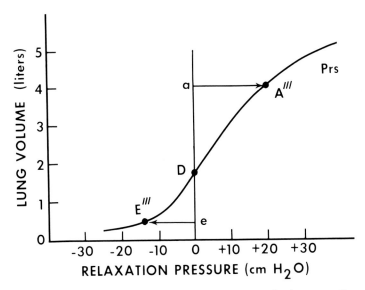

Fig. 7-8. Static pressure-volume curve of lungs and chest together. *Abscissa.* Mouth pressure developed during relaxation against closed airway at different lung volumes. This indicates the total pressure developed by the respiratory system (Prs) under conditions of zero net muscle force. Arrows to *A'''* and *E'''* indicate Prs at volumes equal to those for lines *A' A"* and *E' E"* in Fig. 7-7B. See text for derivation of these pressures.

—the relaxation-pressure curve.[69] When one relaxes all muscles during closure of airways at the mouth, pressure within the alveoli and airways equals the values on the curve of Figure 7-8, while Ppl equals Pst(w).

The work of breathing can be analyzed in detail, starting from the relaxation-pressure curve and the Pst(l) and Pst(w) curves.[62] When one inspires from FRC, work is needed to increase lung volume; part of this work is provided by chest recoil toward a higher volume. Thus, in addition to that performed actively by the muscles, work is provided by the potential energy in the chest cage. During expiration, some of this work is restored to the chest cage, which returns to a smaller volume where its recoil force is larger. In braking expiration, the inspiratory muscles work while they lengthen (so-called negative work). In addition, work is performed to overcome viscous resistances, primarily those in the airways. This portion of the work of breathing can be measured from the surface area of a pressure-volume loop (e.g., *A* in Fig. 7-7C).

The work of respiratory muscles requires oxygen. When ventilation is increased while keeping other muscles at rest, O_2 consumption increases. The increment of O_2 uptake is attributable to the muscles' work of breathing. Thus, the O_2 consumption required for breathing can be measured[52] during inspiration of CO_2-air mixtures (Chap. 10), by increasing the dead space, or by voluntary hyperventilation. However, the experimental errors are large, since the amount of O_2 used for breathing is a small part of the total O_2 consumption. At high ventilation rates, the O_2 uptake of the respiratory muscles increases steeply.[62] When the work of breathing is increased in lung disease, the increased O_2 consumption required for breathing may offset the gain in O_2 consumption derived from increased ventilation rates. Ventilation increases are then useless, since the net supply of O_2 to other working muscles cannot be increased. This limits the exercise performance of patients with ventilatory insufficiency.

The combination of rate and tidal volume chosen to achieve given rates of lung ventilation influences the work of breathing. At low rates, large tidal volumes are required, and as inspiratory lung volume increases, work against elastic recoil increases. Above about 60 percent of VC (Fig. 7-7A), chest and lung recoil both oppose inspiration; the work required to expand them then increases markedly, due to the alinearity of the Pst(l) and Pst(w) curves. At low lung volumes, considerable muscle force is needed to continue expiration against the increasing recoil of the chest cage. During heavy physical exercise, tidal volume rarely exceeds 50 percent of the VC, probably largely because both volume extremes, near TLC and near RV, require too much work. When ventilation is increased through higher breathing rates, work against flow-resistive forces increases. Here, too, the relation between increased flow and increased work is alinear so that considerable energy is required to increase flows to high values (Chap. 8). Thus, extreme values of tidal volume and rate both greatly increase the work of breathing. During spontaneous breathing, tidal volume and rate values keep respiratory work near a minimum.[58] The adjustment may include setting the rate at a value which also corresponds to minimum muscle force.[51] (See, however, Chap. 10.) Work is a complex result of the forces, but the optimal breathing rates for minimum force and work are similar, and neither optimum is sharply defined.

MAXIMUM STATIC PRESSURES

The physiological limits of the pressure-volume diagram are reached when maximum inspiratory and expiratory pressures are exerted against a closed airway (Fig. 7-9). These limits are set by the force of the respiratory muscles and

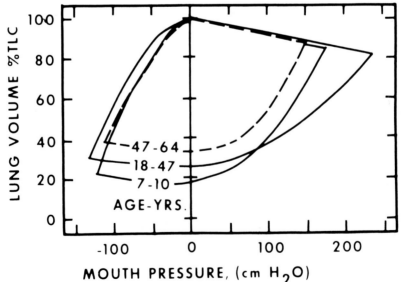

Fig. 7-9. Average maximum inspiratory and expiratory pressures in men of different ages. From reference 23.

the configuration of the chest cage. Near maximum inspiration, the expiratory muscles are stretched and can exert their maximum force. Even at low lung volumes, they can still generate considerable pressure. Optimal conditions for inspiratory muscle contraction exist at lung volumes near RV. As lung volume increases, inspiratory muscle force decreases. In part, this is because the shorter the muscle, the less force it can develop. The muscles probably also work at a mechanical disadvantage near TLC, and contraction of antagonists (particularly abdominal muscles) may further limit their force.

Children can develop high static pressures,[23] and inspiratory pressures can reach 40 to 80 cm H_2O during the newborn's first few breaths.[5] People who use a snorkel during swimming use high inspiratory pressures, too. Prolonged breathing at increased negative pressures in the chest can cause transudation of water from lung blood vessels and may lead to lung edema. Prolonged high expiratory pressures (e.g., during straining movements or when playing wind instruments) may lead to fainting,[29] since the high pressure in the chest hinders venous return of blood to the heart. During exercise, even when ventilation rates are high, the pressures remain below their maximum values.

The large muscle-reserve power permits adequate ventilation even when the muscles are weakened or partially paralyzed. Determination of maximum static pressures is useful to detect respiratory muscle weakness. Since less than maximal pressures are used when performing forced vital capacity maneuvers, VC and expiratory flow rates may be normal while maximum pressures are too low because of muscle weakness.[10]

Breathing efforts against a closed airway do not perform ventilatory work, although the lungs and chest may undergo marked volume changes. The work done in compressing and decompressing gas in the lungs during such maneuvers can be measured with a body plethysmograph.[13] When the airways are partially obstructed, work is spent on gas compression and decompression to the extent that pressures in alveoli behind obstructed airways lag behind those elsewhere. Patients with severe airway obstruction exert considerable effort to breathe, and a large part of this effort is used to generate high alveolar pressures that result in only small flow rates. In such patients, the volume excursions of the chest may be pronounced although tidal volume measured at the mouth may be small. Thus, the observation of chest movements may be misleading.

LIMITS OF INSPIRATION AND EXPIRATION

The limits of maximum inspiratory and expiratory excursions are set by the size of the lungs and chest and by a combination of mechanical factors.

TLC. Near maximum inspiration, compliance of lungs and chest decreases (they become stiffer), while inspiratory muscle force decreases.[56] The limit is reached when the net maximum inspiratory force just balances the combined recoil of lungs and chest. When lung recoil decreases (as in emphysema), the same muscle force can increase volume more; hence, TLC is often increased in emphysema. In addition, long-standing increases in the work of breathing required in emphysema might lead to training of inspiratory muscles; one may speculate that increased inspiratory muscle force may also contribute to increases in TLC.

RV. Near maximum expiration, the alveoli begin to collapse, folding like an accordion (data from cat lungs [17]), but at the end of a maximally forced expiration, the alveoli retain about 20 percent of TLC, the residual volume (RV, Fig. 7-1). Several variables determine whether maximum voluntary expiration is terminated by alveolar collapse,[17] airway closure,[71] or inability to decrease chest cage volume further.[51] Elastic recoil of the chest may set the limit in young persons; their expiratory muscles are unable to compress the chest further, but pressure applied from outside can do so.[51] Contraction of the diaphragm may decrease net muscle force near RV.[4] In older persons and in smokers, airway closure becomes the predominant limiting factor. The two mechanisms—airway closure versus chest recoil and muscle force—can be distinguished from the pattern of MEFV curves (Chap. 9).

In experimental studies, the pressure needed to close small bronchioles is similar to that required to collapse alveoli.[10] Which ones close first depends on the way the lungs are deflated.[20] In dog lungs, airways of about 0.5 mm diameter are likely to close before larger ones;[41] in cat lungs, however, terminal bronchioles, although narrowed and kinked, were not fully closed at low lung volume.[48] Indirect evidence in man suggests that relatively large airways (about 1 mm diameter) may be closed at RV; this results in air trapping, which can be demonstrated by washout of N_2.[16]

CLINICAL APPLICATIONS

The esophageal balloon method for estimating Ppl has been used in many clinical studies on lung elastic recoil. To interpret these data accurately, one should measure thoracic gas volume with a body plethysmograph, so that Pst(l) data can be referred to lung volume in absolute terms.

Airway Obstruction

Measurements of Pst(l), an important driving force for expiratory airflow (Chap. 8), can be used to interpret changes in airway resistance in patients with airway obstruction. In some patients, elastic recoil is normal while resistances are high, suggesting that the obstruction is caused by changes in the airways themselves (smooth muscle contraction, mucus accumulation, mucosal swelling). In other patients, loss of elastic recoil and the concomitant loss of structural support for the small airways can explain the degree of airway obstruction inferred from measurements of flow rates and airway resistance. Different types of pressure-volume-resistance relations have been described in small groups of patients with airway obstruction in the presence of similar values for conventional spirometric measurements.[46] In hemp workers with byssinosis and ventilatory insufficiency, Pst(l) correlated significantly with maximum expiratory flow rates.[36] This suggested that the abnormally low flow rates in these persons were caused, in part, by loss of lung elastic recoil. Thus, measurements of Pst(l) can be used to assess the contribution of reduced elastic recoil to airway obstruction caused by emphysematous lesions.

Emphysema

Loss of elastic lung recoil is a prime feature of the emphysematous lung. The slope of the pressure-volume curve is steep compared to normal, indicating increased lung compliance. Even at maximum inflation, the lungs exert little recoil pressure (Fig. 7-10). Although a low transpulmonary pressure at TLC indicates emphysema,[53] the overlap between normal and abnormal values is considerable, rendering lesser degrees of emphysema undetectable with this method.[46] A genetic abnormality, α_1-antitrypsin deficiency, is associated with an early onset of severe emphysema in young persons.[28] Intermediate degrees of this enzyme deficiency have been attributed to heterozygosity for the relevant gene. Such heterozygous persons have lower Pst(l) values after age 30 than control subjects,[61] which suggests that the more common heterozygous enzyme deficiency may lead to clinical emphysema at a later age.

Lesions similar to those in human emphysema can be produced experimentally in animals with papain, a proteolytic enzyme,[63] and with DL-penicillamine, an agent that inhibits cross-linking between collagen and elastin.[18, 37, 38] Papain acts

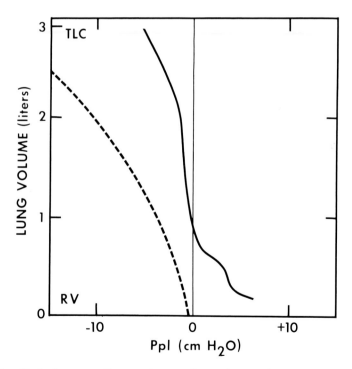

Fig. 7-10. Static lung recoil curve in a patient with emphysema (*drawn curve*) compared to typical normal curve in same volume range (*dashed line*). Static recoil pressure in the patient is minimal even when the lungs are maximally inflated. Lung volume scale in liters above RV.

on the short term, while DL-penicillamine must be administered for 2 or more weeks. The effects of these agents include dilatation of terminal air spaces, increased compliance at small lung volume, and decreased elastic recoil pressures. Such changes also occur in human emphysema, but it is not yet known whether the mode of action of papain or penicillamine is similar to the pathogenetic mechanisms in emphysema. (See also p. 164.)

Asthma

Patients with bronchial asthma (See also Chap. 18) often breathe at increased end-expiratory breathing levels. When data obtained during an asthmatic state were compared with data obtained in a symptom-free interval, several studies [30, 35] showed discreet shifts in the static recoil curves of asthmatic patients, in the sense of decreased elastic recoil. The mechanisms of this change are not clear. In part, it may result from changes in the reference volume: when airway obstruction is severe, the body plethysmograph may slightly overestimate TGV.[12] However, a similar phenomenon has been induced in animals. Pst(l) was decreased and TLC increased in dogs that breathed for 2 weeks with an increased end-expiratory pressure (10–15 cm H_2O). Since liquid-filling of the excised lungs showed no change in pressure-volume curves, the major effect appeared to be on the recoil of the alveolar surface film.[14] In excised dog lungs, a decrease of Pst(l) was induced after only 2–3 hours ventilation at end-expiratory pressure of +7 cm H_2O.[70] Thus, it appears that breathing at increased lung volumes, whether induced by asthma or by breathing against an external expiratory resistance, causes loss of lung recoil. Recovery of recoil pressure in asthma appears to be slow; there is no rapid reversal to normal after isoproterenol or other dilator drugs. The loss of recoil in asthma can account for some decrease of expiratory flow rates and is perhaps one reason why flow rates often remain at slightly less than normal levels for some time, even during adequate drug treatment.

Other Conditions

In *mitral stenosis,* Pst(l) is low at low lung volumes (probably because of vascular congestion) and high near TLC, perhaps due to lung fibrosis.[78] In *obesity,* chest wall compliance is low and the work of breathing is increased;[60] this can explain the reduced vital capacity of obese persons.

SUMMARY

The movements of the chest cage during breathing transmit forces through the pleural space to the lungs, which passively follow all volume changes of the chest cage. The force required to distend the lungs during inspiration is determined by the viscoelastic behavior of lung tissue, which in turn depends on the extensibility of the elastic and collagen fiber network in the lungs. The elastic recoil of the lungs [Pst(l)] can be measured from a pressure-volume curve recorded during stepwise expirations from TLC, relating pleural pressure to lung volume. The elastic recoil of the chest cage [Pst(w)] can be measured from a similar curve recorded during muscular relaxation at different lung volumes. Pst(l) and Pst(w) curves together can be used to determine alveolar pressure and the net pressure developed by the respiratory muscles and to analyze the work of breathing. Maximum pressures developed during forceful inspiration and expiration against a closed airway indicate the limits of respiratory muscle force. The limits of lung volume excursions are set by muscle force, by the size of chest and lungs, by their compliance and, at low lung volumes, by alveolar collapse or airway closure. In patients with lung disease, such as emphysema or airway obstruction, Pst(l) measurements are used to assess the role of lung elastic recoil in reducing lung function.

REFERENCES

1. Agostoni E: Mechanics of the pleural space. Physiol Rev 52:57–128, 1972
2. Agostoni E, D'Angelo E, Roncoroni G: The thickness of the pleural liquid. Respir Physiol 5:1–13, 1968
3. Agostoni E, Mead J: Statics of the respiratory system, in Fenn WO, Rahn H (eds): Handbook of Physiology, Section 3: Respiration, vol I. Washington, D.C., American Physiological Society, 1964, pp 387–409
4. Agostoni E, Sant'Ambrogio G, del Portillo Carrasco H: Electromyography of the diaphragm in man and transdiaphragmatic pressure. J Appl Physiol 15:1093–1097, 1960
5. Avery ME, Wang N-S, Taeusch HW Jr: The lung of the newborn infant; a disorder of prematurity is combatted. Sci Am 228:74–85, 1973
6. Bachofen H, Hildebrandt J: Area analysis of pressure-volume hysteresis in mammalian lungs. J Appl Physiol 30:493–497, 1971
7. Bachofen H, Hildebrandt J, Bachofen M: Pressure-volume curves of air- and liquid-filled excised lungs—surface tension in situ. J Appl Physiol 29:422–31, 1970
8. Bartlett D Jr: Origin and regulation of spontaneous deep breaths. Respir Physiol 12:230–238, 1971
9. Bevan C, McKerrow CB, Morgan EJ: A method of measuring pulmonary compliance without an oesophageal tube. J Physiol (Lond) 217:10P–11P, 1971
10. Black LF, Hyatt RE: Maximal static respiratory pressures in generalized neuromuscular disease. Am Rev Respir Dis 103:641–650, 1971
11. Bouhuys A: Airflow control by auditory feedback; respiratory mechanics and wind instruments. Science 154:797–799, 1966
12. Bouhuys A, Hunt VR, Kim BM, Zapletal A: Maximum expiratory flow rates in induced bronchoconstriction in man. J Clin Invest 48:1159–1168, 1969
13. Bouhuys A, Proctor DF, Mead J: Kinetic aspects of singing. J Appl Physiol 21:483–496, 1966
14. Buhain WJ, Brody JS, Fisher AB: Effect of artificial airway obstruction on elastic properties of the lung. J Appl Physiol 33:589–594, 1972
15. Bull HB: Protein structure and elasticity, in Remington JW (ed): Tissue Elasticity. Washington, D.C., American Physiological Society, 1957, pp 33–42
16. Burger EJ Jr, Macklem PT: Airway closure: demonstration by breathing 100% O_2 at low lung volumes and by N_2 washout. J Appl Physiol 25:139–148, 1968
17. But VI: Contraction of smooth muscle of the bronchial tree and its effects on hysteresis of the lungs. Bul Exp Biol Med (USSR) 73:11–13, 1972
18. Caldwell EJ, Bland JH: The effect of penicillamine on the rabbit lung. Am Rev Respir Dis 105:75–84, 1972
19. Campbell EJM, Agostoni E, Newsom Davis J: The Respiratory Muscles: Mechanics and Neural Control. London, Lloyd-Luke, 1970

20. Cavagna GA, Stemmler EJ, DuBois AB: Alveolar resistance to atelectasis. J Appl Physiol 22:441–452, 1967

21. Cherniack RM, Farhi LE, Armstrong BW, Proctor DF: A comparison of esophageal and intrapleural pressure in man. J Appl Physiol 8:203–211, 1955

22. Colebatch HJH, Mitchell CA: Constriction of isolated living liquid-filled dog and cat lungs with histamine. J Appl Physiol 30:691–702, 1971

23. Cook CD, Mead J, Orzalesi MM: Static volume-pressure characteristics of the respiratory system during maximal efforts. J Appl Physiol 19:1016–1022, 1964

24. D'Angelo E, Michelini S, Agostoni E: Partition of factors contributing to the vertical gradient of transpulmonary pressure. Respir Physiol 12:90–101, 1971

25. Defares JG, Donleben PG: Relationship between frequency-dependent compliance and unequal ventilation. J Appl Physiol 15:166–169, 1960

26. Douglas JS, Dennis MW, Ridgway P, Bouhuys A: Airway dilatation and constriction in spontaneously breathing guinea pigs. J Pharmacol Exp Ther 180: 98–109, 1972

27. Einthoven W: Der Donders'sche Druck und die Gasspannungen in der Pleurahöhle. Pfluegers Arch 44:152–174, 1888

28. Eriksson S: Studies of alpha$_1$-antitrypsin deficiency. Acta Med Scand 177 (suppl 432): 1–85, 1965

29. Faulkner M, Sharpey-Schafer EP: Circulatory effects of trumpet playing. Br Med J 1:685–686, 1959

30. Finucane KE, Colebatch HJH: Elastic behavior of the lung in patients with airway obstruction. J Appl Physiol 26: 330–338, 1969

31. Fisher MJ, Wilson MF, Weber KC: Determination of alveolar surface area and tension from in situ pressure-volume data. Respir Physiol 10:159–171, 1970

32. Forrest JB: The effect of changes in lung volume on the size and shape of alveoli. J Physiol (Lond) 210:533–547, 1970

33. Fukaya H, Martin CJ, Young AC, Katsura S: Mechanical properties of alveolar walls. J Appl Physiol 25:689–695, 1968

34. Glogowska M, Richardson PS, Widdicombe JG, Winning AJ: The role of the vagus nerves, peripheral chemoreceptors and other afferent pathways in the genesis of augmented breaths in cats and rabbits. Respir Physiol 16:179–196, 1972

35. Gold WM, Kaufman HS, Nadel JA: Elastic recoil of the lungs in chronic asthmatic patients before and after therapy. J Appl Physiol 23:433–438, 1967

36. Guyatt AR, Douglas JS, Zuskin E, Bouhuys A: Lung static recoil and airway obstruction in hemp workers with byssinosis. Am Rev Respir Dis 108:1111–1115, 1973

37. Hoffman L, Blumenfeld OO, Mondshine RB, Park SS: Effect of DL-penicillamine on fibrous proteins of rat lung. J Appl Physiol 33:42–46, 1972

38. Hoffman L, Mondshine RB, Park SS: Effect of DL-penicillamine on elastic properties of rat lung. J Appl Physiol 30:508–511, 1971

39. Horie T, Hildebrandt J: Dynamic compliance, limit cycles and static equilibria of excised cat lung. J Appl Physiol 31: 423–430, 1971

40. Hughes JMB, Rosenzweig DY: Factors affecting trapped gas volume in perfused dog lungs. J Appl Physiol 29:332–339, 1970

41. Hughes JMB, Rosenzweig DY, Kivitz PB: Site of airway closure in excised dog lungs: histologic demonstration. J Appl Physiol 29:340–344, 1970

42. Ingram RH Jr, Schilder DP: Association of a decrease in dynamic compliance with a change in gas distribution. J Appl Physiol 23:911–916, 1967

43. Jaeger MJ, Otis AB: Effects of compressibility of alveolar gas on dynamics and work of breathing. J Appl Physiol 19:83–91, 1964

44. Jonson B: A flow-regulating valve for use in respiratory physiology. Scand J Clin Lab Invest 24:127–130, 1969

45. Jonson B: Pulmonary mechanics in normal men, studied with the flow regulator method. Scand J Clin Lab Invest 25: 363–373, 1970

46. Jonson B: Pulmonary mechanics in patients with pulmonary disease, studied with the flow regulator method. Scand J Clin Lab Invest 25:375–390, 1970

47. Klingele TG, Staub NC: Alveolar shape changes with volume in isolated, air-filled lobes of cat lung. J Appl Physiol 28:411–414, 1970

48. Klingele TG, Staub NC: Terminal bronchiole diameter changes with volume in isolated, air-filled lobes of cat lung. J Appl Physiol 30:224–227, 1971

49. Konno K, Mead J: Static volume-pressure characteristics of the rib cage and abdomen. J Appl Physiol 24:544–548, 1968

50. Landowne M, Stacy RW: Glossary of Terms, in Remington JW (ed): Tissue Elasticity. Washington, D. C., American Physiological Society, 1957, pp 191–201

51. Leith DE, Mead J: Mechanisms determining residual volume of the lungs in normal subjects. J Appl Physiol 23:221–227, 1967

52. Liljestrand G: Untersuchungen über die Atmungsarbeit. Skand Arch Physiol 35:199–293, 1918

53. Macklem PT, Becklake MR: The relationship between the mechanical and diffusing properties of the lung in health and disease. Am Rev Respir Dis 87:47–56, 1963

54. Mead J: Control of respiratory frequency. J Appl Physiol 15:325–336, 1960

55. Mead J: Mechanical properties of lungs. Physiol Rev 41:281–330, 1961

56. Mead J, Milic-Emili J, Turner JM: Factors limiting depth of a maximal inspiration in human subjects. J Appl Physiol 18:295–296, 1963

57. Mead J, Takishima T, Leith D: Stress distribution in lungs: a model of pulmonary elasticity. J Appl Physiol 28:596–608, 1970

58. McIlroy MB, Marshall R, Christie RV: The work of breathing in normal subjects. Clin Sci 13:127–136, 1954

59. Milic-Emili J, Mead J, Turner JM, Glauser EM: Improved technique for estimating pleural pressure from esophageal balloons. J Appl Physiol 19:207–211, 1964

60. Naimark A, Cherniack RM: Compliance of the respiratory system and its components in health and obesity. J Appl Physiol 15:377–382, 1960

61. Ostrow DN, Cherniack RM: The mechanical properties of the lungs in intermediate deficiency of α_1-Antitrypsin. Am Rev Respir Dis 106:377–383, 1972

62. Otis AB: The work of breathing, in Fenn WO, Rahn H (eds): Handbook of Physiology, Section 3: Respiration, vol I. Washington, D.C., American Physiological Society, 1964, pp 463–476

63. Park SS, Goldring IP, Shim CS, Williams MH Jr: Mechanical properties of the lung in experimental pulmonary emphysema. J Appl Physiol 26:738–744, 1969

64. Pierce JA: Tensile strength of human lung. J Lab Clin Med 66:652–658, 1965

65. Pierce JA, Ebert RV: Fibrous network of the lung and its change with age. Thorax 20:469–476, 1965

66. Pratt PC: Intrapulmonary radial traction: Measurement, magnitude and mechanics, in Bouhuys A (ed): Airway Dynamics: Physiology and Pharmacology. Springfield, Charles C Thomas Publisher, 1970, pp 109–122

67. Proctor DF, Caldini P, Permutt S: The pressure surrounding the lungs. Respir Physiol 5:130–144, 1968

68. Radford E Jr: Recent studies of mechanical properties of mammalian lungs, in Remington JW (ed): Tissue Elasticity. Washington, D.C., American Physiological Society, 1957, pp 177–190

69. Rahn H, Otis AB, Chadwick LE, Fenn WO: The pressure-volume diagram of the thorax and lung. Am J Physiol 146:161–178, 1946

70. Raimondi AC, Massarella GR, Pride NB: The effects of ventilation on the elastic recoil of excised dogs' lungs. Respir Physiol 12:205–217, 1971

71. Slagter B, Heemstra H: Limiting factors of expiration in normal subjects. Acta Physiol Pharmacol Neerl 4:419–421, 1955

72. Sugihara T, Hildebrandt J, Martin CJ: Viscoelastic properties of alveolar wall. J Appl Physiol 33:93–98, 1972

73. Trop D, Peeters R, van de Woestijne KP: Localization of recording site in the esophagus by means of cardiac artifacts. J Appl Physiol 29:283–287, 1970

74. Turner JM, Mead J, Wohl ME: Elasticity of human lungs in relation to age. J Appl Physiol 25:664–671, 1968

75. van de Woestijne KP: Influence of forced inflations on the creep of lungs and thorax in the dog. Respir Physiol 3:78–89, 1967

76. West JB: Distribution of mechanical stress in the lung, a possible factor in localisation of pulmonary disease. Lancet 1:839–841, 1971

77. West JB, Matthews FL: Stresses, strains, and surface pressures in the lung caused by its weight. J Appl Physiol 32:332–345, 1972

78. Wood TE, McLeod P, Anthonisen NR, Macklem PT: Mechanics of breathing in mitral stenosis. Am Rev Respir Dis 104:52–60, 1971

79. Woolcock AJ, Vincent NJ, Macklem PT: Frequency dependence of compliance as a test for obstruction in the small airways. J Clin Invest 48:1097–1106, 1969

Chapter 8

Pressure-Flow Relations

Airflow through the airways requires a driving pressure generated by changes in alveolar pressure (Chap. 7). When alveolar pressure is less than atmospheric pressure and the airways are open, air flows in; when Palv is greater than Patm, air flows out. In this chapter we relate Palv to the resulting flows and discuss variables that influence these relations.

PHYSICS OF AIRFLOW

Flow Patterns

Airflow patterns through tubes can be laminar or turbulent; special patterns arise when tube diameter varies (orifice flow) and when the tube branches (Fig. 8-1). In long, straight, smooth-walled, rigid cylindrical tubes, airflow increases in proportion to driving pressure (Fig. 8-2A). But when flow increases, this relationship changes and becomes alinear because flow becomes turbulent beyond a limit set by the Reynolds' number—a dimensionless value that depends upon the linear velocity of the gas, the radius of the tube, and the properties of the gas. Linear gas velocity ($\dot{v}$) relates to $\dot{V}$ (flow rate) and the cross-sectional area of the tube:

$$\dot{V} = \dot{v} \cdot A \qquad (1)$$

In the bronchial tree, total cross-sectional area increases greatly toward the periphery (Table 2-1); since flow through each cross section is constant, linear gas velocity decreases and conditions for laminar flow improve.

In the *upper airways,* the complex geometry causes flow patterns that do not fit any of the types shown in Figure 8-1.[25] In the *bronchial tree,* the predominant pattern varies with size (Chap. 3, p. 47): turbulence in trachea and large bronchi,[42] laminar flow in smaller bronchi (down to the 12th generation, approximately), and convective block flow and axial diffusion in the smallest airways. Other patterns

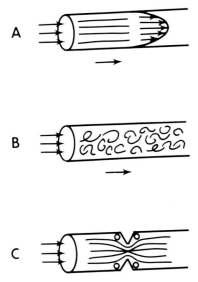

Fig. 8-1. Airflow patterns. *A.* Laminar flow. A flat gas front at the tube entrance is converted to a parabolic velocity front at a point several diameters removed from the entrance of the tube. Length of arrows is proportional to linear gas velocity. Energy is lost in friction between layers of gas; layers nearer to the wall are increasingly slowed down. All molecules move in the direction of flow. *B.* Turbulent flow. Due to increased velocity and a high Reynolds' number, the layers of moving gas (in *A*) have broken up. Gas molecules move in all directions through the lumen of the tube causing extra energy loss. Because of the direction of the driving pressure, there is net motion of gas in the direction of the arrow. *C.* Orifice flow. Gas velocities increase as the lumen of the tube narrows. Vortices may develop in the corners as indicated. In the orifice, kinetic energy of the gas (mv^2) increases and lateral pressure (potential energy) decreases.

are, however, superimposed on these. Vortices, which develop during inspiration and expiration (Fig. 8-3),[52] help mix the gas streams through the cross section of the tubes. In the branchings, the flow profile changes, to a large extent independently of the incoming flow profile (i.e., flat or parabolic). Velocity in the branches is greater near the inside walls (Fig. 8-3). Some authors consider the effect of the branches so important that they see the bronchial tree "as a series of interconnected junctions rather than as a series of branched tubes." [52]

Energy Losses

The relation between driving pressure and flow in tubes depends on the flow pattern. Thus, study of energy losses during flow gives indirect information on the flow pattern. During laminar, or Poiseuille, flow the driving pressure is dissipated in friction between moving layers of air and converted to heat. Airways do not fulfill the strict requirements of laminar flow conditions: they are short, branched, elastic, not quite straight, with uneven wall surfaces, and are not always cylindrical. These deviations from ideal tubes lead to extra losses of energy, in what Rohrer called "extra resistances." [51] Consequently, flow increments decrease as driving pressure increases; the $P\text{-}\dot{V}$ relations are curvilinear (Fig. 8-2B).

Laminar flow depends on gas viscosity, while energy losses in vortices, turbulence, and other flow patterns that deviate from laminar flow are influenced by gas density. Since departures from laminar flow are more pronounced in large than in small airways, gas density affects flow through the former more than flow through the latter (see also Chap. 9, p. 179).

In *upper airways* (airway opening to trachea) air flows through channels of relatively fixed geometry (except during speech). The nose is a high-resistance

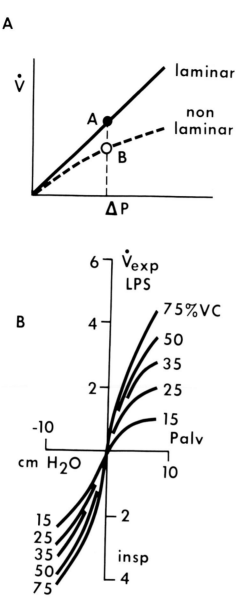

Fig. 8-2. *A.* Linear pressure-flow relation during laminar flow; alinear relation during nonlaminar flow (i.e., turbulence, orifice flow, branching or vortices, etc.). The same driving pressure ΔP yields higher flows during laminar (A) than during nonlaminar (B) flow. *B.* Pressure-flow relations in airways depend on lung volume during inspiration (left lower quadrant) and expiration (right upper quadrant). $\dot{V}_{insp}$ and $\dot{V}_{exp}$ are inspiratory and expiratory flow rates, respectively; Palv=alveolar pressure. From reference 4.

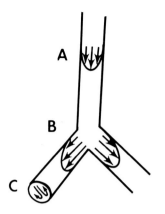

Fig. 8-3. In the daughter branches, a parabolic velocity front (A) is converted to an asymmetrical front with high velocities near the inside wall (B). Vortices also develop (C). Modified from reference 52.

pathway, the mouth a low-resistance one. When the pressure drop across the nasal passages exceeds about 4 cm H_2O, healthy persons begin to breathe through their mouths.[45] Even during mouth breathing, about 50 percent of the total energy loss during breathing (in terms of pressure drop) occurs in the upper airways. Some of this loss is caused by redirection of flow in the pharynx; another part is due to the resistance of the glottal opening to flow. For unclear reasons, both total upper-airway resistance and laryngeal resistance depend on lung volume, increasing as lung volume decreases.[55] Typical pressure drops for 1 liter/sec flow are 0.83 cm H_2O from mouth to trachea, and 0.31 cm H_2O across the larynx, both during quiet breathing at mid-lung volume.[55] The size of the glottal opening decreases with decreasing lung volume and flow rates; it is widest during panting. The mechanisms affecting glottal opening are not clear.[56]

In the *bronchial tree,* about 75 percent of the pressure drop is spent on changing the flow profiles, e.g., from flow with a uniform velocity ("flat front") to a parabolic front.[41] The branches per se and the change in cross-sectional area each account for about 10 percent of the total pressure drop. These losses are not equal in all generations; the largest pressure drop (80 percent of the total) occurs in the first 4 to 6 airway generations, i.e., in the trachea and large bronchi.[41, 47] As air enters the trachea through the narrow glottal chink, secondary turbulences are created in the upper part of the trachea.[42] Otherwise, turbulent flow is not an important source of energy loss. The actual pressure drops are less than would be calculated for turbulent flow; factors related to airway geometry are more important sources of energy loss.[41] During inspiration, gas velocities decrease as gas enters smaller airways with a large total cross-sectional area (divergent flow); during expiration, velocities increase as gas leaves the bronchial tree (convergent flow). The energy losses due to these changes in the kinetic energy of the gas stream are small but increase with flow rate.[23, 41]

Energy losses during flow, other than those in the gas itself, are caused by viscous properties of tissues and by the presence of mucus in airways. Energy losses due to acceleration of the *chest wall* are negligible in healthy persons and are increased in obesity, where they conceivably may limit maximum flows and cough velocities.[53] Viscous losses in *lung tissue* depend more on tidal volume and breathing level than on flow rate.[3] Therefore, lung tissue resistance is in fact a consequence of tissue hysteresis (p. 124). *Airway mucus* is a source of extra energy loss when the thickness of the mucus layer exceeds 300 μm.[12] The shearing forces between air and liquid then agitate the liquid when flow increases, leading to roughness of the liquid surface or even eddies of liquid that may move through the lumen. When this happens, the pressure drop increases sharply since it then depends on the force to move the liquid rather than the air (Fig. 8-4). The liquid's physical properties affect these events: a layer of thin liquid is more easily disturbed than a more tenacious mucus layer. This is an important source of energy loss whenever bronchial secretions are increased, as in bronchitis.

Pressure-Flow Relations

Since energy losses in airways are larger than would be expected if flow were laminar, pressure-flow curves are alinear (Fig. 8-2B). Calculations of pressure drops based on the assumption of laminar flow throughout the bronchial tree [20] yield smaller pressure drops than those actually observed. Equations that correct for nonparabolic flow profiles are more accurate [47] and also account for changes

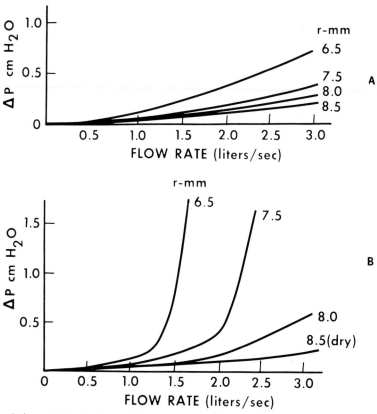

Fig. 8-4. *A, B. Ordinate:* driving pressure for airflow through tubes of different caliber. *Abscissa:* flow rate. The parameter (r) is the radius of several dry tubes (*A*) and the effective radius of a dry tube of 8.5 mm radius in which the caliber is reduced by layers of liquid of varying thickness (*B*). When waves appear in the liquid, resistance increases abruptly. From reference 12.

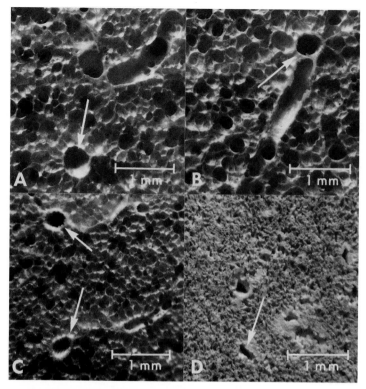

Fig. 8-5. Terminal bronchioles (*arrows*) in freeze-dried cat lungs. Lung volume: *A*, 100%; *B*, 48%; *C*, 23%; *D*, 8% of maximal lobe volume. Airway caliber decreases with lung volume. At the lowest volume (*D*), the terminal bronchioles are thick-walled and kinked but not closed. From reference 29.

in pressure drops when gases of different densities are breathed.[25] Especially in the first 10 airway generations, pressure drops are much greater than would be expected from laminar flow predictions.

Airway caliber increases with lung volume (Fig. 8-5). Therefore, P-$\dot{V}$ relations cannot be described by a single curve but rather by a family of curves, with lung volume as the parameter (Fig. 8-2*B*). At low driving pressures, inspired and expired flows are similar; as they increase, the P-$\dot{V}$ curves for inspiration and expiration diverge. Inspiratory flow continues to increase to a limit set mainly by the ability of the inspiratory muscles to contract rapidly (p. 168). Alveolar and pleural pressures are increasingly subatmospheric during inspiration. Hence, the airways in the chest are exposed to an increasing pull on their outside walls, transmitted through the elastic structure of the lungs and through the pleural space. During expiration, however, alveolar and pleural pressures increase, and Ppl exceeds Patm during fast expirations (Fig. 7-7*C*). The high pressures in the chest cage lead to dynamic compression of airways, which narrows them and limits further increases of expiratory flow.

FORCED EXPIRATION

Dynamic Compression

During forced expiration, airway geometry changes radically. A large segment of the trachea and bronchi in the chest cage is compressed when flow is high (hence "dynamic") due to the high pleural pressures that are developed to generate high alveolar pressures. This phenomenon has been described since 1892 (reference 5 gives a historical survey), but accurate observations have only been made recently. The compressed airway segment may occupy several generations of large intrathoracic airways, and its length varies. At large lung volumes the compressed airway segment is short; its length increases as lung volume decreases. It is important to realize that dynamic compression is a physiologic event occurring in all healthy persons during forced expirations and cough maneuvers.

The anatomical extent of dynamic compression can be seen during bronchoscopy or in suitably timed x-ray films of airways lined with contrast medium. The speed at which flow and pressures change during dynamic compression can be shown with the body plethysmograph (Fig. 8-6), which records the sudden compression of alveolar gas that occurs when its pressure rises.[54] When lung volume is known, Palv can be calculated. Near the end of a forced expiration, alveolar pressure increases sharply and suddenly, while airflow decreases. In about 0.2 seconds (between lines *b* and *c* in Fig. 8-6), Palv increases from about +10 to +25 cm H₂O. These events reflect the onset of dynamic compression of large airways.

Models of Pressure-Flow Relations

During forced expiration, dynamic compression is a predominant factor in determining pressure-flow relations, while other factors, such as the effect of branching, become relatively less important. Thus, the altered airway geometry markedly changes the pressure-flow relations from those during quiet breathing.

During dynamic compression of large airways, expiratory flow reaches maximum values, and P-$\dot{V}$ curves therefore show plateaus—further pressure increases do not yield flow increments (see Fig. 8-10*A*). Many variables that affect flow through airways cannot be measured directly (caliber, length, muscle tone, thickness of mucus layer). Analysis of theoretical models allows one to vary these factors one at a time and to examine the effect of each on simulated flow. In this way, hypotheses concerning airflow dynamics can be formulated and compared with experimental data obtained on the total system. Unfortunately, since many variables needed in model studies have been insufficiently quantitated, the results must be interpreted with caution.

Several formal models [17, 44, 60] include a precise description of the system, in simple or complex form, suitable for insertion of experimental data. These models are complete in the sense that they offer a mathematical description of the system. All assumptions and simplifications made in the model design can be clearly defined. Less complete, more intuitive models concentrate on specific character-

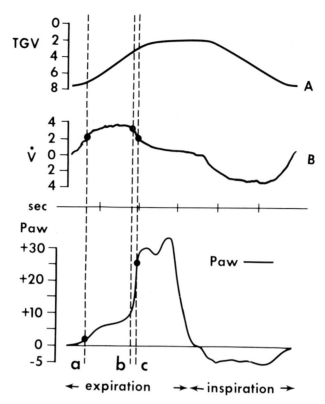

Fig. 8-6. *Upper panel.* From top down, thoracic gas volume (*A*) and airflow rate at mouth (*B*). *Lower panel.* Pressure across airways (alveoli-mouth, Paw, cm H_2O) measured with body plethysmograph. *Abscissa.* Time in seconds. During *inspiration*, the pressure (Paw) and flow (*B*) traces are similar in shape; pressure and flow change in the same direction. During *expiration* this is only true in the initial phase (*a–b*). From *b* to *c*, pressure (Paw) increases sharply, while flow rate decreases. This reflects the onset of dynamic compression of large airways. Modified from reference 6.

istics of the system and use these to derive a theory concerning the whole.[34, 50] Each of these models illustrates important physiological principles.

Many features of pressure-flow curves can be explained with a simple model of airway geometry (Fig. 8-7).[60] The peripheral airways, suspended without cartilage in the structure of the lungs, are represented by a distal airway segment (1); its resistance to flow is a function of lung volume.[29] The intermediate segment (2) is dynamically compressed during forced expirations, and has a resistance determined primarily by the pressure difference across its walls. Finally, the upper airways form a proximal segment (3) with a fixed resistance. In this model[60] the critical variable is the pressure at which segment 2 begins to compress, or the critical transmural pressure, Ptm'.[50] With different values of Ptm', the model predicts many physiological features of pressure-flow relations. Palv is the independent variable that drives the model. Although the model is simple, it can simulate the main features of IVPF curves (p. 156) and MEFV curves (Chap. 9), and it allows qualitative estimates of effects of airway obstruction and loss of lung recoil force.

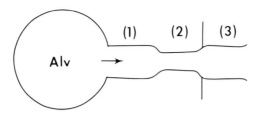

Fig. 8-7. Simple model of expiratory airflow. See text for description of segments 1, 2, and 3. A formal description of this model has been given by Yamabayashi et al.[60]

A much more complex model [44] calculates pressure drops associated with flow based on airway geometry, gas properties, and energy losses in airways. It simulates IVPF and MEFV curves more accurately than the simple model of Figure 8-7. As in other models, lung elastic recoil and airway wall compliance are the main variables affecting pressure-flow relations during forced expirations. Also, beyond a critical driving pressure, corresponding to the pressure at which maximum flows are reached, airways become unstable in this model.[44]

In Fry's model [17] the precise description of transmural stress across the airway walls is crucial in determining the pressure-flow relations. In particular the final configuration of the compliant airways is important, as shown for plastic tubes in Figure 8-8. If the tube closes at infinitely high pressures (1 in Fig. 8-8), the P-$\dot{V}$ curve reaches a plateau. If the tube does not close completely at any pressure, flow first levels off to a plateau, but as driving pressure increases further, flow resumes its increase; this represents flow through a maximally narrowed tube which cannot be further compressed (2 in Fig. 8-8). Finally, if the tube closes at a finite compressing pressure (3 in Fig. 8-8), flow reaches a maximum and then becomes unstable. When the tube closes, flow stops; as a result, dynamic compression is reduced and flow resumes. Hence, airflow oscillates, and conditions in the tube depend on time as an additional variable. Experimental data in man have also suggested unstable airway behavior during maximum flow,[6] similar to that of the plastic tube of Figure 8-8, 3.

Equal Pressure Point Theory

In the airways, pressure decreases in the direction of flow. During expiration at high flow rates, somewhere inside the airways the pressure must equal Ppl (Fig. 8-9). This is because Palv is always greater than Ppl by the amount of Pst(l) (Eq. 7-2, p. 127). The pressure difference between the alveoli and the equal pressure point (EPP) equals Palv – Ppl = Pst(l). Hence, the driving pressure for flow from alveoli to the EPP equals the static lung recoil pressure.[34] The flow rate through the upstream airway segment (U in Fig. 8-9) must equal flow through the downstream segment (D) and the upper airways because the three are in series. Since the model applies to conditions of maximum flow, this flow rate equals $\dot{V}_{max}$. Therefore, the flow resistance of the upstream segment is given by Rus = Pst(l)/$\dot{V}_{max}$[34] and can thus be calculated from two measurable quantities, Pst(l) and $\dot{V}_{max}$.

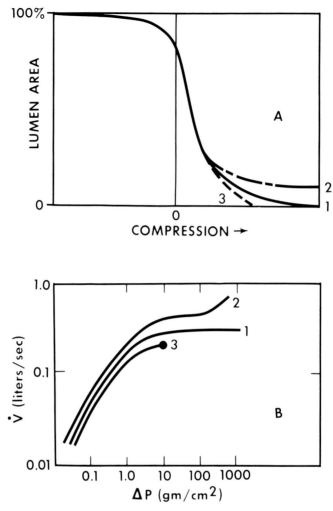

Fig. 8-8. Behavior of plastic tubes (Penrose tubing) at high flow rates. *A.* Pressure-lumen area diagram (100% = wide open; 0% = closed). Zero ordinate = resting position of tube. Lines 1, 2, and 3 indicate different tube configurations under compressing pressures, corresponding to the pressure-flow curves 1, 2, and 3 in *B.* Curve 3 terminates at the black dot; at higher pressures, pressure-flow relations are unstable and cannot be described by a line. See also text. Modified from reference 17.

The EPP model directs attention to the important role of Pst(l) as a driving pressure for airflow. It explains why $\dot{V}_{max}$ decreases when the lungs have lost elastic recoil or when peripheral airways are obstructed (Chap. 9). Confusion can arise, though, from unwarranted extensions of the concept. For instance, while the pressure relations show clearly that there must be an EPP somewhere along the airway, its location cannot be determined accurately in anatomical terms. The EPP does not separate the uncompressed and the compressed airway segment. Dynamic compression probably begins somewhere downstream from the EPP, where a sufficiently strong transmural compressing pressure develops during forced expiration.

As Ppl and Palv increase at a given volume, the EPP travels upstream, begin-

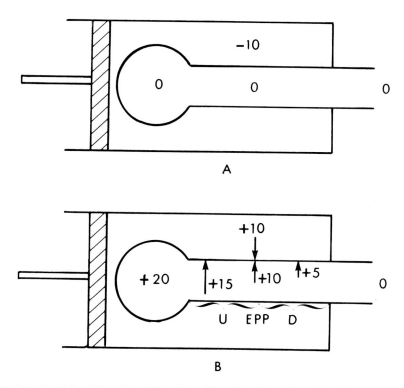

Fig. 8-9. The equal pressure point (EPP) model.[34] *A*. No airflow. Ppl=Pst(*l*) =−10 cm H_2O. Palv = 0. *B*. Maximum expiratory flow. Palv = +20 cm H_2O. Ppl = −10+20 = +10 cm H_2O [Eq. (2), Chap. 7]. At EPP, pressure in airway=Ppl= +10 cm H_2O. *U*=upstream, *D*=downstream segment. A more complete set of similar diagrams has been discussed elsewhere.[4, 57]

ning in the trachea at the chest cage inlet. It stops when dynamic compression is fully established and flow has reached its maximum value at that volume. As lung volume decreases, Pst(*l*) decreases and Ppl for the same Palv must increase (see Fig. 7-6, p. 129). Unless the compressed airway segment is highly compliant, the EPP moves toward the periphery with decreasing lung volume. At the same time, the compressed airway segment lengthens, as can be observed directly in excised lungs where the pressure outside the extrapulmonary airways is known.[31]

The Flow-Limiting Segment

Once the large airways are dynamically compressed, upstream pressure variations no longer affect flow. Rather, flow is determined by the difference between the extrabronchial (compressing) pressure and the pressure at the airway opening. This behavior is that of a Starling resistor.[50] However, the compressed segment is unstable and vibrates,[6, 18] and its behavior is highly complex. Wheezing during forced expirations probably results from the vibrations in the compressed airway segment as well as in the larynx. The concept of a critical transmural pressure at which compression begins is elusive—it is difficult to define in an oscillating airway segment and depends on airway wall compliance. The latter varies as a function of cartilage content and structure and of smooth muscle tone.[40, 43] The Starling resistor theory predicts increased maximum flow after smooth muscle relaxation;[50] in fact, flow rates may remain the same or increase or decrease in healthy persons.[7, 59]

Airway Wall Compliance

During quiet breathing, movements of airway walls are minimal. During deep and forced breathing, their caliber changes to an extent determined by airway wall stiffness. The pressure-diameter curve of isolated airways is S shaped (as in the tubes of Fig. 8-8); most of the caliber change occurs in a narrow range of pressures. In small airways, smooth muscle tone, attachments to lung tissue, and perhaps surface forces in the epithelial lining are the principal factors affecting wall compliance.[36] In large airways, cartilage and muscle tone are its principal determinants. Smooth muscle contraction can change the trachea into a nearly rigid tube, protected against compression by overlapping cartilage edges.[40] Muscle tone itself also changes tracheal compliance, and graded increases in tracheal stiffness can be achieved by electrical stimulation of the nerve in an isolated preparation.[43] Thus, tracheal compressibility might be subject to physiological regulation.

Relaxing muscle tone makes large airways more flaccid and compressible and may lead to decreased maximum expiratory flows in healthy persons.[7] In contrast, reducing muscle tone in small airways leads to increased caliber and higher maximum expiratory flows. An operational definition of small and large airways can be based on this difference in the consequences of muscle tone changes.[4] *Small airways* are unprotected by cartilage and have a thick layer of smooth muscle. Their caliber decreases with increasing muscle tone. *Large airways,* however, are protected against caliber changes by cartilage—during quiet breathing, muscle tone does not greatly affect their caliber; during dynamic compression, their tone provides wall rigidity and thus prevents compression and enhances maximum flows. During dynamic compression, the effects of muscle tone on airway caliber and maximum flows are opposite in small and large airways.[4, 7]

EXPERIMENTAL MEASUREMENTS

Isovolume Pressure-Flow (IVPF) Curves

Since pressure-flow relations depend on lung volume, they cannot be described by a single curve, but rather by a family of curves, with lung volume as the parameter (Fig. 8-2B). These curves differ during inspiration and expiration; they show flow limitation during expiration, and they can be altered by changing the density of the inspired gas.[19]

The three variables (volume, pressure, flow) can be measured with different methods. Flow is recorded with a flowmeter at the mouth; this signal can be integrated to obtain lung volume changes. Alternatively, volume changes can be measured with a body plethysmograph,[14] which can provide lung volume in absolute terms if thoracic gas volume is also measured.[28] Palv can be measured from esophageal pressure (Pes) records or from plethysmographic recordings. The shape of IVPF curves differs when volume is recorded at the mouth or with a body plethysmograph: the latter "sees" the volume change due to both the volume of the gas expired and the volume of the gas compressed, while an instrument at the mouth measures only volume changes due to the volume of expired gas. The two volumes differ whenever Palv is not equal to zero; the difference is important when Palv is high.[6, 24] Measurements of Palv with the esophageal balloon [19, 34] or with the body plethysmograph [6] result in similar curves. The IVPF curves recorded with one method can be transferred into diagrams valid for another method by using the static recoil curve to relate Pes to Palv, and by using Boyle's law to calculate lung volume at Palv from volume measured at the mouth.[6] The choice between volume measurements at the mouth and plethysmographic volume measurements is discussed further in Chapter 9 (p. 183).

Volume-pressure-flow relations are described in graphs with two variables on the x and y axis and the third variable as the parameter. Pressure-flow (Fig. 8-10A) and flow-volume (Fig. 8-10B) diagrams are commonly used; in the first, volume is the parameter, and in the second, pressure. Diagram A is a set of IVPF curves; diagram B includes the MEFV curve (Chap. 9).

Inspiratory IVPF curves depend less on volume than expiratory IVPF curves (Fig. 8-10A). Due to dynamic compression, the expiratory curves have flow plateaus at low volumes. At large volumes, expiratory flow is limited by the velocity of muscle contraction (see below). In normal subjects, plateaus are observed at lung volumes up to about 80% of VC (range, 57–93 percent [58]). As lung volume decreases, the pressure needed to reach maximum flow decreases. At

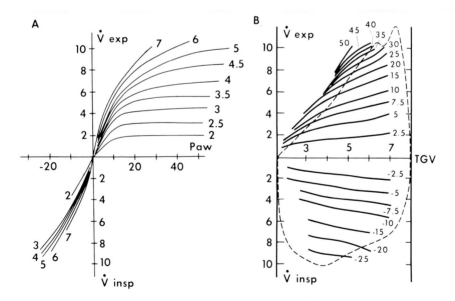

Fig. 8-10. *A.* Isovolume pressure-flow curves in a healthy subject. Thoracic gas volume for each line shown (2–7 liters). Paw = pressure difference between alveoli and mouth (cm H_2O). $\dot{V}_{exp}$ and $\dot{V}_{insp}$ in liters per second. *B.* Flow-volume diagram from same data as *A. Ordinate.* Same as *A. Abscissa.* Thoracic gas volume (TGV) in liters. Isobars for Paw in cm H_2O. *Dashed line.* Single forced inspiratory (below abscissa) and expiratory (above abscissa) vital capacity maneuvers. Modified from reference 6.

small lung volumes, very small alveolar pressures will lead to maximum flow rates. This can also be seen in diagram *B,* where pressure isobars indicate Palv values at different flows and volumes. The slope of these isobars, in particular during expiration, reflects the increased airway resistance (see below) as lung volume decreases.

A more detailed diagram of experimental points on IVPF curves is given in Figure 8-11. During inspiration and during expiration at low flows, the points are grouped closely together around the lines, which were drawn freehand. These data were obtained from large series of breaths recorded at different times and with varying breathing patterns. Thus, these pressure-flow relations appear to vary little with time or breathing pattern. When expiratory flow rates reach maximum values, the variability increases, as indicated by the hatched areas in Figure 8-11. Standardizing volume history (i.e., all expirations made from TLC) does not reduce this variability.[27, 58] Previous flow rates are important—during forced expirations maximum flows are often lower than during more relaxed expirations, with lower initial flows (see also Fig. 9-5, p. 181). In Figure 8-11, optimal IVPF curves were drawn through the highest flow points at each volume. Similar data

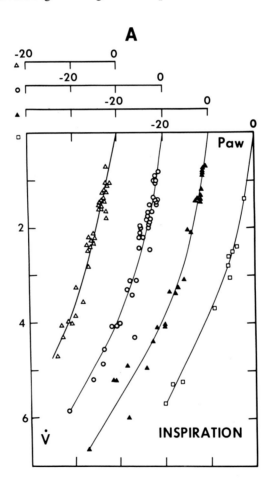

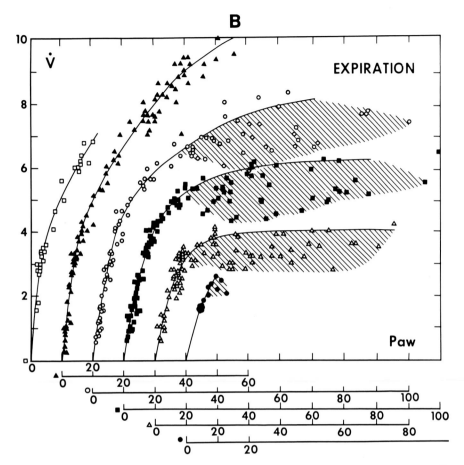

Fig. 8-11. Experimental isovolume pressure-flow data in a healthy subject. Zero points for Paw (see legend to Fig. 8-10) on abscissa are different for each IVPF curve, as indicated by the appropriate symbol next to each zero line, to avoid overlapping curves. Parameter: volume; □ = 6 liters, ▲ = 5 liters, ○ = 4 liters, ■ = 3.5 liters, △ = 3 liters, ● = 2.5 liters (thoracic gas volume at alveolar pressure). From reference 6.

are also shown as Palv isobars in the flow-volume diagram of Figure 8-10. These optimal isobars reach higher maximum flows, at a given volume, than were actually obtained during forced expirations.

Consequently, flow rates are often less than optimal during forced expirations [34] (see also Chap. 9, p. 177). In some subjects there may be a true "negative effort-dependence" of flow. That is, the IVPF curve goes through a maximum flow value and flow decreases when pressure increases further. However, this phenomenon occurs only in a few subjects.[34, 48] Time charts of the same data (e.g., Fig. 8-6) show that optimal flow rates always occur before dynamic compression becomes obvious (i.e., before *b* in Fig. 8-6). Suboptimal flows occur later. It appears that the onset of dynamic compression can vary, perhaps because of subtle differences in airway compliance or in the time course of transmural pressure changes. Thus, the mechanical behavior of large airways may vary subtly from breath to breath. Accurate information on transmural pressure changes during dynamic compression along the airway is not available and the precise course of the mechanical events is difficult to analyze.[48] Models of expiratory flow also suggest unstable conditions during maximum flow (p. 153). In addition, the shape of the compressed segment may vary.[46]

Equations Describing IVPF Curves

Two types of equations have been proposed

$$Palv = K_1 \cdot \dot{V} + K_2 \cdot \dot{V}^2 \qquad (\text{Rohrer's equation})[51]$$

$$Palv = k \cdot \dot{V}^n \qquad (\text{Ainsworth and Eveleigh's equation})[2]$$

Both describe pressure-flow relations accurately at low flows but underestimate Palv as flows increase, particularly for expiratory curves.[6] The constants in both equations vary with lung volume. Therefore, calculations of these constants from pressure-flow curves which have not been obtained under isovolume conditions carry little meaning. The constants have no physiological meaning but can serve to summarize portions of the curves as an empirical description.

Airway Resistance (Raw)

Airway resistance, the ratio of driving pressure to flow rate at any point on an IVPF curve, varies with lung volume and flow rate. The nearly linear initial parts of IVPF curves, near zero flow, represent values for resistance at low flow rates. Their slopes are, however, affected by the variable resistance of the glottis and depend on the exact maneuvers used.[56] Also, these slopes vary with volume and flow, and hence Raw depends on volume. At higher driving pressures, Raw increases owing to the alinearity of IVPF curves. A set of relations between Raw, lung volume, and flow rate is shown in Figure 8-12. Inspiratory resistance depends much less on volume than expiratory resistance, which increases sharply as dynamic compression narrows the large airways. The higher the flow rate, the larger the volume at which Raw begins to increase steeply. This steep increase reflects the plateau of IVPF curves.

Raw and its reciprocal, airway conductance (Gaw), can be measured with a body plethysmograph[14] using either panting breaths[13] or a rebreathing technique.[26, 28] Flow-resistive pressure differences can also be derived from Ppl measurements (Fig. 7-7C, p. 132); the result is then called pulmonary resistance (R1) rather than airway resistance. The total resistance (Rt) of the respiratory system (including chest wall) can be estimated by imposing oscillating flow patterns upon spontaneous breaths, e.g., with a loudspeaker placed in series with a mouthpiece. Like other methods, this technique requires careful control of lung volume levels;[16] it is not sensitive to small variations in resistance.[15]

Measurement of Raw during panting in the body plethysmograph at inspiratory flow rates of 0.5–1.0 liters/sec, and with simultaneous determination of thoracic gas volume (TGV), is the preferred method. The effect of lung volume on Raw is often taken into account by calculating specific conductance (SGaw), i.e., the Gaw/TGV ratio. Although this is sometimes useful for summarizing Gaw data,

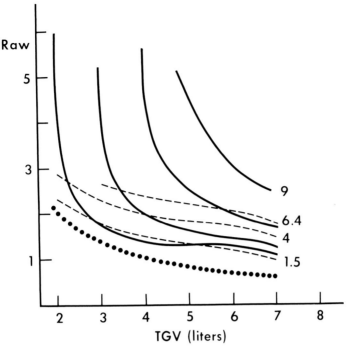

Fig. 8-12. Raw (cm H_2O/liter/sec) as a function of lung volume, with flow rate (1.5–9 liters/sec) as the parameter. *Drawn lines:* expiration; *dashed lines:* inspiration. These data were obtained with a rebreathing method.[28] Typical data for panting Raw (at lower flows) are indicated by the dotted line. After reference 6.

it may be misleading if the slopes and positions of Gaw-TGV curves differ (Fig. 8-13). Measurement of Gaw at different volumes is the preferred method for describing changes in Raw, e.g., after bronchodilator drugs.[4, 7]

Measurements of Raw in man in vivo include the resistance of all airways between airway opening and alveoli. By measuring pressures at points in between, one can partition Raw into portions corresponding to different parts of the airways. For instance, measurement of the pressure below the glottis (Ps [25, 59]) allows determination of the pressure differences (Palv−Ps) and (Ps−Pao) [Pao=pressure at airway opening]. Thus, the resistance of the lower (alveoli to subglottic area) and upper (from there to airway opening) airways can be measured. At large lung volumes, upper airway resistance is minimal (Fig. 8-14); it increases during deflation. Within the bronchial tree, further partitioning of Raw is possible with catheters placed in different bronchi. Such measurements have been performed in patients with lung diseases and in healthy persons.[21, 33] More elaborate experiments are feasible in animal experiments and also in excised human lungs where the pressure outside the airways can be controlled. In dog lungs, the airways of the fourth to ninth generation contribute most to total lower airway resistance.[30] In excised human lungs, pressure measurements in small airways have shown that airways smaller than 2 mm internal diameter contribute little to the resistance of the bronchial tree.[32] These findings agree with theoretical calculations on the distribution of flow resistance in the bronchial tree.[20, 41]

The site of resistance is important for interpretating Raw measurements. Raw

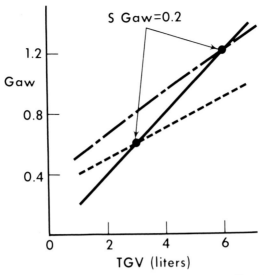

Fig. 8-13. Airway conductance (Gaw, liters/sec/ cm H$_2$O) as a function of thoracic gas volume, TGV. Three Gaw-TGV graphs are shown. Gaw at a given lung volume may differ even though the Gaw/TGV ratio (SGaw) is equal ($= 0.2$) on selected points of each curve.

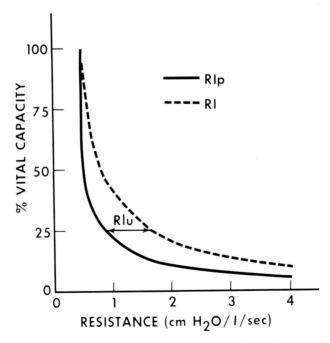

Fig. 8-14. Total lung resistance (Rl), resistance of lower airways (below glottis) and lungs (Rlp), and resistance of upper airways (Rlu) as a function of lung volume (*ordinate*). Deflation curves for healthy subject; data from reference 59.

is chiefly determined by the resistance of upper airways, glottis, trachea, and large bronchi. Thus, resistance changes in more peripheral airways must be large and extensive in order to affect total Raw. Measurements of maximum expiratory flow rates detect small airway obstruction better than Raw measurements [4, 8, 59] (Chap. 9). When Raw changes without significant alterations of maximum flows, the resistance changes probably occur in upper or large airways.

Maximum Expiratory Flow-Volume Curves

These curves are derived from IVPF curves (Fig. 8-10) and are described in Chapter 9.

VARIATION IN AIRWAY CALIBER

Experimental Changes in Airway Caliber

Asthma and several other lung diseases (Chaps. 14–18) are characterized by airway obstruction, often developing slowly over the course of years. Acute changes of airway caliber can be induced by drugs (histamine, choline esters), by dust exposure, and by reflex actions. In vivo, acute changes of airway caliber are usually assessed with indirect measurements, e.g., of Raw or maximum flows. Recently,

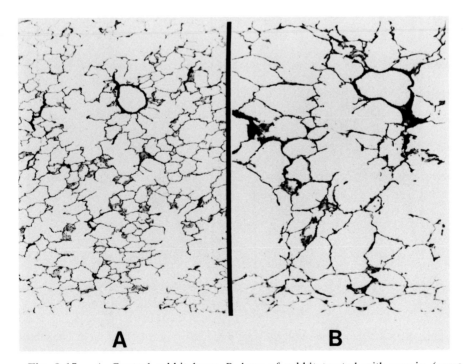

Fig. 8-15. *A.* Control rabbit lung; *B.* lung of rabbit treated with papain (same magnification as *A*). The mean number of alveolar attachments to small airways (< 1.25 mm internal circumference) was 10.1 in the controls and 8.5 in the papain-treated animals. Alveolar and alveolar duct sizes are increased after papain administration. Figure and data from reference 10.

improved radiological techniques using tantalum,[11] or without any contrast medium,[35, 36] have led to direct visualization of airway caliber changes in experimental animals. These methods can demonstrate the site as well as the extent of airway narrowing under various experimental conditions.[11, 35, 37]

The decreased caliber of small airways in emphysema is usually attributed to loss of recoil in the lungs (p. 139). Emphysema can be simulated in rabbits treated with papain, a proteolytic enzyme (p. 139). This treatment resulted in decreased maximum flow rates on IVPF curves in rabbits in which structural lung damage was minimal and lung compliance was normal.[10] The flow decrement appeared to be due to a loss of tethering of small airways by surrounding alveolar attachments (Fig. 8-15). After papain administration, alveolar size increased moderately, but

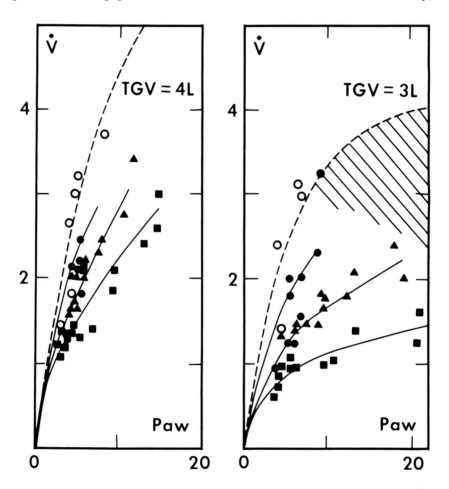

Fig. 8-16. Effect of histamine inhalation on expiratory IVPF data in a healthy subject, at two values of TGV. Paw (see legend to Fig. 8-10) in cm H_2O; $\dot{V}$ in liters per second. Symbols: control inhalation ○; 10 mg histamine base per ml ●; 20 mg histamine base per ml ▲; 30 mg histamine base per ml ■. Hatched area similar to those in Figure 8-11. After histamine inhalation, maximum flow rates at TGV = 3 liters are depressed, in dose-related fashion. The effect is less marked at the higher lung volume. From reference 6.

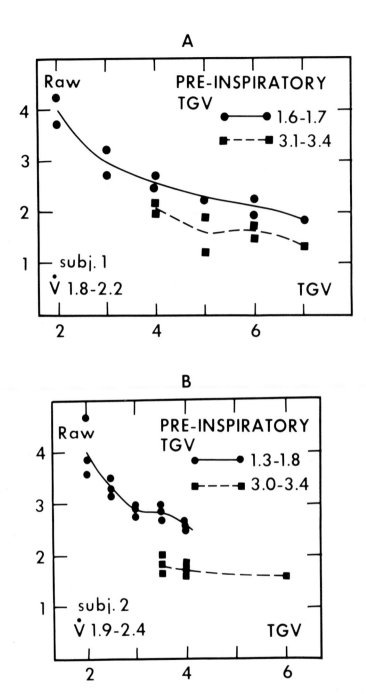

Fig. 8-17. Effect of preinspiratory lung volume on Raw. *Drawn lines.* Inspiration from near RV. *Dashed lines.* Inspiration from higher volumes, as shown in graph. Range of flow rates shown for each subject; the difference between drawn and dashed lines cannot be explained by pressure-flow alinearity. From reference 6.

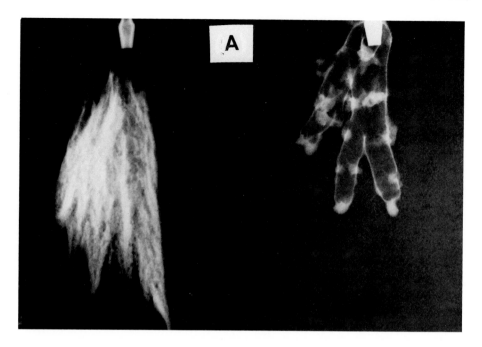

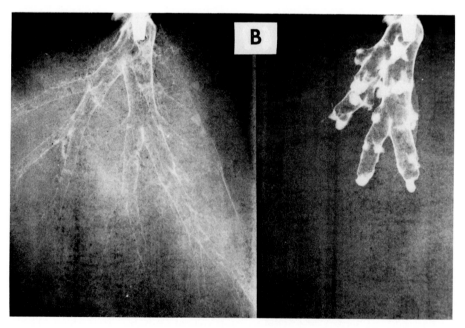

Fig. 8-18. *A.* Roentgenogram of intact dog lung lobe inflated to Ptp = 15 cm H$_2$O (*left*) and dissected bronchial tree at same Ptp (*right*). The airways are much wider when lung tissue is removed. *B.* Inflated dog lung lobe (*left*) and dissected airways (*right*), both at Ptp = 40 cm H$_2$O. At this high inflation pressure, airway caliber is similar in lobe and dissected airways. No contrast medium used. From reference 36.

the airways showed no anatomical changes that could explain the decreased flows. Decreased maximum flows, therefore, may reflect damage to lung structure when more direct measurements of lung elastic recoil do not yet pick up any change (see also Chap. 7, p. 130). Maximum flows on IVPF curves are also sensitive indices of drug-induced small airway obstruction, especially when flows are measured at small lung volumes [4, 6] (Fig. 8-16). The initial slope of IVPF curves may also change, indicating increased resistance at low flows, but this usually happens at higher dose levels of airway constrictor drugs.

Airway Caliber and Lung Volume History

Airway caliber and resistance to flow depend on both momentary conditions and previous history. For instance, at a given volume, Raw is higher if the preceding expiration was to RV than if expiration was less complete [6] (Fig. 8-17). This hysteresis (p. 124) of Raw can be abolished by atropine; [59] it is, therefore, probably caused by smooth muscle tone. However, when breathing at low lung volumes is prolonged, atelectasis appears to develop, and under these conditions Raw decreases during lung inflation.[9] In animal lungs, the state of the tissue surrounding airways affects their caliber. At the same inflation pressure, lobar and segmental bronchi in dog lungs have a smaller caliber when the lobe is atelectatic than during deflation from an inflated condition.[36] When surrounding atelectatic lung tissue is removed, airway caliber increases [36] (Fig. 8-18A); this does not happen with an inflated lobe (B). How atelectatic tissue compresses the airways is not quite clear, but the phenomenon illustrates the important effect of lung inflation on airway caliber. Muscle tone modifies the effect of the surrounding tissue.[36]

MUSCULAR EFFORT

Force-Velocity Relations

The pressures required to produce maximum flows during expiration are far less than those that can be developed during either static or dynamic breathing maneuvers (Fig. 8-19). Some 40 cm H_2O is enough to reach peak flows at large volumes, although the muscles can easily develop much higher pressures. Peak pressures during maximum exercise average -30 cm H_2O during inspiration and $+6$ cm H_2O during expiration in healthy persons.[39] In patients with airway obstruction, maximum flows are lower, while expiratory pressures during exercise are much higher than the levels required to produce maximum flow rates.[49] In addition, these patients usually require less pressure to achieve $\dot{V}_{max}$ at similar lung volumes than normal persons do. They breathe uneconomically during exercise, exerting much expiratory effort but achieving only low flows.

Potter et al.[49] proposed that this inefficient effort pattern results from an inappropriate motor drive to the expiratory muscles. The IVPF diagram of Figure 8-20 contains force-velocity curves for the expiratory muscles,[22] which indicate that the muscles' ability to produce expiratory pressure increases as the speed of contraction (i.e., flow rate) decreases. When flow rate is zero, muscle force is largest (static effort; Fig. 8-19). This inverse relation between flow rate and

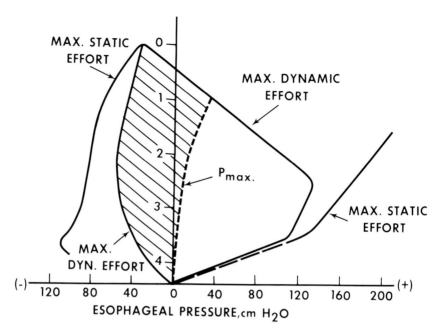

Fig. 8-19. Maximum static and dynamic pressures as a function of lung volume. Static effort = against closed airway. Dynamic effort = during forced vital capacity maneuvers. P_{max} = pressures needed to reach maximum expiratory flow rates. *Ordinate:* lung volume (liters from TLC). *Abscissa:* esophageal pressure, cm H_2O. From reference 22.

pressure is inherent to the physiological properties of striated muscles.[1] During inspiration and at large volumes during expiration, the rate of expiratory flow is limited by the muscles' ability to develop force during rapid contractions.[1, 22] If persons with airway obstruction continued to develop the same muscle force as during health, they would use higher pressures and achieve lower flows (compare points *A* and *B* in Fig. 8-20). If they increased muscle force, in a vain attempt to increase flow, breathing would become even more uneconomical (e.g., point *B* might move to *C*).

Indirect support for this hypothesis comes from acute experiments with unloading of the respiratory system.[38] When healthy subjects breathe a helium-oxygen mixture (80 percent He, 20 percent O_2), their expiratory flow rates increase, and IVPF curves are shifted upward (Fig. 8-20). For the same oxygen uptake, exercise ventilation increases, while peak expiratory pressure decreases. Breathing of helium, a light gas, unloads the respiratory system because less energy is lost in turbulence and other nonlaminar flow patterns, which are density-dependent. This response to unloading is largely a consequence of the force-velocity curve of the muscles.[38] Apparently, respiratory motor drive is only incompletely adapted to the lesser energy losses, since flow increases and P_{CO_2} decreases. Thus, the regulation of breathing fails to keep P_{CO_2} constant (see also Chap. 10, p. 223). Similarly, regulation may fail to decrease motor drive in patients with airway obstruction who seem to continue to use a motor drive appropriate for healthy

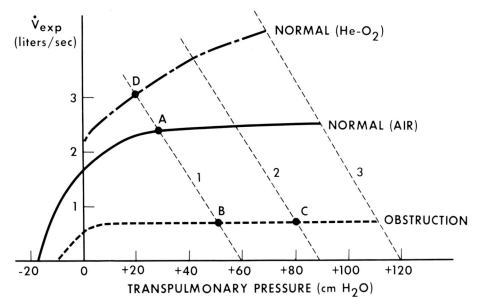

Fig. 8-20. IVPF curves in normal subject breathing air (——) or He-O$_2$ (———),
and in a patient with airway obstruction (– – –). Force-velocity curves of respiratory muscles 1, 2, and 3 describe increasing levels of muscular effort, corresponding
to static transpulmonary pressures of +60, +90, and +120 cm H$_2$O. When the system
is loaded by airway obstruction, flow decreases and pressure increases for the same effort (compare points *A* and *B* on force-velocity curve 1). When the system is unloaded
by He-O$_2$ breathing, flow increases and pressure decreases, again for the same effort, e.g.,
from *A* to *D*. Modified from reference 49; the He-O$_2$ curve indicates the direction of
changes observed by Nattie and Tenney.[38]

lungs. Training these patients to decrease their uneconomical breathing patterns
might result in less energy spent on respiratory muscles and hence more energy
available for physical work by other muscles.

Work Rate of Breathing

The power dissipated during airflow is given by

$$\dot{W} = 0.1 \ P \cdot \dot{V} \tag{2}$$

where $\dot{W}$ = power (rate of work) in watts, P = driving pressure in cm H$_2$O and
$\dot{V}$ = flow rate in liters per second. The equation is strictly valid only when pressure
and flow rate are in phase. In a logarithmic pressure-flow diagram (Fig. 8-21)
instantaneous power values can be read from the diagonal lines of equal power.
During maximally forced expirations, power may reach more than 20 watts for
brief instants. During quiet breathing, power is minimal, and even during heavy
exercise the rate of work remains small. In patients with airway obstruction, it
is usually said that the work of breathing is large. This is true if one looks at
pressure-volume loops (discussed in Chap. 7). However, here we consider only
the power exerted to drive airflow, not the overall effort of breathing. Expiratory

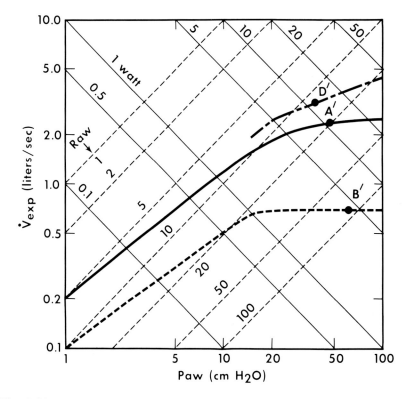

Fig. 8-21. Pressure-flow diagram on logarithmic coordinates. IVPF curves are those also shown in Figure 8-20. Points A', B', and D' correspond to points A, B, and D in Figure 8-20. Drawn diagonal lines are isobars for equal power output [from Eq. (2)]. Dashed diagonal lines are lines for equal Raw ($= Paw/\dot{V}_{exp}$).

power remains low in obstructed patients even though high pressures are used in an effort to overcome the high airway resistance (B'). Unloading the system with helium increases expiratory power only slightly; flows and pressure change reciprocally (e.g., from A' to D' in Fig. 8-21).

SUMMARY

Airflow patterns in airways are complex and do not fit a simple physical model. Pressure-flow relations are alinear and much energy is lost in transforming flow patterns (entrance effects; branches). During forced expiration, the geometry of large airways in the chest is profoundly changed by dynamic compression, which limits expiratory flow rates. The dynamically compressed airways are unstable and vibrate; the degree of compression depends on wall stiffness and smooth muscle tone. Experimentally, pressure-flow relations can be assessed with IVPF and MEFV curves and with airway resistance measurements. Airway-constrictor drugs decrease airway caliber, and this also happens when alveolar structure is damaged with a proteolytic enzyme, papain. Both actions result in lower flow rates on IVPF curves. Muscular effort limits inspiratory flow and, at large lung volumes, expiratory flow. Force-velocity relations of the respiratory muscles can account for the inappropriately high expiratory pressures used by patients with airway obstruction who exert much effort but achieve only a low expiratory flow and a low external work rate of breathing.

REFERENCES

1. Agostoni E, Fenn WO: Velocity of muscle shortening as a limiting factor in respiratory air flow. J Appl Physiol 15: 349–353, 1960
2. Ainsworth M, and Eveleigh JW: A method of estimating lung resistance in humans. Porton, Wiltshire, England, Ministry of Supply, Chemical Defense Experimental Establishment, Porton Tech. Paper No. 320, 1952
3. Bachofen H, Scherrer M: Lung tissue resistance in healthy subjects and in patients with lung disease, in Bouhuys A (ed): Airway Dynamics; Physiology and Pharmacology. Springfield, Charles C Thomas, 1970, pp 123–134
4. Bouhuys A: Airway dynamics and bronchoactive agents in man, in Bouhuys A (ed): Airway Dynamics; Physiology and Pharmacology. Springfield, Charles C Thomas, 1970, pp 263–282
5. Bouhuys A: Relation entre le débit expiratoire maximum et le volume pulmonaire (Maximum flow/volume relationships). Bull Physiopathol Respir (Nancy) 7:303–311, 1971
6. Bouhuys A, Jonson B: Alveolar pressure, airflow rate, and lung inflation in man. J Appl Physiol 22:1086–1100, 1967
7. Bouhuys A, van de Woestijne KP: Mechanical consequences of airway smooth muscle relaxation. J Appl Physiol 30:670–676, 1971
8. Bouhuys A, van de Woestijne KP: Respiratory mechanics and dust exposure in byssinosis. J Clin Invest 49:106–118, 1970
9. Butler J, Caro CG, Alcala R, DuBois AB: Physiological factors affecting airway resistance in normal subjects and in patients with obstructive respiratory disease. J Clin Invest 39:584–591, 1960
10. Caldwell EJ: Physiologic and anatomic effects of papain on the rabbit lung. J Appl Physiol 31:458–465, 1971
11. Clarke SW, Graf PD, Nadel JA: In vivo visualization of small-airway constriction after pulmonary microembolism in cats and dogs. J Appl Physiol 29: 646–650, 1970
12. Clarke SW, Jones JG, Oliver BR: Resistance to two-phase gas-liquid flow in airways. J Appl Physiol 29: 464–471, 1970
13. DuBois AB, Botelho SY, Comroe JH Jr: A new method for measuring airway resistance in man using a body plethysmograph: values in normal subjects and in patients with respiratory disease. J Clin Invest 35:327–335, 1956
14. DuBois AB, van de Woestijne KP (eds): Body Plethysmography, Progress in Respiration Research, 4; Herzog H, Series Editor. Basel, S Karger, 1968
15. Ferris BG Jr: Use of pulmonary function tests in epidemiologic surveys. Bull Physiopathol Respir (Nancy) 6:579–594, 1970
16. Fisher AB, DuBois AB, Hyde RW: Evaluation of the forced oscillation technique for the determination of resistance to breathing. J Clin Invest 47:2045–2057, 1968
17. Fry DL: A preliminary lung model for simulating the aerodynamics of the bronchial tree. Comput Biomed Res 2: 111–134, 1968
18. Fry DL: Theoretical considerations of the bronchial pressure-flow-volume relationships with particular reference to the maximum expiratory flow-volume curve. Phys Med Biol 3:174–194, 1958
19. Fry DL, Hyatt RE: Pulmonary mechanics. A unified analysis of the relationship between pressure, volume and gas flow in the lungs of normal and diseased human subjects. Am J Med 29:672–689, 1960
20. Green M: How big are the bronchioles?, St. Thomas' Hosp Gazette 63:136–139, 1965
21. Herzog H, Keller R, Maurer W, Baumann HR, Nadjafi A: Distribution of bronchial resistance in obstructive pul-

monary disease and in dogs with artificially induced tracheal collapse. Respiration 25:361–394, 1968

22. Hyatt RE, Flath RE: Relationship of airflow to pressure during maximal respiratory effort in man. J Appl Physiol 21:477–482, 1966

23. Hyatt RE, Wilcox RE: The pressure-flow relationships of the intrathoracic airway in man. J Clin Invest 42:29–39, 1963

24. Ingram RH Jr, Schilder DP: Effect of gas compression on pulmonary pressure, flow, and volume relationships. J Appl Physiol 21:1821–1826, 1966

25. Jaeger MJ, Matthys H: The pressure flow characteristics of the human airways, in Bouhuys A (ed): Airway Dynamics; Physiology and Pharmacology. Springfield, Charles C Thomas, 1970, pp 21–32

26. Jaeger MJ, Otis AB: Measurement of airway resistance with a volume displacement body plethysmograph. J Appl Physiol 19:813–820, 1964

27. Jonson B: Pulmonary mechanics in normal men, studied with the flow regulator method. Scand J Clin Lab Invest 25:363–373, 1970

28. Jonson B, Bouhuys A: Measurement of alveolar pressure. J Appl Physiol 22:1081–1085, 1967

29. Klingele TG, Staub NC: Terminal bronchiole diameter changes with volume in isolated, air-filled lobes of cat lung. J Appl Physiol 30:224–227, 1971

30. Macklem PT: Partitioning of the pressure drop in the airways, in Bouhuys A (ed): Airway Dynamics; Physiology and Pharmacology. Springfield, Charles C Thomas, 1970, pp 85–97

31. Macklem PT, Mead J: Factors determining maximum expiratory flow in dogs. J Appl Physiol 25:159–169, 1968

32. Macklem PT, Mead J: Resistance of central and peripheral airways measured by a retrograde catheter. J Appl Physiol 22:395–401, 1967

33. Macklem PT, Wilson NJ: Measurement of intrabronchial pressure in man. J Appl Physiol 20: 653–663, 1965

34. Mead J, Turner JM, Macklem PT, Little JB: Significance of the relationship between lung recoil and maximum expiratory flow. J Appl Physiol 22:95–108, 1967

35. Murtagh PS, Proctor DF, Permutt S, Kelly B, Evering S: Bronchial closure with mecholyl in excised dog lobes. J Appl Physiol 31:409–415, 1971

36. Murtagh PS, Proctor DF, Permutt S, Kelly BL, Evering S: Bronchial mechanics in excised dog lobes. J Appl Physiol 31:403–408, 1971

37. Nadel JA: New technique for studying structural changes of airways in vivo using powdered tantalum, in Bouhuys A (ed): Airway Dynamics; Physiology and Pharmacology. Springfield, Charles C Thomas, 1970, pp 73–83

38. Nattie EE, Tenney SM: The ventilatory response to resistance unloading during muscular exercise. Respir Physiol 10: 249–262, 1970

39. Olafsson S, Hyatt RE: Ventilatory mechanics and expiratory flow limitation during exercise in normal subjects. J Clin Invest 48:564–573, 1969

40. Olsen CR, Stevens AE, McIlroy MB: Rigidity of tracheae and bronchi during muscular constriction. J Appl Physiol 23:27–34, 1967

41. Olson DE, Dart GA, Filley GF: Pressure drop and fluid flow regime of air inspired into the human lung. J Appl Physiol 28:482–494, 1970

42. Owen PR: Turbulent flow and particle deposition in the trachea, in Wolstenholme GEW, Knight J (eds): Circulatory and Respiratory Mass Transport, Ciba Foundation Symposium. Boston, Little, Brown and Company, 1969, pp 236–252

43. Palombini B, Coburn RF: Control of the compressibility of the canine trachea. Respir Physiol 15:365–383, 1972

44. Pardaens J, van de Woestijne KP, Clément J: A physical model of expiration. J Appl Physiol 33:479–490, 1972

45. Patrick GA, Sharp GR: Oronasal distribution of inspiratory flow during various activities. J Physiol (London) 206: 22P–23P, 1970

46. Pedersen OF: Relation entre le débit expiratoire maximum et le volume pulmonaire (Maximum flow/volume relationships). Bull Physiopathol Respir (Nancy) 7:327–331, 1971

47. Pedley TJ, Schroter RC, Sudlow MF: The prediction of pressure drop and variation of resistance within the human bronchial airways. Respir Physiol 9:387–405, 1970

48. Peslin R: Relation entre le débit expira-

toire maximum et le volume pulmonaire
(Maximum flow/volume relationships).
Bull Physiopathol Respir (Nancy) 7:
348–351, 1971

49. Potter WA, Olafsson S, Hyatt RE:
Ventilatory mechanics and expiratory
flow limitation during exercise in patients
with obstructive lung disease. J Clin Invest 50:910–919, 1971

50. Pride NB, Permutt S, Riley RL, Brom-
berger-Barnea B: Determinants of maximal expiratory flow from the lungs. J
Appl Physiol 23:646–662, 1967

51. Rohrer F: Der Strömungswiderstand in
den menschlichen Atemwegen und der
Einfluss der unregelmässigen Verzweigung des Bronchial-systems auf den Atmungsverlauf in verschiedenen Lungenbezirken. Pflueger's Arch 162:225–299,
1915

52. Schroter RC, Sudlow MF: Flow patterns
in models of the human bronchial airways. Respir Physiol 7:341–355, 1969

53. Sharp JT, Henry JP, Sweany SK, Meadows WR, Pietras RJ: Total respiratory
inertance and its gas and tissue components in normal and obese men. J Clin
Invest 43:503–509, 1964

54. Sonne C: Untersuchungen über die relative Weite der Bronchiolen bei der verschiedenen Luftspannung der Lungen.
Beitrag zur Kenntnis der Pathogenese
des Bronchial-Asthmas. Acta Med Scand
58:313–341, 1923

55. Spann RW, Hyatt RE: Factors affecting
upper airway resistance in conscious
man. J Appl Physiol 31:708–712, 1971

56. Stănescu DC, Pattijn J, Clément J, van de
Woestijne KP: Glottis opening and airway resistance. J Appl Physiol 32:460–
466, 1972

57. van de Woestijne KP, Afschrift M,
Bouhuys A: Pressions, débits et volumes
pulmonaires pendant la respiration for-
cée. Poumon Coeur 24:969–987, 1968

58. van de Woestijne KP, Zapletal A: The
maximum expiratory flow-volume curve:
peak flow and effort-independent portion,
in Bouhuys A (ed): Airway Dynamics;
Physiology and Pharmacology. Springfield, Charles C Thomas, 1970, pp 61–72

59. Vincent NJ, Knudson R, Leith DE,
Macklem PT, Mead J: Factors influencing pulmonary resistance. J Appl Physiol
29:236–243, 1970

60. Yamabayashi H, Takahashi T, Tono-
mura S, Takahashi H: An analog model
of the mechanical properties of the lung
and airway, in Bouhuys A (ed): Airway
Dynamics; Physiology and Pharmacology. Charles C Thomas, 1970, pp. 33–41

Chapter 9

Flow Volume Curves

The derivation of maximum expiratory flow-volume (MEFV) curves from iso-volume pressure-flow (IVPF) curves, discussed in the previous chapter, is shown in the schematic diagram of Figure 9-1. Over a large portion of the vital capacity (VC), MEFV curves represent flows that correspond to plateaus on IVPF curves. MEFV curves can be recorded simply during a forced expiration and do not require pressure measurements in a plethysmograph or with an esophageal balloon. MEFV curves were first used by Dayman [14] and by Fry and Hyatt.[19, 23] In recent years they have been used in many experimental and clinical studies. Maximum flow rates on MEFV curves depend on many physiological and mechanical factors, any one of which can alter the curve's configuration. Since the mechanical events during forced expiration are complex and insufficiently understood, interpretation of MEFV curves in terms of lung mechanics is limited.[23] This limitation does not detract, however, from the value of flow-volume curves in detecting and quantitating acute changes in lung function that result from drugs, pollutants, or disease. For this purpose, the partial expiratory flow-volume (PEFV) curve [6] is particularly suitable.

DETERMINANTS OF MAXIMUM FLOW RATES

The dynamics of forced expirations have been described in Chapter 8. Here we discuss these mechanical events as they affect maximum flows and determine the size and shape of the MEFV curve.

Airway Resistance

Increased resistance in upper airways or an added resistance placed at the mouth decreases flow rates. This decrease occurs first at large lung volumes and extends to lower volumes as the resistance increases [Fig. 9-4 (5)].[26, 37a, 41] At high lung volumes, expiratory muscle power sets the limit on expiratory flow; peak

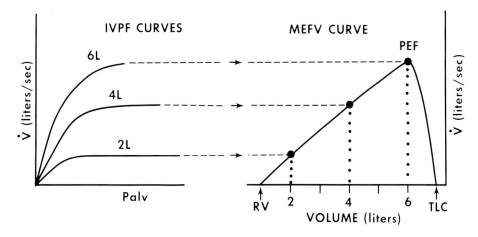

Fig. 9-1. Schematic diagram to illustrate derivation of maximum expiratory flow-volume (MEFV) curve from a family of isovolume pressure-flow (IVPF) curves. *Ordinates:* expiratory flow rate. *Abscissa:* (left) alveolar pressure; (right) lung volume. From reference 2.

flows are determined chiefly by upper airway resistance and muscle power. When, as in tracheal stenosis, upper airway resistance is markedly increased, it limits flow to values lower than those that result from the normal flow-limiting mechanism. The MEFV curve then only reaches its normal contour at volumes where the physiological mechanism sets a lower limit than the resistance in the upper airways. However, upper airway resistance must be significantly increased in order to affect the MEFV curve.

In the upper third of the VC, expiratory effort has a pronounced effect on flow rates (Fig. 9-5). Below about 80 percent of the VC (Chap. 8, p. 157), the MEFV curve represents flows that correspond to plateaus on IVPF curves (Fig. 9-1). The analysis in the previous chapter has shown that maximum flows at these volumes are chiefly determined by the flow resistance of peripheral airways and by lung elastic recoil. Since measurements of airway resistance during quiet breathing or panting primarily reflect the resistance of large and extrathoracic airways (p. 162), it is not surprising that data on airway resistance and MEFV curves may disagree. The discrepancies arise because resistance is chiefly determined by large-airway caliber, while maximum flow mainly reflects the caliber of small airways. Airway resistance increases only when there is extensive narrowing of small airways (Chap. 8).

These discrepancies between resistance and flow rates occur, for instance, when airways are dilated with drugs that relax airway smooth muscle.[9] In healthy persons, these drugs nearly always decrease airway resistance while maximum flows increase slightly, if at all, and may even decrease. The reduced resistance probably reflects an increased large-airway caliber, measured when airflow rates are low and no dynamic compression occurs. Maximum flow changes result from two opposing factors: (1) increased caliber of small airways, leading to increased flow, and (2) decreased stiffness of large airways through smooth muscle relaxation (p. 156), leading to increased dynamic compression and lower flows. Depending on the balance between these opposing factors, maximum flow may increase, decrease, or remain constant. In asthma the increased small-airway caliber following administration of dilator drugs is the preponderant factor and maximum flows usually increase markedly (Fig. 18-4, p. 449).

Lung Elastic Recoil

Lung elastic recoil is the principal driving force for expiratory flow at low lung volumes (p. 154). The relation between maximum flow and elastic recoil can be assessed graphically (Fig. 9-2); their ratio $[Pst(l)/\dot{V}_{max}]$ equals the resistance of the upstream airway segment in Mead's theory (p. 153). In the experiment of Figure 9-2, a constrictor drug decreased maximum flow at equal values of $Pst(l)$. Since $Pst(l)$ did not change, this result indicates a decrease in small airway caliber by smooth muscle contraction.[6] In other conditions, maximum flow and elastic recoil both change while their ratio remains constant. For example, when elastic recoil in hamsters is reduced by a proteolytic enzyme (papain), $Pst(l)$ decreases

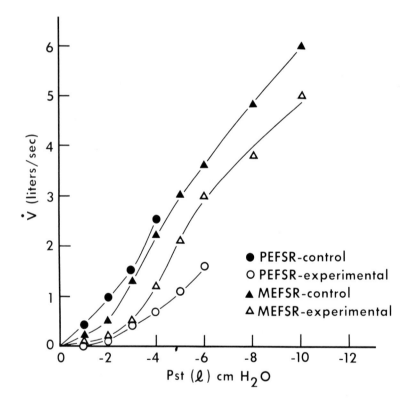

Fig. 9-2. Maximum flow-static recoil curves in a healthy subject, before and after histamine aerosol inhalation. *Abscissa:* static lung recoil pressure [Pst (*l*)]; *ordinate:* expiratory flow rate. PEFSR = partial expiratory flow-static recoil curve, corresponding to PEFV maneuver. MEFSR = maximum expiratory flow-static recoil curve, corresponding to MEFV maneuver. After inhalation of the constrictor aerosol, maximum flows at equal Pst(*l*) are decreased, indicating small-airway narrowing. The difference is greater on the partial (PEFSR) than on the maximum (MEFSR) curves. From reference 6.

but the ratio between maximum flow and Pst(l) is unchanged.[42] In man, chest strapping increases Pst(l) as well as maximum flow, again leaving the relationship between the two unchanged.[49] In these instances, as in parenchymal lung disease, the changes in maximum flow result from changes in lung elastic recoil. In diffuse lung fibrosis, high static recoil pressures are often associated with high maximum flows.[28, 31] In emphysema, low maximum flows are associated with loss of elastic recoil and low values of Pst(l).[14, 50] Since small airways are embedded in the lung parenchyma (Fig. 2-2B; p. 31), parenchymal elastic-recoil forces are transmitted to these airway walls. In this manner, lung structure provides the conditions in which an increase or decrease of elastic recoil force can lead to passive changes in airway caliber and hence to changes in maximum expiratory flow.

Acceleration of Gas

The total cross section of the airways decreases from the alveoli to the trachea (p. 30). Therefore, gas velocity rises as expired gas travels from the alveoli through the increasingly narrow bronchial tree. The acceleration of expired gas may affect maximum flows at high lung volumes;[36] at lower volumes, when flows decrease, this factor is minor.

Limits to Inspiration and Expiration

These limits determine VC, the volume axis of the MEFV curve. When airway closure limits expiration, flow gradually decreases toward the residual volume (RV) point (the "tail" of curve *3* in Fig. 9-4). When chest wall recoil limits expiration, the curve terminates abruptly, as in Figure 9-4, *1* (see also Chap. 7, p. 138).

Flow History

The variability of maximum flows on IVPF curves is discussed on p. 158 (Fig. 8-11). At a given volume, maximum flow is a function of previous flow rates (Fig. 9-5A and C): the lower the preceding flow, the higher the maximum flow. A precise explanation of this phenomenon is not available. The development of dynamic compression probably varies as a function of initial flows during more or less forced expirations.[7, 44] When initial flows are low, dynamic compression is still in progress at low lung volumes. The compression contributes to increased flow but cannot fully explain it.[44] Gas flow from compressing large airways can also lead to short-lasting bursts of flows above the contour of the MEFV curve, e.g., during a cough.[27] Since these transients do not reflect gas expired from alveoli, they should be ignored when assessing maximum flows as an index of ventilatory capacity. In emphysema, alternating compression and decompression of large airways can lead to spuriously high flow rates during maximum breathing capacity maneuvers, thereby overestimating the true capacity of the patient to ventilate the alveoli. Much of the volume displaced during such maneuvers may shuttle back and forth between the atmosphere and the large airways.[50]

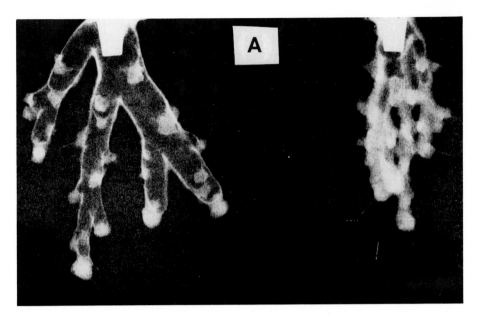

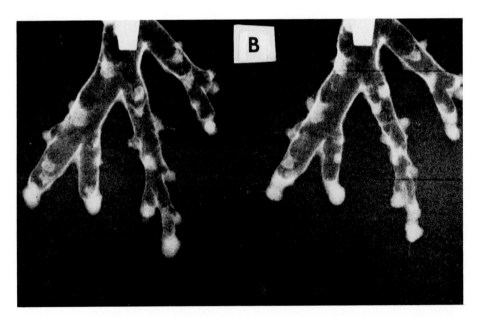

Fig. 9-3. Dissected bronchial tree of dog lung lobe. Left: control; right: after mecholyl. *A:* Inflation to 20 cm H$_2$O transpulmonary pressure. Mecholyl causes marked airway constriction. *B:* Inflation to 40 cm H$_2$O transpulmonary pressure. A similar administration of mecholyl causes no discernible constriction of the passively distended airways. From Murtagh et al.[40]

Inspired Gas Composition

Maximum flow rates on MEFV curves increase with the inspiration of a light gas (80 percent He-20 percent O_2) and decrease as gas density increases.[47] Viscosity of the inspired gas has only a minor effect. With a light gas, the flow increase is most pronounced at large lung volumes. These flows are determined largely by effort and by the caliber of large airways, where the flow pattern is consistent with a major effect of gas density (p. 146). In some patients with airway obstruction, the absence of a flow rate increase upon breathing He-O_2[15] suggests a decreased dependence of expired gas flow on density. In part, this reduced dependence may result from low flow rates and hence a decrease in turbulence and other density-dependent energy losses. The lack of density dependence in these patients' maximum flows might also be explained by small-airway narrowing.[15] In the lower-volume portion of the MEFV curve, the portion most sensitive to small-airway obstruction, breathing He-O_2 has little effect on maximum flow.[15, 47]

Airway Muscle Tone

In isolated dog lung lobes, the effect of constrictor drugs on airway caliber can be observed directly.[40] Figure 9-3 shows that this effect depends markedly on lung inflation. At a low inflation pressure (A), airway narrowing and closure are pronounced, while the length of these lobar and segmental bronchi changes much less. High inflation pressures are required to open the airways again. Surface tension of the mucosa may contribute to closure once caliber is reduced. At a high inflation pressure (B), almost no narrowing occurs after the constrictor drug is applied. This experiment demonstrates phenomena quite similar to those seen in flow-volume curves in man (Figs. 9-8, 9-9): constrictor agents lead to much more significant reductions of airway caliber at low lung volumes than at high volumes. In addition, airway closure in man may occur at an increased volume (e.g., the increased RV after histamine exposure on the PEFV curves in Fig. 9-8), and a maximum inspiration can reopen these airways, at least temporarily (RV is lower at the end of the MEFV curves in Fig. 9-8). The effects of changes in smooth muscle tone in man are described in more detail on p. 199.

For practical purposes, the most important determinants of maximum flows on MEFV curves, at lung volumes less than about 70 percent of VC, are small-airway caliber and lung static recoil pressure. In several instances, increased or decreased elastic recoil leads to changes in maximum flows. In other conditions, small-airway caliber is the principal variable.

PATTERNS OF MEFV CURVES

The shape and size of the MEFV curve vary considerably among normal subjects and patients with lung disease—in fact, no simple mathematical expression fits all the variations.[12] Three main patterns account for the majority (Fig. 9-4). In healthy young persons, the descending portion of the curve is approximately linear (2) or concave to the volume axis (1). In older persons, the tail end of the curve, near RV, is often convex to the volume axis (3). Some subjects have

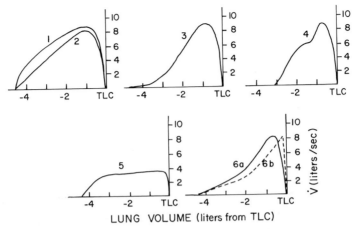

Fig. 9-4. MEFV curve patterns. *1* and *2*. Healthy young subjects. *3*. Older subject; this pattern is also frequent among young smokers.[48] *4*. Curve with intermediate
plateau ("shoulder"). *5*. Typical curve pattern in upper airway obstruction, e.g., tracheal stenosis. *6*. A slow response of the volume-recording instrument distorts the true
form of the curve (*a*) into the pattern of curve *b*.

an intermediate plateau ("shoulder") on the curve (*4*). MEFV curve patterns
in growing children have been discussed in Chapter 1 (p. 16 and Fig. 1-9). The
shape of MEFV curves may be distorted by technical factors, e.g., when the response time of the flow channel exceeds that of the volume-recording channel
(Fig. 9-4, 6).

In series of successive blows, the shape of the MEFV curve varies as a function
of effort (Fig. 9-5*A*). Flow rates at lower lung volumes are often similar in spite
of considerable variation in initial effort (Fig. 9-5*B*). Although this phenomenon
has prompted the description of the descending portion of the curve as effort-
independent, this term should not be taken literally, as the example of Figure 9-5*A*
indicates. At any volume, a certain minimal effort is required to achieve maximum
flow, but at low lung volumes flow is independent of further effort once this
minimum has been attained. At high volumes, IVPF curves do not show plateaus,
and flow continues to increase until the limit of expiratory muscle power has been
reached.

Fig. 9-5. MEFV curves recorded with computer system (Fig. 9-7). Each graph
shows five consecutive blows. The dashed lines in *A* and *C* indicate the maximum flow
contour (see text). The examples chosen are from subjects whose expiratory effort
varied considerably, as appears from the large differences in PEF between individual
blows. The $FEV_{1.0}$ is less sensitive to differences in effort than PEF, partly because
flows at midlung volumes are often higher when effort is less (see *C*). This phenomenon
is observed also when lung volume changes are measured with a body plethysmograph.[7]
In *C*, $FEV_{1.0}$ varied only between 1.88 and 2.00 liters in the five blows shown, in spite
of large differences in peak flow between the blows.

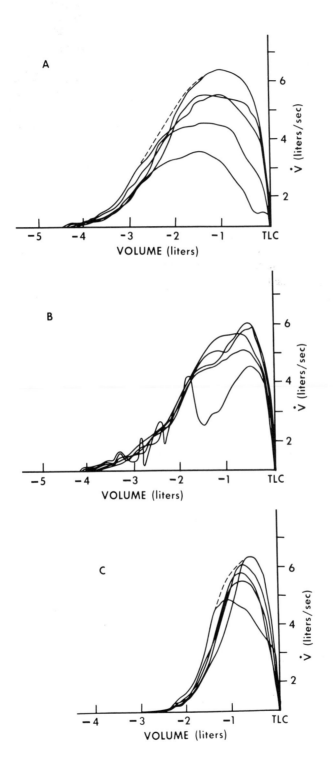

Maximum flows at lower lung volumes often show reverse effort-dependence, with a reduction in flows following an increase in initial effort and initial flow rates (Fig. 9-5*A* and *C*). In these instances, the curve recorded during maximally forced expiration shows lower flows than the curve obtained by superimposing a number of curves recorded during less forced expirations.[24] The contour of this set of curves is indicated by the dashed lines in Figure 9-5*A* and *C*. For practical purposes, the maximum-effort curve is easier to perform and to standardize.

Gross changes in MEFV curve patterns occur in obstructive as well as restrictive lung diseases (Fig. 9-6*A*). In obstructive disease, flow rates are low, especially near RV, and the curve is convex to the volume axis. In restrictive function loss, VC is decreased and flow rates are relatively high, resulting in a pronounced concave descending portion of the curve. Comparison of these curves with the normal pattern should take TLC into account. In obstructive disease, TLC is often abnormally large, while it is decreased in restrictive disease. Comparison on an absolute volume scale (Fig. 9-6*B*) shows better how much the mechanical characteristics of airways and lungs differ in the two types of patients. The patient with restrictive disease reaches high flow rates at thoracic gas volumes less than the residual volume of the patient with severe airway obstruction.

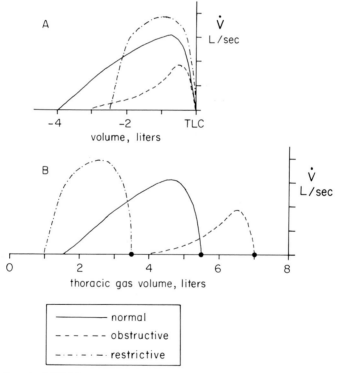

Fig. 9-6. *A.* MEFV curves plotted on volume scale relative to total lung capacity (TLC). Typical curves of a healthy person, a patient with severe airway obstruction, and a patient with restrictive function loss. *B.* The same curves plotted on an absolute lung volume scale, based on measurements of thoracic gas volume; ● = TLC for each curve. From reference 5. Used with permission of McGraw-Hill Book Co. (copyright 1974).

The visual pattern of MEFV curves allows major changes, in the sense of obstruction or restriction, to be recognized at a glance. Observer error in distinguishing the three main shapes is infrequent.[48] Recognition of inconsistent or faulty "blowers" is easy. Since the curve provides a picture of ventilatory reserves that can be understood without much explanation, it is often helpful in the clinical management of patients with lung disease. In asthma patients, the curves can be used to demonstrate effects of drugs, and a smoker's obstructive curve pattern can help convince him to stop smoking. In these respects, the MEFV curve is superior to the spirogram, which does not facilitate visualization of flow rates. Because MEFV curves are increasingly used as lung function tests in clinical and epidemiological studies, the following sections of this chapter focus on the methods for recording the curves, the measurements provided, and the clinical applications.

METHODS FOR RECORDING MEFV CURVES

Recordings of maximum expiratory flow versus lung volume can be obtained with respiratory flowmeters (pneumotachographs), or with spirometers, or with a combination of the two.

SPIROMETERS

Spirometers provide a record of expired volume versus time. By differentiating this record with respect to time, one can obtain flow rates, but this is a laborious, error-prone task when done manually.[3] Although electrical differentiating circuits can simplify the job, they suffer from low signal-to-noise ratios and signal distortion.[1] A specially designed spirometer[46] records MEFV curves directly, but its insufficient response characteristics distort the high initial flows.

PNEUMOTACHOGRAPHS

A pneumotachograph consists of a mechanical resistance placed in the airstream (a wire mesh screen, orifice, or, in Fleisch's instrument, a bundle of narrow tubes). To avoid instrumental reduction of flow rates, its resistance should be minimal, yet sufficient to produce a measurable pressure difference as a function of flow rate. This pressure difference is sensed by a transducer and amplified to a voltage suitable to drive a pen recorder or oscilloscope beam. The output should be a linear function of flow rate; otherwise the flow recording requires correction for alinearity. In addition, the instrument needs to have adequate frequency response and minimal phase shift. With Fleisch pneumotachographs,[18] frequency response is adequate and phase shift minimal up to frequencies of about 20 Hz.[45] This is sufficient since higher frequencies are insignificant during forced expirations.[32] The tubing attached to Fleisch pneumotachographs can affect their calibration;[17] hence, they should be calibrated and used with the same tube configuration.

VOLUME EXPIRED VERSUS PLETHYSMOGRAPHIC
VOLUME CHANGES

The volume measurement needed for the MEFV curve can be obtained with (1) a spirometer at the mouth, (2) integration of expiratory airflow rate to volume, or (3) a body plethysmograph. The choice is a matter of principle as well as practice. The simplest method is to measure the volume expired at the mouth (methods 1 or 2) under atmospheric pressure. During a forced expiration, alveolar gas is compressed from atmospheric to a higher pressure. Consequently, the alveolar gas volume decreases (according to Boyle's law) even if no air is expired. The body plethysmograph measures the chest's volume decrease, which during flow exceeds the amount of gas expired; the difference is the volume decrement of alveolar gas that results from gas compression.[25] Therefore, MEFV curves obtained with methods 1 or 2 differ from those obtained with the plethysmograph. Peak flows are closer to TLC on the former. In healthy persons the difference is small, and MEFV curves recorded with the plethysmograph and a spirometer at the mouth, from the same expiration, can almost be superimposed.[10] In patients with airway obstruction the difference is larger, since alveolar pressures are often high.[25]

The choice of method depends on one's purpose. To relate maximum flow rates to lung static recoil, one needs plethysmographic volume measurements since static recoil pressure depends on the actual lung volume, regardless of alveolar gas compression. The plethysmograph is also preferable if one wants to compare flow rates measured under conditions in which gas compression may vary markedly, e.g., when comparing spontaneous flow rates during exercise with forced expiratory flows.[20] However, to assess airway obstruction, volume measurement at the mouth may be preferable. The "compression artifact" in MEFV curves recorded at the mouth [23] is in fact a consequence of airway obstruction. At apparently equal lung volumes, volume measurement at the mouth yields lower flow rates because of alveolar gas compression, which increases with the degree of airway obstruction. Hence, this method reflects airway obstruction more completely than the plethysmographic method.[59] In restrictive lung disease, high flows are reached with minimal effort and the effect of gas compression should therefore be minimal. For assessing maximum expiratory flow rates in lung disease, measuring volume changes at the mouth is a valid procedure. We have adopted this procedure in routine recording of MEFV curves in the laboratory and in epidemiological studies; the plethysmographic procedures used in our laboratory have been described previously.[4]

INTEGRATION OF FLOW

For measuring volume changes at the mouth we favor integration of a flow signal (method 2) over volume recording with a spirometer (method 1). In method 2 a single signal (flow rate) acts as input to obtain both volume and flow at the output; furthermore, there are no mechanical moving parts, maintenance is minimal, and the electronic signal is easy to handle. Integration can be done by digital computer or with stable integrating circuits. The inaccuracies of differentiating circuits are thus avoided, as is the need to match the response characteristics of a separate flowmeter and spirometer. A compact and portable instrument using integrating circuitry has been developed in our laboratory.[53] The instrument provides internal digital outputs of forced vital capacity (FVC), peak expiratory flow rate (PEF), and timed forced expiratory volumes ($FEV_{0.5}$, $FEV_{1.0}$, and $FEV_{3.0}$), as well as flow and volume outputs for MEFV curve display on a storage oscilloscope or XY-recorder. For measuring $FEV_{0.5}$, $FEV_{1.0}$, and $FEV_{3.0}$, it is useful to superimpose time pulses on the recording.[21]

REFERENCE VOLUMES

Measurement of total lung capacity is often required for a comparison of MEFV curves on an absolute volume scale rather than relative to the point of maximum inspiration (Fig. 9-6B). Absolute lung volumes are used for comparing MEFV curves in some patients with asthma whose TLC (determined with the plethysmograph) decreases during treatment with bronchodilator drugs (see Fig. 7 in Bouhuys et al., reference 6). RV is less satisfactory as a reference volume,[26] since it varies more than TLC breath-to-breath during a series of forced expirations. When absolute volume data are not available, it is better to superimpose curves of an individual subject on the assumption that TLC is constant, as in Figures 9-5 and 9-10.

COMPUTER SYSTEM

For routine clinical use and for epidemiological studies, processing MEFV curve data with a digital computer allows integration of flow to volume, standardization of recording and data processing, and immediate availability of numerical values and computer-compatible data output. The system * used in our mobile facility for epidemiological studies (Fig. 9-7) employs a Fleisch #4 pneumotachograph as the flow sensor and a pressure transducer and electronic hardware to

SYSTEM CONFIGURATION FOR THE MOBILE LABORATORY

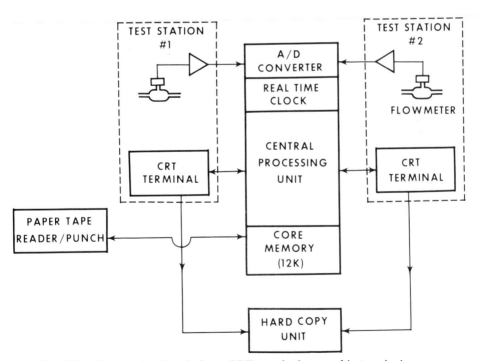

Fig. 9-7. See text for description. CRT terminal = graphic terminal.

* The system was developed by R. W. Tuttle, J. Virgulto, A. Huang, and D. Altieri of the Yale University Lung Research Center.

generate a signal suitable for analog-to-digital conversion. Two such systems are linked to a PDP-8E computer via an analog-digital converter. Two graphic terminals suitable for oscilloscopic display of alphanumeric data and graphs are also linked to the computer in an interactive mode. A time-sharing program allows simultaneous use of both terminals with minimum waiting times for data processing. The software includes special calibration and zero drift correction subroutines. In using the system, the test operator first enters identification data and administers a questionnaire (Chap. 13). Next, the subject is instructed to perform the MEFV curve test. Upon command from the operator, the computer starts sampling flow signals to establish a zero flow baseline. Flow is sampled every 5 msec, and the baseline value is subtracted from each sample. When expiratory flow exceeds 0.5 liters/sec, all counting elements in the computer are set at zero and accumulation of expiratory flow data begins. All successive flow signals, at 5-msec intervals, are added to obtain volume change; at each 50-ml volume increment, the corresponding flow value is stored. The number of 50-ml volume increments is counted. Special subroutines are used to store values for PEF, $FEV_{1.0}$, and $FEV_{3.0}$ during the forced expiration. (For definitions of these terms see Table 9-1). Flow sampling continues as long as flow exceeds 0.05 liters/sec. At the end of the blow the total volume expired is added up and stored (FVC). Thus, at the end of the first blow the computer has stored FVC, PEF, $FEV_{1.0}$, and $FEV_{3.0}$, as well as instantaneous flow points at 50-ml intervals over the full FVC range. Immediately after the blow, both the key data (FVC, $FEV_{1.0}$) and the MEFV curve are displayed on the terminal. The process is started anew for the following blows with the same data storage. After the third blow, a subroutine compares the $FEV_{1.0}$ values of the three blows and eliminates the data from the blow with the lowest $FEV_{1.0}$ from the computer memory. This comparison is repeated after the fourth and fifth blows. At the end of five blows, the terminal displays all five MEFV curves and their FVC and $FEV_{1.0}$, values, while the computer memory contains an array of flow points, at 50-ml intervals, for the two blows with the highest $FEV_{1.0}$, as well as the FVC, PEF, $FEV_{1.0}$, and $FEV_{3.0}$ values for these two blows. Next, the operator initiates a computation routine that uses all data from the two blows with the highest $FEV_{1.0}$ values. Their average FVC, PEF, $FEV_{1.0}$, and $FEV_{3.0}$ are computed, and the stored flow points are averaged at each 50-ml interval. These points are displayed as an average MEFV curve on the terminal, and MEF50% and MEF25% (Table 9-1) are computed and displayed. From prediction equations stored in the computer, predicted values for FVC, $FEV_{1.0}$, and flow rates are computed and used to display the actual data as a percentage of the predicted values.

The software includes several quality-control features. A blow is automatically rejected if it lasts 1 second or less. If a blow was delivered in a faulty manner, the operator may reject it, thereby eliminating the data from the computer memory. So that the operator can monitor the consistency of blows, the percentage difference between the highest and next highest $FEV_{1.0}$ is displayed on the terminal. At the end of the test all data are displayed on the terminal screen. The operator then activates (1) a hard copy unit that produces a sheet with all data and the MEFV curve as they appear on the screen (Fig. 13-2), and (2) a paper tape punch unit that stores the same data in computer-compatible format for later processing. The hard copy makes possible immediate review of data and, if necessary, initiation of medical care; the paper tape is essential for processing grouped data. A somewhat simpler system used in our clinical routine function laboratory since 1970 provides a condensed output report on a Polaroid ® print, which is convenient for permanent filing in a patient's record.

PARTIAL EXPIRATORY FLOW-VOLUME (PEFV) CURVE

In studies of airway constrictor and dilator agents, the measurement of flow rates at low lung volumes is of special interest (p. 167). The PEFV curve is a recording of maximum expiratory flow rates at volumes less than about 50 percent of VC, during a forced expiration starting at about 60 percent VC rather than at TLC (Figs. 9-8 and 9-9). Thus, the PEFV curve records maximum flows at low lung volumes without a previous inspiration to TLC. To compare PEFV curves before and after drugs or environmental inhalants, one needs a reference volume. Residual volume (RV) is not suitable, since it often increases during airway obstruction and is therefore not constant. TLC is more suitable since it usually remains constant unless constriction is severe. If the subject inspires to TLC

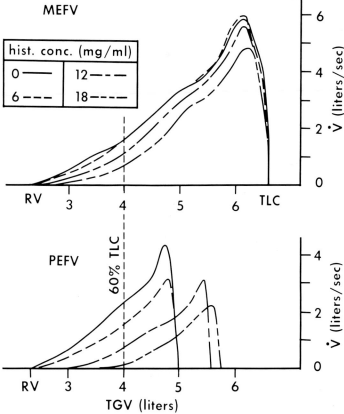

Fig. 9-8. Increasing dosage of histamine aerosol inhalations in a healthy subject. *Ordinate:* expiratory flow rate; *abscissa:* thoracic gas volume (TGV). Upper curves: MEFV curves; lower curves: PEFV curves. Flow measurements at 60% TLC can be used to quantitate the response (vertical dashed line; 60% TLC = 4 liters). From reference 6.

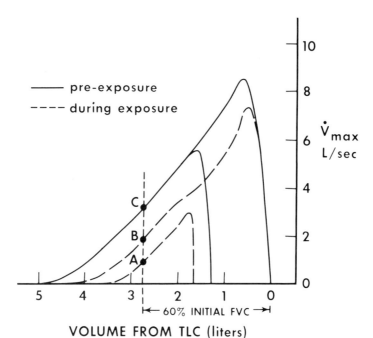

VOLUME FROM TLC (liters)

Fig. 9-9. MEFV and PEFV curve in a healthy subject before and during exposure to flax dust. The vertical dashed line indicates MEF40% (at TLC −60% of the initial FVC). MEF40% decreases from C to A on the PEFV curve and from C to B on the MEFV curve. From reference 8.

directly after the PEFV curve recording, TLC can be established as a reference volume point on the record. This procedure allows serial PEFV curves to be superimposed, using TLC as a common reference (Fig. 9-9). Separate determinations of TLC with the body plethysmograph can be used to demonstrate whether the assumption of a constant TLC is valid. Alternatively, one can record PEFV curves with the subject in the body plethysmograph and determine thoracic gas volume (TGV) at the beginning of each PEFV curve (Fig. 9-8).[6] For this procedure the subject inspires to about 60 percent VC; a shutter in the mouthpiece is then closed and TGV determined while the subject pants against the closed shutter.[16] Next, the shutter is opened and the subject expires forcefully to RV to record the PEFV curve. Although we used this method initially, later work has confirmed the validity of the simpler procedure, using TLC as the reference volume, under different experimental conditions.[8, 38, 56, 57, 58]

MEASUREMENTS FROM MEFV AND PEFV CURVES

All conventional spirometric measurements (FVC, $FEV_{1.0}$, and $FEV_{3.0}$) can be obtained from MEFV curve recordings. The definitions and preferred abbreviations of these terms are given in Table 9-1. As a single measurement of ventilatory capacity, the $FEV_{1.0}$ has several advantages.[22] It is relatively independent of effort (see Fig. 9-5 and its legend), and it includes sufficient flows at low lung volumes to be sensitive to airway obstruction. In contrast, $FEV_{0.5}$ is too effort-dependent,

Table 9-1.
Nomenclature and Definitions

Measurements	Recommended Name	Abbreviations	Comments and Synonyms
1. Maximum volume measured on expiration after the deepest inspiration	Vital capacity	VC	
(a) during a slow expiration	Slow vital capacity	SVC	Fast vital capacity; forced expiratory vital capacity
(b) during a forced expiration	Forced vital capacity	FVC	
2. Volume of gas expired over a given time interval during a forced expiration	Forced expiratory volume	FEV_T * ($_T$ = time interval in sec)	Timed vital capacity; fast vital capacity; forced expiratory vital capacity
3. Peak expiratory flow	Peak expiratory flow	PEF	
4. Mean expired flow during specified segments of the forced expiratory volume; e.g., between 25% and 75% of FVC †	Mean maximum expiratory flow, qualified by volume range	MMEF MMEF 25%–75%	
5. Instantaneous maximum expiratory flow at specified lung volumes, e.g.:	Maximum expiratory flow, qualified by volume at which measured	MEF	
(a) at 50% FVC ‡		MEF 50% §	
(b) at 25% FVC ‡		MEF 25% §	
(c) at TGV = 5 liters		MEF 5 liters	
(d) at 60% TLC		MEF 60% TLC	
6. Instantaneous maximum expiratory flow rates at specified lung volumes, from PEFV curves, e.g., at 40% FVC ‡	As 5	As 5 a-d, add (P) MEF 40% (P) §	

* When computing the FEV_T/VC ratio, specify whether SVC or FVC is used in the denominator, e.g., $FEV_{1.0}$/FVC. Use of FVC is preferred since it is obtained from the same blow as $FEV_{1.0}$.
† Percentages of VC are expressed on a scale where TLC=100% and RV=0%; use FVC to determine volume segments.
‡ I.e., TLC-50% FVC (5a), TLC-75% FVC (5b), and TLC-60% FVC (6). In serial experiments where FVC varies, control FVC values should be used to determine volume levels for all flow measurements (see Fig. 9-9).
§ The abbreviation presumes that percentage FVC is the most common volume reference; further qualification is only needed when another reference is used, as in 5c and d.
This table is a modified and expanded version of Hyatt's table.[22]

189

while $FEV_{2.0}$ and $FEV_{3.0}$ always include low flows near the end of the FVC and are therefore less sensitive to airway obstruction than the $FEV_{1.0}$. From spirometric recordings of forced expirations, one can calculate the mean mid-expiratory flow rate (MMFR [29]), i.e., the average flow rate between 25 and 75 percent of the FVC. This excludes the flows at large lung volumes, which are high even in patients with airway obstruction, as well as those near RV which are usually low even in normal subjects. Hence, the MMFR averages flow over a portion of the MEFV curve that is most sensitive to airway obstruction. However, the MEFV curve allows more detailed interpretation of these flow rates. Now that accurate flowmeters are widely available, there seems little reason to continue the use of average flows like the MMFR.

The slope of the effort-independent portion of the MEFV curve shows individual differences related to lung disease—it is steep in patients with restrictive disease and flat in patients with airway obstruction. Early studies concluded that this slope contains the most useful clinical information, since it reflects the time constants of the peripheral portions of the airways and lungs.[47] The slope of the effort-independent portion is, however, often nonlinear. It can be expressed quantitatively by taking the average slope over a defined portion of the curve, e.g., between 50 and 75 percent of VC, or between 50 and 25 percent of VC [28] (Fig. 9-10). These slope indices discriminate between healthy subjects and persons with airway obstruction,[28] but they are not sensitive to minor changes in airway caliber. In many experiments with constrictor and dilator drugs, we have found that the slope remains unchanged even though maximum flows at a given lung volume decrease.[6] Figures 9-8, 9-9, and 9-10 show examples. Measurement of flow rates at 1 liter above RV has also been proposed,[30] but this procedure is unsatisfactory because it uses RV as a reference volume (see p. 185). In our

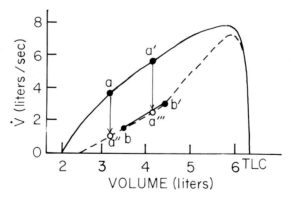

Fig. 9-10. Quantitation of MEFV curve data. A straight line *aa′* is the slope of the drawn MEFV curve between 25% and 50% of FVC. *bb′* is the slope over the same volume segment, after airway constriction, on the dashed curve. The slope remains nearly unchanged (*bb′* parallels *aa′*), while MEF25% (at TLC − 75% control FVC) decreases from *a* to *a″* and MEF50% (at TLC − 50% control FVC) decreases from *a′* to *a‴*. The change of peak flow is minimal.

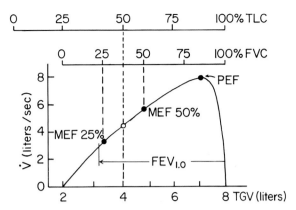

Fig. 9-11. Quantitation of MEFV curve data. One-second mark on the curve indicates the end point of the FEV$_{1.0}$. Maximum flows are referred to three different lung volume scales: %TLC, %FVC, and liters thoracic gas volume. PEF, MEF25%, MEF50%, MEF50% TLC, and MEF 5 liters are indicated on the curve; the last two are identical. See Table 9-1 for definition and nomenclature of these measurements.

experience this index does not reflect changes in airway caliber with sufficient sensitivity.[6] Any measurement based on the last portion of the curve depends on the endpoint of vital capacity, which is often variable and difficult to determine, especially in patients with airway obstruction.

Measuring instantaneous flow rates is more satisfactory than assessing the slopes of MEFV curves. Since inhalation of low doses of histamine aerosol decreases plateau flow rates on IVPF curves (Fig. 8-16), particularly at low lung volumes,[7] we studied these flow rates on MEFV and PEFV curves.[6] First, we had to decide what volume levels were suitable for flow measurements. Figure 9-11 indicates the main choices. A volume level in terms of percentage of VC is most practical, since this value is always available. Measuring MEF values at different percentages of FVC and of TLC has been useful in clinical studies where patients were compared with healthy subjects (p. 198). For assessing airway obstruction on MEFV curves we have found useful MEF50%, MEF40%, and MEF25%. On PEFV curves we usually measure MEF40%(P) (i.e., flow at TLC minus 60 percent of the control FVC), which avoids the transients that may be present near the peak of the PEFV curve.

The most commonly measured flow rate on the MEFV curve is the peak expiratory flow rate (PEF). Since it can be measured with simple devices, the PEF is often used as a separate lung function test. Unfortunately, PEF is highly sensitive to effort (Fig. 9-5) and varies considerably within the same subject.[3] In addition, PEF reflects the conductance of large and upper airways rather than that of small airways; in fact, PEF may depend largely on the size of the subject's trachea.[36] It is insensitive to slight degrees of airway obstruction (Fig. 9-10). Thus, a normal PEF does not exclude significant lung disease, and PEF underestimates airway obstruction. In patients with severe airway obstruction, PEF may include significant contributions of transients (p. 177) which do not reflect

Table 9–2.
Prediction Equations

Measurement	Males	Females	Coefficients for Height in cm *	
			Males	Females
VC	$0.12102H† − 0.01357A‡ − 3.18373$	$0.07833H − 0.01539A − 1.04912$	0.30981	0.20052
FEV$_{1.0}$	$0.09107H − 0.02320A − 1.50723$	$0.06029H − 0.01936A − 0.18693$	0.23314	0.15434
MEF75%	$0.09030H − 0.01987A + 2.72554$	$0.06876H − 0.01926A + 2.14653$	0.23117	0.17603
MEF50%	$0.06526H − 0.03049A + 2.40337$	$0.06220H − 0.02344A + 1.42640$	0.16707	0.15923
MEF25%	$0.03583H − 0.04142A + 1.98361$	$0.02334H − 0.03450A + 2.21596$	0.09172	0.05975
PEF	$0.14393H − 0.02403A + 0.22544$	$0.09130H − 0.01776A + 1.13160$	0.36846	0.23373

* Insert in corresponding equation if height is measured in cm.
† Height in inches.
‡ Age in years.
From Cherniack and Raber,[11] based on data from 859 nonsmoking men and 452 nonsmoking women. FVC and FEV$_{1.0}$ in liters. BTPS; flow rates in liters per second, ATPS.

airflow from alveoli. For these reasons, PEF should be discarded as a separate
lung function test.

In studies in which each subject serves as his own control, one needs to
compare flows at a constant lung volume under different conditions. MEF50%
is not suitable for this purpose since its volume level varies with the vital capacity.
If TLC is constant, it can be used as the reference volume, and MEF can be
measured at TLC minus a constant volume (e.g., 60 percent of the control FVC:
Fig. 9-9). If thoracic gas volume measurements are available for all measurements,
serial curves can be superimposed on an absolute lung volume scale (Fig. 9-8).
When comparing changes of flow rates, e.g., after drugs, in different subjects,
the results can be expressed in terms of percentage change (Fig. 9-16). One can
also use a correction factor for lung size, e.g., by expressing flow rates in units
of TLC/sec (Fig. 1-9, p. 16) or of FVC/sec.

NORMAL VALUES

Prediction equations for flows on MEFV curves based on a study of nonsmoking residents of a low-pollution area (Manitoba, Canada [11]) are shown in
Table 9-2. Average normal MEFV curves constructed from these equations are
shown in Figure 9-12. To emphasize the similarity in the shape of the curve's
descending portions in all women and in young men, these curves have been
superimposed at RV. Only the curve for older men is markedly convex toward

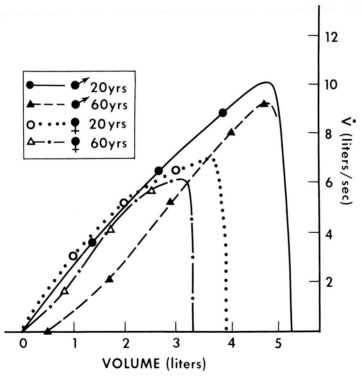

Fig. 9-12. Normal MEFV curves computed from the prediction equations in
Table 9-2 [11] using height = 72 in. for men and 68 in. for women. See text for discussion.

Table 9–3.
Variability of Maximum Expiratory Flow Rates in Healthy Subjects

	Subject 1	Subject 2	Subject 3	Subject 4
FVC (liters)				
n	50	52	50	23
$\bar{x}$	6.35	2.94	3.90	4.60
S.D.	0.148	0.242	0.161	0.164
C.O.V.(%)	2.3	8.2	4.1	3.6
S.E.	0.020	0.034	0.022	0.034
S.E./$\bar{x}$(%)	0.3	1.2	0.6	0.7
$FEV_{1.0}$ (liters)				
n	28	—	17	10
$\bar{x}$	5.31	—	3.04	3.66
S.D.	0.141	—	0.151	0.109
C.O.V. (%)	2.7	—	5.0	3.0
S.E.	0.026	—	0.036	0.035
S.E./$\bar{x}$ (%)	0.5	—	1.2	1.0
MEF40% (liters per second)				
n	50	52	50	23
$\bar{x}$	5.16	1.74	2.54	3.22
S.D.	0.420	0.228	0.292	0.301
C.O.V. (%)	8.1	13.1	11.5	9.3
S.E.	0.059	0.032	0.041	0.063
S.E./$\bar{x}$ (%)	1.1	1.8	1.6	2.0
MEF40% (P) (liters per second)				
n	48	51	51	15
$\bar{x}$	4.66	1.98	2.24	3.32
S.D.	0.738	0.420	0.348	0.347
C.O.V. (%)	15.8	21.2	15.5	10.5
S.E.	0.106	0.059	0.049	0.090
S.E./$\bar{x}$ (%)	2.3	3.0	2.2	2.7

Data from control experiments over a period of several months in laboratory workers (subjects 1–3) and in one untrained subject (4) on a single day. All were nonsmokers. The timemarker on MEFV curves (for $FEV_{1.0}$ determination) was used only part of the time, and not at all in subject 2; hence the smaller number of $FEV_{1.0}$ values. n=number of blows; $\bar{x}$= mean values; S.D.=standard deviation; C.O.V.=coefficient of variation ($=S.D. \times 100/\bar{x}$); S.E. =standard error. The variability of FVC and $FEV_{1.0}$ values (C.O.V. 2.3%–8.2% and S.E. 0.3%–1.2% of mean) is less than that of MEF values (C.O.V. 8.1%–21.2% and S.E. 1.1%– 3.0% of mean). Unpublished material, Yale University Lung Research Center.

the volume axis. This difference between older men and women is unexplained, especially since the men did not include persons with known occupational expo- sures (R.M. Cherniack, personal communication, 1973). It may reflect differences in the aging process in male and female lungs, or undetected environmental exposures in the men. Since the methods to obtain MEFV curves are as yet insufficiently standardized, these data still need to be confirmed by results from other population groups.

VARIABILITY OF MAXIMUM EXPIRATORY FLOW RATES

The between-blows variability of MEF measurements has been discussed on p. 180; it is largely a function of flow history and effort. If all data are taken from maximum-effort blows, this source of variability can be reduced. Data on a large number of forced expirations were obtained in healthy persons (Table 9-3). The MEF40% and MEF40% (P) values varied more than $FEV_{1.0}$ and FVC. Although such variations may not be random (e.g., some values might be low because of an undetected pollutant exposure), inpractice, they constitute "noise" in the measurement. The method's ability to detect changes depends on the signal-to-noise ratio, rather than on the variability of control values per se, as Table 9-4 illustrates. MEFV curves were recorded in 17 teen-age smokers, before and after smoking a cigarette.[57] The standard error of the mean MEF50% was about twice that of the mean FVC and $FEV_{1.0}$, both before and after smoking. However, the decrease in MEF50% after smoking was much larger than the decrease in FVC and $FEV_{1.0}$, both as a percentage of the mean control value and as a percentage of the standard error of the mean control value. The latter percentage relates the effect of smoking (the signal) to the variability of the control data (the noise) and is hence analogous to a signal-to-noise ratio. Thus, even though the MEF values vary more than FVC and $FEV_{1.0}$, they are more sensitive to changes even in the presence of this variability.

Under less controlled conditions, as when comparing individual results to an average norm derived from group data in healthy persons, there are additional sources of variability. It is likely that known or unknown pollutants subtly but significantly affect flow rates and influence the data from any normal group of persons. Data from one large group of male and female nonsmokers in a low-pollution area (Table 9-2 [11]) show standard errors for the estimate of MEF50% and MEF25%, from their multiple regressions on age and height, which are 1.7 to 2.6 times larger than those for $FEV_{1.0}$. Extension of such studies to persons in urban environments may show whether MEFV curves are able to quantitate pollutant effects against the background of the other variables involved.

CLINICAL APPLICATIONS

Functional Assessment of Lung Disease

MEFV curves, which can detect obstructive as well as restrictive lung function changes,[28, 31] provide a quantitative assessment of ventilatory function suitable for routine use in any person capable of delivering a few forced expirations. The curves can be used (1) as a diagnostic test in individual patients, (2) to provide objective data on the effects of treatment, (3) to study the natural course of disease, (4) to detect subclinical function disturbances, and (5) to assist in the assessment of ventilatory limitations on exercise performance.

Use of MEFV curves in diagnosing asthma, bronchitis, emphysema, and other obstructive diseases is based on recognition of the obstructive curve pattern (Fig. 9-6) and on measurement of flow rates. In children and adolescents, an MEFV curve which is convex to the volume axis is nearly always associated with

Table 9–4.
Changes in Lung Function After Cigarette Smoking

Measurement	Mean ± S.E.		Difference (liters or liters per sec)	Difference (% of mean control)	Difference (% of S.E.)
	Before	After			
FVC (liters)	5.38 ± 0.15 (2.8%) *	5.37 ± 0.17 (3.2%)	−0.01 (NS)	−0.2	7%
FEV$_{1.0}$ (liters)	4.57 ± 0.13 (2.8%)	4.51 ± 0.12 (2.7%)	−0.06 (NS)	−1.3	46%
MEF50% (liters per sec)	5.8 ± 0.34 (5.9%)	5.4 ± 0.31 (5.7%)	−0.40 (p < 0.001)	−6.9	118%

* In parentheses: S.E. as a percentage of mean value (columns 2 and 3). Difference between before and after values in absolute units (column 4), as a percentage of the mean control value (column 5), and as a percentage of the standard error of the control data before smoking (column 6). NS=not significant.

Data from 17 teenagers before and after smoking one cigarette (from reference 57).

a history of smoking, asthma, or other lung disease. Recognition of the restrictive curve pattern assists in the diagnosis of different forms of lung fibrosis. Treatment procedures (drugs, mist therapy) can be assessed from curves recorded before and after treatment, using appropriate controls.[6, 9, 34, 55, 37, 54, 56] If a standardized method is used, MEFV curves can help define the natural course of lung function changes in such diseases as sarcoidosis and cystic fibrosis, and in long-term observations of groups of patients during periods on and off therapy. MEFV curves are particularly appropriate for detecting subclinical disease in epidemiological studies on population groups outside hospitals (Chap. 13). The use of MEFV curves to assess limits on exercise performance is shown in Figure 12-1 (p. 279) and its legend. Many patients with emphysema reach maximum expiratory flow rates during tidal breathing at rest.[50] Such persons have little or no reserve for ventilation increases during exercise, and attempts to increase ventilation result in unduly high expiratory pressures (Chap. 8, p. 168). Although this does not explain the subjective symptom of dyspnea, it does provide an objective explanation of severely limited exercise tolerance. Other chapters in this book describe the applications of MEFV and PEFV curves to studies of smoking (Chap. 14), occupational lung diseases (Chaps. 15, 17), air pollution (Chap. 16), and bronchial asthma (Chap. 18). Clinical studies in our laboratories have used MEFV curves to assess lung function in cancer patients treated with bleomycin [43] and in children with congenital heart disease.[39] The use of MEFV and PEFV curves in the assessment of small airway obstruction warrants a more detailed discussion.

Assessment of Small-Airway Obstruction

Maximum flow rates at low lung volumes are decreased when small-airway caliber is reduced by drugs or dust [6, 52] and in bronchial asthma and cystic fibrosis.[54] In experiments with drugs, cigarette smoke, or textile dust, maximum flow rates decrease more on PEFV than on MEFV curves [6, 38, 56, 57] (Figs. 9-8, 9-9, 9-16). In patients with asthma, maximum flows on MEFV curves are often decreased at a time that airway resistance is within normal limits.[6, 41] The improvement of asthma patients after treatment with dilator drugs is best seen in the increase of flow rates in the lower half of the VC.[37] It is not yet possible to draw a definite conclusion concerning the relative sensitivity of different function tests in detecting small-airway obstruction. Several studies suggest, however, that maximum flows at low lung volumes are highly sensitive to changes in small-airway caliber. In smokers, maximum flows at low lung volumes often decrease when other tests (nitrogen washout, "closing volume," and frequency dependence of dynamic compliance) show normal results or less significant changes.[13, 33] In a group of 10 men, measurable closing volumes were found in only 5 men with "tails" on the MEFV curve.[51] The relation between closing volume and flow rates on MEFV curves is further discussed on page 71 (Fig. 4-9).

Figure 9-13 illustrates the difference between measurements of peak flow and of MEF25% in children with cystic fibrosis or asthma; MEF25% was much more frequently abnormal than PEF. Measurements of MEF also correlated with an independent assessment of the children's condition, as expressed in a clinical score (Fig. 9-14). An example of airway obstruction in a cotton cardroom worker, partially reversed by inhalation of an isoproterenol aerosol, is shown in

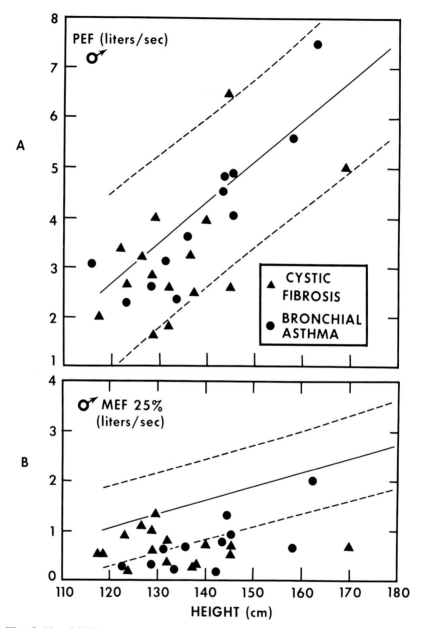

Fig. 9-13. MEFV curve data in children with cystic fibrosis or asthma. Drawn and dashed lines: mean normal values ± standard error.[55] *A*. Only a few patients have abnormally low peak flows; *B*. many more have abnormally low flow rates at 25% VC. Modified from reference 54.

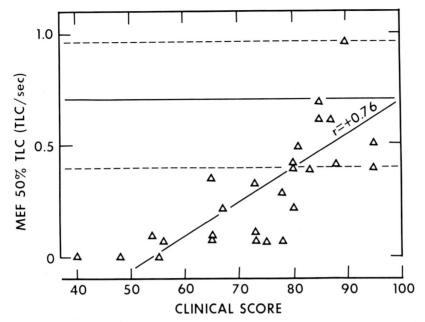

Fig. 9-14.   MEFV curve versus clinical evaluation in children with cystic fibrosis. *Ordinate:* MEF50% TLC expressed in units of TLC per second to eliminate effect of variation in lung size between patients. *Abscissa:* clinical score assessed independently by a pediatrician. The correlation is significant at the 1% level. Drawn and dashed lines: mean normal values ± SE.[55] From reference 54.

Figure 18-21, p. 480. These curves were recorded with the computer system of Figure 9-7. After isoproterenol inhalation, flow rates increase, while the slope of the effort-independent portion of the curve is unchanged. Post-isoproterenol flows are still abnormally low, suggesting significant irreversible airway obstruction (see also Chap. 17, p. 432).

In experiments with constrictor agents, the decrease in flow rates on MEFV and PEFV curves is related to the drug's concentration in the inhaled aerosol. In some subjects, adequate dose-response relations can be obtained from measurements of $FEV_{1.0}$ as well as of MEF40% and MEF40% (P) (Fig. 9-15A). In other subjects, the deep inspiration required for measurement of $FEV_{1.0}$ and MEF40% appears to abolish the constrictor effect; only the PEFV curve then provides a dose-related response of flow rates (Fig. 9-15B). This experience suggests that subtle effects of inhaled agents may be missed if one relies exclusively on forced expirations after a maximal inspiration. The sensitivity of PEFV curves to induced small-airway obstruction is also shown by the experiment of Figure 9-16 in which a healthy subject is exposed to flax dust:[8] MEF values on the PEFV curve decreased more than those on the MEFV curve, while the change in $FEV_{1.0}$ was minimal. In patients with bronchial asthma, PEFV curves are highly sensitive to the effect of bronchodilatation with isoproterenol.[6] In healthy persons, flow rates on PEFV curves increase significantly after administration of atropine,[52] demonstrating the existence of a normal degree of airway muscle tone in small airways. In other studies, PEFV curves have been used to demonstrate airway obstruction after

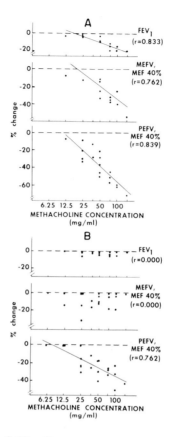

Fig. 9-15. Dose-response curves with methacholine aerosol inhalations. Each graph represents all data obtained from MEFV and PEFV curves in one subject. *Abscissa:* methacholine concentration in nebulized fluid. Duration of all inhalations—30 seconds. Subject *B* has no decrease of $FEV_{1.0}$ at any dose level, while flow decreases on the MEFV curve are erratic. Only MEF40% on the PEFV curve shows a dose-related decrease. In this subject, the drug effect is seen on the PEFV curve, but not consistently on the MEFV curve which was recorded immediately afterward. Thus, a single maximum inspiration often abolished the effect of the constrictor drug, at least temporarily. In subject *A,* the effect of the maximum inspiration was less and all three measurements show dose-related responses. As a percentage of control values, the PEFV curve showed the largest changes. Data contributed by Dr. C.A. Mitchell.[38]

inhalation of 1 ppm SO_2 in air (Chap. 16), after smoking one or two cigarettes,[57] and after 30 seconds' exposure to hairspray aerosols [58] (Fig. 18-3). In addition, these curves have provided evidence on the interaction between different airway-constrictor drugs [38] (Fig. 18-16).

Changes in flow rates on MEFV or PEFV curves do not reveal the cause of airway obstruction; they merely indicate its degree. In experiments with agents that alter smooth muscle tone acutely, this effect can explain the changes in airway caliber. In other instances, such as cigarette smoking, the nature of the obstruction is less clear since the biological effects of many pollutants on small airways have not been adequately studied. Inflammation of the mucosa and accumulation of secretions may play a role, while reduced elastic recoil must be considered in long-standing flow rate decreases. The evidence concerning the site of obstruction is likewise indirect. Such evidence rests in part on models of expiratory airflow, which indicate that small-airway caliber is a major determinant of maximum flow (p. 154); further evidence comes from concurring results of tests that measure other aspects of small-airway function, such as nitrogen clearance (Chap. 4), frequency-dependence of compliance (Chap. 7), and airway closing volume

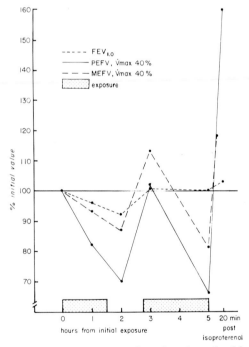

Fig. 9-16. Exposure to flax dust in a healthy subject. MEFV and PEFV curves as well as $FEV_{1.0}$ recorded with maneuver of Figure 9-9. *Ordinate:* percentage change from control values = 100%. The MEF measurements show constrictor responses to dust exposure, with recovery between exposures and, at the end of the experiment, after isoproterenol. See text for further comments. From reference 8.

(Chap. 4). For practical purposes, the PEFV curve has the advantage of being both simple to perform and highly sensitive to small changes in airway caliber.

SUMMARY

Maximum and partial expiratory flow-volume (MEFV and PEFV) curves describe maximum flows as a function of lung volume during forced expirations. Maximum expiratory flow rates are determined mainly by the flow resistance of peripheral airways and by lung elastic recoil; previous flows and inspired gas composition also affect flow rates. Lung size and age influence the shape and size of MEFV curves, and obstructive and restrictive lung disease produce abnormal curve patterns. To record MEFV curves, one uses a flowmeter to sense flow rate and integrating circuits to provide volume excursions. Data processing can be done on-line by computer. With similar equipment, PEFV curves can be recorded in reference to the point of maximum inspiration. Measurements of instantaneous flows at specified lung volumes (for nomenclature see Table 9-1) allow assessment of flow changes in comparison with normal values and with individual control data in acute experiments with inhaled agents. MEFV curves aid in diagnosis and management of asthma, bronchitis, cystic fibrosis, emphysema, and lung fibrosis. They are particularly suitable for detecting subclinical disease in industrial and community population groups, and for assessing effects of therapy on lung function in obstructive diseases of the airways. MEFV curves, and even more, PEFV curves, offer a highly sensitive, objective, and simple means of assessing small airway obstruction induced by smoking, dust, and air pollutants.

REFERENCES

1. Bargeton D, Florentin E, Menier R, Vardon G: Recording of second time derivative $\ddot{V}$ of displaced volume V in breathing. J Appl Physiol 34:259–262, 1973

2. Bouhuys A: Airways dynamics and bronchoactive agents in man, in Bouhuys A (ed): Airway Dynamics; Physiology and Pharmacology. Springfield, Charles C Thomas, 1970, pp 263–282

3. Bouhuys A: The clinical use of pneumotachography. Acta Med Scand 159:91–103, 1957

4. Bouhuys A: Recent applications of volume displacement body plethysmographs. Progr Respir Res 4:24–38, 1969

5. Bouhuys A, Gee JBL: Environmental lung disease, in: Harrison's Principles of Internal Medicine, ed 7. New York, McGraw-Hill, 1974, pp 1310–1320

6. Bouhuys A, Hunt VR, Kim BM, Zapletal A: Maximum expiratory flow rates in induced bronchoconstriction in man. J Clin Invest 48:1159–1168, 1969

7. Bouhuys A, Jonson B: Alveolar pressure, air flow rate and lung inflation. J Appl Physiol 22:1086–1100, 1967

8. Bouhuys A, Mitchell CA, Schilling RSF, Zuskin E: A physiological study of byssinosis in colonial America. Trans NY Acad Sci 35:537–546, 1973

9. Bouhuys A, van de Woestijne KP: Mechanical consequences of airway smooth muscle relaxation. J Appl Physiol 30:670–676, 1971

10. Bouhuys A, van de Woestijne KP, with the technical assistance of Kane G, van Wayenburg J: Respiratory mechanics and dust exposure in byssinosis. J Clin Invest 49:106–118, 1970

11. Cherniack RM, Raber MB: Normal standards for ventilatory function using an

automated wedge spirometer. Am Rev Respir Dis 106:38–46, 1972

12. Clément J, van de Woestijne KP: Validity of simple physical models in interpreting maximal expiratory flow-volume curves. Respir Physiol 15:70–86, 1972

13. Da Silva AMT, Hamosh P: Effect of smoking a single cigarette on the "small airways." J Appl Physiol 34:361–365, 1973

14. Dayman H: Mechanics of airflow in health and in emphysema. J Clin Invest 30:1175–1190, 1951

15. Despas PJ, Leroux M, Macklem PT: Site of airway obstruction in asthma as determined by measuring maximal expiratory flow breathing air and a helium-oxygen mixture. J Clin Invest 51:3235–3243, 1972

16. DuBois AB, Botelho SY, Bedell GN, Marshall R, Comroe JH Jr: A rapid plethysmographic method for measuring thoracic gas volume: A comparison with a nitrogen washout method for measuring functional residual capacity in normal subjects. J Clin Invest 35:322–326, 1956

17. Finucane KE, Egan BA, Dawson SV: Linearity and frequency response of pneumotachographs. J Appl Physiol 32:121–126, 1972

18. Fleisch A: Der Pneumotachograph; ein Apparat zur Geschwindigkeits registrierung der Atemluft. Pfluegers Arch 209:713–722, 1925

19. Fry DL, Hyatt RE: Pulmonary Mechanics. A unified analysis of the relationship between pressure, volume and gasflow in the lungs of normal and diseased human subjects. Am J Med 29:672–689, 1960

20. Grimby G, Stiksa J: Flow-volume curves and breathing patterns during exercise in patients with obstructive lung disease. Scand J Clin Lab Invest 25:303–313, 1970

21. Hankinson JL, Lapp NL: Time-pulse generator for flow-volume curves. J Appl Physiol 29:109–110, 1970

22. Hyatt RE: Dynamic lung volumes, in: Fenn WO, Rahn H (eds): Handbook of Physiology, Section 3: Respiration, vol II. Washington, D.C., American Physiological Society, 1965, pp 1381–1397

23. Hyatt RE, Black LF: The flow-volume curve: a current perspective. Am Rev Respir Dis 107:191–199, 1973

24. Hyatt RE, Schilder DP, Fry DL: Relationship between maximum expiratory flow and degree of lung inflation. J Appl Physiol 13:331–336, 1958

25. Ingram RH Jr, Schilder DP: Effect of gas compression on pulmonary pressure, flow, and volume relationship. J Appl Physiol 21:1821–1826, 1966

26. Jordanoglou J, Pride NB: A comparison of maximum inspiratory and expiratory flow in health and in lung disease. Thorax 23:38–45, 1968

27. Knudson RJ, Mead J, Leith DE: Flow transients from the respiratory system. Fed Proc 27:227a, 1968

28. Lapp NL, Hyatt RE: Some factors affecting the relationship of maximal expiratory flow to lung volume in health and disease. Chest 51:475–481, 1967

29. Leuallen EC, Fowler WS: Maximal midexpiratory flow. Am Rev Tuberc Pulm Dis 72:783–800, 1955

30. Lloyd TC Jr, Wright GW: Evaluation of methods used in detecting changes of airway resistance in man. Am Rev Respir Dis 87:529–537, 1963

31. Lord GP, Gazioglu K, Kaltreider N: The maximum expiratory flow-volume in the evaluation of patients with lung disease. Am J Med 46:72–79, 1969

32. McCall CB, Hyatt RE, Noble FW, Fry DL: Harmonic content of certain respiratory flow phenomena of normal individuals. J Appl Physiol 10:215–218, 1957

33. McFadden ER Jr, DeGroot WJ: An assessment of closing volumes and maximum mid-expiratory flow rates as tests of small airway disease. Clin Res 21:667, 1973

34. McFadden ER Jr, Lyons HA: Serial studies of factors influencing airway dynamics during recovery from acute asthma attacks. J Appl Physiol 27:452–459, 1969

35. McFadden ER Jr, Newton-Howes J, Pride NB: Acute effects of inhaled isoproterenol on the mechanical characteristics of the lungs in normal man. J Clin Invest 49:779–790, 1970

36. Mead J, Turner JM, Macklem PT, Little JB: Significance of the relationship between lung recoil and maximum expiratory flow. J Appl Physiol 22:95–108, 1967

37. Mellins RB, Lord GP, Fishman AP:

Dynamic behavior of the lung in acute asthma. Med Thorac 24:81–98, 1967

37a. Miller RD, Hyatt RE: Obstructing lesions of the larynx and trachea: clinical and physiologic characteristics. Mayo Clin Proc 44:145–161, 1969

38. Mitchell CA, Piscitelli D, Bouhuys A: Interaction of humoral agents on airway smooth muscle responses (ASMR) in man. Physiologist 15:219, 1972

39. Motoyama EK, Goto H, Wu B, de Leuchtenberg N: Evidence of lower airway obstruction in children with heart disease. American Pediatric Society Annual Meeting. May 19, 1973

40. Murtagh PS, Proctor DF, Permutt S, Kelly B, Evering S: Bronchial closure with mecholyl in excised dog lobes. J Appl Physiol 31:409–415, 1971

41. Overrath G, Konietzko N, Matthys H: Die diagnostische Aussagekraft des expiratorischen Flussvolumendiagramms. Pneumonologie 146:11–25, 1971

42. Park SS, Goldring IP, Shim CS, Williams MH Jr: Mechanical properties of the lung in experimental pulmonary emphysema. J Appl Physiol 26:738–744, 1969

43. Pascual RS, Mosher MB, Sikand RS, De Conti RC, Bouhuys A: Effect of bleomycin on pulmonary function in man. Am Rev Respir Dis 108:211–217, 1973

44. Peslin R, Mead J: Influence de l'histoire antérieure de débit sur la relation débit expiratoire maximum/volume pulmonaire. Unpublished manuscript

45. Peslin R, Morinet-Lambert J, Duvivier C: Étude de la réponse en fréquence de pneumotachographes (Frequency response of pneumotachographs). Bull Physiopathol Respir (Nancy) 8:1363–1376, 1972

46. Peters JM, Mead J, van Ganse WF: A simple flow-volume device for measuring ventilatory function in the field. Am Rev Respir Dis 99:617–622, 1969

47. Schilder DP, Roberts A, Fry DL: Effect of gas density and viscosity on the maximal expiratory flow-volume relationship. J Clin Invest 42:1705–1713, 1963

48. Seely JE, Zuskin E, Bouhuys A: Cigarette smoking: Objective evidence for lung damage in teen-agers. Science 172:741–743, 1971

49. Stubbs SE, Hyatt RE: Effect of increased lung recoil pressure on maximal expiratory flow in normal subjects. J Appl Physiol 32:325–331, 1972

50. Takishima T, Grimby G, Graham W, Knudson R, Macklem PT, Mead J: Flow-volume curves during quiet breathing, maximum voluntary ventilation, and forced vital capacities in patients with obstructive lung disease. Scand J Respir Dis 48:384–393, 1967

51. Takishima T, Takahashi K: "Closing volumes" and decreased maximum flow at low lung volumes in young subjects. J Appl Physiol 34:188–193, 1973

52. Vincent NJ, Knudson R, Leith DE, Macklem PT, Mead J: Factors influencing pulmonary resistance. J Appl Physiol 29:236–243, 1970

53. Virgulto J, Bouhuys A: Electronic circuits for recording of maximum expiratory flow-volume (MEFV) curves. J Appl Physiol 35:145–147, 1973

54. Zapletal A, Motoyama EK, Gibson LE, Bouhuys A: Pulmonary mechanics in asthma and cystic fibrosis. Pediatrics 48:64–72, 1971

55. Zapletal A, Motoyama EK, van de Woestijne KP, Hunt VR, Bouhuys A: Maximum expiratory flow-volume curves and airway conductance in children and adolescents. J Appl Physiol 26:308–316, 1969

56. Zuskin E, Lewis AJ, Bouhuys A: Inhibition of histamine-induced airway constriction by ascorbic acid. J Allergy Clin Immunol 51:218–226, 1973

57. Zuskin E, Mitchell CA, Bouhuys A: Interaction between effects of beta blockade and cigarette smoke on airways. J Appl Physiol (in press)

58. Zuskin E, Bouhuys A: Acute airway responses to hairspray preparations. N Engl J Med (in press)

59. Zamel N, Kass I, Fleischli GJ: Relative sensitivity of maximum expiratory flow-volume curves using spirometer versus body plethysmograph to detect mild airway obstruction. Am Rev Respir Dis 107:861–863, 1973

Chapter 10

Control of Breathing

The respiratory control system regulates a series of usually complementary but sometimes competitive or even incompatible activities. It must (1) maintain, through involuntary controls, a regular rhythmic breathing pattern; (2) adjust the tidal volume and the rate of breathing so that the minute volume of ventilation is sufficient to meet the demands for gas exchange in the lungs; and (3) adjust the breathing pattern so that it is consistent with other activities that use the same muscles, such as speech and the control of posture. Under most circumstances, breathing is controlled so well that the arterial partial pressures of oxygen and carbon dioxide remain constant within narrow limits.

Breathing is a motor act and its control resembles that of other movements. According to Luria, "The system is self-regulating: the brain judges the result of every action in relation to the basic plan and calls an end to the activity when it arrives at a successful completion of the program. This mechanism is equally applicable to elementary, involuntary forms of behavior, such as breathing and walking, and to complicated, voluntary ones such as reading, writing, decision-making and problem-solving." [76] The output of the breathing apparatus can be measured by recording respiratory muscle activity, lung volume changes, and arterial or alveolar gas tensions. In addition, many components of the control system have been studied in detail. However, we have as yet no adequate concept of how the control system fits all incoming signals together to determine the required motor output pattern. This chapter attempts a synthesis insofar as that is possible with our current knowledge. The following reviews offer more detailed discussions as well as access to the voluminous literature on the control of breathing: References 14, 17, 22, 27, 32, 34, 62, 69, 73, 86, 98, 99, 110, 114, and 116.

ORGANIZATION OF THE CONTROL SYSTEM

Breathing is usually involuntarily controlled. Networks of nerve cells in the brain stem ("respiratory centers") initiate the involuntary rhythmic breathing movements. The autonomous activity of the centers is modified by nervous and

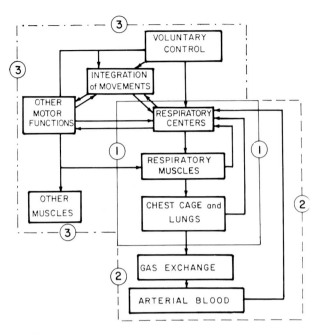

Fig. 10-1. Organization of respiratory control system. Blocks *1, 2,* and *3* contain the elements concerned
with the three main goals of the control system (see text).

chemical stimuli and is regulated in the framework of a complex control system
which has three main functional components (Fig. 10-1).

Control of the Breathing Pattern (block 1 in Fig. 10-1)

The periodic motor output of the centers, which leads to regular rhythmic
breathing, is conducted to the diaphragm via the phrenic nerves, to the intercostal
nerves via nerve roots from the 1st to 6th thoracic segment of the spinal cord,
and to abdominal muscles via nerve roots of the 7th to 12th thoracic and 1st
lumbar segment.

The actions of these individual muscles must be coordinated. For this purpose,
the motor output of the centers is modified by coordination centers in the spinal
cord, which determine the precise timing and the dosage of the impulses to each
muscle. The respiratory as well as the coordinating centers monitor the result
of their motor output. The former receive information on lung volume from receptors in the lungs, via vagal afferent fibers. The coordination centers receive
signals from the muscle spindles in the respiratory muscles which indicate
the state of muscle contraction.

Control of Ventilation (block 2 in Fig. 10-1)

The motor output of the respiratory centers (the ventilatory drive) must be
adjusted to meet the metabolic demands for gas exchange. For this adjustment,
the centers use information on the arterial partial pressures of O_2 and CO_2 and on

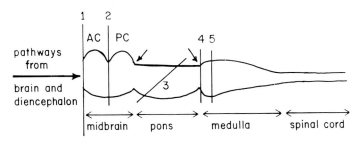

Fig. 10-2. Schematic diagram of brain stem structures, with levels of transections discussed in text. AC and PC = anterior and posterior colliculus, respectively. Between arrows: floor of the 4th ventricle. Distance between transections *4* and *5*—about 2 mm.

the H$^+$ ion concentrations in arterial blood, information provided by chemoreceptor cells near the centers themselves as well as in strategic sites in major arteries (carotid body, aorta). Appropriate modification of the motor output requires processing, storage, and integration of this information with other signals received by the centers. In this way, the ventilation of the lungs, per unit time, is regulated to maintain arterial O$_2$ and CO$_2$ tensions constant within narrow limits under most physiological conditions.

Integrative Control of Breathing (block 3 in Fig. 10-1)

The control of breathing must be integrated with the control of other motor functions using the same muscles: posture, speech, singing, swallowing, laughing. Hence, the respiratory centers must have links to other motor centers in the central nervous system, as well as connections to higher coordinating centers and to brain centers which initiate voluntary movements.

THE RESPIRATORY CENTERS

The brain stem contains an intricate network of neurons which maintains coordinated rhythmic breathing independent of afferent inputs. When the connection between the brain and the brain stem is severed in animals (transection *1* in Fig. 10-2), normal breathing resumes after the animal recovers from the operation. When the pons is separated from the medulla oblongata (transection *4* in Fig. 10-2), breathing is irregular and gasping. When the medulla is sectioned 2 mm lower (transection *5*), breathing stops. Thus, the centers crucial for rhythmic breathing appear to be situated between transections *4* and *5* in the upper part of the medulla. Regular coordinated breathing requires, however, that these centers have connections with other centers in the midbrain and pons.

Anatomically, the respiratory centers are not precisely defined. Cellular action potentials synchronous with breathing have been recorded from different sites in the pons and medulla.[21] Inspiratory discharges often occur at sites other than those of expiratory discharges. The ventilatory drive of the centers may be due to inherent automaticity of their nerve cells or may result from interconnections between these cells in a network. The centers may function like an electrical circuit in which a

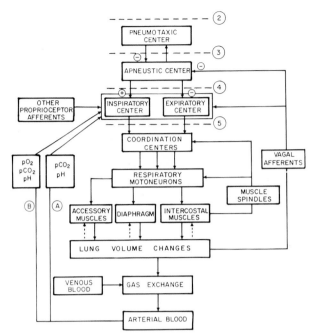

Fig. 10-3. Main functional components of the control system and the breathing apparatus. Dashed lines 2, 3, 4, and 5 indicate the corresponding transections in Figure 10-2. Facilitatory (+) and inhibitory (−) effects in the brain stem shown where appropriate. Dashed arrows indicate mechanical effect of lung volume changes on muscles (p. 209). *A:* central chemoreceptors; *B:* peripheral chemoreceptors.

rhythmic, oscillating output is caused by time delays in certain components and their connections.[79] Indirect support for this view comes from experiments with active and passive hyperventilation in cats.[38] When their ventilatory drive is actively increased (by stimulating the carotid body nerve), ventilation continues after the stimulation ceases. Presumably, internal feedback loops with time delays enable the centers to keep firing after the stimulus stops. With passive hyperventilation (by a respirator) the centers are not activated, and hence breathing stops because of lack of appropriate stimuli when the artificial ventilation ceases.[38]

The precise arrangement of the respiratory neuronal network in the midbrain and pons is unknown. After transection 2 (Fig. 10-3), breathing usually remains normal; therefore, the crucial network appears to be situated in the lower part of the midbrain and in the pons. After transection 3 combined with vagotomy, respiratory arrest occurs in an inspiratory position (apneusis). Breathing resumes, although it is irregular, when transection 4 is made. Thus, the lower part of the pons appears to contain a center which, when isolated from higher centers and from vagal afferents, promotes inspiration and inhibits expiration (apneustic center). When the apneustic center is connected to the midbrain, the action of the former is inhibited and breathing is rhythmic, even when the vagi have been cut. When the vagi are intact after transection 3, apneusis does not occur either. Hence, both vagal afferents and stimuli from a center in the midbrain (pneumotaxic center) affect the function of the apneustic center; apneusis occurs only when both sources of stimuli have been removed. However, even vagotomized cats with midbrain lesions may regain a normal breathing pattern when awake, suggesting that higher centers may compensate for the loss of stimuli from the midbrain and vagus.[105] Figure 10-3 schematically depicts the relations between the pneumotaxic, apneustic, inspiratory, and expiratory centers. These relations represent functional links in a complex network rather than distinct pathways between anatomically defined groups of neurons.

CONTROL OF THE BREATHING PATTERN

Mechanical Factors

To inspire and expire a tidal volume requires inspiratory and expiratory muscle activity, adapted to the lung volume and to the chest cage configuration. The recoil forces of the chest and lungs determine how much force is needed, and in which direction. For instance, inspiring a small tidal volume from FRC requires only inspiratory muscle activity; expiration is mainly passive, through elastic recoil. At higher lung volumes, the same tidal volume requires more inspiratory force to counteract the increased recoil force of the lungs and chest (Figs. 7-1, 7-8). At lung volumes below FRC, expiration always requires active muscle force. During breathing against positive pressure, inspiration may be passive (since inspiratory force is supplied), while expiration must be active. The respiratory motoneuron output must be adapted to meet these varying demands. Hence, the relation between muscle force and tidal volume is not constant.

In addition, the relation between the nervous stimuli that reach the muscles and the force developed depends on the initial length of the muscles. For the same degree of stimulation, muscles develop more force when they are stretched. Thus, to develop a similar inspiratory force, the inspiratory muscles require more stimulation when they are shortened (at high lung volumes).

The regulation of the division of labor between inspiratory and expiratory muscles is not clear but may require vagal afferent signals.[7] In cats, pressure breathing leads to contraction of abdominal muscles, which provide added expiratory force to overcome the load. This response is abolished by vagotomy, even when breathing is stimulated by CO_2.[6] However, responses to pressure breathing in man are probably more complex (see below).

Because of the complex relations between motoneuron output, muscle force, and tidal volume, the latter is a reliable measure of total motoneuron output only when the mechanical conditions are constant. Additional information on motoneuron output can be obtained from recordings of phrenic nerve discharge and of intercostal muscle electromyograms, which reflect important components of the motor drive but do not indicate its integral. Thus, none of these measurements provides a full picture of the output of the controlling system.

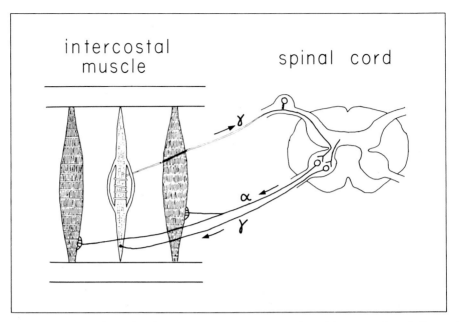

Fig. 10-4. Schematic diagram of respiratory muscle, with a muscle spindle, and its main neural connections with the spinal cord. γ-afferent fibers to the spinal cord and α- and γ-efferent fibers to the muscle fibers and the spindles, respectively, are shown. The γ-afferent fibers have their cell bodies in the dorsal root ganglion and synapse with α-motoneurons in the spinal cord (interneurons not shown). The termination of a motor pathway descending from higher centers is also shown.

Proprioceptive Control by Muscle Afferents

The respiratory muscles contain two kinds of proprioceptive receptors—muscle spindles and tendon receptors—which sense their state of contraction. These sensors can initiate reflex changes in muscle tension via coordinating centers in the spinal cord. The nerve fibers from the sensors (γ-afferents) reach the spinal cord via the dorsal roots (Fig. 10-4). When these roots are cut, the electrical activity in the external intercostal muscles decreases, in man [87] as well as in adult cats.[77] Thus, inputs from the γ-afferents affect inspiratory muscle activity.

Muscle spindles and tendon receptors influence muscle contraction in opposite directions. Stretching the intercostal muscles (which contain many spindles) increases muscle force (facilitation), while stretching the diaphragm (which contains mainly tendon receptors) inhibits its contraction.[31] The motor control of the intercostal muscles differs from that of the diaphragm; they also influence each other via mechanical and nervous linkages. Movement of the rib cage exerts force on the diaphragm, which is attached to it. More indirectly, movements of the rib cage affect the position of the diaphragm via changes in pleural pressure, and vice versa (see p. 239). In addition, contraction of intercostal muscles influences the diaphragm via nervous reflexes. In cats, contraction of the diaphragm can reinforce itself via an intercostal-to-phrenic nerve reflex, elicited by the pull of the diaphragm on the chest cage.[29] While this reflex may help to coordinate posture control and straining maneuvers,[30, 31] its role in breathing per se is uncertain.

Although the proprioceptive control system appears particularly well suited for rapid adaptations of muscle forces to changing demands, its importance in the control of breathing is not clear. Section of dorsal roots in man causes only temporary respiratory muscle paralysis.[87] When sudden loads (e.g., positive pressure at the mouth) are imposed on the breathing apparatus, proprioceptive stimuli elicit a "load-compensating reflex," which alters muscle activity appropriately. However, this response lasts so briefly that it can hardly affect ventilation.[88] In addition, responses to loading in man are influenced by anticipation of its effects and by learning in successive experiments.[48, 89, 108] Furthermore, changes in lung volume due to positive mouth pressures can explain at least some responses mechanically (via changes in elastance) without the need to invoke nervous control mechanisms.[45, 81]

Thus, the physiological function of proprioceptive muscle control in the control of breathing is not established. Since the muscles, chest cage, and lungs form a slow-responding mechanical system, which receives its motor input from fast-traveling nerve signals, afferent signals from sensors in the muscles would seem to be indispensable for control. Yet, perhaps the afferent signals have a less direct function, since their control function does not appear to influence ventilation under conditions (loading) in which it would seem most needed. The linkage of a fast nervous system to a slow-responding mechanical system is reminiscent of the linkage of a high-speed computer to a slow output device, such as a teletype. If the computer gave its output at its own rate to the teletype, only a fraction of the information would be recorded. In computer technology this problem is solved by buffers and flags. That is, the computer stores its information temporarily in a memory unit (buffer) and waits for a signal (a flag), indicating that the teletype is ready to produce an output signal. Thus, information is transferred sequentially at a discontinuous rate that the teletype can handle. If the analogy has any value, the muscle afferents may function as flags that signal the state of the muscles to the coordination centers. Such a function would not necessarily affect the motor output but merely facilitate its transmission to the muscles.

Proprioceptive Control by Vagal Afferents

More than 100 years ago, Hering and Breuer[98] proposed that inspiration is self-limiting because lung inflation stimulates receptors in lung tissue (stretch receptors) which, via vagal afferent fibers, lead to cessation of inspiration. This concept was based on the finding that intact animals stop breathing when their airway is closed after the lungs have been inflated. With the vagi cut, they attempt to inspire against the closed airway. Thus, vagal afferents appear to inhibit inspiration.

In a recent, more detailed concept of vagal control,[20] the ventilatory drive of the respiratory centers sets the rate of inspiratory muscle contraction and hence inspiratory flow rate (the slope of lines _1, 2,_ and _3_ in Fig. 10-5). This drive terminates after a time interval set by the centers (about 1.7 seconds in Fig. 10-5). However, this interval limits inspiration only when the ventilatory drive is minimal and inspiration therefore is slow (_3_ in Fig. 10-5). The greater the ventilatory drive (_1_ and _2_), the sooner inspiration ends (i.e., earlier in _1_ than in _2_). After vagotomy, inspiration lasts equally long in all three instances, presumably when the respiratory centers stop firing of their own accord. It is likely that the hyperbolic relation

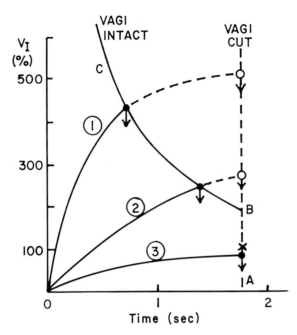

Fig. 10-5. Effect of vagotomy on relation between inspired volume (V_I; tidal volume during quiet breathing $= 100\%$) and duration of inspiration (time). Lines *1, 2,* and *3* represent three inspirations with different ventilatory drives, before (*drawn lines*) and after (*drawn + dashed lines*) vagotomy. The slope of these lines indicates inspiratory flow rate. The arrows indicate the end of inspiration in each instance, before and after vagotomy. Clark and Euler [20] place the normal tidal volume level (X) in the range AB. As discussed in the text, it may lie close to B. A comparison of lines *1* and *2* shows how vagal control amplifies the effect of increased ventilatory drive. Flow rate in *1* is about three times larger than in *2;* since inspiration lasts only half as long, tidal volume is about twice as large in *1* as in *2*. Because the rate has doubled, ventilation increases about fourfold. After vagotomy, rate is low and fixed; both tidal volume and ventilation are twice as large in *1* as in *2*. After reference 20.

between inspired volume (V_I) and the duration of inspiration, represented by curve BC in Figure 10-5, is related to firing of vagal afferent fibers from the lungs.

Vagal afferent signals from the lungs do not alter the centers' ventilatory drive [39] but influence the combination of tidal volume and breathing rate chosen for a given minute ventilation. After vagotomy in cats, tidal volume increases and rate decreases, while minute ventilation remains constant.[7] Conditions that normally affect breathing rate (e.g., breathing of CO_2-enriched air, airway obstruction) do not do so after vagotomy. In intact humans, too, breathing rate usually increases when tidal volume increases (with V_T up to about half the VC [58]). Hence, large inspirations are brief, in accordance with the hyperbolic relation between V_I and time in Figure 10-5.

In man at rest, vagal block does not affect the breathing pattern.[55] On the other hand, vagal afferent signals have been recorded in man at FRC, and these signals increase at larger lung volumes.[53, 56] Also, breathing rate increases as soon as tidal volume increases when the vagi are intact.[58] During normal breathing in man the control system appears to operate close to point B in Figure 10-5. As long as inspiration ends close to point B on the hyperbolic curve BC, vagal block would have little effect on the breathing pattern; yet, detectable afferent firing might occur. When ventilatory drive increases, the inspiratory point moves up the hyperbolic curve, and the breathing rate increases because of vagal inhibition. Thus, the principle of self-limited inspiration proposed by Hering and Breuer seems to be well established as an important mechanism that limits lung volume changes during breathing.[7] Even though the consequences of the vagal afferent activity on ventilation are imperceptible during quiet breathing, this activity appears to be largely responsible for the increase in rate when tidal volume increases, during exercise, hypercapnia and hypoxia.[20, 94, 95, 104]

Hering and Breuer also proposed that expiration is self-limiting, due to receptors which respond to decreases in lung volume (deflation receptors). Yet, there is no evidence for a role of deflation reflexes in the control of breathing patterns,[65] and it is not known at precisely which lung volume, presumably below FRC, they are activated. Deflation reflexes may be important under abnormal conditions where inspiratory efforts counteract collapse of peripheral lung units, as in pneumothorax or guinea pig anaphylaxis.[64, 65]

The concept of vagal control over tidal volume and rate appears to conflict with mechanical theories suggesting that the breathing rate is adjusted to optimal values in terms of the work or force of breathing (Chap. 7, p. 136). The mechanisms which accomplish this goal are not clear, and since the minima are far from critical, the fact that work and force are close to optimal may be just a useful but fortuitous consequence of the total system design. In fact, it has been suggested that minimal work would require a square wave inspiratory flow pattern and an exponentially decaying expiratory flow pattern,[118] while apneustic breathing at a constant minute ventilation causes a higher Pa_{O_2} and a lower Pa_{CO_2} than a sinusoid breathing pattern (Chap. 5, p. 86). None of these patterns occurs in man at rest or during moderate hyperventilation. The vagal control represents a more precise mechanism of rate control that may have developed independently or may have become adapted to the mechanical system design.[20]

Synthesis

The breathing pattern reflects mechanical conditions of the lungs and chest as well as the ventilatory drive provided by the respiratory centers in the medulla, modified by afferent inputs from vagal nerve fibers which signal changes in lung volume. Coordination of the respiratory muscle action may involve vagal afferent stimuli at the level of the centers as well as proprioceptive input from the muscles at the spinal level. Two types of sensors in the muscles provide afferent information to the spinal cord centers, and the muscles' proprioceptive control system can adjust muscle action to changes in loads and in other mechanical conditions. However, the physiological function of this system remains elusive. The role of vagal control is better established. Vagal afferents from stretch receptors in the lungs inhibit inspiration during lung inflation (Hering-Breuer reflex) and determine the end point of inspiration when tidal volume is increased during breathing. This rate control of the vagal nerve afferents amplifies the chemical control of ventilation. When an increase in chemical stimuli enhances the inspiratory drive, tidal volume increases. At the same time, vagal control leads to a rate increase (Fig. 10-5), which multiplies the effect of the increased respiratory drive on minute ventilation. Hence, the centers controlling ventilatory drive need only vary the rate of inspiratory drive in order to increase or decrease minute ventilation.[20]

CONTROL OF VENTILATION

The cells in the medullary respiratory centers can increase the ventilatory drive by firing more frequently, by increasing the number of firing cells, or both. Inspiratory drive is usually the only output, expiration being passive. The inspiratory drive is modulated by many different inputs into the centers, including inputs from (1) chemoreceptor cells near the centers sensitive to P_{CO_2} and H^+ concentration; (2) peripheral chemoreceptors sensitive to P_{O_2}, P_{CO_2}, and H^+ concentration in arterial blood; (3) higher centers in the midbrain; and (4) cerebral centers: (a) voluntary stimuli, as during breath holding or voluntary hyperventilation; and (b) in the context of other motor acts, including complex reflex events like posture control and swallowing, as well as learned patterns of motor behavior such as speech and singing (Chap. 11).

Central Chemoreceptors

After interruption of all known afferents, the respiratory centers still respond to a local increase of P_{CO_2} with increased discharge, leading to increased ventilation. The classical interpretation of this finding was that the centers' cells were sensitive to P_{CO_2} or to the change in local H^+ concentration resulting from changes in P_{CO_2}. However, the CO_2-sensitive cells, or chemoreceptors, most likely are separate from the centers themselves. They are probably located near the ventrolateral surface of the medulla, about 0.1–0.2 mm below the surface, and relatively far from the respiratory centers. Stimulation of these cells depends on the composition of the brain's interstitial fluid, specifically its pH and P_{CO_2}.[73, 84, 92] In turn, these values depend on the composition of blood perfusing the medulla and of cerebrospinal fluid (CSF). When the composition of CSF is kept constant, CO_2 breathing can still cause large ventilation increases acting via increased blood P_{CO_2}.[92] In cats, the ventilatory responses to inhaled CO_2 and to changes in CSF P_{CO_2} occur at about the same speed,[10] suggesting that the chemoreceptor cells are about equally accessible to CSF and to blood P_{CO_2} changes. Thus, the stimuli that the central chemoreceptors provide to the centers are determined both by CSF and blood levels of P_{CO_2} and pH, with bicarbonate as an important determinant of pH in CSF and in the chemoreceptors (Fig. 10-6).

The composition of CSF may differ from that of arterial blood, since the blood-brain barrier is easily permeable to CO_2 but not to bicarbonate, lactic acid, and

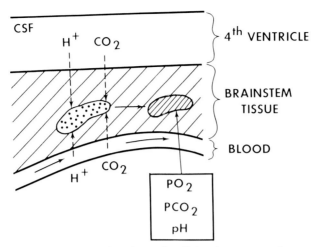

Fig. 10-6. Chemical stimuli impinge upon the central chemoreceptors (*stippled area*) by diffusion of H⁺ ions and CO_2 (*1*) from the bloodstream, and (*2*) from CSF. Stimuli from the central chemoreceptors are conducted to the respiratory centers (*dark hatching*), and these also receive stimuli from afferent fibers from chemoreceptors (*block and arrow below*).

other fixed acids. Hence, CSF P_{CO_2} follows the P_{CO_2} changes in arterial blood while levels of CSF bicarbonate and thus CSF pH may differ appreciably from those of blood. This explains why a similar degree of acidosis affects ventilation differently when it is caused by CO_2 breathing than when it is caused by lactic acid accumulation, as during heavy exercise. In the case of CO_2, CSF P_{CO_2} increases rapidly, and hence CSF pH decreases. Consequently, the centers are exposed to a high P_{CO_2} and a low pH both in blood and in CSF. In the case of lactic acid, no primary change in CSF pH occurs since this ion does not penetrate the blood-brain barrier. However, the resulting decrease in blood pH stimulates ventilation via the peripheral chemoreceptors (see below)—arterial P_{CO_2} decreases, followed rapidly by a decrease of CSF P_{CO_2} and a resulting increase of CSF pH, exposing the centers to opposing stimuli. Peripheral chemoreceptor stimulation and a decrease in blood pH near the centers lead to increased ventilation, while the increased CSF pH exerts an opposite effect. This mechanism explains the long-standing observation that, for the same blood pH change, CO_2 is a more effective stimulus to breathing than other acids.

Peripheral Chemoreceptors

Peripheral chemoreceptors are located in the carotid bodies, near the bifurcation of the common carotid artery and near the arch of the aorta (aortic bodies). The carotid bodies weigh only 1–2.5 mg and have a disproportionately large blood flow (1–2 liters/min/100 gm tissue at 130 mm Hg pressure [78]). Hence, their O_2 consumption is negligible compared to the amount of O_2 flowing through them, and their cells may be exposed to close to arterial P_{O_2} values. The chemoreceptor cells of the carotid and aortic bodies discharge in response to a decrease in arterial P_{O_2} and pH and an increase in arterial P_{CO_2}. The stimuli from these cells reach the central nervous system via the glossopharyngeal nerve (from the carotid bodies) and via the vagus nerve (from the aortic bodies). The resulting change in the centers' ventilatory drive ordinarily activates inspiratory, but not expiratory, muscles.[6] Stimulation of chemoreceptor cells also changes heart rate and vascular tone. Peripheral chemoreceptor cells at other sites [22] probably do not play as important a role as the carotid and aortic bodies.

The mechanism of chemoreceptor-cell sensitivity is unknown. Chemical transmission may be involved,[40] or the effect of hypoxia may be mediated through respiratory chain enzymes.[83] Some authors suggest that the hypoxia response, which depends on arterial P_{O_2} and not on O_2 content, is mediated through pH changes within the carotid body.[8] Chemoreceptor stimulation occurs in CO poisoning through its effect on the shape and position of the Hb-dissociation curve (Fig. 6-9, p. 114), which may decrease the local P_{O_2} in the chemoreceptor tissues even if the arterial P_{O_2} is unchanged.[82] In human adults, the hypoxia response is chiefly mediated through the carotid bodies, since bilateral resection of the carotid bodies [59, 75] and denervation of the carotid body [115] abolish or greatly reduce the hypoxia response. Blockade of the vagal and glossopharyngeal nerves in man has the same effect.[54] Neurological disease involving the afferent pathways from the chemoreceptors may abolish the hypoxia response while leaving the centers' CO_2 response intact.[9]

Ventilatory Responses to CO_2

Both central and peripheral chemoreceptors are sensitive to changes in local P_{CO_2}. The peripheral chemoreceptors act rapidly but contribute only a small portion of the total ventilatory drive; the central chemoreceptors are slower but, in dogs, provide about 80 percent of the total ventilatory drive.[5]

When healthy persons breathe 3–7 percent CO_2 in air, tidal volume, breathing rate, and minute ventilation increase. Graphs of minute ventilation versus arterial or alveolar P_{CO_2} (Fig. 10-7) describe the sensitivity of the control system to CO_2, but their interpretation is complex. In principle, the slope of the curve ($\Delta \dot{V}_E / \Delta P_{CO_2}$) reflects the "gain" or sensitivity of the CO_2 controller, but the curves are often alinear and determination of their slopes is inaccurate.[36] In addition, ventilatory response may be affected by mechanical factors. For instance, during pressure breathing in cats, minute ventilation responds less to CO_2, while phrenic nerve motoneuron activity increases as usual.[6] The decreased compliance of the lungs and chest due to the increased lung volume prevents ventilation from increasing in response to increased motoneuron output. An analogous condition occurs in patients with severe airway obstruction (p. 226).

At near-normal alveolar gas tensions, ventilation responds to a small increase in CO_2 tension (Fig. 10-7). When the arterial P_{CO_2} is decreased by hyperventilation, minute ventilation is temporarily reduced and often stops briefly (apnea).[3] During breathing of CO_2-enriched air, the increased ventilation reduces the increase of arterial P_{CO_2} but cannot prevent Pa_{CO_2} from rising markedly when the inspired CO_2 tension is higher than the initial Pa_{CO_2}. At still higher levels,

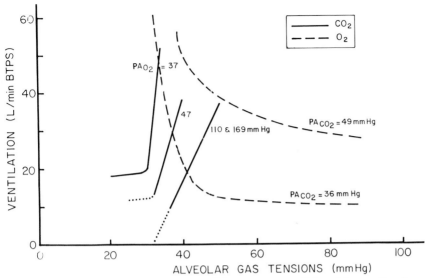

Fig. 10-7. Ventilatory responses to CO_2 at constant PA_{O_2} (*drawn lines*) and to O_2 at constant PA_{CO_2} (*dashed lines*). Data for CO_2 responses from reference 90 and for O_2 responses from reference 74.

the narcotic effect of CO_2 reduces ventilation and causes rapid retention of CO_2 in blood and tissues. The centers' sensitivity to CO_2 may depend on impulses from higher centers. In patients with bilateral cerebral lesions, CO_2 responses were often increased,[97] suggesting that stimuli from the brain normally inhibit the CO_2 response (cf. also reference 113).

Ventilatory Responses to Hypoxia

When one breathes room air, the chemoreceptors are active and they increase their activity when the inspired P_{O_2} is decreased. Inspiration of a single breath of pure oxygen leads to temporary reduction of minute ventilation (Fig. 10-8), suggesting that hypoxic drive contributes to ventilation during room-air breathing. With prior breathing of a hypoxic gas mixture, the O_2 breath reduces ventilation more, reflecting an increased hypoxic drive in hypoxia. At near-normal alveolar gas tensions, small changes in alveolar P_{O_2} affect ventilation much less than changes in alveolar P_{CO_2} (Fig. 10-7). The ventilatory responses to hypoxia lead to secondary changes in arterial P_{CO_2}. Since the controlling system is very sensitive to CO_2, the response to hypoxia per se can only be studied adequately when Pa_{CO_2} is kept constant (see next section).

Athletes respond less to hypoxia and to CO_2 than do untrained healthy persons; both hypoxic and hypercapnic responses correlate negatively with the maximum working capacity.[16] Whether these diminished ventilatory responses are related to chemoreceptor function or to differences in central processing of chemoreceptor information is not known.

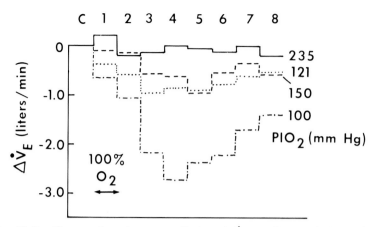

Fig. 10-8. Changes in minute ventilation ($\Delta \dot{V}_E$, *ordinate*) induced by a single breath of 100 percent O_2 (breath 1) in subjects who breathed different O_2 mixtures (O_2 partial pressures at right) during the control period (*C*) and during breaths 2–8. Average data from 3 subjects of Dejours et al., J Physiol (Paris) 49:115–119, 1957. Inspired O_2 tensions calculated assuming that atmospheric pressure was 760 mm Hg (altitude, 50 meters).

Interaction Between CO_2 and O_2 Stimuli

By carefully manipulating inspired gas concentrations, one can keep alveolar and arterial P_{O_2} tensions constant while changing P_{CO_2}, and vice versa. This procedure yields graphs of minute ventilation versus P_{CO_2} at constant P_{O_2}, and of minute ventilation versus P_{O_2} at constant P_{CO_2} (Fig. 10-7). Clearly, the level of alveolar P_{O_2} influences the response to CO_2-tension changes, and vice versa.[24, 50, 74, 90] At low values of P_{O_2}, the response to CO_2 is alinear; there appears to be a threshold below which P_{CO_2} changes do not affect ventilation. Above the threshold, ventilation increases steeply with increased P_{CO_2}, more so than when the alveolar P_{O_2} is normal or increased. Conversely, at near-normal alveolar P_{CO_2}, large decreases of P_{O_2} are required before ventilation increases markedly. At a higher alveolar P_{CO_2}, lesser degrees of hypoxia elicit a response, and the sensitivity to P_{O_2} changes in the range between 50 and 80 mm Hg appears to increase. The mechanism of the interaction between CO_2 and hypoxic stimuli is not known. At least in part, interaction takes place in the carotid bodies,[44] but the cellular events involved in the interaction have not been identified.

Physiological Events Involving the Control of Ventilation

In this section the foregoing discussions of the components of the ventilatory control system are applied to conditions during breath holding, exercise, and sojourn at high altitude.

Breath holding. Man can voluntarily suspend breathing for periods of less than a minute to over 10 minutes, depending on his motivation, his initial lung volume, and his alveolar gas tensions at the beginning of breath holding. Both the CO_2 stimulus and the hypoxic stimulus influence the "breaking point" at which the subject can no longer resist the urge to breathe. After someone quietly breathes room air, he commonly reaches the breaking point when PA_{CO_2} is about 50 mm Hg and PA_{O_2} about 70 mm Hg.[62] Breath holding can be prolonged (1) by first hyperventilating, (2) by first inspiring a breath of 100 percent O_2, and (3) maximally by first hyperventilating while inspiring 100 percent O_2. When P_{O_2} is high, alveolar P_{CO_2} determines the breaking point and vice versa, when P_{CO_2} is low, alveolar P_{O_2} is the limiting factor. At the end of a voluntary breath hold, breathing a gas low in O_2 and high in CO_2 can enable the subject to hold his breath again, even though alveolar gas composition has not improved.[47] This suggests that chest movements play a role in determining the end point of breath holding.

Exercise. Ventilation may increase from its resting value of about 5 liters/ min to 60 liters/min or more during exercise. This adaptation to the increased demand for oxygen and to the need to excrete more CO_2 is so effective that arterial P_{O_2} need not decrease even during maximum work, while arterial P_{CO_2} need not increase.

Ventilation increases upon the onset of exercise (Fig. 10-9) [34, 35] so rapidly that flow rate increases during the phase of the breath in which work begins.[60] This immediate response must be due to nervous stimuli, since it occurs too rapidly to be explained by blood-borne chemical stimuli. Since ventilation also increases when the limbs are passively exercised, these nervous stimuli to breathing may be elicited by proprioceptors in the limb muscles or joints,[23, 34] which sense muscular contraction, particularly the rate of movement.[2] For instance, passive stretching

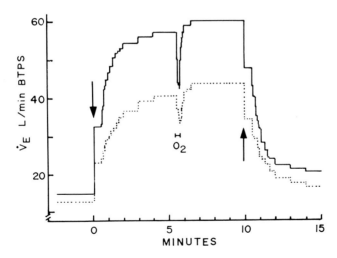

Fig. 10-9. Mean ventilatory responses to exercise in lowlanders (*solid line*) and highlanders (*dotted line*) at 3660 meters (12,300 ft) altitude. Arrows indicate beginning and end of work (load: 120 watts). Both the initial and steady-state responses are less in highlanders than in lowlanders. Three inspirations of 100 percent O_2 were given in the sixth minute of exercise. The ensuing decrease of $\dot{V}_E$ indicates the contribution of hypoxic drive to ventilation before and after the O_2 breaths. The hypoxic drive is less in the highlanders than in the lowlanders. Modified from reference 71.

of a leg muscle increases phrenic nerve discharge in dogs.[63] However, ventilation increases more during active than during passive exercise, and, in addition, the initial response may be too rapid to be explained by afferent neural stimuli.[93] Hence, the increased neurogenic ventilatory drive at the start of exercise may originate centrally, as a set of impulses from the brain to the respiratory centers, concomitant with motor impulses to the exercising muscles. The abrupt increase in ventilatory drive might be a learned response rather than part of a feedback control system.[4, 61]

After its rapid initial increase, ventilation increases further, slowly, before it levels off during the steady state of exercise. The neurogenic drive (see above) continues to provide a large fraction of the total ventilatory drive during this phase.[28, 34] When one suddenly stops exercising, the neurogenic drive stops and ventilation decreases within a few seconds (Fig. 10-9). Another part of the total ventilatory drive is contributed by hypoxic stimuli, since a breath of 100 percent O_2, taken during exercise, abruptly reduces ventilation (Fig. 10-9).

Since arterial P_{CO_2} is often unchanged during transition from rest to work, and usually decreases during heavy work, CO_2 stimuli were long thought to be unimportant in increasing ventilation during exercise.[43] However, the relation between P_{CO_2} and ventilation may be obscured by other stimuli, in particular the increased neurogenic drive when work begins. When these other stimuli are kept constant (as when changing from light to heavier exercise in unanesthetized dogs, increasing treadmill grade, and keeping rate of leg movements constant), the relation between changes in P_{CO_2} and ventilation is similar to that obtained with CO_2 inhalation.[2] Under these conditions, changes in P_{CO_2} during exercise can account for the ventilatory increase. During heavy exercise, arterial P_{CO_2} and pH decrease due to accumulation of lactic and pyruvic acid in blood. Peripheral chemoreceptor stimulation by increased blood acidity then provides additional ventilatory drive.

High altitude. When a sea-level resident first arrives at high altitude, his ventilation at rest and during work increases in response to the acute hypoxia. Without hyperventilation, P_{CO_2} would remain constant and the alveolar point would be situated at 1″ in Figure 10-10. Due to hyperventilation, P_{CO_2} decreases, and P_{O_2} increases about 6 mm Hg (to point 1′, at 4600 meters = 15,000 feet). The gain in alveolar P_{O_2} continues when ventilation increases further during continued stay at altitude (arrows in Fig. 10-10). Thus, acclimatization results in increases in alveolar P_{O_2} at the expense of increased ventilation and decreased alveolar P_{CO_2}.

Acclimatization of sea-level residents ("lowlanders") involves increased sensitivity and a decreased threshold to CO_2, which occur within 3 days after arrival at altitude (4540 meters [66]). Responses to hypoxia remain unchanged during the first 11 days at this altitude.[66] The increased CO_2 sensitivity is probably due to changes in the composition of brain extracellular fluid (ECF). Initially alveolar P_{CO_2}, and concurrently CSF P_{CO_2}, decrease due to the hypoxic drive via the arterial chemoreceptors.[13] The decreased CSF P_{CO_2} leads to an increase in ECF pH, which inhibits the ventilatory drive. Gradually, CSF bicarbonate concentration is adjusted to the low P_{CO_2}, and ECF pH decreases. Thus, the initial inhibitory effect of the high ECF pH on ventilatory drive is removed, and ventilation increases further.[109]

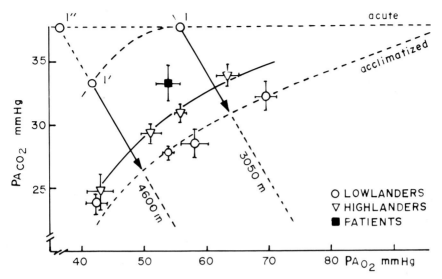

Fig. 10-10. O_2-CO_2 diagram (see Chap. 5) with R lines for two altitudes (3050 meters = 10,000 feet; 4600 meters = 15,000 feet). Inspired P_{O_2} = 100 and 80 mm Hg, respectively (note that the ordinate has been interrupted so that the R lines do not intersect the abscissa at the PI_{O_2} value). Line labeled "acute" shows changes in alveolar gas tensions during an acute transfer from sea level to altitude (alveolar point 1 at 3050 meters; point 1' at 4600 meters). Point 1" is the alveolar point that would occur at 4600 meters without hyperventilation. Arrows indicate changes in alveolar gas during acclimatization. In highlanders, especially those with airway obstruction (see p. 226), PA_{O_2} is lower and PA_{CO_2} higher than in acclimatized lowlanders. The point for the patients is an average of 9 patients (mean age 52 years). Bars indicate 2 SE for PA_{O_2} and PA_{CO_2}. Modified from reference 70.

The increased ventilation of lowlanders at altitude improves their oxygenation at the expense of increased work of breathing. Native highlanders ventilate less at the same oxygen uptake than recently acclimatized lowlanders.[68] Since they utilize a smaller portion of their ventilatory capacity for the same work, they are less dyspneic than lowlanders. However, their reduced ventilatory response leads to lower alveolar O_2 tensions (Fig. 10-10). In one study, PA_{O_2} averaged 56 mm Hg in highlanders and 61 mm Hg in acclimatized lowlanders at similar work loads.[71] Highlanders may tolerate hypoxia better than acclimatized lowlanders, and can therefore work harder, but the mechanisms of this tolerance are ill understood. Short-term acclimatization to altitude (weeks or months) does not lead to an adaptation that equals that of native highlanders.

Native highlanders have a smaller ventilatory response to hypoxia than acclimatized lowlanders (Fig. 10-9). This "blunted hypoxic drive" occurs in persons native to altitudes of 2900 meters and higher, and in persons of widely varying ethnic origins, living in the Andes, in Colorado, and in the Himalayas.[46, 68, 111] Animals native to high altitude (yaks, heifers, and sheep in the Himalayas; dogs and llamas in the Andes) have a normal response to hypoxia.[15, 67, 70] The decreased hypoxic response may explain why highlanders ventilate less and have a lower PA_{O_2} and a higher PA_{CO_2} than acclimatized lowlanders (Fig. 10-10).

The blunted hypoxic response of highlanders has been attributed to failure of the peripheral chemoreceptors, which might also account for the slower response of highlanders to CO_2.[72, 117] However, in cats, development of the blunted hypoxic response appears to require intact connections between the brain stem and higher brain centers. In these animals, a blunted hypoxic response can be evoked during stays of up to 4 months in a low-pressure chamber (atmosphere equivalent to 5500 meters = 18,000 feet altitude).[113] Experiments with decerebration or removal of the cerebral cortex in cats suggest that cortical centers inhibit the response to hypoxia at altitude, while centers in the diencephalon facilitate it.[113]

Synthesis. Central chemoreceptor cells in the medulla respond to CO_2 with increased chemoreceptor drive, leading to increased ventilation. The local P_{CO_2} near these cells is determined by the composition of blood and of CSF. Peripheral chemoreceptor cells in carotid bodies and aortic wall respond to decreased arterial P_{O_2} and pH and to increased arterial P_{CO_2}, leading to afferent nervous stimuli, which increase ventilatory drive. The relations between increased ventilatory drive induced by central and peripheral chemoreceptor stimuli on the one hand, and lung ventilation on the other hand, are complicated by (1) the mechanical properties of muscles, chest wall, and lungs and (2) interaction between CO_2 and hypoxic stimuli. The breaking point of *breath holding* may be determined by the CO_2 or by hypoxic stimuli. The increased ventilation during *exercise* is elicited by (1) rapid-acting neurogenic stimuli from muscle or joint receptors in the limbs or from brain centers, or both; (2) responses to increased P_{CO_2}, which can be detected when other stimuli are kept constant; and (3) responses to decreased arterial pH during heavy exercise. At *high altitude,* the hypoxic stimulus increases ventilation in newly arrived lowlanders; further hyperventilation results from increased CO_2 sensitivity, probably a result of changes in the pH of brain extracellular fluid. Native highlanders ventilate less and respond less to hypoxia than acclimatized lowlanders.

INTEGRATIVE CONTROL OF BREATHING

"The course of events in the organism forms a network, with circular or net-like connections between several chains of events. . . . the existence of such networks provides the general conditions for regulation of an event."[103] Thus, in 1921 Rohrer introduced the principle of the control of breathing as a regulatory system involving positive and negative feedback ("Hin- und Rückkoppelung von Teilvorgängen"). In recent years, mathematical models have been used extensively to describe quantitatively how feedback loops can regulate the output of the controller (i.e., the ventilatory drive of the respiratory centers) so that the controlled quantities (arterial gas tensions) remain close to constant.[19, 37, 80, 100, 102]

In addition, breathing movements must be coordinated with other motor functions using the same muscles, which necessitates nervous connections between respiratory and other motor centers. For instance, pathways from the cerebellum to the phrenic nerve center may provide a means for integrating diaphragmatic contraction in the control of posture.[30] In the cerebral cortex, an area close to Broca's speech center may help integrate speech and breathing (Chap. 11).

Electrical stimulation of the motor area in the cortex causes individual muscles to contract but does not lead to coordinated breathing movements. Voluntary changes in coordinated breathing probably involve indirect (extrapyramidal) pathways from the cerebral cortex to the spinal cord, with coordination occurring at a subcortical level.

The integration of breathing with the control of speech, singing, and wind-instrument playing (Chap. 11) poses special problems, as for the trumpet player who marches in a band, especially uphill! Marching bands generally prefer brass instruments, which require higher flow rates than most woodwinds and are therefore more compatible with exercise requirements. Integrative control of breathing during these activities has its limits; for instance, it is impossible to speak normally during heavy exercise, since the flow rate requirements for the two activities differ too much. The integration between swallowing and breathing has been discussed in Chapter 2. In several animals, heat loss through the respiratory system helps regulate body temperature. When placed in a hot environment, they hyperventilate, thus increasing heat loss through the respiratory passages. An increase in body temperature in cats leads to an increased ventilatory drive of the respiratory centers.[39] In unanesthetized goats, breathing rate increased from about 40 breaths per minute to 270 breaths per minute during thermal polypnea, with an increase in rectal temperature of only 1° C.[57] This response was accompanied by a decrease of arterial P_{CO_2} from 39 to 25 mm Hg. Dogs, too, depend to a large extent on respiratory heat elimination for their body temperature control. In conscious, trained dogs, arterial P_{CO_2} decreases by 4–7 mm Hg during exercise on a treadmill.[1] Apparently, the thermoregulatory process requires goats and dogs to ventilate in excess of their requirements for gas exchange.

Thus, the needs of other regulatory processes sometimes appear to take precedence over ventilation control for purposes of gas exchange. In man, too, the ventilatory control system does not always ideally fulfill its task of keeping blood gas tensions within normal limits. During exercise, ventilation depends on the ventilatory load rather than on the oxygen uptake.[85] When the breathing apparatus is unloaded by breathing a light gas (He-O_2; see also Chap. 8), ventilation increases for the same oxygen uptake, and P_{CO_2} decreases from 35 to 30 mm Hg. During the same work, with the subject breathing room air, P_{CO_2} remained constant at 35 mm Hg. The control system seems to set the level of ventilation in accordance with expected requirements and fails to adjust the ventilatory drive under the unusual condition of a decreased ventilatory load. Apparently, the low P_{CO_2}, which should act as an error signal, is ignored. This also happens during prolonged pressure breathing, which leads to hyperventilation and a decreased arterial P_{CO_2}.[45] During heavy exercise, too, the control system appears to abandon its function of keeping blood gas tensions constant. Arterial P_{CO_2} may decrease to 30 mm Hg or less when O_2 uptake is more than 3 liters/min,[12, 34] due primarily to the metabolic acidosis of exercise. Hyperventilation may occur in part because the inspiratory muscles participate in the work itself, for instance, by moving and stabilizing the shoulder girdle. To some extent, hyperventilation during exercise is advantageous because it allows higher alveolar oxygen tensions.

DEVELOPMENT OF THE CONTROL OF BREATHING

When the infant begins to breathe after birth, the control system does not yet function optimally and develops further during the first stages of postnatal development.

Initiation of Breathing

The fluid which fills the lungs in utero is expelled during delivery (Chap. 1). Some air may enter the infant's lungs as his chest and lungs recoil to a resting position immediately after his chest has passed through the birth canal. However, forceful inspiratory maneuvers are needed to expand the lungs during the first few breaths and to keep them inflated (see p. 137, Chap. 7). Some studies suggest that the ventilatory drive required to produce this force is largely initiated by changes in the newborn's blood gas tensions, i.e., an increase in P_{CO_2} and a decrease in P_{O_2}. For instance, in fetal lambs delivered by cesarean section, the circulation can be maintained by cross-perfusion. If the arterial blood gases are controlled at close to normal levels in such animals, they do not begin to breathe.[91] Lowering P_{O_2} or increasing P_{CO_2} in their arterial blood, or both, invariably triggers breathing, while clamping the cord does not. The low P_{O_2} and high P_{CO_2} stimuli interact much as they do in adults (p. 218).

Several elements of the respiratory control system function at birth. Newborn infants decrease their ventilation when breathing 100 percent O_2 during 8–15 seconds, or during 5 breaths,[25, 101] suggesting that the peripheral chemoreceptors are tonically active, as they are in adults (p. 217). In newborn animals, ventilatory responses to hypoxia are not sustained more than a few minutes, although the carotid nerve afferents keep firing.[106] Thus, exhaustion of immature central or effector neurons [107] rather than immaturity of receptors or afferent fibers may be involved. In the highly immature newborn opossum, responses to CO_2 and hypoxia occur in 5-day-old animals (weighing 350 mg; age from conception 18 days).[42] In 15–20-day-old opossums, interaction between CO_2 and hypoxic stimuli occurs as described on p. 218. In newborn infants an inflation reflex can be elicited, presumably through activation of stretch receptors in lungs; this reflex disappears after a few days.[26] Newborn infants are highly sensitive to CO_2 during the first weeks of life.[112]

In spite of the presence of functional vagal afferents and chemoreceptors for CO_2 and hypoxia, rhythmic control of breathing is not fully developed at birth. In particular, higher integrative control appears to be lacking. For instance, the human newborn swallows air and inspires air into the lungs at the same time;[11] he must learn to integrate swallowing and breathing as they occur in the adult (see Chap. 2). It has even been suggested that the first few breaths are in fact modified swallows, similar to the breathing maneuvers of frogs.[11]

Early Development of Control Mechanisms

In human infants during the first weeks of life, responses to CO_2 decrease [112] while responses of tidal volume to 100 percent oxygen (5 breaths) increase.[25] The roles of vagal afferents and of proprioceptive control also appear to change during development.

Vagal afferents. The newborn's most important need is to maintain lung inflation. In particular, insufficient development of lung surfactant (Chap. 1, p. 9) may lead to alveolar collapse in premature newborns. Thus, it is not surprising that ventilatory responses to changes in lung volume are well developed at birth, even in the highly immature opossum.[11] These responses differ, at least in opossums, from those in adults and include gasping and prolonged inspirations. In some immature animals, vagal input is critical for the control of breathing. Newborn kittens survive decerebration only if the vagi are intact—they stop breathing and die when the vagi are cut. The mature (21 days) decerebrated rabbit develops increased inspiratory force when the trachea is occluded, even after the vagi have been cut. The immature newborn rabbit, also decerebrated, shows this response only when the vagi are intact.[106] Thus, input from vagal afferents appears to be critical for maintaining breathing in these immature animals, and this may be related to their prime need to maintain lung inflation. The adult animal's lungs are mechanically more stable and hence less susceptible to collapse. For adults, vagal afferent input appears to be less critical during quiet breathing as well as during exercise, and deflation reflexes play a role only under pathological conditions with lung collapse.[65]

Proprioceptive control. In comparison with vagal input, proprioceptive input from the respiratory muscles appears to be relatively unimportant for the young animal. In the mature cat (28 days), sectioning 7 adjacent dorsal roots on both sides decreases EMG activity in external intercostal muscles. In the newborn kitten, the same muscles show unchanged activity after the same dorsal root section.[106] Hence, proprioceptive control of the respiratory muscles functions in the mature cat but not in the newborn kitten. Integration of the control of breathing with proprioceptive muscle control [31, 39] may be essential for integrating breathing with other motor acts (walking, running, posture control). But while this integration is essential for the mature animal, it is less important for the newborn whose motor abilities are immature.

CLINICAL APPLICATIONS

While breathing-control disorders as separate clinical entities are relatively rare, many pharmacological substances affect the central control mechanisms, and depression of breathing by anesthetics and other drugs is a common clinical problem.[69] Decreased ventilation as a result of structural damage to the central nervous system usually occurs together with other signs of neurological disorders. In clinical practice, depressed ventilatory control is usually detected only when it leads to overt ventilatory failure, requiring artificial ventilation.

Decreased ventilation caused by failure of control mechanisms must be distinguished from that caused by parenchymal lung disease and airway obstruction. Since lung disease and failure of control may coexist, this is not always easy. A patient with decreased minute ventilation, reduced vital capacity, and forceful chest movements during breathing usually has severe airway obstruction. In case of doubt, one can use esophageal pressure recordings (Chap. 7) to distinguish between lack of respiratory drive and ventilatory failure due to lung disease. When the respiratory drive and the respiratory muscles are intact, pleural-pressure swings during the breathing cycle are usually normal or increased, reflecting adequate forces applied to the lungs. In patients with respiratory muscle paralysis or insufficient ventilatory drive, the inadequate force is reflected by decreased pleural-pressure swings. Electromyography of respiratory muscles, using surface or needle electrodes for the intercostal and abdominal muscles and an intraesophageal electrode for the diaphragm,[17] may be used to record individual muscle function. In patients with normal lungs and depressed ventilatory drive, measurements of ventilation at rest, during voluntary breathing maneuvers (VC; hyperpnea), exercise, or inspiration of CO_2, low oxygen mixtures and 100 percent O_2 can yield information on the control system. Single-breath tests with 100 percent O_2, during a period of breathing 13 percent O_2, can indicate the presence of a hypoxic ventilatory drive.[33] Vital capacity breaths of 5 percent or 15 percent CO_2 in N_2 or O_2, with subsequent measurement of ventilation, also permit assessment of chemoreceptor drive.[49] However, these tests have been insufficiently standardized, and the variability of normal responses is large. Nevertheless, in selected patients and in the context of other diagnostic information, they may help to determine the role of ventilatory control mechanisms in ventilatory failure.

Ventilatory Control in Airway Obstruction

In patients with severe chronic airway obstruction, responses of ventilation to low P_{O_2} or increased P_{CO_2} are often less than in normal persons. Ventilatory drive may be inappropriately strong (Chap. 8, p. 168), but the increased work of breathing leads to insufficient ventilation even though the forces applied by the respiratory muscles are normal or increased. The hypercapnia which sometimes occurs during O_2 breathing in these patients has been attributed to lack of central response to CO_2. Thus, ventilation would be driven largely by the hypoxic drive from the peripheral chemoreceptors, and administration of oxygen would abolish this input. However, increased airway resistance at the mouth, combined with an added dead space, causes a similar response to O_2 in healthy subjects, suggesting that hypercapnia in patients may also be explained on the basis of the increased work of breathing [18] (see also p. 137). Although the responses to CO_2 and O_2 in patients with obstruction are low in absolute terms (measured in liters per minute), they equal those of normal persons when measured as a fraction of the maximum voluntary ventilation.[52] Thus, both patients and healthy persons use a similar proportion of their ventilatory capacity when responding to similar CO_2 and hypoxic stimuli. In patients with airway obstruction and ventilatory failure, relief of obstruction is obviously the more important treatment goal, for when this is achieved, the response to ventilatory stimuli improves.

At altitude, even a person with moderate airway obstruction may have severe dyspnea, polycythemia, and hypercapnia [70] (Fig. 10-10). In part, his higher P_{CO_2} and lower P_{O_2}, in comparison with a healthy highlander, may be caused by relative lack of ventilatory response to low P_{O_2} and high P_{CO_2}.[72]

During sleep, ventilatory drive is normally reduced, resulting in increases in arterial P_{CO_2} from 2–10 mm Hg. Similar increases occur in patients with airway obstruction and are accompanied by decreases in arterial P_{O_2} (avg. 7.4 mm Hg [96]). These changes are, however, not much greater than those in healthy sleepers. When ventilation is depressed and cardiac output is normal, the average $\dot{V}_A/\dot{Q}$ ratio decreases. Since recumbency by itself leads to decreased $\dot{V}_A/\dot{Q}$ ratios in parts of the lungs (p. 91; Chap. 5), one might expect that during sleep, patients with severe airway obstruction and a nonuniform distribution of $\dot{V}_A/\dot{Q}$ would have appreciable decreases in P_{O_2} combined with some increases in P_{CO_2}, according to the shape of the $\dot{V}_A/\dot{Q}$ lines (Fig. 5-6, p. 88). In fact, the distribution of $\dot{V}_A/\dot{Q}$ ratios in these patients may already be large due to the disease itself, and the incremental distribution abnormality due to sleep may be difficult to detect.

Central Hypoventilation

Reduced ventilatory drive in the presence of normal lung and respiratory muscle function occurs in patients with neurological disease, e.g., encephalitis or brain stem lesions. Some patients with insufficient ventilatory drive are thought to be "lazy breathers." Rohrer described two physicians who thought that they had temporarily lost ventilatory control during a severe illness, "so that only the conscious will to continue to breathe had brought them through this critical condition." [103] Such observations have been made in other patients who lack central ventilatory drive and may require admonitions to breathe. They often ventilate normally during the day but develop ventilatory failure during sleep. They may need artificial ventilation every night to prevent hypoxemia and CO_2 retention. In recent years, unilateral stimulation of the phrenic nerve (electrophrenic respiration) has been used successfully to supplement the inspiratory drive and to normalize gas exchange in these patients [51] (Fig. 10-11). Since at least some patients with central hypoventilation appear to have a localized neurological defect with few symptoms other than failure of ventilatory drive, one wonders whether the plasticity of the brain would permit re-education through a conditioning approach, perhaps using rhythmic sensory stimulation.

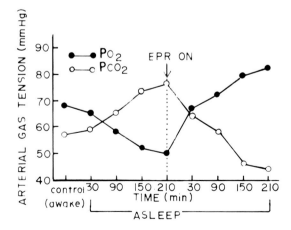

Fig. 10-11. Normalization of blood gas tensions by electrophrenic respiration (EPR) in a patient with encephalitis. During sleep, PA_{O_2} decreased and PA_{CO_2} increased, until EPR was initiated. From reference [51].

Cheyne-Stokes Breathing [19]

Cheyne-Stokes breathing is a pattern of waxing and waning breathing, in which periods with large tidal volumes alternate with apnea or minimal breathing lasting 15–60 seconds. An oscillating output can occur in any control system involving feedback (Rohrer, 1921 [103]), for instance, when the temporal relation between the feedback and the output signal is disrupted, or when the system is insufficiently damped. The oscillating ventilatory drive in Cheyne-Stokes breathing is promoted by time delays in the feedback signals, for instance, prolongation of the circulation time. In disease of the central nervous system, where inhibitory impulses from higher centers are removed, the CO_2 controller may become less stable, or its response may be so depressed that the alinear O_2 controller takes over. This promotes output oscillations, since O_2 stores in the body are small and the O_2 controller is therefore less damped and inherently less stable than the CO_2 controller.

SUMMARY

A complex nervous control system—with humoral as well as nervous inputs—regulates the rhythmic pattern of breathing, adjusts ventilation to match the needs for gas exchange, and coordinates breathing with other motor activities. Respiratory centers in the brain stem initiate the nervous ventilatory drive; coordinating centers in the spinal cord ensure appropriate dosage and timing of nervous impulses to participating muscles. Respiratory muscle force depends on muscle length and hence on lung volume. Muscle force, along with the mechanical state of the chest and lungs (lung volume, airway caliber, airway pressure), determines the tidal volume which results from a given level of ventilatory drive.

The respiratory centers in the brain stem receive feedback information concerning the output of the control system from (1) proprioceptive muscle afferents, (2) vagal afferents from the lungs, (3) central chemoreceptors sensitive to P_{CO_2} and pH levels in brain extracellular fluid, and (4) peripheral chemoreceptors (in carotid and aortic bodies), which respond to decreases in arterial P_{O_2} and pH and to increases of arterial P_{CO_2}. CO_2 and O_2 stimuli interact in their effect on ventilation. The physiological importance of the control system becomes clear from experiments on breath holding in man, and from studies on responses to exercise and high-altitude hypoxia in man and animals.

Integration of breathing with other motor acts (speech, swallowing, thermal polypnea in animals, postural control) requires nervous connections between nerve centers subserving breathing and those subserving other motor activities. Under some conditions, the requirements of other motor acts appear to prevail over the main goal of the breathing apparatus, i.e., to keep arterial blood gas levels constant within narrow limits.

The respiratory control system functions at birth but undergoes further development during maturation. In newborn animals, vagal afferents from the lungs are essential to maintain breathing, while proprioceptive muscle control is as yet undeveloped.

In assessing disease states with ventilatory failure, one must differentiate between (1) lack of ventilatory drive (due to drugs or central nervous system damage), (2) respiratory muscle paralysis, and (3) inability to ventilate the lungs because of lung disease in spite of adequate ventilatory drive and muscle force. Central hypoventilation, often a result of brain stem lesions, can now be treated by implanting an electrode that stimulates the phrenic nerve and supplements the efferent motor stimuli to the diaphragm.

REFERENCES

1. Bainton CR, Mitchell RA: Effect of skin cooling on exercise ventilation in the awake dog. J Appl Physiol 30:370–377, 1971

2. Bainton CR: Effect of speed vs. grade and shivering on ventilation in dogs during active exercise. J Appl Physiol 33:778–787, 1972

3. Bainton CR, Mitchell RA: Posthyperventilation apnea in awake man. J Appl Physiol 21:411–415, 1966

4. Beaver WL, Wasserman K: Tidal volume and respiratory rate changes at start and end of exercise. J Appl Physiol 29:872–876, 1970

5. Berger AJ, Davies DG, Dutton RE: Transient ventilatory responses in intact and chemodenervated dogs. Fed Proc 32:356a, 1973

6. Bishop B, Bachofen H: Comparison of neural control of diaphragm and abdominal muscle activities in the cat. J Appl Physiol 32:798–805, 1972

7. Bishop B, Bachofen H: Vagal control of ventilation and respiratory muscles during elevated pressures in the cat. J Appl Physiol 32:103–112, 1972

8. Black ASM, McCloskey DI, Torrance RW: The responses of carotid body chemoreceptors in the cat to sudden changes of hypercapnic and hypoxic stimuli. Respir Physiol 13:36–49, 1971

9. Bokinsky GE, Hudson LD, Weil JV: Impaired peripheral chemosensitivity and acute respiratory failure in Arnold-Chiari malformation and syringomyelia. N Engl J Med 288:947–950, 1973

10. Borison HL, McCarthy LE: CO_2 ventilatory response time obtained by inhalation step forcing in decerebrate cats. J Appl Physiol 34:1–7, 1973

11. Bosma JF, Truby HM, Lind J: Studies of neonatal transition: Correlated cineradiographic and visual-acoustic observations. Acta Paediatr Scand [Suppl] 163: 93–109, 1965

12. Bouhuys A, Pool J, Binkhorst RA, van Leeuwen P: Metabolic acidosis of exercise in healthy males. J Appl Physiol 21:1040–1046, 1966

13. Bouverot P, Candas V, Libert JP: Role of the arterial chemoreceptors in ventilatory adaptation to hypoxia of awake dogs and rabbits. Respir Physiol 17: 209–219, 1973

14. Brooks McC, Kao FF, Lloyd BB (eds): Cerebrospinal Fluid and the Regulation of Ventilation. Oxford, Blackwell Scientific Publications, 1965

15. Brooks JG, Tenney SM: Ventilatory response of llama to hypoxia at sea level and high altitude. Respir Physiol 5: 269–278, 1968

16. Byrne-Quinn E, Weil JV, Sodal IE, Filley GF, Grover RF: Ventilatory control in the athlete. J Appl Physiol 30:91–98, 1971

17. Campbell EJM, Agostoni E, Newsom Davis J (eds): The Respiratory Muscles; Mechanics and Neural Control, ed 2. Philadelphia, WB Saunders Co, 1970

18. Cherniack RM, Chodirker WB: Hypercapnia with relief of hypoxia in normal individuals with increased work of breathing. J Appl Physiol 33:189–192, 1972

19. Cherniack NS, Longobardo GS: Cheyne-Stokes breathing: An instability in physiologic control. N Engl J Med 288: 952–957, 1973

20. Clark FJ, von Euler C: On the regulation of depth and rate of breathing. J Physiol (Lond) 222:267–295, 1972

21. Cohen MI: How respiratory rhythm originates: evidence from discharge patterns of brain stem respiratory neurones, in Porter R (ed): Breathing: Hering-Breuer Centenary Symposium. Ciba Found Symp, London, J & A Churchill, 1970, pp 125–150

22. Comroe JH Jr: The peripheral chemo-

receptors, in Fenn WO, Rahn H (eds):
Handbook of Physiology, Section 3:
Respiration, vol I. Washington, D.C.,
American Physiological Society, 1964,
pp 557–583

23. Comroe JH Jr, Schmidt CF: Reflexes
from the limbs as a factor in the hyperpnea of muscular exercise. Am J
Physiol 138:536–547, 1943

24. Cormack RS, Cunningham DJC, Gee
JBL: The effect of carbon dioxide on
the respiratory response to want of
oxygen in man. Q J Exp Physiol 42:
303–319, 1957

25. Crance JP, Becquart P, Bouverot P,
Arnould P: Réponses ventilatoires du
nouveau-né au test oxygène. J Physiol
(Paris) 63:32A, 1971

26. Cross KW, Klaus M, Tooley WH,
Weisser K: The response of the new-
born baby to inflation of the lungs. J
Physiol (Lond) 151:551–565, 1960.

27. Cunningham DJC, Lloyd BB (eds):
The Regulation of Human Respiration.
Philadelphia, FA Davis Company, 1963

28. D'Angelo E, Torelli G: Neural stimuli
increasing respiration during different
types of exercise. J Appl Physiol 30:
116–121, 1971

29. Decima EE, von Euler C: Excitability
of phrenic motoneurones to afferent input from lower intercostal nerves in the
spinal cat. Acta Physiol Scand 75:580–
591, 1969

30. Decima EE, von Euler C: Intercostal
and cerebellar influences on efferent
phrenic activity in the decerebrate cat.
Acta Physiol Scand 76:148–158, 1969

31. Decima EE, von Euler C, Thoden U:
Intercostal-to-phrenic reflexes in the
spinal cat. Acta Physiol Scand 75:568–
579, 1969

32. Dejours P: Chemoreflexes in breathing.
Physiol Rev 42:335–358, 1962

33. Dejours P: Control of respiration by
arterial chemoreceptors, in: Regulation
of Respiration. Ann NY Acad Sci 109:
682–695, 1963

34. Dejours P: Control of respiration in
muscular exercise, in Fenn WO, Rahn
H (eds): Handbook of Physiology,
Section 3: Respiration, vol I. Washington, D.C., American Physiological Society, 1964, pp 631–648

35. Dejours P: The regulation of breathing during muscular exercise in man. A
neurohumoral theory, in Cunningham

DJC, Lloyd BB (eds): The Regulation
of Human Respiration. Philadelphia,
Blackwell Scientific Publications, FA
Davis Company, 1963, pp 535–547

36. Dejours P, Puccinelli R, Armand J,
Dicharry M: Concept and measurement
of ventilatory sensitivity to carbon dioxide. J Appl Physiol 20:890–897, 1965

37. Duffin J: A mathematical model of the
chemoreflex control of ventilation.
Respir Physiol 15:277–301, 1972

38. Eldridge FL: Posthyperventilation
breathing: different effects of active
and passive hyperventilation. J Appl
Physiol 34:422–430, 1973

39. Euler C von, Herrero F, Wexler I:
Control mechanisms determining rate
and depth of respiratory movements.
Respir Physiol 10:93–108, 1970

40. Eyzaguirre C, Koyano H: Origin of
sensory discharges in carotid body
chemoreceptors. Cold Spring Harbor
Symposia on Quantitative Biology 30:
227–231, 1965

41. Farber JP: Development of pulmonary
reflexes and pattern of breathing in the
Virginia Opossum. Respir Physiol 14:
278–286, 1972

42. Farber JP, Hultgren HN, Tenney SM:
Development of the chemical control
of breathing in the Virginia Opossum.
Respir Physiol 14:267–277, 1972

43. Fenn WO: Introductory remarks, in
Nahas GG (ed): Regulation of Respiration. Ann NY Acad Sci 109:415–417,
1963

44. Fitzgerald RS, Parks DC: Effect of
hypoxia on carotid chemoreceptor response to carbon dioxide in cats. Respir
Physiol 12:218–229, 1971

45. Flenley DC, Pengelly LD, Milic-Emili
J: Immediate effects of positive-pres-
sure breathing on the ventilatory response to CO_2. J Appl Physiol 30:7–11,
1971

46. Forster HV, Dempsey JA, Birnbaum
ML, Reddan WG, Thoden J, Grover
RF, Rankin J: Effect of chronic exposure to hypoxia on ventilatory response
to CO_2 and hypoxia. J Appl Physiol
31:586–592, 1971

47. Fowler WS: Breaking point of breath-
holding. J Appl Physiol 6:539–545,
1954

48. Freedman S, Weinstein SA: Effects of
external elastic and threshold loading

on breathing in man. J Appl Physiol 20:469–472, 1965

49. Gabel RA, Kronenberg RS, Severinghaus JW: Vital capacity breaths of 5% or 15% CO_2 in N_2 or O_2 to test carotid chemosensitivity. Respir Physiol 17: 195–208, 1973

50. Gee JBL: Some factors in the control of respiration in man. BSc Thesis, Oxford University, 1949

51. Glenn WWL, Holcomb WG, Gee JBL, Rath R: Central hypoventilation; long-term ventilatory assistance by radiofrequency electrophrenic respiration. Ann Surg 172:755–773, 1970

52. Godfrey S, Edwards RHT, Copland GM, Gross PL: Chemosensitivity in normal subjects, athletes, and patients with chronic airways obstruction. J Appl Physiol 30:193–199, 1971

53. Guz A, Noble MIM, Eisele JH, Trenchard D: The role of vagal inflation reflexes in man and other animals, in Porter R (ed): Breathing: Hering-Breuer Centenary Symposium. Ciba Found Symp, London, J & A Churchill, 1970, pp 17–40

54. Guz A, Noble MIM, Widdicombe JG, Trenchard D, Mushin WW: Peripheral chemoreceptor block in man. Respir Physiol 1:38–40, 1966

55. Guz A, Noble MIM, Widdicombe JG, Trenchard D, Mushin WW: The effect of bilateral block of vagus and glossopharyngeal nerves on the ventilatory response to CO_2 of conscious man. Respir Physiol 1:206–210, 1966

56. Guz A, Trenchard DW: Pulmonary stretch receptor activity in man. A comparison with dog and cat. J Physiol (Lond) 213:329–343, 1971

57. Heisey SR, Adams T, Hofman W, Riegle G: Thermally induced respiratory responses of the unanesthetized goat. Respir Physiol 11:145–151, 1971

58. Hey EN, Lloyd BB, Cunningham DJC, Jukes MGM, Bolton DPG: Effects of various respiratory stimuli on the depth and frequency of breathing in man. Respir Physiol 1:193–205, 1966

59. Holton P, Wood JB: The effects of bilateral removal of the carotid bodies and denervation of the carotid sinuses in two human subjects. J Physiol (Lond) 181:365–378, 1965

60. Ingemann Jensen J, Vejby-Christensen H, Petersen ES: Ventilatory response to work initiated at various times during the respiratory cycle. J Appl Physiol 33:744–750, 1972

61. Ingemann Jensen J, Vejby-Christensen H, Petersen ES: Ventilation in man at onset of work employing different standardized starting orders. Respir Physiol 13:209–220, 1971

62. Kellogg RH: Central chemical regulation of respiration, in Fenn WO, Rahn H (eds): Handbook of Physiology, Section 3: Respiration, vol I. Washington, D.C., American Physiological Society, 1964, pp 507–534

63. Kindermann W, Pleschka K: Phrenic nerve response to passive muscle stretch at different arterial CO_2 tensions. Respir Physiol 17:227–237, 1973

64. Koller EA, Ferrer P: Discharge patterns of the lung stretch receptors and activation of deflation fibers in anaphylactic bronchial asthma. Respir Physiol 17:113–126, 1973

65. Koller EA, Ferrer P: Studies on the role of the lung deflation reflex. Respir Physiol 10:172–183, 1970

66. Lahiri S: Dynamic aspects of regulation of ventilation in man during acclimatization to high altitude. Respir Physiol 16:245–258, 1972

67. Lahiri S: Unattenuated ventilatory hypoxic drive in ovine and bovine species native to high altitude. J Appl Physiol 32:95–102, 1972

68. Lahiri S, Milledge JS, Sørensen SC: Ventilation in man during exercise at high altitude. J Appl Physiol 32:766–769, 1972

69. Lambertsen CJ: Effects of drugs and hormones on the respiratory response to carbon dioxide, in Fenn WO, Rahn H (eds): Handbook of Physiology, Section 3: Respiration, vol I. Washington, D.C., American Physiological Society, 1964, pp 545–555

70. Lefrançois R, Gautier H, Pasquis P: Ventilatory oxygen drive in acute and chronic hypoxia. Respir Physiol 4: 217–228, 1968

71. Lefrançois R, Gautier H, Pasquis P, Vargas E: Factors controlling respiration during muscular exercise at altitude. Fed Proc 28:1296–1300, 1969

72. Lefrançois R, Gautier H, Pasquis P, Cevaer AM, Hellot MF, Leroy J: Chemoreflex ventilatory response to CO_2

in man at low and high altitudes. Respir Physiol 14:296–306, 1972

73. Leusen I: Regulation of cerebrospinal fluid composition with reference to breathing. Physiol Rev 52:1–56, 1972

74. Loeschcke HH, Gertz KH: Einfluss des O_2-Druckes in der Einatmungsluft auf die Atemtätigkeit des Menschen, geprüft unter Konstanthaltung des alveolaren CO_2-Druckes. Pflueger's Arch 267: 460–477, 1958

75. Lugliani R, Whipp BJ, Seard C, Wasserman K: Effect of bilateral carotid-body resection on ventilatory control at rest and during exercise in man. N Engl J Med 285:1105–1111, 1971

76. Luria AR: Functional organization of the brain. Sci Am 222:66–78, 1970

77. Lynne-Davies P, Couture J, Pengelly LD, Milic-Emili J: Immediate ventilatory response to added inspiratory elastic loads in cats. J Appl Physiol 30: 512–516, 1971

78. McCloskey DI, Torrance RW: Autoregulation of blood flow in the carotid body. Respir Physiol 13:23–35, 1971

79. Merton PA: Discussion, in Porter R (ed): Breathing: Hering-Breuer Centenary Symposium. Ciba Found Symp, London, J & A Churchill, 1970, pp 156–157

80. Milhorn HT Jr, Benton R, Ross R, Guyton AC: A mathematical model of the human respiratory control system. Biophys J 5:27–46, 1965

81. Milic-Emili J, Pengelly LD: Ventilatory effects of mechanical loading, in Campbell EJM, Agostoni E, Newsom-Davis J (eds): The Respiratory Muscles; Mechanics and Neural Control, ed 2. Philadelphia, WB Saunders Company, 1970, pp 271–290

82. Mills E, Edwards MW Jr: Stimulation of aortic and carotid chemoreceptors during carbon monoxide inhalation. J Appl Physiol 25:494–502, 1968

83. Mills E, Jöbsis FF: Simultaneous measurement of cytochrome a_3 reduction and chemoreceptor activity in the carotid body. Nature 225:1147–1149, 1970

84. Mitchell RA, Loeschcke HH, Massion WH, Severinghaus JW: Respiratory responses mediated through superficial chemosensitive areas on the medulla. J Appl Physiol 18:523–533, 1963

85. Murphy TM, Clark WH, Buckingham IPB, Young WA: Respiratory gas exchange in exercise during helium-oxygen breathing. J Appl Physiol 26:303–307, 1969

86. Nahas GG (ed): Regulation of respiration. Ann NY Acad Sci 109:411–948, 1963

87. Nathan PW, Sears TA: Effects of posterior root section on the activity of some muscles in man. J Neurol Neurosurg Psychiat 23:10–22, 1960

88. Newsom Davis J: Spinal control, in Campbell EJM, Agostoni E, Newsom Davis J (eds): The Respiratory Muscles; Mechanics and Neural Control, ed 2. Philadelphia, WB Saunders Company, 1970, pp 205–233

89. Newsom Davis J, Sears TA: The proprioceptive reflex control of the intercostal muscles during their voluntary activation. J Physiol (Lond) 209:711–738, 1970

90. Nielsen M, Smith H: Studies on the regulation of respiration in acute hypoxia. Acta Physiol Scand 24:293–313, 1951

91. Pagtakhan RD, Faridy EE, Chernick V: Interaction between P_{O_2} and P_{CO_2} in the initiation of respiration of fetal sheep. J Appl Physiol 30:382–387, 1971

92. Pappenheimer JR, Fencl V, Heisey SR, Held D: Role of cerebral fluids in control of respiration as studied in unanesthetized goats. Am J Physiol 208: 436–450, 1965

93. Paulev P-E: Cardiac rate and ventilatory volume rate reactions to a muscle contraction in man. J Appl Physiol 34: 578–583, 1973

94. Phillipson EA, Hickey RF, Bainton CR, Nadel JA: Effect of vagal blockade on regulation of breathing in conscious dogs. J Appl Physiol 29:475–479, 1970

95. Phillipson EA, Murphy E: Vagal control of respiratory rate and depth independent of lung inflation in conscious dogs. Fed Proc 32:355 (abstract), 1973

96. Pierce AK, Jarrett CE, Werkle G Jr, Miller WF: Respiratory function during sleep in patients with chronic obstructive lung disease. J Clin Invest 45:631–636, 1966

97. Plum F: Neurological integration of behavioural and metabolic control of breathing, in Porter R (ed): Breathing:

Hering-Breuer Centenary Symposium. Ciba Found Symp, London, J & A Churchill, 1970, pp 159–175

98. Porter R (ed): Breathing: Hering-Breuer Centenary Symposium. Ciba Found Symp, London, J & A Churchill, 1970

99. Porter R, Knight J (eds): High Altitude Physiology: Cardiac and Respiratory Aspects. Edinburgh, Churchill Livingstone, 1971

100. Priban IP, Fincham WF: Self-adaptive control and the respiratory system. Nature 208:339–343, 1965

101. Reinstorff D, Fenner A: Ventilatory response to hyperoxia in premature and newborn infants during the first three days of life. Respir Physiol 15:159–165, 1972

102. Reynolds WJ, Milhorn HT Jr, Holloman GH Jr: Transient ventilatory response to graded hypercapnia in man. J Appl Physiol 33:47–54, 1972

103. Rohrer F: Die Regulation der Atmung. Schweiz Med Wochenschr 4:73–79, 1921

104. Rosenstein R, McCarthy LE, Borison HL: Constancy of the relationship between respiratory frequency and tidal volume with respect to alveolar carbon dioxide and oxygen in decerebrate cats. Fed Proc 32:356a, 1973

105. St. John WM, Glasser RL, King RA: Rhythmic respiration in awake vagotomized cats with chronic pneumotaxic area lesions. Respir Physiol 15:233–244, 1972

106. Schwieler GH: Some aspects of respiratory regulation during the postnatal development in cats and rabbits. Life Sci [II] 6:1803–1810, 1967

107. Schwieler GH, Douglas JS, Bouhuys A: Postnatal development of autonomic efferent innervation in the rabbit. Am J Physiol 219:391–397, 1970

108. Sears TA: Breathing: a sensori-motor act. Sci Basis Med 7:129–147, 1971

109. Severinghaus JW, Mitchell RA, Richardson BW, Singer MM: Respiratory control at high altitude suggesting active transport regulation of CSF pH. J Appl Physiol 18:1155–1166, 1963

110. Sørensen SC: The chemical control of ventilation. Acta Physiol Scand [Suppl] 361: 1–72, 1971

111. Sørensen SC, Severinghaus JW: Irreversible respiratory insensitivity to acute hypoxia in man born at high altitude. J Appl Physiol 25:217–220, 1968

112. Stahlman M: Respiratory regulation in the newborn, in Nahas GG (ed): Regulation of Respiration. Ann NY Acad Sci 109:882–891, 1963

113. Tenney SM, Scotto P, Ou LC, Bartlett D Jr, Remmers JE: Suprapontine influences on hypoxic ventilatory control, in Porter R, Knight J (eds): Ciba Found Symp on High Altitude Physiology: Cardiac and Respiratory Aspects. Edinburgh, Churchill Livingstone, 1971, pp 89–102

114. Torrance RW (ed): Arterial Chemoreceptors. Oxford, Blackwell Scientific Publications, 1968

115. Wade JG, Larson CP Jr, Hickey RF, Ehrenfeld WK, Severinghaus JW: Effect of carotid endarterectomy on carotid chemoreceptor and baroreceptor function in man. N Engl J Med 282: 823–829, 1970

116. Wang SC, Ngai SH: General organization of central respiratory mechanisms, in Fenn WO, Rahn H (eds): Handbook of Physiology, Section 3: Respiration, vol 1. Washington, D.C., American Physiological Society, 1964, pp 487–505

117. Weil JV, Byrne-Quinn E, Sodal IE, Filley GF, Grover RF: Acquired attenuation of chemoreceptor function in chronically hypoxic man at high altitude. J Clin Invest 50:186–195, 1971

118. Yamashiro SM, Grodins FS: Optimal regulation of respiratory airflow. J Appl Physiol 30:597–602, 1971

Chapter 11

Voluntary Breathing Acts: Speech, Singing, and Wind-Instrument Playing

Man's breathing apparatus is essential to his ability to speak. Although other animals can communicate through voice sounds, only man can speak at a rate that exceeds the flicker fusion frequency of the eye.[44] Man's speaking facility is made possible by a detailed coding system. Only human speech sounds have the characteristics that allow coding as well as decoding; hence, human language requires human speech.[44] Individual speech sounds do not stand alone, but rather derive meaning from a context of phonemes, syllables, words, and sentences. The respiratory bellows provide the power, with a pressurized stream of air, for the vocal apparatus. Man's upper airways include a number of specialized organs for speech —a larynx for voicing sounds, a mobile pharynx for varying those sounds, and the soft palate, tongue, and lips, which further alter the resonant properties of the supravocal tract and help form consonants (e.g., /p/ with the lips; /k/ with the soft palate).

These adaptations of the supravocal tract and the larynx for speech also allow other forms of human communication. Singing and wind-instrument playing use the respiratory tract to express a wide range of emotions in a highly organized fashion. In contrast with the songbird's small, species-specific repertoires,[48] man's music covers the total range of his religious, historical, and cultural experience. As in speech, individual sounds in music derive their meaning from a context of phrases, movements, and compositions.

In this chapter I discuss the respiratory aspects of speech, singing, and wind-instrument performance. These include the generation of pressure and airflow and the coordination of muscular events; breathing patterns and control mechanisms are discussed also. Some attention is given to the relationship between respiratory and speech disorders and to the development of speech and language. Detailed discussions of the physiology of the larynx and of phonetic and linguistic aspects of speech are available elsewhere.[15, 28, 30, 39, 44, 53, 55]

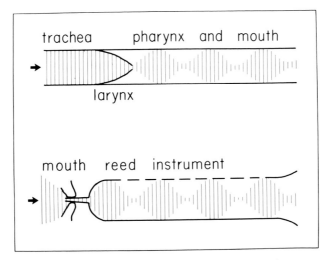

Fig. 11-1. Generation of sound waves in the larynx and in a reed instrument. From reference 5.

RESPIRATORY MECHANICS

Generation of Sound

Sound waves are produced when (1) mechanical systems—such as the strings of violins, the membranes of drums, and the vocal folds of the human glottis—create vibrations in the surrounding air, or (2) an airstream in a fixed mechanical system is disturbed, as in the flute and the organ pipe.

During speech and singing, the vocal folds in the larynx transform a pressurized stream of air from the lungs into a series of air pulses (Fig. 11-1). This process (phonation) generates the fundamental frequency of the voice. The supravocal tract then lets energy through at certain multiples of this frequency (harmonics), while other frequencies are damped. The resonance of the supravocal tract determines which sounds pass through with minimum loss. The characteristics vary with the tract's length and shape. The frequencies at which energy maxima occur (the formants) are characteristic for each speech sound, vowel or consonant. Vowels are voiced sounds produced while the supravocal tract assumes a fixed shape and is open to the atmosphere. Consonants involve either constriction or abrupt changes in the shape of the supravocal tract; consonants may be voiced (e.g., /m/, /b/) or unvoiced (e.g., /p/, /s/).

In brass instruments, the human lips form a vibrating reed; in most woodwinds, the instrument's mouthpiece contains a reed. In both instances, the player's expiration creates an air column which causes the reed to vibrate. Flutes have no reeds and belong to the class of "aerodynamic whistles" [13]—the tone is formed by blowing an airstream across a hole in the mouthpiece. In all wind instruments, the horn functions as a resonance chamber; its length and thus its resonating frequency can be altered. The vibrations set up in the horn in turn determine the vibrating frequency of the reed. The reed and the horn are interdependent and the horn "enslaves the reed" (Benade, in discussion of reference 6). In wind instruments the fundamental frequency of the reed corresponds to one tone at that frequency, with its harmonics. The human voice is much more versatile. Since the glottis is only loosely coupled with the supravocal tract,[27] we can speak or sing different vowels by altering the configuration of the supravocal tract, independent of the glottal fundamental.

Voice Input and Output

The flow rate and the pressure head of the expiratory airstream during speech or singing are the input characteristics of the vocal apparatus. Its output can be measured with acoustical methods (sound pressure, frequency spectrogram, i.e., a recording of dominating voice frequencies versus time).

Driving Pressure

During speech and singing, the pressure drop across the glottis or supravocal tract provides the driving pressure for sound generation. During phonation, the principal pressure drop occurs across the phonating glottis, since the supravocal tract is open to the atmosphere. During articulated speech, the site of the main pressure drop shifts, depending on the speech sounds. For instance, explosive consonants like /p/ are preceded by increased pressure on the alveolar side of an occlusion in the upper airway. In any case, the pressure difference between the subglottal area and the atmosphere is the total pressure drop across the vocal apparatus.

Although tracheal puncture provides a safe, direct measurement of subglottal pressure (Ps), many persons find this method unacceptable. Indirect measurements of Ps, such as those derived from esophageal pressure measurements (Fig. 7-6), are therefore preferred. By recording the lung static recoil curve separately, one can measure Ps as the horizontal distance between the esophageal pressure points on a pressure-volume curve and the static recoil curve (Fig. 11-2). Although this method ignores the pressure drop contributed by lower-airway resistance, this is usually minimal compared to the pressure drop across the vocal apparatus.[9] Comparisons with the direct (tracheal puncture) method, during speech, have validated the esophageal pressure method.[42] Another indirect measurement of Ps is based on the compression of alveolar gas which results from increased alveolar pressure (Palv). This method, which requires a body plethysmograph to record the chest volume changes due to gas compression,[33] eliminates the need for an esophageal balloon and may also respond faster to rapid pressure changes than the esophageal pressure method.

During wind-instrument playing, driving pressures can be measured directly by inserting an air-filled balloon[4] or a miniature pressure transducer[59] into the mouth. The indirect methods discussed above can also be used. Since the pressure drop across the lips or reed is usually much larger than other pressure drops in the airways, one may assume that mouth pressure, Pm, equals Palv.

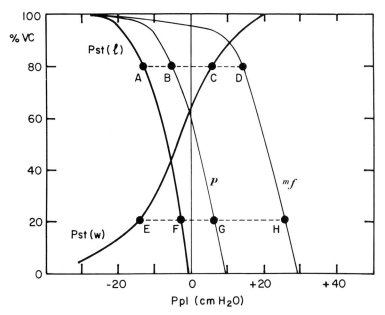

Fig. 11-2. Pressure-volume diagram of the lungs and chest. Pst(l) = static recoil curve of the lungs. Pst(w) = static recoil curve of chest wall. Lines marked p and mf show pressure-volume curves during singing of a soft (p) and a louder (mf) tone. AB = FG = subglottic pressure for soft tone. AD = FH = subglottic pressure for louder tone. Pmus shown at 80% and 20% VC. At 80% VC, Pmus is negative (inspiratory) for the soft tone (BC) and positive for the louder tone (CD). At 20% VC, Pmus is positive for both tones (EG and EH, respectively). Modified from reference 8.

Generation of Driving Pressures

The pressures needed to drive the vocal apparatus or a horn result from (1) the elastic recoil forces of the lungs and the chest cage, (2) active contraction of expiratory muscles, and (3) relaxation of inspiratory muscles. The analysis of recoil and muscular pressures [Pst(l), Pst(w), and Pmus] in Chapter 7 (pp. xx and Fig. 7-7) helps explain the complex mechanical problem faced by speakers, singers, and wind musicians. For example, to maintain a constant sung tone throughout the vital capacity, the singer must maintain a constant subglottic pressure even though his lung and chest recoil forces change as lung volume decreases. An analogy with the bow of a violin may be useful. The length of the bow limits the duration of a tone on the violin; similarly, the vital capacity limits the duration of tones during singing. But the violinist can hold the bow against the strings at any point, while the singer must continuously work with or against the elastic forces of the lungs and chest. "Imagine the difficulties a violinist would have sustaining a steady tone with strings attached to his bow!" [51]

The contributions of elastic and muscular forces are analyzed quantitatively in Figure 11-2, which is similar to Figure 7-7. The graph shows pressure-volume curves recorded while the subject sang two constant tones and relates these to the Pst(l) and Pst(w) curves. The subject inspired to TLC, initiated the tone, and

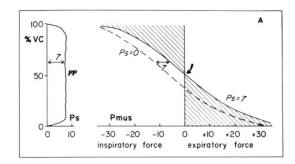

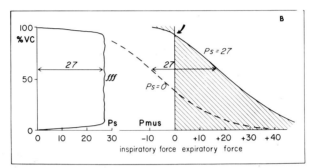

Fig. 11-3. Inspiratory and expiratory force (*right-hand graphs*) during singing of tones at constant subglottic pressures, Ps (*left-hand graphs*), as a function of lung volume (ordinate). Dashed lines represent forces required to hold the breath at all lung volumes (Ps = 0). Drawn lines labeled Ps = 7 (*A*) and Ps = 27 (*B*) represent net muscle force during singing. At curved arrows, net muscle force is zero. From reference 51.

maintained it at constant pitch and loudness throughout the VC. The first part of each curve reflects the compression of alveolar gas required to increase alveolar (=subglottic) pressure. Both curves lie to the right of the Pst (*l*) curve, indicating that Palv is positive throughout, and they run at equal horizontal distances from the Pst(*l*) curve. Thus, subglottic pressure was maintained constant once the proper level to produce the tone had been reached. The curve for the soft tone (*p*) runs to the left of the Pst(w) curve until lung volume reaches about 60 percent of the VC. In this portion of the curve, Pmus is negative; i.e., the subject exerts a net inspiratory muscle force. Below 60 percent VC, Pmus becomes positive —the subject now exerts net expiratory muscle force to sustain the tone at equal loudness. The louder tone (*mf*) required net expiratory force almost immediately after the tone was initiated. The legend of Figure 11-2 indicates how to read the numerical values of Ps and Pmus from the graph. Each curve intersects with the Pst(w) curve; at this point Pmus=0.

By plotting Pmus versus lung volume (Fig. 11-3), one can visualize the direction and degree of muscular effort. In general, inspiratory muscles maintain low subglottic pressures at high lung volumes, while higher subglottic pressures, at lower lung volumes, require contraction of the expiratory muscles. Hence, near

TLC, to maintain a low subglottic pressure in *A,* the inspiratory muscles must literally "brake" the expiratory flow. As the tone continues, inspiratory effort gradually relaxes in order to keep Ps constant. At about 50 percent VC, net muscle force is zero, since the elastic recoil of the lungs and chest exactly balance one another at the required subglottic pressure level ($+7$ cm H_2O). Lower lung volumes require increasing net expiratory force to maintain the tone. A louder tone requires expiratory muscle action at high lung volumes; the inspiratory muscle brake is then only necessary near TLC (*B*). At 90 percent VC, the combined chest and lung recoil force provides the required subglottic pressure ($+27$ cm H_2O). At all lower volumes expiratory force is used. Higher subglottic pressures (or mouth pressures, in the case of wind instruments) require expiratory muscle force as soon as the tone is initiated.

Pmus indicates the net inspiratory or expiratory muscle force that results from different combinations of inspiratory and expiratory muscle effort. For instance, when Pmus $=0$, all respiratory muscles may be relaxed, or the contractions of the inspiratory and expiratory muscles (agonists and antagonists) may just balance one another. An electromyogram (EMG—a recording of electrical activity in individual muscles) indicates which participating muscles are contracted. The EMG therefore complements the information provided by the pressure-volume diagram: while the former indicates which muscles are active, the latter shows the net forces developed by muscle contraction. During speech, EMG recordings indicate inspiratory muscle activity (external intercostal muscles) at high lung volumes.[23] As lung volume decreases, inspiratory muscle activity decreases, while that of the expiratory muscles (internal intercostals) increases.[57] Even though considerable inspiratory force is required to produce soft tones at high lung volumes (Fig. 11-3*A*), EMG recordings suggest that the strongest inspiratory muscle, the diaphragm, does not contribute to this force. The diaphragm remains electrically silent, while the external intercostal muscles show marked EMG activity. The diaphragm's inactivity probably results from its lack of muscle spindles (see p. 210). Fortunately, since the mechanical interaction between the intrapleural and intra-abdominal pressures regulates the position of the diaphragm (see next section), contraction of the diaphragm is not needed to regulate subglottic pressure.

Intra-abdominal Pressure

When man is upright, the weight of the abdominal organs contributes to the mechanical control of intrapleural pressures.[9] The elasticity of the external abdominal wall provides the primary support for the viscera. The diaphragm is subject to an upward pull exerted by the negative intrapleural pressure. Hence, lung elastic recoil tends to pull the diaphragm and the abdominal viscera upward. This tendency is counteracted by the weight of the abdominal viscera, an opposing force which is greater the larger the hydrostatic pressure gradient in the abdominal cavity. Hence, the opposing force increases with elevation of the diaphragm. A person who begins to sing a soft tone near TLC expands the rib cage by contracting inspiratory muscles and relaxing the abdominal muscles. Although the negative intrapleural pressure pulls the diaphragm upward, this force is checked by the weight of the abdominal contents, which tends to pull it downward. In this way, the weight of the abdominal viscera replaces active contraction of the diaphragm with a passive inspiratory force and makes possible the production of soft sung tones at high lung volumes while the diaphragm remains relaxed. Analysis of intra-abdominal (intragastric) and intrapleural pressures suggested that this maneuver required an elevated rib cage and relaxed abdominal muscles.[9] Direct measurements of rib cage and abdominal wall displacements during singing have confirmed this conclusion.[37]

Airflow Rate

The driving pressure and the resistance of the vocal apparatus together determine the expiratory airflow rate during speech and singing. With wind instruments, mouth pressure and the resistance of the opening between the lips or in the reed determine flow. Since sound is produced by alternately closing and opening the vocal folds or the reed, or by periodic occlusions at other sites during articulated speech, instantaneous flow rate varies as a function of these rapid changes in the glottis, supravocal tract, or mouthpiece. During stable events (singing of constant tones), the mean expiratory flow rate remains approximately constant and can be measured from the slope of a recording of lung volume versus time, with the subject seated in a body plethysmograph.[9] This method is not suitable when flows are more variable, as during articulated speech. Instantaneous flow rates can then be measured with face masks incorporating a wire mesh flowmeter screen [33, 36] (p. 183). When correctly designed, these masks impede articulation only minimally. Flow measurements are best interpreted in relation to simultaneous driving pressure and sound output measurements (see below).

Lung Volume

Lung volume changes during production of speech or other sounds reflect alveolar gas compression and expiratory airflow rates. Sounds can be produced at all lung volume levels within the constraints of the pressure-volume diagram (see below). Thus, lung volume recordings are chiefly of indirect interest—they allow construction of pressure-volume diagrams (Fig. 11-2), visualization of breathing patterns (Fig. 11-9), and measurement of total ventilation during speech (Fig. 11-12). Their slopes also indicate inspiratory and expiratory flow rates. When the subject is seated in a body plethysmograph with his head out and a seal around the neck, lung volumes during speech, singing, and wind-instrument playing can be recorded and studied without attaching measuring devices to the subject's mouth.[6, 9] These recordings reflect alveolar gas compression as well as expiratory airflow and thus can help relate lung recoil pressures to pressures during sound production. Since the latter pressures may vary from near-static values to maximum expiratory pressures, alveolar gas compression varies considerably, a fact not reflected in volume recordings made with instruments connected to the mouth (Chap. 9, p. 184).

Relations Between Driving Pressure, Airflow Rate, and Sound Level

Singing. Simultaneous measurements of airflow, subglottic pressure, and sound levels during singing of tones of constant pitch and loudness are plotted as a function of lung volume in Figure 11-4. One subject (DFP) is trained and the

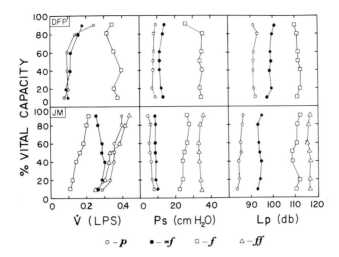

Fig. 11-4. Airflow rate ($\dot{V}$, *left graphs*), subglottic pressure (Ps, *middle graphs*), and sound level (Lp, *right graphs*) in a trained amateur singer (DFP, *upper row of graphs*) and in an inexperienced and untrained singer (JM, *lower row of graphs*). All data are plotted versus lung volume in percent of vital capacity. Symbols indicate different sound levels for the same tone (Bb3) in both subjects. Lung volume measured with body plethysmograph, $\dot{V}$ from slope of volume recording, Ps with esophageal balloon (as in Fig. 11-2), and sound level with microphone in front of the mouth. From reference 8.

other (JM) untrained in singing. In both subjects, sound level increases with increasing subglottic pressures. The latter vary within narrow limits during each tone; flow rates vary more and often decrease with lung volume, especially in JM. Moreover, the relation between flow rate and sound level differs between the subjects. The trained singer (DFP) uses minimal flow rates when he sings softly; flow increases when he sings louder tones. JM, on the other hand, uses high flow rates for the softest tone; with increasing sound level, flow rate decreases, except at the highest sound level, where higher flows again appear. This difference between the two singers is clearer in Figure 11-5, in which subglottic pressures and flow rates are plotted against one another. Each data point represents a tone sung at constant pitch and loudness; the symbols indicate tones of different pitch. The trained singer (*A*) increases flow as well as pressure when he sings a tone louder; the untrained singer (*B*) usually decreases flow while increasing pressure for tones of increasing loudness.

Differences in the pressure-flow behavior of the two subjects in Figure 11-5 suggest differences in the mechanical efficiency of the phonating glottis. With louder tones, the untrained singer's mechanical efficiency increases much more than that of the trained singer. The two sets of lines in Figure 11-5 illustrate this phenomenon. One set of diagonal straight lines indicates equal values of the product Ps · $\dot{V}$, which is the power spent in producing the constant tones (see Fig. 8-21, p. 170). At right angles with these lines are the lines of equal resistance,

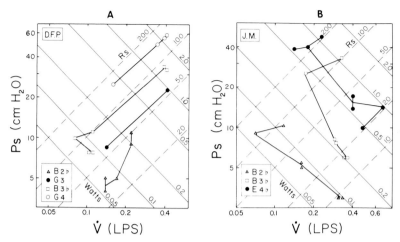

Fig. 11-5. Subglottic pressure (Ps, *ordinate*) and flow rates ($\dot{V}$, *abscissa*) for different tones in a trained (A) and an untrained (B) singer. The lines connect points at different sound levels for each tone. Ps increases with sound level in both graphs. Drawn diagonal lines are lines of equal power ($= Ps \cdot \dot{V}$) in watts. Dashed diagonal lines indicate equal values of the equivalent dc resistance of the glottis (Rs). From reference 8.

i.e., the ratio Ps/$\dot{V}$, which represents the equivalent dc resistance values of the phonating glottis. The trained singer (A) spends increasing amounts of power, up to more than 2 watts, when he increases loudness. Except for the tone with the lowest pitch, the dc resistance of his glottis remains nearly constant. The untrained singer, on the other hand, sings softly with high flow rates; as he sings louder, flow decreases while Ps increases, and the product Ps $\cdot$ $\dot{V}$ remains nearly constant except for the loudest tones. Hence, this subject produces louder tones while spending the same power; i.e., the mechanical efficiency of his glottis increases with loudness. At the same time, the equivalent dc resistance of his glottis increases about tenfold. Other studies have shown that experienced singers, too, may increase the mechanical efficiency of their glottides when singing louder, but to a lesser extent than untrained singers.[12]

Analysis of the harmonic contents of tones produced by the inexperienced and the trained singers of Figures 11-4 and 11-5 [8] helps explain the differences in mechanical efficiency. The frequency spectra of the trained singer suggest that the air pulses through his glottis have a similar waveform for soft and loud tones (Fig. 11-6). The untrained subject's louder tones are richer in high frequencies (i.e., they are harsher sounds), and the glottal air pulse becomes more peaked as loudness increases. When subject JM sings softly, a substantial portion of the central airstream through the glottis does not participate in sound production. Apparently, the vocal folds do not close at any time during the cycle. Thus, there is a constant expired airstream through the glottis, or a "dc air leak." When JM sings louder tones, the dc leak decreases and disappears. Then all of the airstream participates in sound production, which explains why the mechanical efficiency of sound production increases so dramatically. The trained subject DFP may have a small dc leak when he sings softly, but there is no marked change in

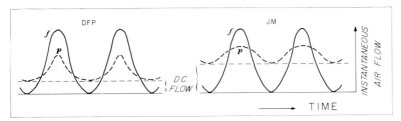

Fig. 11-6. Schematic representation of glottal waveforms (instantaneous airflow rate versus time) in subjects DFP (trained) and JM (untrained). *Dashed lines:* soft tones (*p*). DC flow: constant airstream through glottis, larger in JM than in DFP. *Solid lines:* loud tones (*f*). From reference 8.

waveform as he increases loudness. Figures 11-5 and 11-6 suggest that there are important differences in the control of vocal fold vibrations in trained and untrained singers. The untrained singer is apparently unable to adduct the vocal folds completely, or nearly so, when he sings softly. This results in a "breathy" character of these soft tones.

Speaking. While tones sung at constant pitch and loudness help demonstrate the mechanical events during phonation and speech, they have no linguistic meaning and display few of the complexities of articulated speech. The combination of consonants and vowels in phonemes, the elementary building blocks of speech, causes complex changes in pressure and flow which are often out of phase with one another. In Figure 11-7, subglottal pressure is high and flow rate low when the vowel /a/ is spoken. The high mechanical efficiency of the phonating glottis leads to a high sound-output level. In contrast, one produces the consonant /h/ with the nonphonating glottis wide open. Since there is little resistance in the supravocal tract, subglottal pressure is low and flow rate is high. In spite of the high flows, little sound is produced. Thus, the relation between sound output, on the one hand, and pressures and flows, on the other hand, is much more complex during speech than during singing of constant tones.

Figure 11-7 shows that the speaker exerts rapid, precise control over the glottis and supravocal tract. Each time the glottis narrows for vowel production, the vocal folds vibrate at exactly the same pitch as they did during the previous vowel (as when saying ha-ha-ha). High-speed movies indicate that the folds actually begin to vibrate, at nearly the correct pitch, even before the glottal chink is fully closed, while the folds still "flutter in the wind." [36] As a consequence, it is difficult to decide where the consonant ends and the vowel begins.

When short-lasting sounds are spoken at approximately constant loudness, subglottic pressures vary only slightly (see Figs. 3 to 5 in Lieberman [12]). In contrast, flow rates vary considerably, and different phonemes have characteristic flow rate patterns. [36] Phonemes with voiceless consonants (Fig. 11-7) are associated with high flow rates (/hah/, /pap/), while phonemes with voiced consonants generally have low flows (/zaz/, /vav/). As a result, speech material that includes many high-flow phonemes requires larger amounts of expired air than material with many low-flow phonemes. [10, 60]

Thus, variations in flow rate are a prominent respiratory feature in articulated

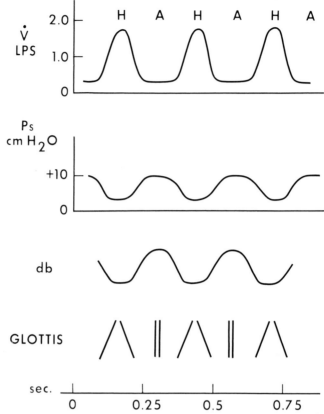

Fig. 11-7. Schematic diagram of flow rate, subglottic pressure, and sound level during utterance ha-ha-ha. See text for discussion. Modified from reference 3.

speech; different classes of speech sounds have distinct flow rate patterns. Variations in flow rate, at constant subglottic pressure, reflect the resistance of the glottis and supravocal tract, and therefore depend upon the neuromuscular control of these organs. Subglottic pressure usually increases with loudness, as in singing and during stress of syllables.[38, 42] Consequently, one must integrate control of respiratory muscles (which control subglottal pressure) and laryngeal and articulatory muscles (which control the syllable). In some languages, e.g., in Swedish, stress has linguistic significance; precise coordination between respiratory and laryngeal muscles then assumes special importance.

The interaction between subglottal pressure and laryngeal control therefore largely determines the pitch, loudness, and quality of voiced speech sounds. One can study this interaction with excised human larynges,[52, 58] in which vocal-fold tension and subglottal pressure can be controlled independently. At constant vocal-fold tension, pitch rises with increased subglottic pressure. Thus, if one increases subglottic pressure in order to produce a louder tone, vocal-fold tension must be adjusted to maintain a constant pitch. To sing a tone progressively louder or softer while maintaining constant pitch, singers must learn this fine control of

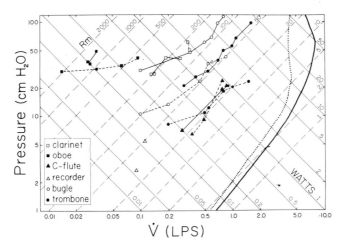

Fig. 11-8. Pressure-flow data for different wind instruments, with broken lines indicating a low tone and solid lines a high tone on each instrument. The solid and the dotted curves at the right are isovolume pressure-flow curves at two different lung volumes during expiration in a healthy subject. Drawn diagonal lines indicate power input values (as in Fig. 11-5); dashed diagonal lines indicate equivalent dc resistance values across lips and instrument (Rm = mouth pressure/flow rate). From reference 6.

respiratory and laryngeal muscles. Public speakers also need this control to express emotional content (e.g., in reading poetry) or simply to avoid monotony by varying pitch, loudness, and voice quality.

Wind-instrument playing. The requirements for mouth pressures and flow rates on wind instruments vary with the type of instrument and with pitch and loudness (Fig. 11-8). In some instruments, such as the oboe, the vibrating reed has a high resistance, and tone production (Fig. 11-1) requires relatively high pressures at low flow rates. In others, both pressure and flow are small (e.g., the recorder). For brass instruments and flutes, pressure and flow rise with increasing loudness, while resistance across the opening between the lips remains close to constant. High tones on brass generally require higher pressures than low tones. A brass player's power input (Pm · $\dot{V}$) may reach up to about 20 watts, compared with up to 2 watts in singers (Fig. 11-5A). Measurements of sound level, pressure, and flow indicate that the singing voice and wind instruments have similar levels of efficiency in converting airflow pulses into sound waves, i.e., up to about 1 percent.[7, 8]

BREATHING PATTERNS

For all types of sound production, breathing patterns are determined by (1) the pressure and flow requirements of the sound output and (2) the ventilatory requirements for gas exchange.

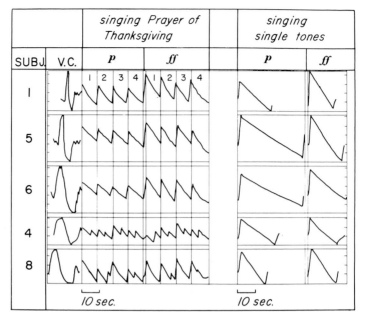

SUBJ.	V.C.	singing Prayer of Thanksgiving			singing single tones	
		p	*ff*		*p*	*ff*
1						
5						
6						
4						
8						

Fig. 11-9. Good-quality (subjects 1, 5, 6) and poor-quality (subjects 4, 8) volume recordings during singing of a song ("Prayer of Thanksgiving"). At left, vital capacity recording with volume scale in liters. At right, volume traces during singing of constant tones by the same subjects. The steeper their slopes, the higher the rate of flow during the tone. See text for discussion. From reference 8.

Singing

Breathing movements during singing consist of rapid inspirations followed by prolonged expirations (Fig. 11-9). The exact pattern adopted for the same song varies among individuals and may be related to singing proficiency.[9] Presumably, good phrasing (i.e., no inspirations in midphrase) and using most of the vital capacity without expiring to near RV are desirable from a standpoint of breathing economy. The three subjects in Figure 11-9, who had good-quality volume traces by such standards, increased total expired volume when a song was rendered loud (ff) rather than soft (p). These subjects also increased flow rates when singing tones louder. On the other hand, singers with poor-quality volume traces used high rates for single soft tones. These subjects appeared to behave like the untrained singer of Figure 11-5, in that they used excessive flow rates for soft tones. The breathing pattern adopted by trained singers depends greatly on the composition. Prolonged phrases, especially those sung forte, often require using nearly the full vital capacity (see Fig. 3 in Bouhuys et al.[9]).

Speaking

When one reads aloud, increasing voice volume calls for larger lung volume excursions; airflow rates may increase or remain the same.[9] Expiration often continues until lung volume decreases below functional residual capacity. As with singing, phrasing depends on the speech content and purpose; good public speakers use phrasing in conjunction with other mechanisms to achieve maximum impact. For one to read poetry, and perhaps even to write it, breath control is especially important. The American poet Charles Olson regarded poetry lines as elements shaped, in part, by the pattern of the poet's breath: "The line comes (I swear it) from the breath, from the breathing of the man who writes, at the moment that he writes . . . for only he, the man who writes, can declare, at every moment, the line, its metric and its ending—where its breathings shall come to termination." [41] When an experienced reader seated in a body plethysmograph read Olson's poetry, his volume recordings indeed showed that the breathing pattern helped to structure and define the lines and phrases, to clarify the intent of the poet, and to improve rhythm.[41]

Wind-Instrument Playing

The breathing pattern during wind-instrument playing resembles that during speech and singing—rapid inspirations are followed by prolonged expirations (see Figs. 2 and 3 in reference 4). The length of the expiration varies with the composition. By specifying when the player may inspire, many composers control their performers' breathing patterns. Since composers usually do not take into account ventilatory constraints, experienced instrumentalists should tell them whether their specifications can be met in practice.

Wind-instrument players often use nearly the full vital capacity and close to maximum expiratory pressures (Fig. 11-10). During prolonged expiration, alveolar

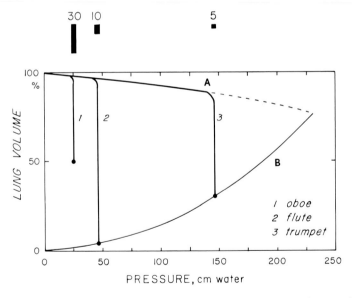

Fig. 11-10. Maximum expiratory pressure-volume diagram; lung volume in percentage VC. Curve *B* (beginning at lung volume 0) represents highest expiratory pressures at any lung volume. Lines 1, 2, and 3 represent pressure-volume events when playing single tones on different instruments (duration of each tone, in seconds, indicated above diagram). Continuous and dashed line *A* beginning at lung volume 100 percent represents pressure-volume events when air in the lungs is compressed by expiratory effort while no air leaves the lungs. Modified from reference 5.

CO_2 tension rises, with an additional increment caused by the elevated alveolar pressures. Thus, more than the singer or speaker, the horn player faces mechanical as well as gas-exchange constraints. The restrictions imposed by the instrument sometimes lead to special breathing patterns. For instance, typical flow rates for the oboe range from 50 to 150 ml/sec, far less than is needed to meet ventilatory requirements. Therefore, the player learns to perform additional quick expirations and inspirations between phrases (Fig. 11-12). In addition, some oboe players learn to breathe through their noses while continuing to produce tones. Apparently, they keep mouth pressure elevated by closing the oral cavity with the tongue, the epiglottis, and/or the soft palate.[4] Oriental snake charmers and players of the zurnah, a shawnlike instrument used in Turkey, reportedly also use this technique.[2]

RESPIRATORY CONSTRAINTS

The vital capacity determines the maximum volume that can be expired for a prolonged utterance or musical phrase. If driving pressures and flow rates are low, one may use nearly the full VC. However, a high pressure or flow, or both, prevents use of the full VC. Although the size of the vital capacity is presumably unrelated to musical aptitude, a performer with large VC may have a selective advantage. Brass players have larger than predicted vital capacities,[4] a fact more apt to reflect initial selection than training. Although some wind-instrument teachers recommend special breathing exercises to increase VC in their students, there is no evidence that the exercises are effective.

Maximum expiratory pressure. Figure 11-10 shows pressure-volume curves during playing of single tones on wind instruments, and these are compared with maximum expiratory pressures (p. 136; Fig. 7-9). Since the flute tone requires a mouth pressure of 50 cm H_2O, a value that can be maintained over most of the VC, the player can use nearly the full VC. Trumpet players, however, use much higher pressures for playing high and loud tones. Part of the VC is spent in compressing alveolar gas from 100 percent VC to about 90 percent VC. The resulting pressure level can be maintained from about 90 to about 30 percent of VC (Fig. 7-9). Below 30 percent VC, the trumpet player can no longer maintain the required pressure because it exceeds the maximum expiratory pressure at lower lung volumes. Hence, the player can effectively use only about half the VC for high or loud tones. Maximum expiratory pressures depend on age and sex,[17] but even young children (7–10 years) are able to produce pressures higher than 100 cm H_2O over about half the VC. Since only the high and loud tones require such high pressures on brass, children can play these instruments quite well. Maximum expiratory pressures decrease slightly with age.[17] Although, theoretically, this decrease could limit the older brass performer, superior musical skill may compensate for the loss.

Maximum expiratory flow rates. During speech and singing, average expiratory flow rates rarely exceed 0.5 liters/sec. While healthy subjects can maintain flows of this order over nearly the full VC (Chap. 9), patients with severe airway obstruction may have difficulty (see Fig. 9-6). Such patients often break speech

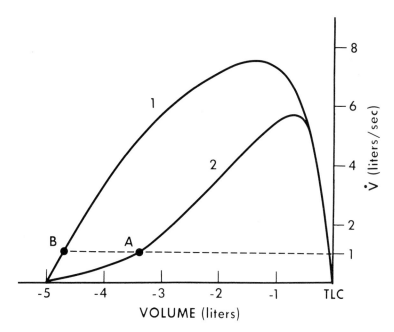

Fig. 11-11. Typical MEFV curves of young (*1*) and old (*2*) wind-instrument players. Dashed line indicates flow of 1 liter/sec required for tone. See text for discussion.

phrases frequently, probably because they can maintain the required flow rate only at higher lung volumes. Gas-exchange limitations may also contribute to the halting speech of dyspneic patients.

Older brass-instrument players frequently complain that they "run out of breath" sooner than they used to. This complaint may reflect flow limitations, as illustrated in Figure 11-11. Brass players frequently use flow rates of 1–2 liters/sec (Fig. 11-8). The player with MEFV curve *1* can maintain a flow of 1 liter/sec over nearly the full VC; this flow is maximal at point B, which is near RV. The player with MEFV curve *2*, on the other hand, can sustain a 1 liter/sec flow for only 3.4 seconds (i.e., not at volumes less than at A), while player *1* can play this tone for 4.7 seconds, i.e., 38 percent longer. Curves *1* and *2* typify MEFV curves of younger and older men, respectively (compare Fig. 9-12, p. 193). They might also represent MEFV curves for nonsmoking and smoking players of similar age (compare Fig. 14-2, p. 321). Since many wind players smoke heavily,[2,4] smoking as well as age may reduce performance by decreasing maximum flows at low lung volumes.

Breath-holding time. The oboe player often uses flow rates as low as 50 ml/sec. To expire to a full VC of 5 liters at this flow would take 100 seconds, much longer than most people can hold their breath. Therefore, the oboe player usually plays over only a portion of the VC before inspiring again, or he performs a rapid expiration followed by a deep inspiration (Figs. 11-10 and 11-12). The need for gas exchange restricts his performance.

Hyperventilation. High flow rates at low pressures are used for low tones on brass instruments, e.g., the bass tuba.[4] During prolonged passages with such tones, these players may complain of dizziness, presumably caused by hyperventilation.

Circulatory limitations. High alveolar pressures impede the flow of venous blood to the heart and cause arterial blood pressure to drop.[25] Because of diminished cerebral blood supply, this drop in pressure may lead to dizziness and fainting. Since the coronary blood supply might also decrease, strenuous brass performance may pose risks for older players. The effects of hyperventilation and of high pressures may potentiate one another with respect to symptoms of dizziness during playing (Campbell, in discussion of reference 6).

CONTROL OF BREATHING

To speak, sing, or play a horn requires fine control over respiratory, laryngeal, pharyngeal, oral, and facial muscles. Even a simple act like singing a tone of constant pitch and loudness requires continuous, precise adjustments of inspiratory and expiratory muscle contraction (Fig. 11-3). At the same time, these muscles must be used to control ventilation for gas exchange (Chap. 10). For adequate performance, all participating muscles must contract to the correct degree, at the right time, and in proper sequence. Hence, the central nervous system must not only coordinate these elaborate sets of motor impulses, but also integrate them with those required for other motor acts involving the same muscles (breathing, swallowing, facial expression, posture). These sets of instructions and their mutual coordination develop during a process of trial and error. The learning process is guided by regular progress reports, or feedback information, from the moving structures as well as auditory and sometimes visual cues. We shall first discuss the sources of feedback information and, next, a concept of the integrated control system.

Sources of Feedback

The child learning to speak and the student of voice or wind instruments both require *auditory feedback* from their own sounds and those made by others. Birds do not learn to sing if they grow up in isolation.[48] When the initial learning process is complete, auditory feedback becomes less essential. Human speech begins to deteriorate markedly only over a year after the onset of nerve deafness,[19] and adult birds, when deafened, maintain normal song performance.[48] Additional sources of feedback include afferent signals from *muscle spindles* [11, 57] and from *sensory receptors* in laryngeal joints [35] and in the supravocal tract.

Muscle spindles indicate the relative state of muscle contraction. This information is integrated in the spinal cord, with impulses which travel down from higher centers in the brain and brainstem—together these assure the proper degree of muscle contraction. Muscle spindles are numerous in the intercostal muscles, the most important muscles in regulating subglottic pressure. The diaphragm, which has few muscle spindles, performs no active role during speech or singing (see p. 239). Perhaps surprisingly, the laryngeal muscles, which adjust the vocal-fold tension needed to control voice pitch precisely, contain no muscle spindles. In the cat, sensory receptors in the cricothyroid joint can signal changes in joint position to the central nervous system, resulting in efferent motor signals to intrinsic laryngeal muscles.[35] Since the relative positions of the thyroid and cricoid cartilages affect the length of the vocal folds and hence their tension, feedback from the cricothyroid sensory receptors may influence pitch control. Whether these particular receptors are present in man is not known. But the paucity of suitable laryngeal receptors suggests that auditory feedback is more important than other feedback sources for pitch control. Lastly, superficial sensory receptors along the supravocal tract, including the lips, probably help control articulation and wind-instrument performance.

Central Control Mechanisms

Although many nerve centers and pathways contribute to speech control,[24] its organization remains a mystery. Human language is one of the most highly organized outputs of the brain. However, since language is the main tool for studying the brain, no one has found a way to study how the brain controls speech.[62] Nevertheless, some general concepts of brain function can be derived from the study of language and other precise motor acts such as writing.[21, 30, 40]

Motor acts are often thought to result from a sequence of reflex events, involving efferent motor signals to the muscles and afferent signals to the central nervous system from muscles and other structures, which modify the efferent signals. However, many skilled motor acts preclude this explanation, since they are performed too rapidly to allow time for nerve conduction of afferent signals and processing of feedback information.[40] To sing a tone at nearly correct pitch, or to speak a word intelligibly, one has no time to conduct a complex series of reflex maneuvers (Fig. 11-7). Rather, one must perform such skilled motor acts according to preprogrammed instructions. The advance programming, or learning, also permits these acts to be performed in sequence. Thus, to speak even a single phoneme, the barest rudiment of human language, requires a predetermined, precisely quantitated and sequenced set of motor signals to the muscles; the impulses required to make the initial sound depend on the subsequent sounds within the phoneme.

Lashley[40] has emphasized that most skilled motor tasks require an "organized temporal order" for their execution. Individual parts of a set of events must occur in a prescribed sequence; they are part of a preprogrammed set of motor impulses. The instructions for each phoneme form a sort of subroutine for larger programs; phonemes are structured into syllables and words, and words into sentences and messages. The programming of human speech and language involves linguistic formulation as well as coordination of motor control per se.[30] Similarly, in music the performer develops a set of motor instructions that reflects the hier-archical and rhythmic order of notes, chords, measures, themes, parts, movements, and symphonies. Forty phonemes are used in English, incorporating only nine distinctive features.[14] Hence, a small number of basic instructions is enough to build up the elaborate structure of human language. Simpler organized sounds produced by animals may differ from human language mainly in the absence of higher levels of organization. In the katydid, the motor output for singing is emitted by a neuronal pacemaker that fires at the singing frequency; transmitting signals to the forewing muscles involves only a few neuronal elements.[34] Like human speech the purring of cats also involves coordination of vocal and respiratory muscles. Since purring persists even after afferent nerves from lungs and muscles have been cut, the alternating contractions of laryngeal muscles and diaphragm which cause purring must originate centrally. Thus, purring seems to be a good example of a stereotyped, programmed motor act.[56]

Even though programmed instructions may largely determine speech events, feedback information is also important. Feedback contributes to the ongoing assessment of performance, by detecting errors and modifying motor instructions. Feedback is particularly important for timing speech events and adjusting speech volume in relation to ambient noise levels.[30] When a subject's speech output is fed back to his ears via a delaying electronic circuit, speech is disrupted, primarily because of difficulties in articulation.[30] When loud random noise masks the sound of a wind instrument to the player's ear, he can usually remain on pitch, probably because he still receives tactile sensory input from his lips. However, ambient noise can make it impossible to produce a constant tone on the recorder, played through a tube inserted in the mouth, because the player receives neither auditory nor tactile information about tone production (personal observation).

The concepts of speech and language discussed in this section have practical importance not only in speech therapy, but also in efforts to synthesize speech artificially ("talking computers" [29]) and to understand and improve learning processes in children and music students.

Learning to Speak

The human infant learns to speak in response to speech sounds from those around him. Children born deaf do not develop speech without considerable special training. Although human language includes several added levels of complexities, the principles involved in human learning may be similar to those in songbird's learning.[48, 49] Young birds pick up selected auditory cues from their environment. Since they learn only their own song, and not those of other species, their brains must have some genetically determined pattern or template, which guides the selection process. Training may increase this template's precision, enabling the bird to improve vocalization, guided by auditory feedback from its own song and from others of the same species. This feedback information in turn further increases the template's precision.

Deaf-mute children lack appropriate control over breathing when they attempt to speak.[61] Yet, they have no trouble performing other coordinated acts, such as masticating and swallowing, which use the same muscle groups. Hence, since the children's lower coordination centers appear to function well, their speech defects must reflect a lack of central organization, rather than a lack of muscle coordination. The child that learns to speak develops a steadily increasing number of programmed sets of motor instruction, as well as the ability to organize these into an infinitely varying set of larger speech structures (words, sentences, messages). The early acquisition of speech apparently has a lasting effect on speech habits, and this often interferes with later acquisition of a new language. This is remarkable since man retains the capacity to learn many other skilled motor acts throughout his life. Perhaps the very early development of speech leads to fixed habits that inhibit the development of new patterns.

Integration With Ventilatory Control

The airflow requirements for speech must be reconciled with the ventilatory requirements for gas exchange. When one breathes room air at rest, ventilation per minute increases slightly during speech. The increase is greater when the speech material includes many high-flow consonants such as the /h/.[10] Significant hypocapnia has been observed in one study.[20] When ventilatory demands are increased, as during exercise or breathing of 3 percent CO_2, minute ventilation increases even though speech requires lower flows. Under these conditions, speech usually decreases the average minute ventilation (e.g., from an average of 18.9 to 16.0 liters/min during exercise; personal observation). Similarly, the speaker breathing 3 percent CO_2 in air has a minute ventilation which is less than the minute ventilation at rest during CO_2 breathing.[10] Thus, the speaker appears to achieve a compromise between ventilatory and speech demands on flow rates. How can he increase minute ventilation while maintaining flows compatible with intelligible speech? Figure 11-12 shows the solution to this problem schematically. Suppose that minute ventilation at rest is 7.5 liters/min, and the breathing rate is 15 breaths per minute. During speech, breathing rate declines to 12 breaths per

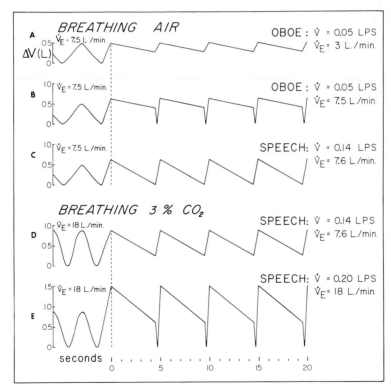

Fig. 11-12. Schematic diagram of breathing pattern during oboe playing (A, B), speech while breathing room air (C), and speech during breathing of 3% CO_2 in air (D, E). Resting pattern and minute ventilation ($\dot{V}_E$) at left in each graph. At right, average expiratory flow rates ($\dot{V}$) and minute ventilation ($\dot{V}_E$) during play or speech. Patterns A and D are incompatible with gas-exchange requirements ($\dot{V}_E$ too low). Hence, the player or speaker adopts pattern B or E to meet these demands. After data from references 4 and 10. Further discussion in text.

minute, tidal volume increases, and expiration is prolonged (C). Expiratory flow rate is assumed constant at 0.14 liters/sec. During 3 percent CO_2 breathing at rest, minute ventilation increases to 18 liters/min (D). If the subject maintained the same breathing pattern for speech while breathing CO_2, the minute ventilation would be only 7.6 liters/min and CO_2 would be retained. Two mechanisms that prevent this are [10] (1) the mean expiratory flow rate increases during speech, resulting in a more "breathy" but still intelligible voice, and (2) the speaker superimposes rapid expirations followed by deep inspirations upon the speech breathing pattern. The schematic curve E includes both mechanisms; actually, the minute ventilation decreases when speaking at rest during CO_2 breathing, so that compensation is incomplete.[10] The curves A and B show that oboe players adopt a similar breathing pattern to maintain ventilation (see p. 249).

RESPIRATION AND SPEECH IN DISEASE

There have been few quantitative studies of subglottic pressures, airflow rates, and breathing patterns in patients with speech abnormalities. Recordings of these events might help develop objective standards for diagnosing speech disorders and for assessing the effect of therapy. In re-educating patients with speech disorders, visualization of airflow rates and breathing patterns might help the patient correct malcoordination of respiratory muscle effort. For instance, a deaf-mute student might benefit from watching the normal flow pattern for various phonemes on an oscilloscope screen and trying to match this pattern. Such methods might also help stutterers and singers. Since "waste of air" seems to be common to several speech disorders and to untrained singers, visualization of airflow control might teach them how to use minimal flow rates. Monitoring muscle effort with electromyographic recordings might also be useful. Feedback from the EMG of laryngeal muscles helps to "unlearn" the habit of subvocal speech while reading.[32]

Dysarthria and aphasia. In disorders of articulation (dysarthria), muscle coordination is impaired. In patients with brain lesions, the ability to speak is often impaired while coordination of the muscles remains intact (aphasia). Recordings of subglottic pressure and flow may help to distinguish between malcoordination (dysarthria) and programming disorders (aphasia). In the latter, if there is residual speech, one would expect normal flow and pressure patterns. Such patients might be able to sing steady tones at constant loudness and pitch, while patients with dysarthria would probably have lost this ability.[18] Unfortunately, there are few reports of detailed physiological studies of speech in patients with dysarthria (parkinsonism, multiple sclerosis).[31] Hence, it is not clear how much this speech defect results from poor coordination of respiratory, laryngeal, and articulatory muscle contraction. The hypokinetic speech—reduced voice volume, monotonous voice, and dysarthria—of patients with parkinsonism relates to the delayed onset of movements and to their slowness and small amplitude. Airflow and subglottic pressure recordings might provide objective data on the effectiveness of treating this disease with drugs like L-dopa, which alter the duration of phonation and the length of pauses between utterances.[50]

Substitute vocal apparatus.   Aphasia, in which speech is impossible in spite of an intact vocal apparatus, clearly demonstrates the importance of the central control system to speech. Conversely, patients who have undergone a laryngectomy for cancer learn to speak with a different effector apparatus, the entrance to the esophagus.[22] Apparently, once central speech control is fully developed, one can learn to use it to operate another peripheral apparatus. Other damage to the vocal apparatus is also compatible with good performance. For example, a patient with permanent unilateral paralysis of a vocal fold became a good choir singer after training,[1] and injecting Teflon into atrophied or paralyzed vocal folds can help restore the normal voice, even though the injected fold has no means of adjusting its tension by muscle contraction.[16]

DEVELOPMENT OF SPEECH AND LANGUAGE

Human speech is a relatively recent phylogenetic development.[44] When man assumed the upright posture, the altered position of his head led to the development of a bend in the upper airway. This increased airway resistance, as well as the dangers at the crossroads between food and air passages (Chap. 2). A more sophisticated swallowing mechanism became imperative to prevent food from entering the trachea and air from entering the stomach, even though both passed through a long pharynx. This modification required improved pharyngeal musculature and a coordinated reflex mechanism, integrated with respiratory control. The descent of the larynx to its position in modern man took place concurrently.[26] Hence, while the swallowing mechanism had obvious immediate survival value, the use of the mobile, muscular pharynx for speech may have followed almost accidentally.

The development of the articulatory capability in the supravocal tract was crucial to modern man's acquisition of speech. Monkeys can alter the shape of the supravocal tract only within narrow limits, mainly because their pharynx is short and immobile.[47] Newborn infants, too, have a short pharynx, and the configuration of their supravocal tract resembles that of nonhuman primates.[46] Analyses of the skulls of Neanderthal and Cro-Magnon man [45] indicate that the former had a short pharynx, while that of the latter resembles modern man's. Thus, Cro-Magnon man may have been able to speak, while Neanderthal man had at best very limited speech capabilities. The development of the motor apparatus for speech may be more crucial to the acquisition of speech than was formerly thought. This explains why it is impossible to teach chimpanzees to speak English. Although they have sufficient brainpower to learn language [e.g., they can learn to communicate and understand messages in other code systems (sign language) using colored plastic objects [54] or computer-controlled word symbols [56a]], they lack the vocal equipment.

The upright posture also provided another advantage for speech—it facilitated more precise regulation of subglottic pressure with the intercostal muscles and the hydraulic pull of the abdominal contents on the diaphragm.[9] Given these various structural possibilities, primitive man probably began to notice his ability to produce a larger variety of sounds that could be used to communicate with others. As he used his hands increasingly to manipulate tools, communication by gesture alone became less practical. In addition, he soon found that the voice could transmit messages to people whom he could not see. Central organization probably took place concurrently. The "improved vocalization apparatus, like the use of tools, served . . . to give the brain more to think about." [26] In turn, improved central control probably led to refined vocal output. In primates, the laryngeal output is noisy and irregular; [43] pitch control in man is much more precise.

The ontogenesis of speech in infants may represent an abbreviated form of the phylogenetic development. In newborn infants, the vocal apparatus is not suitable for speech, [46] and the central organization of speech does not function. As the vocal apparatus improves through structural changes in the supravocal tract, the infant generates some speech sounds, which in turn elicit feedback from people around him. This improves the speech "templates" [48] and stimulates the infant to make more and different sounds (see p. 252).

I speak, therefore I am? Lieberman and Crelin [45] have commented on the historical background of our concepts of speech development. Descartes' cogito ergo sum (I think, therefore I am) identified the mind as the central feature of being human. In this context, apes were nonhuman because they were not supposed to think and therefore had nothing to say. But in fact, apes can learn language, [54, 56a] although they cannot speak. Unlike Descartes, Lieberman and Crelin suggest that "Man is human because he can say so," [45] and they stress the importance of the vocal apparatus to our ability to speak. Yet, speech, language, and thought are closely associated. The act of thinking requires some mode of expression in language. To the extent that the Premacks' chimpanzee, Sarah, interprets messages in a plastic symbol code and responds to them with an appropriate answer, she may be said to think. [54] Although man uses nonverbal modes of communication to express feelings, we cannot assess his rational thoughts unless he speaks or writes about them. Perhaps what makes us human is that we listen to others, we think, and we speak our minds.

SUMMARY

The respiratory bellows supplies power to the vocal apparatus and drives wind instruments. This power is generated by the elastic recoil of chest and lungs and by the respiratory muscles. Expiratory muscles supply driving pressure; inspiratory muscles brake the recoil forces so that low driving pressures can be maintained even at large lung volumes. Simultaneous recordings of driving (subglottal) pressure and airflow show that experienced speakers and trained singers exert precise control over their glottides and supravocal tracts. To achieve control of pitch, loudness, and quality of the voice, the muscular control of the glottis and supravocal tract is integrated with that of the respiratory muscles. Breathing patterns during speech, singing, and wind-instrument playing consist of rapid inspirations and prolonged expirations; the patterns depend on the pressure and flow requirements of the voice or instrument as well as on the need to ventilate the lungs. Volume, pressure, and flow constraints of the respiratory bellows set limits to performance, especially with wind instruments. The control of speech and similar voluntary acts requires programming of nerve impulses to the muscles in precisely quantitated and sequenced sets of motor instructions. Feedback control (auditory, proprioceptive, and tactile) helps develop these sets during learning and monitors performance afterwards. Under some conditions, special breathing patterns are used to reconcile incompatible requirements of sound production and gas exchange. The recording of respiratory events may prove helpful in diagnosing and treating speech disorders.

Human speech may have developed when man adopted the upright posture, which led to structural changes in the supravocal tract. Similar changes, including the formation of a long, mobile pharynx, occur in young children; newborn infants lack the articulatory apparatus for coordinated speech. These recent findings have a profound impact on our concepts of human language and thought and their phylogenetic and ontogenetic development.

REFERENCES

1. Aherne G: Singing with a paralysed cord. Lancet 2:1313, 1970
2. Akgün N, Özgönül H: Lung volumes in wind instrument (zurna) players. Am Rev Respir Dis 96:946–951, 1967
3. Bouhuys A: Concluding remarks, in: Sound production in man. Ann NY Acad Sci 155:379–381, 1968
4. Bouhuys A: Lung volumes and breathing patterns in wind instrument players. J Appl Physiol 19:967–975, 1964
5. Bouhuys A: Physiology and musical instruments. Nature 221:1199–1204, 1969
6. Bouhuys A: Pressure-flow events during wind instrument playing, in: Sound production in man. Ann NY Acad Sci 155:264–275, 1968
7. Bouhuys A: Sound-power production in wind instruments. J Acoust Soc Am 37:453–456, 1965
8. Bouhuys A, Mead J, Proctor DF, Stevens KN: Pressure-flow events during singing, in: Sound production in man. Ann NY Acad Sci 155:165–176, 1968
9. Bouhuys A, Proctor DF, Mead J: Kinetic aspects of singing. J Appl Physiol 21:483–496, 1966
10. Bunn JC, Mead J: Control of ventilation during speech. J Appl Physiol 31:870–872, 1971
11. Campbell EJM, Agostoni E, Newsom Davis J: The Respiratory Muscles: Mechanics and Nerve Control, ed 2. Philadelphia, WB Saunders Co Inc, 1970
12. Cavagna GA, Margaria R: An analysis of the mechanics of phonation. J Appl Physiol 20:301–307, 1965
13. Chanaud RC: Aerodynamic whistles. Sci Am 222:40–46, 1970
14. Cherry C: On Human Communication, ed 2. Cambridge, Massachusetts Institute of Technology Press, 1966
15. Chomsky N, Halle M: The Sound Pattern of English. New York, Harper and Row, 1968
16. Cole R: Speech, in: Patterns of Orofacial Growth and Development, ASHA Reports No. 6. Washington, D.C., American Speech and Hearing Association, 1971, pp 79–95
17. Cook CD, Mead J, Orzalesi MM: Static volume-pressure characteristics of the respiratory system during maximal efforts. J Appl Physiol 19:1016–1022, 1964
18. Davis JN: Discussion remarks, in: Sound production in man. Ann NY Acad Sci 155:203, 1968
19. Dedo HH: Discussion remarks, in: Sound production in man. Ann NY Acad Sci 155:203, 1968
20. Dejours P, Wagner S, Dejager M, Vichon M-J: Ventilation et gaz alvéolaire pendant le langage parlé. J Physiol (Paris) 59:386, 1967
21. Denier van der Gon JJ, Thuring JPh: The guiding of human writing movements. Kybernetik 2:145–148, 1965
22. Diedrich WM: The mechanism of esophageal speech, in: Sound production in man. Ann NY Acad Sci 155:303–317, 1968

23. Draper MH, Ladefoged P, Whitteridge D: Expiratory pressures and air flow during speech. Br Med J 1:1837–1843, 1960

24. Dunker E: The central control of laryngeal function, in: Sound production in man. Ann NY Acad Sci 155:112–121, 1968

25. Faulkner M, Sharpey-Schafer EP: Circulatory effects of trumpet playing. Br Med J 1:685–686, 1959

26. Fenn WO: Perspectives in phonation, in: Sound production in man. Ann NY Acad Sci 155:4–8, 1968

27. Flanagan JL: Source-system interaction in the vocal tract, in: Sound production in man. Ann NY Acad Sci 155:9–17, 1968

28. Flanagan JL: Speech Analysis, Synthesis, and Perception. New York, Springer, 1965

29. Flanagan JL: The synthesis of speech. Sci Amer 226:48–58, 1972

30. Fry DB: The control of speech and voice, in Kalmus H (ed): Regulation and Control in Living Systems. London, John Wiley and Sons, 1966

31. Grewel F: Classification of dysarthrias. Acta Psych Neurol Scand 32:325–337, 1957

32. Hardyck CD, Petrinovich LF, Ellsworth DW: Feedback of speech muscle activity during silent reading: rapid extinction. Science 154:1467–1468, 1966

33. Hixon TJ: Some new techniques for measuring the biomechanical events of speech production: one laboratory's experiences. ASHA Reports No. 7. Washington, D.C., 1972, American Speech and Hearing Association, pp 68–103

34. Josephson RK, Halverson RC: High frequency muscles used in sound production by a katydid. I. Organization of the motor system. Biol Bull. 141:411–433, 1971

35. Kirchner JA, Suzuki M: Laryngeal reflexes and voice production, in: Sound production in man. Ann NY Acad Sci 155:98–109, 1968

36. Klatt DH, Stevens KN, Mead J: Studies of articulatory activity and airflow during speech, in: Sound production in man. Ann NY Acad Sci 155:42–55, 1968

37. Konno K, Mead J: Measurement of the separate volume change of ribcage and abdomen during breathing. J Appl Physiol 22:407–422, 1967

38. Ladefoged P: Linguistic aspects of respiratory phenomena, in: Sound production in man. Ann NY Acad Sci 155:141–151, 1968

39. Ladefoged P: Three Areas of Experimental Phonetics. New York, Oxford University Press, 1967

40. Lashley KS: The problem of serial order in behavior, in Jeffress LA (ed): Cerebral Mechanisms in Behavior. New York, Wiley, 1951, pp 112–136

41. Lieberman MR, Lieberman P: Olson's "projective verse" and the use of breath control as a structural element. Language and Style 5:287–298, 1973

42. Lieberman P: Direct comparison of subglottal and esophageal pressure during speech. J Acoust Soc Am 43:1157–1164, 1968

43. Lieberman P: Primate vocalizations and human linguistic ability. J Acoust Soc Am 44:1574–1584, 1968

44. Lieberman P: The Speech of Primates. The Hague, Mouton and Co, 1972

45. Lieberman P, Crelin ES: On the speech of Neanderthal man. Linguistic Inquiry 2:203–222, 1971

46. Lieberman P, Crelin ES, Klatt DH: Phonetic ability and related anatomy of the newborn and adult human, Neanderthal man, and the chimpanzee. American Anthropologist 74:287–307, 1972

47. Lieberman P, Klatt DH, Wilson WH: Vocal tract limitations on the vowel repertoires of rhesus monkey and other non-human primates. Science 164:1185–1187, 1969

48. Marler P: A comparative approach to vocal learning: Song development in white-crowned sparrows. J. Comp Physiol Psychol (Monograph 71, No. 2, Part 2): 1–25, 1970

49. Marler P: Birdsong and speech development: could there be parallels? Am Sci 58:669–673, 1970

50. Mawdsley C, Gamsu CV: Periodicity of speech in Parkinsonism. Nature 231: 315–316, 1971

51. Mead J, Bouhuys A, Proctor DF: Mechanisms generating subglottic pressure, in: Sound production in man. Ann NY Acad Sci 155:177–181, 1968

52. Müller J: Von der Stimme und Sprache, in: Handbuch der Physiol. des Menschen, Vol II, Book 4, Part 3. Coblenz, J. Holscher, 1837

53. Negus VE: The Comparative Anatomy and Physiology of the Larynx. New York, Hafner, 1949

54. Premack AJ, Premack D: Teaching language to an ape. Sci Am 92–99, 1972

55. Pressman JJ, Kellemen G: Physiology of the Larynx, ed 2, revised by JA Kirchner, Rochester, Minn., American Academy of Ophthalmology and Otolaryngology, 1970

56. Remmers JE, Gautier H: Neural and mechanical mechanisms of feline purring. Respir Physiol 16:351–361, 1972

56a. Rumbaugh DM, Gill TV, Glasersfeld EC von: Reading and sentence completion by a chimpanzee (Pan). Science 182:731–733, 1973

57. Sears TA, Davis JN: The control of respiratory muscles during voluntary breathing, in: Sound production in man. Ann NY Acad Sci 155:183–190, 1968

58. Van den Berg J: Myoelastic-aerodynamic theory of voice production. J Speech Hearing Res 1:227–234, 1958

59. Vivona PM: Mouth pressures in trombone players, in: Sound production in man. Ann NY Acad Sci 155:290–296, 1968

60. Warren DW, Wood MT: Respiratory volumes in normal speech: a possible reason for intraoral pressure differences among voiced and voiceless consonants. J Acoust Soc Am 45:466–469, 1969

61. Woldring S: Breathing patterns during speech in deaf children, in: Sound production in man. Ann NY Acad Sci 155: 206–207, 1968

62. Young, JZ: What can we know about memory? Br Med J 14:647–652, 1970

PART II

Environment and Lung Disease

Part II focuses on the environmental and occupational causes of lung disease. Dust, smoke, and polluted air are "a matter of life and breath," according to the American Lung Association. In a broader context, most lung disease, including infections and allergic diseases, result from interaction between agents inhaled from the environment and the tissues of airways and lungs. Chapters 12-18 deal primarily with diseases that could be largely prevented by better management of the environment. That these diseases remain prevalent reflects, in part, the difficulties of organizing and performing the required multidisciplinary research and of implementing the results into engineering and legal control procedures.

Chapters 12-13 present some basic approaches to the study of environmental lung disease. Chapter 12 introduces the disciplines, a conglomerate including medicine, engineering, physics, biochemistry, and many others. The risks of lung disease caused by environmental inhalants need to be assessed in studies of population groups rather than individuals. For this reason, the epidemiology of lung diseases is singled out for a more elaborate discussion in Chapter 13.

With the basic principles of environmental lung disease study thus outlined, Chapters 14-16 focus on specific environmental exposures. More people's lungs are endangered by cigarette smoke than by any other single inhaled substance. However, many industrial workers face the additional risk of occupational exposure to potentially dangerous dusts, gases, or fumes; and some of these exposures endanger people living near factories as well (Chap. 15). Community air pollution from a variety of other sources may also affect the lungs and airways (Chap. 16). This section summarizes current knowledge concerning the effects of these exposures on airways and lungs, and the mechanisms of action involved, with special emphasis on prevention and control measures.

The final chapters concentrate on two clinical syndromes of environmental lung disease. Chapter 17 discusses the epidemiology, pathophysiology and prevention of byssinosis among textile workers, while Chapter 18 deals with physiological and pharmacological aspects of bronchial asthma. This choice of material is based on personal interest and, in the case of asthma, on the thought that epidemiology and knowledge of environmental exposures have as yet suffered from benign neglect in their application to this prime cause of lung disease among nonsmokers. The use of physiological and pharmacological tools in epidemiological surveys on asthma may help clarify the prevalence of asthma and the role of diverse environmental exposures in its pathogenesis.

Chapter 12

A Framework of Disciplines

Few research problems are the domain of a single academic discipline. In the life sciences, physics and chemistry are the basic supporting disciplines from which methods and concepts derive. Particular categories of life scientists have formed new disciplines with specialized approaches to life phenomena. Biochemists explore the chemistry of life; biophysicists its physical phenomena. Pharmacologists study the actions of drugs on the body—one form of interaction between host and environment. With its heavy dependence on physiological methods to measure responses to drugs, and on statistics to evaluate the results, pharmacology is already a problem-oriented multidiscipline. The toxicologist is even more problem oriented and environment conscious; details of the interaction between toxic agents and biological systems are his main concerns.

The study of environmental lung disease draws heavily on toxicological expertise: precise definition of toxic agents, their dosage and port of entry, as well as their fate in the body. But the study of lung disease also requires medical input and new hygienic and engineering methods to eliminate the risk of exposure to environmental toxins. Furthermore, this field of study offers a full-time challenge to many physicists and engineers who are trying to determine the exact conditions of airflow and the way in which inhaled agents reach lung and airway tissue. These factors directly affect the amounts of inhaled agent that reach effector cells and thus indirectly influence the nature and degree of responses. Thus, the study of environmental lung disease requires more than a multidisciplinary approach; the complexities of the field are rapidly converting it into a multidiscipline of its own, with protagonists coming from medicine, toxicology, physics, engineering, statistics, industrial hygiene, and many other fields.

This chapter introduces only some areas of concern in this multidisciplinary framework. First, I discuss the transport of matter in the lungs and airways, next the responses in the tissues and how these are detected and diagnosed. The last section deals with prevention and control.

TRANSPORT OF MATTER

Physics

Gas molecules, droplets, and dust particles are transported into the airways and lungs, where they elicit responses when they reach the tissues of these structures' walls. The first concern, then, is how matter gets into the lungs and where it is deposited or absorbed.

INHALATION OF GASES AND VAPORS

Uptake. A volatile substance can be absorbed from inspired air at a maximum rate $F_I \cdot \dot{V}_I$, where F_I is the fractional inspired concentration and $\dot{V}_I$ is the volume of inspired gas per unit time. Its actual absorption is usually less than maximum, and its ultimate effect depends on solubility, metabolic fate, excretion, and toxicity.[28] A nonmetabolized, nontoxic substance is absorbed at an exponentially decreasing rate until it saturates tissues and body fluids. When absorption and excretion (or metabolic breakdown) occur simultaneously, some equilibrium concentration will eventually be established. The transport mechanisms for gases may be rate-limited at different steps. For instance, for a heavy gas (SF_6; Chap. 4), diffusion in alveolar gas may limit its uptake; for lighter molecules, diffusion through the alveolocapillary barrier (e.g., CO) or solubility in blood (e.g., many anesthetic gases) may be rate-limiting. At the tissue level, distribution between plasma and tissue is a variable that affects concentrations in different tissues. Transport and distribution mechanisms within the body are crucial for understanding the effects of gases on organs and systems; our discussion will concentrate chiefly on the effects on the lungs.

Absorption in upper airways. Upon inspiration, highly soluble gases are immediately absorbed by the mucus and mucosa of nose and upper airways. Since the nose acts as a "scrubbing tower," little gas reaches the lower airways. The nose removes ozone as well as sulfur dioxide efficiently:[11] when 1 ppm SO_2 was delivered to the nose of dogs, only 0.1 percent of the inspired concentration reached the trachea. For 1 ppm ozone, 100 percent was removed by the nose, and with 8 ppm ozone, only 25 percent reached the trachea. During mouth breathing, this scrubbing action of the nose is bypassed. Perhaps this may explain some reports of decreased performance and acute illness among athletes during air-pollution episodes (p. 403). Track runners who must breathe through their mouths might be at a disadvantage in polluted air—given the same pollutant concentration, their lower airways and lungs might be exposed to much higher effective concentrations than would people during rest or light exercise who breathe through their noses.

Site of effect. This depends largely on the relative solubility of the molecule in mucus of upper airways and in lung tissue. Ammonia is highly soluble in mucus and also very irritating; its effect on upper airways usually leads to withdrawal from the polluted atmosphere. On the other hand, phosgene is not very soluble in watery media;[42] it is also hydrolyzed in mucus to HCl and Cl_2, but this takes time. Therefore, phosgene has little effect on the upper airways. On the other hand, phosgene or its hydrolysis products have major effects on the lung parenchyma. Chlorine occupies an intermediate position. It is not as soluble as ammonia but still exerts some effects in upper airways; parenchymal responses are frequent since much chlorine reaches lower airways as well. Oxygen is not absorbed in upper airways; its toxic effects (from prolonged administration of 100 percent O_2 at 1 atm, or of hyperbaric O_2) include severe parenchymal reactions.[13]

AEROSOL PARTICLES

Transport mechanisms. Droplets or solid particles in air are transported chiefly by bulk flow (Chap. 3). Diffusional transport is important only for very small particles (<0.1 μm diameter). There is an upper limit to the size of particles that can be inhaled, determined, among other factors, by their settling velocity in the atmosphere—particles with a high falling speed are unlikely to be inspired. Once inspired, many large particles are deposited by inertial impaction in the nose, where linear air velocity and hence the kinetic energy of the particles is high, and to a lesser extent elsewhere in the upper airways. Within the bronchial tree, sedimentation due to gravity (or settling) may be important. In peripheral lung units, where only very small particles can penetrate, brownian movement is the main cause of particle deposition. The kinetic energy of the particles is negligible in this zone, and terminal settling velocities are relatively small for these minuscule particles.

The deposition of particles depends on their size, shape, and density. Droplets are generally round; aerosols of uniformly sized droplets can be generated by special equipment in the laboratory (spinning-disk generator). Proponents of "mist therapy" in medicine and pediatrics believe that inhalation of water droplets is a significant therapeutic tool. However, the air within the lungs is already saturated with water vapor, and it is not clear how the "wetness" of airway walls could be increased. In fact, calculations have shown that negligible amounts of water are inhaled with such mists.[55] Liquid aerosols are often used as a vehicle for drugs. The use of a narrow range of particle sizes is important for that application; otherwise, a few large particles may contain nearly all the mass of the drug. If such solutions are hypertonic, or the particles hygroscopic, the droplets may increase in size during transport through the airways.

Models of particle deposition. For theoretical calculations, it is often useful to consider spherical particles with a density of 1. Unfortunately, the anatomy of the airways is not so readily simplified and needs to be formalized in more or less complex mathematical models such as that of Beeckmans.[5] The subject has been summarized by Morrow,[39] and a recent symposium volume provides further details.[37]

The dimensions of particles entering the bronchial tree depend on the breathing pattern as well as on the anatomy of the airways. During quiet nose breathing, most particles larger than 10 μm diameter are probably deposited in the nose. As tidal volume is increased, the nose filters out progressively smaller particles: at higher flow rates, the kinetic energy of smaller particles increases so that more of them impact with the mucosa in the nose. In the bronchial tree, particles are deposited by a combination of impaction (mainly in large airways) and sedimentation (in small airways). Beeckmans [5] has shown that most particles between 0.3 and 1.0 μm diameter are deposited in alveoli and terminal bronchioles. For particles above 1 μm, larger-airway deposition increases. Maximum deposition in the alveoli occurs with particles between 0.3 and 2.0 μm diameter. Since gravity is one important force in particle deposition, less inhaled matter is expected to deposit in airways of astronauts on the moon.[6, 40] The size of infectious organisms, which helps determine their site of deposition, may be related to the location of airborne infections in the lungs and airways.[31]

In spite of their simplifying assumptions, the theoretical models of particle deposition have practical significance for radiological protection and industrial hygiene. For round particles there is reasonable agreement between theoretical and experimental data. However, neither the models nor the experimental data describe the local patterns of deposition. Also, no deposition model available deals with the airways as a set of branching tubes, similar to Weibel's or Cumming's models (Chap. 2). The existing models deal only with aggregates of airways of different sizes; one model, for instance, distinguishes only between tracheobronchial and pulmonary deposition.[50]

Experimental observations. The amount of material deposited in the respiratory tract can be estimated by measuring inspired and expired concentrations of the aerosol.[14, 15] A more direct method is to inhale a labeled aerosol and to determine the amount of label in the lungs of the experimental animal. Inulin is a suitable label, since it is not readily absorbed and can be measured with chemical methods after homogenization of lung tissue. This method has been useful in calibrating inhalation procedures with drugs, so that absolute amounts of various drugs administered by aerosol could be estimated.[16]

In recent years, several investigators have used aerosols of radioactive-labeled particles to describe deposition as well as clearance of particles from the lungs and airways in man. The deposition of these particles can be detected with counters around the chest or with a scintillation camera. The anatomical definition of deposition is rather imprecise; for instance, one can describe deposition in terms of outer, middle, and inner lung zones [43] and assume that the inner zone corresponds roughly to large airways and the outer zone to peripheral portions of lung parenchyma. These methods have indicated that about 50 percent of particles 2 μm in diameter are deposited in ciliated airways in man, and 50 percent in nonciliated ones (alveoli, alveolar ducts, and respiratory bronchioles).[35]

Particle shape. Dust particles often deviate considerably from the uniform, round particle used in model computations. In particular, the settling velocity of long and thin fibers is much less than would be expected from the total fiber mass. Such fibers behave to a large extent as a chain of round particles, so that their falling speed is determined by the diameter rather than by length.[51] This accounts, for instance, for the deep penetration of asbestos fibers into the lung parenchyma and the pleura.

Actions of dust particles. These are much less understood than the actions of substances transported in liquid droplets. So-called inert dusts may cause reflex airway constriction,[17] but how the particles stimulate subepithelial receptors is not clear. Other actions of dust involve biochemical events in macrophage cells which phagocytize—or ingest—the particles. Yet other particles, e.g., carbon,[9] can act as carriers for gaseous air pollutants, which in turn may cause lung damage. (see further p. 390.)

Physiology

Clearance of dust particles. Hatch and Gross [27] calculated the accumulation of dust in man's lungs over a lifetime of dust exposure. If air contains 1 mg fine dust per cubic meter, and one inspires 10 cu m air per day (including some degree of exercise hyperpnea), 10 mg of dust would be inhaled per day, over 3 gm per year, and more than 100 gm during a working life of 30 or more years. Yet, at autopsy one finds only a few grams mineral ash in the lungs. Hatch and Gross quote data on South African gold miners, with a lifetime dust intake of well over 1000 gm; at autopsy the lungs contain only about 20 gm dust. Since a large fraction of the inspired dust is deposited in the airways and lungs, large amounts of dust are obviously removed from the lungs during life. This raises two questions: what are the clearance mechanisms, and what determines the effect on the lungs—the amount inhaled or the amount permanently deposited? The clearance mechanisms include mucociliary clearance assisted by cough (see Chap. 2) and phagocytosis.

The amount of dust required to elicit a biological response depends on the time course for dust action versus the time course for dust clearance. Obviously, a particle that requires 24 hours to act but which is cleared within 1 hour has no chance to affect the lungs. On the other hand, a particle that acts within 1 hour and is cleared only after 24 hours has every opportunity to act. We have some information on clearance times, but data on the time course of many responses are lacking. The clearance time depends on particle size (because deposition depends on size), and its rate decreases with time. At the end of 24 hours, about 20 percent of particles 3 μm in diameter are retained.[39] Silica can kill phagocytic cells, and if this requires 24 hours, the effective dose of silica would be about 20 percent of the inhaled amount. If the time needed for silica to act is about 1 rather than 24 hours, the same data [39] suggest that about 40–50 percent of the total amount inhaled would be the effective dose.

These data remind us that even dust that is cleared from the lungs can cause damage. Some dust particles, while being cleared, can successively enter and kill alveolar macrophage cells, and this may initiate a long-term response such as pulmonary fibrosis. The particles may be removed long before the permanent effect becomes obvious. For dusts that exert their effects in less than 1 hour, such as textile dusts, nearly all material inhaled and deposited in the bronchi would have a chance to act, even though all dust may eventually be cleared from the lungs. The recently revised definition of pneumoconiosis by a working group of the International Labor Organization retains the concept of dust accumulation as an essential feature of this group of diseases.[18] I believe that the term accumulation itself is difficult to define and may not always be relevant.

Mucociliary clearance (see Chap. 2). This mechanism is effective in airways down to the first generation of bronchioles. Beyond these, the ciliary beat becomes ineffective and mucus production is lacking. In that region, phagocytosis is the essential clearance mechanism.

Phagocytosis. In the healthy lung, the alveolar macrophage is the predominant phagocytic cell. During acute inflammation, polymorphonuclear cells are also mobilized. All particles deposited in alveoli are probably engulfed by phagocytic cells within a few hours. Considerable mobilization of macrophages takes place in response to a subacute stimulus, such as prolonged dust exposure; macrophages are also active in delayed hypersensitivity reactions. The process of phagocytosis involves surface phenomena as well as biochemical events in the cell. For instance, both O_2 consumption and glucose oxydation increase; oxydative phosphorylation is an important source of energy for phagocytozing cells.[21] Other biochemical processes may lead to destruction of the particle within the macrophage, for instance, through degradation by lysosomal hydrolases. On the other hand, some particles, including silica, make the lysosome membrane permeable and thus cause release of lysosomal enzymes within the cell. This causes autodigestion, and the products of the dead macrophage cell may be an important element in initiating further tissue reactions in silicosis.[1a] Thus, although macrophages provide important protection against some inhaled particles (microbes), in other instances they become active mediators in the initiation of disease: a true two-edged sword.

The fate of the phagocytic cells varies. They may migrate to lymphatics and reach regional lymph nodes, where they may die and deposit the ingested material. Other cells are removed via the mucociliary ladder. The ease with which alveolar macrophages can be harvested in large numbers from the lungs of rodents by lavage have led to many important studies on the function of these cells. These will be discussed in conjunction with specific exposures (p. 351ff).

Cough. Cough is an efficient bulk-transport mechanism that in a single movement can clear several milliliters of accumulated mucus, foreign matter, and infectious cellular debris from the airways. Although mainly elicited by stimuli in large airways, increased air velocities during cough extend to small airways as well. Thus, cough removes material from a large part of the bronchial tree (see also p. 151).

RESPONSES OF AIRWAYS AND LUNG TISSUE

Physiology

Some responses to inhaled agents have protective value, including some which may be adaptive responses. Also, physiological factors influence responses caused by inhaled agents.

Protective reflexes. These reflexes, elicited by irritant gases from receptors in upper airways, trachea, and large bronchi,[54] cause sneezing, glottal closure, apnea (or rapid shallow breathing), and cough. Some also cause reflex bronchoconstriction, which has no obvious protective value. The other responses assist in either limiting exposure or clearing inhaled matter. Although the protective value of these reflexes is short term, they also act as warning signals to terminate exposure. For some substances, the sense of smell and other subjective sensations are also important warning signals. The absence of such sensations and reflexes may lead to serious lung injury because the individual is not aware of being exposed (e.g., exposure to phosgene).

Increased mucus production. SO_2 and other irritant gases cause an acute increase in mucus production, which may help protect the mucosa and facilitate gas absorption. The longer-term response, which includes hypertrophy of mucous glands and multiplication of goblet cells may have some protective value as well, but also leads to airway obstruction and cough.

Individual sensitivity.   Individuals differ widely in their responses to inhaled agents—exposures that severely affect one individual may leave another person free from any effect. While some miners never get demonstrable pneumoconiosis, many others have extensive dust deposits and lung disease. The reasons for this variability are not understood, but some anatomical and physiological mechanisms are probably involved. For instance, structural and functional differences in upper-airway filter function and in effectiveness of mucociliary clearance may play a role. In fact, the rate of mucociliary transport of particles in the nose varies widely, even when climatic factors are controlled.[3] Responsiveness of effector cells to stimuli may also vary. All these properties are probably distributed randomly among members of a population and contribute to a distribution of sensitivity according to a gaussian function, with a few highly sensitive and a few very insensitive persons at either end of the range, and the majority distributed around a median.

Some experience has suggested the existence of bimodal distributions of sensitivity, with some individuals (reactors) responding and others not (non-reactors). There is no clear evidence of a qualitative difference between such groups, and even the difference between allergic and nonallergic individuals may involve quantitative as well as qualitative factors. The fact that autonomic drugs can modulate airway smooth muscle sensitivity to certain agents (Chaps. 17 and 18) suggests that, at least for some agents, reactor-status is not invariable. It appears that the balance between vagal and sympathetic stimuli to the smooth muscle is important in regulating the muscle's sensitivity to environmental agents. Thus, neural as well as humoral stimuli may interact with inhaled agents at the smooth-muscle cell level. Much work is needed to describe human response patterns to well-known agents, preferably in subjects who belong to an epidemiologically defined group. This enables one to relate the data to experience in a group, which is difficult with the usual, much simpler approach relying on volunteer subjects who happen to be handy around the laboratory.

Adaptation.   Adaptive responses to environmental stimuli have great protective value. At high altitudes, adaptive changes in breathing limit the consequences of oxygen deficiency (Chap. 10). The prime example of a useful adaptive response, however, is that of temperature regulation: both cold adaptation and heat acclimatization help man survive in environments considerably warmer or colder than his body. Most of the common responses of the lungs and airways (airway obstruction, inflammation) to environmental agents do not have adaptive value, in the sense of a physiological change that limits or mitigates the response to the environmental agent. One could consider tachyphylaxis (temporary insensitivity) to inhalation of textile dust a useful adaptive response, because it decreases the dust effect on airways on days of exposure that follow an initial response. In fact, tachyphylaxis is probably an expression of mediator-substance depletion and does not lead to any lasting change in response (Chap. 17). Increased numbers of macrophages (p. 273) are a useful response in the case of microbes but not necessarily in the case of inhaled particles (see p. 268).

Biochemistry

All responses of lungs and airways to inhaled agents involve crucial biochemical events. Few of these have been described in detail. Undoubtedly, some of the basic events are similar to those well known in other cells and tissues; hence, the biochemist who studies the lungs looks mainly for processes of special interest. Respiratory epithelium lends itself to detailed studies of the ciliary beat, its sources of energy, and the cellular events that affect it. The biochemistry of mucus production has been mentioned in Chapter 2. The chemical reactions that lead to the formation of pulmonary surfactant are of special significance (Chap. 1). In phagocytic cells, complex biochemical events involve both energy production for phagocytosis and digestion of the phagocytosed particles. The formation of reticulin and collagen in lung tissue is not understood, nor are the chemical events that lead to alveolar wall destruction in emphysema. The chemical interactions with several pollutants are another important area for the biochemist.

It is obvious that most research in lung biochemistry remains to be done. The heterogeneity of lung tissue cells is a major stumbling block, since events in chopped or homogenized lung tissue cannot be traced to a specific cell type unless other evidence is available. However, some cells can be studied in relatively pure form; alveolar macrophages are a prime example.[41] Airway smooth muscle can be obtained in about 90 percent pure preparations from guinea pig trachea by removing the mucosa and the cartilage (J. S. Douglas, personal communication). Although type II alveolar cells have not yet been isolated, they may be soon; their lamellar bodies can be obtained in nearly pure form.[41]

Pharmacology

Many principles that the pharmacologist uses in the study of interactions between drugs and biological systems are applicable to the study of environmental exposures—for instance, in the construction of dose-response curves from observations of graded responses to different amounts of an agent. Several specific contributions of pharmacologists to environmental lung disease are important.

Airway constriction. This has been studied mainly in connection with asthma (Chap. 18); its role as a component of more complex responses, e.g., to cigarette smoking, is not well known. There is evidence that cigarette smoke, SO_2, and inert dusts cause constriction of airway smooth muscle, possibly transmitted via reflex pathways and abolished by atropine.[17, 54] Others have observed that cigarette smoke [47] and inert dust particles (Al_2O_3, Fe_2O_3, Cr_2O_3) [12] release histamine from lung tissue [47] or degranulate peritoneal mast cells.[12] This provides a mechanism for airway constriction via local release of histamine. This mechanism is also a part of the acute response to textile dust exposure (Chap. 17). Some of the responses in human subjects last only minutes, and these may be of reflex nature. Constriction induced by mediator release begins more slowly, usually after a latent interval, and may last several hours.

Airway dilatation. Beta-stimulant drugs (isoproterenol, epinephrine) are often administered by aerosol. In a double-blind trial, asthma patients showed a significantly greater improvement of $FEV_{1.0}$ when the drug was administered in a fairly uniform, small-sized aerosol (from a pocket nebulizer) than when it was inhaled with a hand nebulizer which produced an inhomogeneous aerosol.[10] With the latter, a few large particles may contain 90 percent or more of the mass, and thus most of the drug; the drug effect then depends mainly on the site where the large particles are deposited. This is likely to be the upper airways (pharynx), where isoproterenol is readily absorbed into the systemic circulation. Thus, only small amounts of the drug reach the intended effector organ, the bronchial muscle, while the systemic absorption causes side-effects (e.g., palpitations).

It would be interesting to know the differences, if any, in the local and systemic effects of similar amounts of isoproterenol or other bronchoactive drugs given in aerosols with uniform droplets, e.g., 1 μm, 3 μm, or 10 μm in diameter. The optimal size of aerosol droplets for use with bronchodilator drugs is important for therapeutic purposes. Correct sizing of aerosol droplets may provide maximum drug effects on airway smooth muscle with minimum systemic absorption and side-effects.

New developments. There is considerable scope for development of new drugs in the prevention and treatment of environmental lung diseases. Even though environmental control should have priority over medical control, suitable pharmacological protection would help in several instances. At present we have no acceptable drugs that inhibit excessive mucus production, nor drugs that protect lung tissue against the development of emphysema. Pharmacological inhibition of fibrous tissue formation, as in silicosis and asbestosis, would be invaluable to prevent progression of these diseases.

Toxicology

Although many acute and chronic effects of toxic agents on the lungs are well known in a descriptive sense, the uptake, metabolism, and removal of toxic agents are poorly understood. Individual differences in these processes may contribute to variability of responses, just as in the physiological mechanisms discussed earlier. Interaction of environmental agents during simultaneous or consecutive exposures is another problem for the toxicologist. But the main challenge in this discipline is probably the development of suitable models for the study of agents that cause toxic effects only after prolonged exposures at relatively low levels.

Such models are important for studies of the natural history of disease in experimental animals, and also for an understanding of the relationship between early injury and chronic disease. This could lead to predictions about potential long-term health hazards, based on short-term observations.

Immunology

The allergic response is perhaps the best-understood source of individual variation in sensitivity to environmental agents. The reaginic antibody system that develops when persons become sensitized to agents like flour or castor oil has been studied extensively (Chap. 18). The lungs are the effector organ in several immunological responses to inhaled agents. The relations between animal models of immunological responses and human disease are still quite uncertain. This is particularly true in conditions where the antigens are relatively ill defined, as in farmer's lung and bird fancier's lung, in which the type of response is still a matter of discussion (see Chap. 15, p. 373).[53] Progress in this field may require careful immunological studies in subjects from defined population groups, which would include healthy persons as well as persons with allergic responses.

Pathology

The morbid anatomy and classical histology of responses of human lungs to inhaled matter are well known; these are reviewed only briefly. We lack knowledge, however, on many early disease states in man. Animal experiments provide some information, but they are not always applicable to man, and for several human diseases we have no animal model.

Lung edema. Acute lung edema (e.g., phosgene or chlorine exposure) begins usually a few hours after exposure. The differences, if any, between edema induced by irritants and that caused by cardiac insufficiency have not been studied in detail. Yandell Henderson[28] suggested that irritant-induced edema would be located primarily in areas that receive a large fraction of inspired air—the dependent lung zones—which are also primarily affected by edema when circulation fails. A significant difference may be that inhaled irritants probably induce obstruction of small airways, with edematous mucosal swelling. This should lead to signs of small-airway obstruction, but alveolar edema usually dominates the clinical picture and, since vigorous treatment is called for, few controlled observations are available.

Emphysema. This term describes a condition including destruction of alveolar septae, confluence of alveoli, formation of large blebs or bullae, loss of alveolar surface area, and loss of lung elastic recoil. Two main forms are distinguished— *centrilobular* and *panacinar emphysema.* In centrilobular emphysema, the terminal airways in the center of a lobule are mainly affected and the more peripheral alveoli may be relatively intact, while in panacinar emphysema, alveolar units are involved. Mechanical factors influence the distribution of emphysematous lesions throughout the lungs, and there is a predilection for the lung tops (see p. 63). In recent years, the ability of certain proteolytic enzymes (papain) to cause a similar pathological entity in the lungs of animals has received much attention.[23] The histological end result of treatment of rats with papain, intratracheally or by aerosol, is very similar to human emphysema (see p. 139). Similar results have been obtained with proteases from alveolar macrophages and blood leucocytes.

Also in recent years, a genetically determined enzyme deficiency in man has been detected, which is associated with early development of emphysema, at least in homozygotic individuals.[33, 49] In this condition, there is a lack of an enzyme that inhibits the proteolytic action of trypsin (α_1-antitrypsin deficiency). How this enzyme deficiency leads to destruction of lung tissue remains a matter for speculation. It may be that shortage of factors which inhibit endogenous proteolytic enzymes can lead to breakdown of lung tissue and formation of emphysematous lesions. This hypothesis has many interesting angles—for instance, why is only lung tissue destroyed when there is a general shortage of the antitryptic enzyme?

Homozygous alpha-1-antitrypsin deficiency (see also Chap. 7, p. 139) is rare and accounts for at most 1–2 percent of all cases of emphysema. Even in these, the role of environmental factors cannot be neglected: most of these patients are also cigarette smokers. Adequate population data on the distribution of the defect are not yet available, but in any case, the majority of emphysema cases must be caused (1) by other agents or processes, or (2) by other as yet unidentified enzyme deficiencies that also unleash proteolytic enzymes. Both hypotheses may be correct. Emphysema may well result from different disease processes, even though histological appearances at the end-stage are the same.

An action of proteolytic enzymes is suspected in laundry-detergent workers who have decreased elastic recoil after prolonged exposure.[38] Older textile workers with decreased ventilatory capacities have decreased elastic recoil pressures.[24a] Loss of lung elastic recoil is characteristic of emphysema, but it can only be recognized during life when it is severe (Chap. 7, p. 139). Thus, emphysema in man is usually diagnosed only in its advanced stages, and the natural history of this important cause of premature death in man remains quite ill understood. In most instances, it is associated with cigarette smoking, but how smoke induces emphysema is not known.

Early cellular responses. The initial events in cellular responses of lung tissue vary according to the toxic agent. With oxygen, alveolar epithelium is damaged and replaced by type II alveolar cells, which form a cuboidal epithelial layer.[52] High partial pressures of O_2 inactivate enzymes and can cause peroxidation of lipids; this results in cell damage. In Weibel's experiments with rats (1 atm, 100 percent O_2),[52] cyanosis and death occurred within 72 hours. Edema formation, destruction of vascular endothelium, and damage to alveolar epithelium were found at 48 hours. The repair response, with cuboid epithelium in alveoli, occurred in monkeys; these were the only animals to survive exposure long enough. Apparently, type II cells with their many organelles have a much better repair capability than type I cells, which lack these.

In paraquat poisoning, the lungs become infiltrated with macrophage cells.[19] This response also occurs with other irritant gases (phosgene, chlorine, SO_2, NO_2, O_3, croton aldehyde), and the pathology of tissue proliferation in the alveoli appears qualitatively rather similar, at least in animal experiments.[24] Activation and accumulation of macrophage cells is probably a first step in many responses to foreign matter or to cell injury. In subsequent stages, granulomatous infiltrates are formed, frequently with giant cells.

Granuloma formation and fibrosis. In several mineral dust-induced diseases granulomatous and fibrous tissues are formed in the lungs. In beryllium disease, the granulomatous response predominates and fibrosis is secondary. With silica and asbestos, the initial response is an accumulation of various cells in the interstitial tissue; this is soon followed by formation of collagen and fibrous tissue. First, fine reticular fibers are formed, and later coarse collagen fiber bundles appear. With hard metals (tungsten, cadmium) an initial inflammatory response is followed by fibrosis. Fibrosis also occurs in certain diseases—e.g., farmer's lung—caused by biological materials. Thus, fibrosis, like emphysema, is an end-stage response which may result from a variety of initial tissue responses.

For the initial formation of fibrotic tissue, destruction of the alveolar basement membrane appears to be a prerequisite. In some cases, as in asbestosis, it is likely that macrophage cells are transformed directly into fibroblasts; in other instances the process is more indirect. The action of silica particles, leading to autolysis of macrophages, has already been discussed (p. 268). Collagen may be formed as a response to specific chemical products from autolyzed macrophages. However, collagen formation may be a rather nonspecific response to several types of low-grade tissue inflammation, and it is uncertain whether dead macrophage cells are directly involved in the process.

In silicosis, fibrous tissue is formed in nodules; in asbestosis, fibrosis is a more diffuse process. Perhaps long asbestos fibers elicit a more widespread response than the smaller silica particles. The original deposition pattern may also be important. Many asbestos fibers, especially curled chrysotile, may be intercepted in small airways, while quartz dust particles are more likely to settle mainly in alveoli and alveolar ducts. The "fibrogenicity" of different mineral dusts varies. Whether a mineral dust causes formation of lung fibrosis depends primarily on its quartz or asbestos content. In addition, the physical state of quartz is important: for the same mass, smaller particles appear to elicit more fibrosis. The prevalence of siliceous rocks in many mines has made it difficult to discern fibrogenetic properties of other substances such as coal. Cases of pure carbon exposure [34] have made it clear, however, that carbon can cause fibrosis in the absence of free silica.

Oncology

Cigarette smoke is the principal inhaled carcinogen. Although several constituents of the smoke may be potential carcinogens, there is no agreement on their relative importance (Chap. 14). An increased risk of lung cancer has also been documented for workers exposed to asbestos, chromates, nickel, arsenic, and radioactive dusts (uranium mines), and it has been suggested for others such as beryllium. Interaction between carcinogens, with more frequent tumor induction resulting from exposure to more than one agent, has been observed in man (smoking and asbestos exposure, Chap. 15) and in animals (low levels of SO_2 in air and benzo-a-pyrene exposure in mice [30]).

DETECTION AND DIAGNOSIS OF ENVIRONMENTAL
LUNG DISEASE

The description of human responses to environmental agents has two principal aspects—detection of disease, which may consist only of demonstrating an increased prevalence of disease among people who have some exposure in common, and accurate clinical diagnosis of the type of disease. For prevention and control purposes, it is often more important to know that an excess of disease exists among a population group, and how large the excess is, than to know the detailed clinical diagnosis in each patient. For treatment of the individual, and for studies on pathogenesis of the disease, complete clinical studies are usually essential. The emphasis in this and other chapters is on detection of disease and on certain detailed studies that have special relevance to environmental factors in lung disease. More complete discussions of the clinical and pathological aspects of many environmental lung diseases are available in several textbooks.[26, 48]

Disease detection in population groups is based on identification of the disease's clinical features. Unfortunately, these features are often not clearly seen until the late stages of disease, and opportunities for clinical study of early responses to environmental agents are rare. It is difficult to design methods to detect disease in early stages unless one knows what to look for. The currently unsatisfactory definition of early stages of many lung diseases (Chap. 13) can be improved by longitudinal epidemiological studies of population groups with exposure risks, using suitable diagnostic methods to detect either the clinical features of the late disease in minor form, or special characteristics of early responses to the exposure. Such work will lead to a clearer picture than we now have of the natural history of chronic bronchitis, emphysema, and several other lung diseases. At the present time, sophisticated diagnostic methods are usually applied at a stage of the disease where the pathological process is largely irreversible.

The clinician is at a disadvantage in discerning the environmental causes of lung diseases. The patient in a hospital or clinic often is incapable of defining environmental hazards to which he may have been exposed. The only part of the environmental history that is often available to the clinician is the history of smoking habits. In the individual patient it is often impossible to weigh smoking against other exposures in terms of respective contributions to lung disease. To understand the environmental factors in lung disease, one needs to study not only the individual patient, but also others similarly exposed; in addition, one must study their environment in detail.

The main tools in detection and diagnosis are the patient's history and physical examination, chest x-ray film, lung function tests, and epidemiological studies (Chap. 13).

History and physical examination. A complete medical history, the key to diagnosing environmental lung diseases, should include details of the patient's smoking, occupation, hobbies, and residence. In population studies, standard questionnaires are essential to elicit this information (Chap. 13; Appendix), and they are also of great help in clinical diagnosis. Physical examination is usually much less helpful than the history, since many physical signs are nonspecific. Signs of ventilatory insufficiency (cyanosis, labored breathing) may be obvious. Wheezing and other abnormal breath sounds may indicate airway obstruction or parenchymal disease. In individual diagnosis, these observations are helpful: an asbestos worker with bilateral basal rales after 20 years' dust exposure probably has asbestosis; a cotton worker with bilateral wheezing on Monday afternoon after work most likely has byssinosis. In studies of groups, physical examinations are usually neither practical nor necessary. More objective data on airway obstruction can be obtained from function tests, and data concerning parenchymal disease from x-ray films. Physical signs are mostly nonspecific, difficult to quantitate, and subject to errors in observation. For these reasons, physical examination is usually omitted in epidemiological studies.

Chest X-ray Films

In mineral dust pneumoconiosis, either the dust deposit or the tissue responses it induces, or both, are radiopaque. Together with a history of exposure, the chest x-ray film is crucial for the diagnosis of these diseases. Detailed descriptions of radiological changes in pneumoconiosis are available elsewhere.[20] International agreement on standardization of techniques and interpretations of chest x-ray changes in pneumoconiosis has been reached.[8] A standard set of x-ray films is available, together with the description of technique and of classification.[8, 29] Lesions are graded according to size and profusion. Gilson[22] has shown that this grading system correlates well with the dust content of the lungs, as determined post mortem (Table 12-1). Because of clearance (p. 267), residual deposits found post mortem are much smaller than the amounts originally inhaled. Nevertheless, the amount of dust retained at the time of death appears to be related to the radiological extent of disease, and the x-ray classification appears to be useful as a semiquantitative guide to dust retention. Gilson has estimated that about 16 gm coal dust, 5 gm mineral dust, or 1.6 gm iron oxide is required to increase the x-ray grade by one unit (e.g., from 0 to 1, or from 2 to 3).[22] These data are based on correlations in large numbers of workers at risk and obviously do not take into account individual variability.

Unfortunately, the x-ray findings sometimes bear little relation to the patient's disability, loss of function, or the severity of other symptoms. Miners with extensive lesions detected on x-ray examination may have few symptoms, while severely disabled miners may have no convincing roentgenographic signs. This problem arises in coal workers' pneumoconiosis as well as in silicosis. In these diseases, it is likely that disability is chiefly associated with bronchial lesions, which do not show on x-ray films (Chap. 15, p. 367). Also, there may be coexisting emphysematous lesions, which cause hypertranslucent areas on the x-ray film, and dust deposits which are radiopaque; these may cancel out if they are superimposed on one another, so that the resulting radiotranslucency of the lungs may be about normal despite extensive lesions.

Individual judgments about x-ray film shadows often differ, in particular about the presence or absence of minor lesions. Systematic studies show large margins of error in roentgenographic assessment. For compensation purposes, the judgment of a single observer should therefore not be decisive. Films should be read independently by at least 2 observers. Their individual judgments should be quantified, according to international classification, and the results then graded and averaged.

Table 12-1
Correlation Between Dust Content of Lungs and X-ray Findings

	X-Ray Category	Weight of Dust in Both Lungs (gm)
Non-miners	0	1.0
Coal miners	0	4.2
"	1	10.0
"	2	13.2
"	3	19.1

0=no pneumoconiosis on chest x-ray film. Categories 1–3 indicate increasing degree of simple pneumoconiosis. Data from reference 22.

The roentgenogram remains an important tool in studies of mineral dust pneumoconiosis, but the almost exclusive reliance on this tool in the past has contributed to our present confusion concerning the functional implications of these diseases.

Lung Function Tests

The physiological bases for function tests are discussed in Chapters 3 through 9. To detect disease, a sensitive test—not necessarily specific for some disease category—is needed; first, those who are normal must be distinguished from those who have some degree of disease. For diagnosis, the tests must also be specific for some functional abnormality that can be interpreted in terms of specific disease processes. Several investigators have recently summarized their views on the choice of tests for epidemiological studies.[4]

In epidemiological studies, the discriminating power of function tests is often better than in individual diagnosis. When judging function loss in a patient, one often compares the data to normal values, which can have a considerable range. In epidemiological studies, one can often compare groups at risk with control groups, and relatively small differences can then be both significant and meaningful. In longitudinal studies, each subject can serve as his own control, and again this allows detection of small differences in function over a span of time.

Two main patterns of function loss occur in environmental lung disease. In silicosis and other fibrotic diseases there is *restrictive function loss*. The functional size of the lungs is decreased: total lung capacity, vital capacity, and residual volume are all reduced. The airways are not obstructed and elastic recoil may be increased because of the abundance of stiff fibrous tissue throughout the lungs. Hence, expiratory flow rates are often high, and the ratio of $FEV_{1.0}$ to VC may be close to 100 percent. The small volume combined with high flow rates results in a typical MEFV curve pattern (Fig. 9-6, p. 182). *Obstructive function loss* occurs when small airways are partially occluded but air entry remains possible. Its effect is best seen during expiration—forced expiratory flow rates are reduced but vital capacity may be normal. Flow reduction is usually most severe at small lung volumes, since airway caliber decreases with lung volume. This results in another typical MEFV curve pattern, with a curvature opposite in direction from that in restrictive function loss (Fig. 9-6, p. 182). Obstructive function changes can be detected even in minor degrees with recordings of MEFV and PEFV curves (Chap. 9) and with methods to detect unequal degrees of gas distribution or increased airway-closure volume (Chap. 4).

In addition to spirometric tests, certain other function tests have been used in epidemiological studies of environmental lung disease. The single-breath diffusion capacity test (Chap. 6) is a suitable, noninvasive test of gas exchange for routine use in epidemiological studies of diseases in which gas exchange may be limited in early stages (asbestosis). Automation and electronic data processing may make these and other relatively complex tests more widely available.

Severe lung function loss limits a person's ability to do physical work and provides a basis for disability. The criteria that are used by the Social Security Administration are shown in Table 12-2. Patients with this degree of function loss are usually short of breath during minimal exertion and can perform only desk work or similar activities. Disability for jobs involving physical exercise may exist with less severe degrees of function loss. Unfortunately, objective criteria for decreased work performance in lung disease are as yet unsatisfactory. Hyatt and associates [46] have shown that patients with obstructive lung disease have a limited exercise capacity because of their limitation in ventilatory capacity. A comparison of exercise ventilation with maximum ventilatory performance as described by the MEFV curve could be a practical test for objective disability evaluation (Fig. 12-1). Other indices of disability can be derived from measurements of diffusing capacity or arterial blood gases. For instance, if the diffusion capacity does not increase during exercise, this implies inability to increase gas exchange and thus provide for sufficient oxygen uptake to meet the requirements of the exercise. A

Table 12-2
Criteria for Disability (S.S.A.) *

Height		$FEV_{1.0} \leq$	$VC \leq$
(in.)	(cm)	(liters)	(liters)
57 or less	146.0 or less	1.0	1.2
58	148.5	1.0	1.3
59	151.0	1.0	1.3
60	153.5	1.1	1.4
61	156.0	1.1	1.4
62	158.5	1.1	1.5
63	161.5	1.1	1.5
64	164.0	1.2	1.6
65	166.5	1.2	1.6
66	169.0	1.2	1.7
67	171.5	1.3	1.7
68	174.0	1.3	1.8
69	176.6	1.3	1.8
70	179.0	1.4	1.9
71	182.0	1.4	1.9
72	184.5	1.4	2.0
73 or more	187.0 or more	1.4	2.0

* Social Security Disability Evaluation, A Handbook for Physicians. U.S. Dept. Health, Education, and Welfare, Social Security Division, July 1970, p 16–17.

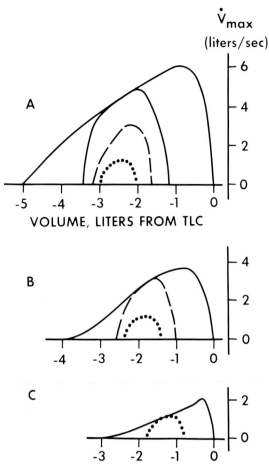

Fig. 12-1. Use of expiratory flow-volume curves to assess disabling loss of ventilatory function. *Dotted line:* tidal expiration (V_T) at rest; *dashed line:* V_T during moderate exercise; *solid line:* V_T during heavy exercise. All expiratory FV loops drawn in contour of MEFV curves in a healthy person (*A*) and in 2 patients with moderate (*B*) and severe (*C*) obstructive disease. Limits of expiratory flow are reached at rest in *C*, during moderate exercise in *B*, and during heavy work in *A*. Patient *C* is dyspneic at rest, and patient *B* during moderate exercise. From reference 26. Used with permission of McGraw-Hill Book Co. (copyright 1974).

low arterial oxygen tension implies deficient oxygenation of body tissues; this may be considered evidence of disability if it occurs during light work or at rest.

Other Methods

The identification and description of materials and organisms that damage the lungs may require help from organic chemists to identify natural products derived from plants, from mineralogists to identify mineral dusts and fibers, from

botanists to identify vegetable matter, and from microbiologists to identify micro-
bial material. For instance, identification of asbestos fibers or of silica in lung
tissue proves exposure to these agents. However, when the source of exposure is
known, identification of the material in the environment is easier and less traumatic
to the patient than the performance of a lung biopsy. While the biopsy may
confirm exposure, it does not indicate the extent of lung disease. In fact, asbestos
can be found in lungs of city dwellers who have no demonstrable lung disease.[32]
For most environmental lung diseases, the epidemiological evidence which links
exposure with increased risk of disease should carry far greater weight than the
results of a single lung biopsy. However, in some cases lung biopsy is essential
for diagnosis.

The use of biochemical and pharmacological methods in the recognition of
responses to environmental agents is still limited. In the future these may become
much more important. Recognition of enzyme deficiencies or alterations in serum
enzyme levels [33, 45] may lead to new diagnostic methods. Improved methods of
detecting inhaled substances or their metabolites in body fluids and tissues are
being developed. Pharmacological tests may aid physicians in detecting persons
likely to be affected by certain exposures (potential reactors), which would be
invaluable in prevention programs.

PREVENTION AND CONTROL

Environmental Hygiene

The prime task of environmental hygiene is to describe the environment and
determine how environmental risks can be prevented or controlled. Many potentially hazardous substances are continually released into the atmosphere, outdoors
and indoors, and chemically pure air is a rarity. In fact, few people would want to
breathe air devoid of pleasant odors, and personal preferences in this respect are
quite individualistic. Thus, aesthetics as well as health effects may help to determine which pollutants should be removed from the atmosphere, and which can
be tolerated.

Threshold limit values. The response to inhaled agents is a function of the
duration of exposure and the concentration of the inhaled agent. The form of
the dose-response relationship is of crucial importance. With some substances,
effects are observed even with minimal doses: the dose-response curve passes
through zero (e.g., certain carcinogens). Thus, any exposure needs to be avoided.
For other substances, environmental hygienists use the concept of a threshold limit
value, which refers to "the airborne concentrations of substances and represent(s)
conditions under which it is believed that nearly all workers may be repeatedly
exposed day after day without adverse effect."[2] Threshold limit values (TLV)
thus refer to occupational exposures only, not to community air pollution. The
organization (the American Conference of Governmental Industrial Hygienists)
that publishes the yearly list of TLV values recognizes their limitations; this group
states specifically that even exposures below TLV levels to some substances may
result in discomfort in highly sensitive individuals, and that a small number of
persons may develop disease at these lower levels.

As our methods of detecting responses to toxic agents have improved, it has become clear that for most substances there is no absolute threshold of exposure below which no response ever occurs. Slight effects of low-level exposures may or may not be medically significant. If they are, even stringent environmental controls may not prevent all illness or acute responses to inhaled agents. Thus, other methods must be used, in addition to environmental control, if all significant disease is to be prevented. In industry, these other methods include (a) detection of highly sensitive individuals and assignment of these persons to nonrisk jobs; (b) periodic examination of persons at risk to detect any environmentally induced disease at an early stage and, if possible, to prevent its progression; this, too, will often include reassignment to another job. Until now, implementation of environmental control measures has to a large extent been the domain of hygienists, and few physicians have taken an active interest in this field. In the future, physicians must work together with hygienists, because adequate control of environmental lung disease, particularly in industry, will require control of the environment as well as surveillance of the individual at risk. The federal standard for asbestos dust (1972) includes a requirement for specified medical examinations and lung function tests, and such requirements may also become a part of other standards to be issued under the Williams-Steiger Occupational Safety and Health Act of 1970.

Measurement of dust concentrations.[1] The crucial criterion in designing an instrument to monitor dust is that it collect all particles likely to be inhaled and deposited in the lungs of people who breathe in that atmosphere. Thus, ideally, the instrument would have some deposition characteristics that resemble those of human airways and lungs. One well-known instrument (Unico high-volume sampler) has an air inlet that leads to a cyclone. In the cyclone, air velocities are increased and large particles settle by impaction, a process not too dissimilar from what happens in the human nose. Next, the air passes through a filter paper that traps the finer dust. Thus, large particles and respirable dust are collected separately and can be weighed. A more recently developed instrument, the vertical elutriator,[36] uses gravity to separate small and large particles. The air inlet of this instrument points downward, and a pump draws in air at a slow rate of flow. Small particles travel upward with the airstream and are collected. The force of gravity predominates for large particles; these travel downward and are not collected. Thus, this instrument collects only particles below a certain size (usually 15 μm). The exact size limit is determined by the rate of airflow—with larger flow rates, larger particles are collected. The vertical elutriator has been used in studies of byssinosis in the cotton textile industry and is recommended for use in control programs. In all dust-sampling studies, the location, number, and timing of measurements are crucial for optimal interpretation of data. The measurements can be designed only with full knowledge of the work practices and the workroom ventilation systems.

For most purposes, the mass of respirable dust is the important criterion for environmental control. To improve accuracy and to average conditions during a typical workshift, measurements are usually made over 8-hour periods. The airflow rate through the sampling instrument must be measured accurately so that the amount of dust collected can be related to the total amount of air passed through the sampler. The measurement is usually expressed in milligrams of dust per cubic meter of air. For certain dusts, measurement of the number of fibers in air rather than the total mass of dust is required for control purposes. In asbestos plants, for instance, asbestos fibers are often mixed with other dust particles which are not a health hazard. Therefore, asbestos fibers are collected on filters and counted under a microscope; with suitable standardization, the fibers counted can be used to compute the number of fibers per milliliter of air.

Personal dust samplers. Rather than characterizing the air in a workroom, the aim of personal-sampling methods is to determine the individual's exposure by sampling the air close to his mouth and nose. Although this appears ideal theoretically, the use of such samplers in practice is subject to errors caused by lack of supervision, accidents, or even tampering. One must also make sure that the person wearing the sampler indeed spends nearly all working time in the area where exposure occurs. No adequate personal sampler for respirable dust is available at this time. Therefore, the methods described in the previous section remain preferable for the time being. Together with approximate data on the amount of time workers spend in various locations, these can be used to evaluate each worker's individual exposure.[7]

Engineering

In the final analysis, control of most environmental lung diseases must come from better engineering methods. These are as diverse as improved farming procedures (to prevent farmer's lung), safer methods for handling toxic gases, prevention of pollutant emission into indoor or outdoor atmospheres, and removal of pollutants from indoor atmospheres when emission controls are insufficient or fail. In most instances, economical as well as environmental and medical aspects must be taken into account. Thus, the control engineer must ask to what extent emission control of pollutant removal is required to meet health standards, which methods are most suitable to accomplish adequate control, and how much installation and proper maintenance are likely to cost.

Control of respirable dust is a good example. Here, the engineer must match wits with the biological designs of our creator: he must design an even better trap for fine dust than the human lungs. For small volumes of air, this can be done with close to 100 percent effectiveness with an electrostatic precipitator. For the amounts of air circulating through large factory workrooms, the capacity of such an instrument would have to be extremely large. Also, the required capacity would be much greater if one wishes to remove 100 percent of all fine dust rather than, say, 99 percent. The question of how much control is needed becomes very important in terms of technical feasibility as well as cost. Another solution to the fine-dust problem would be to enclose all machines and exhaust the dust-laden air to the outside atmosphere, perhaps through a filter to avoid community air pollution. This air would be drawn from the workrooms and would have to be replaced with outside air. In most climates, heating or cooling, or both, of such large air masses would be very costly. Therefore, it is customary to recirculate already cooled or heated air and to remove dust by installing filters or dust traps in the ductwork.

The engineer has to find methods to provide workers with air that is cleaned to the maximum extent required for adequate protection. From a purely medical perspective, cost considerations should not matter; in industrial practice, they always do. Since precise exposure limits are difficult to establish, there is usually a margin of uncertainty concerning control requirements in which economical or technical considerations tend to push the tolerable dust level upward, while health considerations provide arguments to decrease the tolerable levels. The latter should prevail in all instances of highly dangerous (e.g., carcinogenic) exposures. In other cases, engineering controls should at least decrease the prevalence of ill effects to a low level, so that medical surveillance (p. 301) can adequately protect the small number of sensitive individuals who are still affected. In instances where short-term effects can be measured, increased use of medical surveillance can provide relatively rapid feedback of information concerning effectiveness of controls to the engineers. Improved controls can then be designed on the basis of the additional medical information available.

There is a need for increasing cooperation between industrial hygienists, control engineers, and physicians, each of whom has a task in providing a safe environment for the worker in industry. Much of this experience is also useful in dealing with problems of community air pollution (Chap. 16). This cooperation can succeed only when hygienists, engineers, and physicians recognize the constraints under which each of them works and when they understand and respect each other's outlook on the problems.

Legislation

In many states, workmen's compensation laws provide financial compensation to workers injured in their jobs or suffering from occupational diseases. In some states, so-called statutes of limitation deny compensation for injuries if application is made longer than 1 year after the injury. This often leads to denial of claims for chronic occupational illnesses, since the original injury occurred years ago. Disabled workers also may apply for disability benefits under the Social Security Act, but the definition of disabling respiratory disease under that act limits these benefits in practice to severely and permanently disabled persons. The only federal compensation act at this time is the Black Lung Act of 1969 (amended in 1972), which provides compensation for miners disabled by coal workers' pneumoconiosis.

Compensation laws in their usual form do not include incentives to develop prevention and control programs. They only provide some minimal financial security to persons who suffer from end-stage lung disease after years of exposure. With the enactment of the Occupational Safety and Health Act of 1970, the federal government has committed itself to the provision of a safe place of employment, free from recognized hazards, for all Americans. Adequate implementation of this law can go far in developing a more positive approach to problems of environmental lung disease. The Act provides procedures and resources to develop adequate health standards in order to limit exposures, and it also provides mechanisms to enforce the implementation of these standards. The principal agency that provides the research base for standards and enforcement procedures is the National Institute for Occupational Safety and Health, which recommends standards to the U.S. Department of Labor, based principally on the health effects of exposure. The Department of Labor has final authority in setting and enforcing the standards. The success of the Act in terms of workers' health will to a large extent depend on the interest and expertise of the professional workers in the field. It is already clear that one of the main factors limiting the Act's implementation is the lack of medical and industrial hygiene manpower as well as insufficient expertise in the field of engineering-control methods. A major reevaluation of professional priorities, in particular for physicians and engineers, will be necessary to insure that industrial production can continue to develop without damaging the workers' health.

SUMMARY

Environmental inhalants are transported into the airways and lungs during inspiration. Gases are dissolved and particles are deposited in the tissues and may evoke physiological or pathological responses. Dust particles are removed by cough, mucociliary clearance, phagocytosis, and lymphatic transport. The tissue responses include protective reflexes, mucus production, airway constriction or dilatation, lung edema, lung fibrosis, granuloma formation, emphysema, and lung cancer. The early stages of chronic airway and tissue responses are ill defined. The detection of environmentally induced lung diseases requires epidemiological studies with standardized clinical and laboratory methods (history, chest x-ray film, lung function tests) to identify disease states and to describe their prevalence, together with environmental measurements to quantitate exposures. The many disciplines that contribute to understanding physiological and pathological responses to inhaled matter, and to detection, prevention, and control of environmental lung disease are briefly discussed. Coordinated multidisciplinary efforts are required to abolish the varied and widespread risks of lung disease caused by smoking, occupational exposures, and air pollution.

REFERENCES

1. Aerosol Technology Committee, American Industrial Hygiene Association: Respirable mass sampling. Am Ind Hyg Assoc J 31:133–137, 1970

1a. Allison AC, Harington JS, Birbeck M, Nash T: Observations on the cytotoxic action of silica on macrophages, in Davies CN (ed): Inhaled Particles and Vapours II. Oxford, Pergamon Press, 1967, pp 121–131

2. American Conference of Governmental Industrial Hygienists. Threshold limit values of airborne contaminants, 1973

3. Andersen I, Lundquist GR, Proctor DF: Human nasal mucosal function in a controlled climate. Arch Environ Health 23: 408–420, 1971

4. Becklake MR (ed): Respiratory function tests in epidemiologic surveys. Bull Physiopathol Respir (Nancy) 6:533–680, 1970

5. Beeckmans JM: The deposition of aerosols in the respiratory tract. I. Mathematical analysis and comparison with experimental data. Can J Physiol Pharmacol 43:157–172, 1965

6. Beeckmans JM: Alveolar deposition of aerosols on the moon and in outer space. Nature 211:208, 1966

7. Belin L, Bouhuys A, Hoekstra W, Johansson M-B, Lindell S-E, Pool J: Byssinosis in cardroom workers in Swedish cotton mills. Br J Ind Med 22:101–108, 1965

8. Bohlig H, Bristol LJ, Cartier PH, Felson B, Gilson JC, Grainger TR, Jacobson G, Kiviluoto R, Lainhart WS, McDonald JC, Pendergrass EP, Rossiter CE, Selikoff IJ, Sluis-Cremer GK, Wright GW: Special Report: UICC/Cincinnati classification of the radiographic appearances of pneumoconioses. A cooperative study

by the UICC Committee. Chest 58:57–67, 1970

9. Boren HG: Carbon as a carrier mechanism for irritant gases. Arch Environ Health 8:119–124, 1964

10. Bouhuys A: Isoprenaline-inhalatie bij astma bronchiale. Ned Tijdschr Geneesk 107:1739–1742, 1963

11. Brain JD: The uptake of inhaled gases by the nose. Ann Otol Rhinol Laryngol 79:529–539, 1970

12. Casarett MG, Casarett LJ, Hodge HC: An in vitro study of mast cell response to particulate materials. Pharmacology 1:271–282, 1968

13. Clark JM, Lambertsen CJ: Pulmonary oxygen toxicity: A review. Pharmacol Rev 23:37–133, 1971

14. Davies CN, Muir DC: Deposition of inhaled particles in human lungs. Nature 211:90–91, 1966

15. Dennis WL: Deposition of inhaled particles in human lungs. Nature 214:908, 1967

16. Douglas JS, Dennis MW, Ridgway P, Bouhuys A: Airway dilatation and constriction in spontaneously breathing guinea pigs. J Pharmacol Exp Ther 180:98–109, 1972

17. DuBois AB, Dautrebande L: Acute effects of breathing inert dust particles and of carbachol aerosol on the mechanical characteristics of the lungs in man. Changes in response after inhaling sympathomimetic aerosols. J Clin Invest 37:1746–1755, 1958

18. Editorial: Pneumoconiosis redefined. Br Med J 2:552, 1972

19. Fletcher K, Wyatt I: The composition of lung lipids after poisoning with paraquat. Br J Exp Pathol 51:604–610, 1970

20. Fraser RG, Paré JAP: Diagnosis of Diseases of the Chest, vols I & II. Philadelphia, WB Saunders Co Inc, 1970

21. Vogt MT, Thomas C, Vassallo CL, Basford RE, Gee JBL: Glutathione-dependent peroxidative metabolism in the alveolar macrophage. J Clin Invest 50:401–410, 1971

22. Gilson JC: The first Wade lecture: The changing pattern of pneumoconiosis, in: Health Conditions in the Ceramic Industry. International Symposium, Stoke-on-Trent, March, 1968, Oxford, Pergamon Press, 1969, pp 11–28

23. Gross P, Pfitzer E, Tolker E, Babyak MA, Kaschak M: Experimental emphy-sema: its production with papain in normal and silicotic rats. Arch Environ Health 11:50–58, 1965

24. Gross P, Rinehart WE, deTreville RTP: The pulmonary reactions to toxic gases. Am Ind Hyg Assoc J 28:215–321, 1967

24a. Guyatt, AR, Douglas JS, Zuskin E, Bouhuys A: Lung static recoil and airway obstruction in hemp workers with byssinosis. Am Rev Respir Dis 108:1111–1115, 1973

25. Hanna MG Jr, Nettesheim P, Gilbert JR (eds): Inhalation carcinogenesis. U.S. Atomic Energy Commission, Division of Technical Information, 1970

26. Harrison's Principles of Internal Medicine, ed 7. Wintrobe MM, Thorn GW, Adams RD, Braunwald E, Isselbacher KJ, Petersdorf RG (eds). New York, McGraw-Hill, 1974

27. Hatch TF, Gross P: Pulmonary Deposition and Retention of Inhaled Aerosols. New York, Academic Press, 1964

28. Henderson Y, Haggard HW: Noxious Gases and the Principles of Respiration Influencing their Action. New York, Reinhold Publishing Corp, 1943

29. Jacobson G, Bohlig H, Kiviluoto R: Essentials of chest radiography. Radiology 95:445–450, 1970

30. Kuschner M, Laskin S: Experimental models in environmental carcinogenesis. Am J Pathol 64:183–196, 1971

31. Landahl HD: The effect of gravity, hygroscopicity, and particle size on the amount and site of deposition of inhaled particles with particular reference to hazard due to airborne viruses, in Mercer TT, Morrow PE, Stöber W (eds): Assessment of Airborne Particles. Springfield, Charles C Thomas, 1972, pp 421–428

32. Langer AM, Selikoff IJ, Sastre A: Chrysotile asbestos in the lungs of persons in New York City. Arch Environ Health 22:348–361, 1971

33. Laurell CB, Eriksson S: The electrophoretic α_1-globulin pattern of serum in α_1-antitrypsin deficiency. Scand J Clin Lab Invest 15:132–140, 1963

34. Lister WB, Wimborne D: Carbon pneumoconiosis in a synthetic graphite worker. Br J Ind Med 29:108–110, 1972

35. Lourenço RV, Klimek MF, Borowski CJ: Deposition and clearance of 2 μ particles in the tracheobronchial tree of normal subjects—smokers and non-

smokers. J Clin Invest 50:1411–1420, 1971

36. Lynch JR: Air sampling for cotton dust. Trans National Conference on Cotton Dust and Health, University of North Carolina, May 22, 1970, p 33

37. Mercer TT, Morrow PE, Stöber W (eds): Assessment of Airborne Particles. Springfield, Charles C Thomas, 1972

38. Mitchell CA: Loss of pulmonary elastic recoil in workers heavily exposed to proteolytic enzymes in the detergent industry. Submitted for publication.

39. Morrow PE: Dynamics of dust removal from the lower airways; measurements and interpretations based upon radioactive aerosols, in Bouhuys A (ed): Airway Dynamics; Physiology and Pharmacology. Springfield, Charles C Thomas, 1970, pp 299–312

40. Muir DC: Aerosol deposition in the lungs of space travellers. Nature 209: 921, 1966

41. Myrvik QN, Leake ES, Fariss B: Studies on pulmonary alveolar macrophages from the normal rabbit: A technique to procure them in a high state of purity. J Immunol 86:128–136, 1961

42. Nash T, Pattle RE: The absorption of phosgene by aqueous solutions and its relation to toxicity. Ann Occup Hyg 14:227–233, 1971

43. Newhouse MT, Wright FJ, Dolovich M, Hopkins OL: Clearance of RISA aerosol from the human lung, in: Bouhuys A (ed): Airway Dynamics; Physiology and Pharmacology. Springfield, Charles C Thomas, 1970, pp 313–317

44. Page-Roberts BA: Preparation and partial characterization of a lamellar body fraction from rat lung. Biochim Biophys Acta 260: 334–338, 1972

45. Pascual RS, Gee JBL, Finch SC: Usefulness of serum lysozyme measurement in diagnosis and evaluation of sarcoidosis. N Engl J Med 289:1074–1076, 1973

46. Potter WA, Olafsson S, Hyatt RE: Ventilatory mechanics and expiratory flow limitation during exercise in patients with obstructive lung disease. J Clin Invest 50:910–919, 1971

47. Saindelle A, Flavian N, Guillerm R, Hée J: Libération d'histamine par la fumée de cigarette et ses constituants. CR Acad Sci [D] (Paris) 264:2926–2928, 1967

48. Spencer H: Pathology of the Lung, ed 2. Oxford, Pergamon Press, 1968

49. Talamo RC, Allen JD, Kahan MG, Austen KF: Hereditary alpha$_1$-antitrypsin deficiency. N Engl J Med 278:345–351, 1968

50. Task Group on Lung Dynamics: Deposition and retention models for internal dosimetry of the human respiratory tract. Health Phys 12:173–208, 1966

51. Timbrell V: Inhalation and biological effects of asbestos, in Mercer TT, Morrow PE, Stöber W (eds): Assessment of Airborne Particles. Springfield, Charles C Thomas, 1972, pp 429–445

52. Weibel ER: Oxygen effect on lung cells. Arch Intern Med 128:54–56, 1971

53. Wenzel FJ, Emanuel DA, Gray RL: Immunofluorescent studies in patients with farmer's lung. J Allergy Clin Immunol 48:224–229, 1971

54. Widdicombe JG: Respiratory reflexes, in Fenn WO, Rahn H (eds): Handbook of Physiology, Section 3: Respiration, vol. I. Washington, D.C., American Physiological Society, 1964, pp 585–630

55. Wolfsdorf J, Swift DL, Avery ME: Mist therapy reconsidered: An evaluation of the respiratory deposition of labelled water aerosols produced by jet and ultrasonic nebulizers. Pediatrics 43:799–808, 1969

Chapter 13

Epidemiology

Potential hazards in the environment must be assessed from their effects on the health of people who live and work in that environment. Since both environments and populations are constantly changing, this task is not easy. When an inhaled agent is suspected of causing lung disease, one must determine who is exposed to it and whether these people have lung disease. The disease may be limited to the exposed group, or it may also occur, much less frequently, in the general population. Starting from medical observations, one may ask whether certain environmental exposures are common to groups of people with a specific lung disease and, if so, how these exposures cause disease. Well-documented observations on a single case thus can provide invaluable clues, leading to the study of a group of people exposed to a common hazardous agent. The study of such population groups requires the tools of epidemiology, together with the medical and physiological methods discussed in the previous chapter.

The epidemiologist observes disease patterns among populations, deriving clues on etiology and natural history of diseases. He must extract significant information on a few variables from inherently "noisy" data, which reflect the many unknowns that influence the development of disease. By studying random groups of subjects, comparing cases with control subjects, and performing follow-up studies of defined groups of people with common characteristics (cohorts), the epidemiologist is frequently able to draw significant conclusions about a selected variable. Of course, independent experimental findings can often strengthen the epidemiologist's conclusions. The epidemiological association between smoking and lung disease, for example, has led to laboratory studies on agents in cigarettes and in cigarette smoke that biologically affect the airways and lungs (Chap. 14). In spite of these efforts, however, the case against smoking still depends largely on the overwhelming evidence obtained from epidemiological studies. Because epidemiological studies are time consuming and difficult to organize, they have been relatively neglected in the study of many lung diseases. Many experimental observations on the etiology and pathogenesis of lung disease need to be supplemented by epidemiological studies. Bronchial asthma is an example of a disease studied intensively in the laboratory (Chap. 18), while relatively little is known about its prevalence in different population groups and about the distribution of predisposing factors.

Epidemiology deals with the phenomena of diseases as they occur in nature; the uncontrolled character of the raw data sometimes raises doubt about its status as a scientific tool. However, "The simple observation of a natural phenomenon, which happens without our intervention, is much more important than the phenomena of the experiment, determined by our will. The first always reflects the image of reality, while the experiment reflects our limited understanding." Although this statement from Justus von Liebig * referred to chemical phenomena rather than to disease, it could well be applied to the "natural experiment" the epidemiologist observes and tries to explain.

Epidemiologists often collect data about large numbers of people, but the significance of their studies is not merely a function of numbers. In attempting to assess specific risk factors, a comparison of large groups may even be counterproductive—too many extraneous factors may conceal the true risk. It is often useful to compare smaller groups, which may be virtually homogeneous except for the risk factor under study. As for results, it is not enough to find that a disease is no more prevalent among the risk group than among the nonrisk population. In addition, the methods of study must be sensitive enough to detect a difference in disease prevalence. Thus, negative conclusions from group data are not always meaningful, while positive findings about a few cases may be highly significant. One must always be alert for specific risk groups that may be hidden within a large population, and it is therefore not enough to study only the mean data for a group. A close look at the distribution of the data among group members may indicate the existence of subgroups with special characteristics.

Many theoretical and practical problems in epidemiology are discussed in a recent book [12] that provides guidance in organizing surveys and handling data. It also shows the increasing need for epidemiological concepts and methods to monitor health care and to promote prevention of chronic diseases. An excellent introduction to surveys of respiratory disease has been published in 1969 by the American Thoracic Society.[30] In this chapter, I will discuss a number of epidemiological tools, including mortality and morbidity statistics, population studies, and data analysis, as well as some areas where these tools are needed.

Mortality Statistics

Standardized statistical data, using an international classification system, provide national and regional data on the principal causes of death. Although the diagnostic categories are standardized, the judgments of the individual physicians who certify the causes of death are not. Often several diseases coexist, and only the most immediate cause of death may be recorded as the cause. Thus, diseases which lead to death within a short time span, such as myocardial infarctions, are likely to be recorded with fair accuracy, especially in areas with high autopsy rates. On the other hand, victims of such diseases as emphysema and chronic bronchitis can survive many years, and death is often ascribed to intercurrent or

---

* I am indebted to Professors D. Bargeton and H.H. Loeschcke for this quotation.

unrelated diseases. These chronic diseases are therefore easily underestimated as causes of death, as a comparison of autopsy data with death certificates in more than 600 persons (over 40 years old) who died in two university hospitals in Denver has confirmed.[18] Standard sources of mortality data lack sufficient data on the deceased person's environment, including his smoking habits. In retired persons, occupational information may be unavailable or unreliable. In specially designed studies such information can sometimes be obtained from relatives or from union or company records.

The finding of a few deaths attributed to rare diseases may be of great importance in identifying environmental hazards, even when the risk group has not yet been fully identified. When dealing with common diseases, mortality data should be related to the total population at risk, particularly when the excess mortality is small. For instance, a study of the mortality of workers in the newspaper printing industry in Great Britain [19] showed excess lung-cancer deaths among 3485 men who died in the period 1953–1966. Actual deaths were 30–40 percent higher than expected, but the size of the total population at risk was not known. Therefore, mortality rates (number who died per year per 1000 persons at risk) could not be computed. Under these conditions, mortality can be compared only to the proportion of deaths from other causes. Such mortality data are obviously less than perfect, but they nevertheless point to the need for an investigation of environmental risks that could cause an excess of lung cancer in the printing industry.

Mortality data often become more meaningful if they can be related to some prior knowledge of the population among which the deaths occurred. Between 1961 and 1967, Ferris et al.[9] traced 113 deaths among 1167 subjects of a 1961 survey in Berlin, New Hampshire. Mortality was higher among those who had chronic lung disease and a low $FEV_{1.0}$ in 1961, but only 3 deaths were actually attributed to respiratory disease. Cigarette smoking, exposure to gas at work, and heart disease were other predictors of higher mortality risks. In the Staveley survey in Great Britain,[11] mortality was high among foundry workers, smokers, and men with a low FEV value when first seen. Both smoking and a low FEV value had considerable prognostic significance. The prognostic value of low FEV values also appeared from a small-scale study among hemp workers in Spain (Zuskin and Bouhuys, unpublished data). Among 146 men aged 50 to 69 years who were included in a 1967 survey, 7 died between 1967 and 1970 (Table 13-1). All except 1 of the deaths occurred in a subgroup of 27 individuals who suffered from severe disabling byssinosis, with an $FEV_{1.0}$ of 1 liter or less. As in Ferris et al.'s study, a low $FEV_{1.0}$ was associated with a high mortality rate during the follow-up period. These examples show that mortality data collected systematically by individual researchers can yield more pertinent information than is available from vital statistics records; the latter are further complicated by changes in styles of diagnosing and classifying diseases.

In the future, ongoing health surveillance among the living should decrease our dependence on mortality rates as an indicator of environmental health risks. In the first place, environmental control should be geared toward preventing disease, not just to providing countermeasures after the fact. Furthermore, the time lag in collecting and assessing mortality data and their inherent inaccuracies render them useless in many instances that call for environmental control. The errors may go

Table 13-1
Male Hemp Workers (50–69 Years Old in 1967)

	1967 n	1970 † (%)	1967 FEV$_{1.0}$ < 1 liter	1970 † (%)	1967 FEV$_{1.0}$ > 1 liter	1970 † (%)
With history of Monday chest tightness	133	7 (5.3)	27	6 (22)	106	1 (0.9)
No history of Monday tightness	13	0	0	—	13	0
Total	146	7	27	6	119	1

n = total number of men seen in each category. † = number of men who had died between 1967 and 1970. Data of E. Zuskin and A. Bouhuys, 1970 (unpublished).

either way. The finding of excess cancer deaths in newspaper-printing workers (p. 289) may be real or a statistical artifact. On the other hand, mortality may be within normal limits in instances involving known environmental hazards. Enterline[5] found mortality from respiratory disease below expected values in cotton textile workers, although it is well known that disabling byssinosis occurs among textile workers (Chap. 17). Death in retired textile workers may be attributed to heart disease, lung infection, or intercurrent illness, and the former occupation may not be detected from mortality statistics.

Morbidity Statistics

There are several sources of data on morbidity from specified diseases in the United States. The National Health Survey collects data on illness in a representative sample of American families, but these are based upon the person's own understanding of the diagnosis. With respect to chronic respiratory disease, at least some of these data suggest serious underestimation of true prevalence (Table 14-2, p. 317). Data on sickness absence in industry are not suitable for studies on chronic diseases. The disease itself might lead to increased absence, but fears about job security may counteract this trend. The Social Security Administration publishes data on the number of disability awards made for a large number of specific disease conditions, classified according to occupation.[21] These indicate the approximate incidence of severely and permanently disabling diseases and allow comparison of the relative incidence of disability in different occupational groups. Registries of specific diseases can provide important clinical data if all, or nearly all, cases are reported. If the data can be linked to the population at risk, trends in prevalence and incidence can be followed. For instance, the data on cancer deaths in Connecticut's cancer registry[3] allow mortality to be calculated for the population of the state as a whole. But since these data are not related to environmental and occupational characteristics of the patients, the influence of these variables on cancer mortality cannot be examined. Registries of twins in Sweden and in the United States have provided data on smoking and respiratory symptoms in smoking-discordant twins.[32] Registries can focus attention on diseases linked with specific environmental hazards, but the total population at risk cannot easily be identified, and environmental data must be obtained separately. If 20 cases of an occupational lung disease are reported each year, it is crucial to know whether 100, 1000 or 100,000 people are at risk, and whether the population at risk is increasing or decreasing. Reporting of specific diseases can yield morbidity data and indicate trends of disease incidence. The main source of error is under-reporting. In West Germany, 9100 cases of sarcoidosis were reported but another 7,000–21,000 cases were probably not reported. Neumann's study of case loads in 3 cities showed prevalence rates 2 to 3 times higher than the national average based on the reported cases.[20]

Population Surveys

To obtain reliable morbidity data, special studies are necessary to find out who is ill as a result of environmental exposure. Usually, a population at risk is compared with a control population. Questionnaires as well as objective diagnostic tools can be used to detect disease.

Survey methods. The initial approach to the problem is often a cross-sectional survey of the population at risk. If the population is small, all members can be studied; otherwise, one may study a sample of the total population. The definitions of small and large populations depend on the goals and methods of the study. Questionnaire surveys have been done in populations of more than 10,000, while surveys with complex measurements may be limited to fewer than 100 subjects. In addition to the group at risk, one needs to study a control population, not subject to exposure, with exactly the same methods as the population at risk. Ideally, the control population should differ from the population at risk only in its lack of exposure; in practice this is never so. The following fictitious example of a cross-sectional survey illustrates some of the pitfalls that one may encounter.

Two workers at X company have chronic bronchitis and claim that irritant gases at their place of work caused the disease; both were healthy before they worked there. One smokes 10 cigarettes per day; the other has never smoked. To investigate their claims, all 100 workers at X company are studied (Table 13-2). Fifteen percent have chronic bronchitis. As a control group, all 100 workers at A company are studied. Here, too, 15 persons have chronic bronchitis. Thus, the crude prevalences of bronchitis are similar in both companies; at A, no irritant gases are used, and thus it seems that there is no excess of disease at X that could be attributed to irritants. However, this conclusion is premature. At the X company there are strict rules against smoking, since the irritant gases are also highly flammable. As a result, most workers at X are nonsmokers. At A, on the other hand, most employees perform closely scheduled and mentally stressful desk work; there are no restrictions on smoking and 80 percent of A's work force are cigarette smokers. When the nonsmokers at both companies are considered separately, the prevalence of bronchitis is 3.5 times greater among nonsmokers at X than among nonsmokers at A (Table 13-2). Furthermore, 12 out of the 14 nonsmokers with bronchitis at X are in a job with much higher concentrations of the irritant than are the other workers. There are a total of 20 men in that job. Thus, among a group specifically at high risk, the prevalence

Table 13-2
Epidemiological Survey of Lung Disease

Factory	Number	Men With Chronic Bronchitis & Emphysema	Non-smokers	Non-smokers With Chronic Bronchitis & Emphysema	% Non-smokers With Chronic Bronchitis & Emphysema
A (control)	100	15	20	1	5.0
X (suspected risk)	100	15	80	14	17.5

This is an example based on fictitious data; see text. The crude prevalence of chronic bronchitis and emphysema is equal in factories A and X. However, the alleged irritant gas in factory X is highly flammable; therefore most of X's workers are nonsmokers. The prevalence of disease is in fact 3.5 times higher among the nonsmokers in X than in A.

of disease is $12/20 = 60$ percent. The first impression suggested that there was no special bronchitis risk at X company; thus, the clinical observations of 2 patients, both with that company, might be a coincidence. In fact, the main risk at X was inhalation of an irritant; at the A company, the main risk was smoking, and crude bronchitis prevalences were equal. Eventually, it turned out that a small group of persons in one specific job at X had a very high risk of bronchitis. To establish this required examination of the workers, evaluation of their smoking habits, and an investigation of their jobs and working environment. Hence, to ensure valid data, a cross-sectional survey should include at least 90 percent of the defined groups; a larger percentage of absentees and refusals leads to uncertain conclusions since those not seen may either be healthier or sicker than the others.

A cross-sectional survey, as in Table 13-2, shows disease prevalence at the time of study. Follow-up studies can provide data on the incidence of new cases as well as on the natural course of the disease among a defined population group. If the environment is monitored, such data can be related to change in environmental exposures. A main problem of such longitudinal surveys is the high lapse rates, resulting from population mobility and administrative and other factors. Lapse rates increase with the duration of follow-up, but, fortunately, relatively short periods (3–5 years) can often give valuable information. Such studies are difficult and few have been done. In the future, by easing data collection and processing and by ensuring standardization of procedures, computerized methods may facilitate adequate follow-up studies of groups of people exposed to various risks of lung disease.

If the inhaled substance causes disease only after a long delay, one can perform a "longitudinal study in the past," defining a group of people who were at risk at some previous point in time. Selikoff and associates identified all members of a union of asbestos workers in 1942, traced their fate into the 1960s, and determined the cause of death of those who died in the interval.[28] This study established the greatly increased risk of death from lung cancer among asbestos workers.

Choice of populations. If exposure is known, it dictates the choice of population. In choosing the appropriate control groups, age and sex distribution, smoking habits, social status, and possible occupational factors (such as the need for heavy physical labor) must be taken into account. Differences between the population at risk and the control group need not always be a survey drawback; sometimes they reinforce the conclusions. In The Netherlands, I once used a group of long-term prison inmates as controls for a study on nearby flax workers. The prisoners included many heavy smokers, while few of the flax workers smoked as much. The flax workers had more respiratory symptoms and significantly lower $FEV_{.75}$ values; the fact that they smoked less than the controls strengthened the argument that their respiratory disease was caused by flax dust inhalation, not by smoking.[2]

Groups of hospital patients may be suitable populations for the study of agents that cause severe and immediate responses, leading to hospital admission. Extension of such studies to the occupational group to which the patients belong can reveal instances of less severe disease and also clues for prevention. For the study of longer-term risks, occupational groups are indispensable. This is true for occupational diseases as well as for diseases prevalent in the general population. Groups of firemen and telephone workers have been invaluable in international comparisons of cardiovascular diseases as well as chronic bronchitis. However, occupational groups by definition exclude those disabled or diseased persons who retire prematurely from the work force; hence, a study group limited to active workers may not accurately reflect the occupational hazards.

On the other hand, a survey of workers who apply for disability benefits can be biased in the opposite direction. In one such group (miners who applied for benefits in Great Britain [16]), a chest x-ray film and $FEV_{1.0}$ data were obtained before death, and these were correlated with autopsy findings. The final $FEV_{1.0}$ correlated well with the emphysema count of the lungs, but the relation between $FEV_{1.0}$ and roentgenographic category was more complex (Fig. 13-1). These data suggest that, with respect to lung function, miners without roentgenographic evidence of pneumoconiosis are worse off than miners with extensive simple pneumoconiosis (grades 2 & 3). In fact, in those miners whose x-ray films showed severe, complicated pneumoconiosis, the $FEV_{1.0}$ was only slightly lower than that of miners with no roentgenographic changes. It is crucial that these data came from men who applied for disability benefits. Perhaps miners with x-ray changes applied to some extent regardless of symptoms and function loss. Among the total group of miners without x-ray changes, men with symptoms and function loss are more likely to apply, so that the group without x-ray changes was probably biased in favor of disabled individuals. Before drawing any further conclusions one would have to exclude this source of bias. Clearly, data interpretation must take into account the fact that persons who apply for disability awards are a selected group.

In surveys of community population groups, one can use geographical selection criteria (all inhabitants of a town or circumscribed area), or one can use groups with special age, social, or religious characteristics. To study lung disease in nonsmokers, one may turn to special groups such as Seventh-Day Adventists or active sportsmen. However, one is never certain that the health of people in such groups is unrelated to initial selection factors. Sportsmen certainly are a biased group, with better than average physical fitness. The uncertainty decreases when similar disease patterns occur among several unrelated groups of nonsmokers, such as Seventh-Day Adventists, track runners, and women in areas of the world where social custom prohibits their smoking. Another approach is to study the total population of a town and identify the nonsmokers. This avoids the selection bias

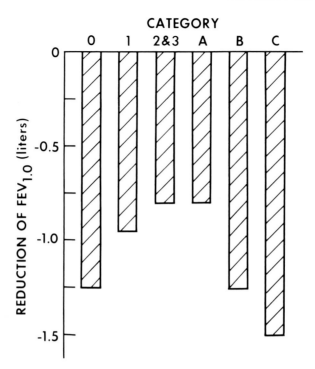

Fig. 13-1. X-ray classification and lung function of miners who applied for disability benefits in Great Britain. *Abscissa:* x-ray category. 0 = absence of x-ray changes due to pneumoconiosis; 1, 2, and 3 = increasing degrees of simple pneumoconiosis; A, B and C = increasing degrees of complicated pneumoconiosis (progressive massive fibrosis). See also Chapter 15, p. 364. *Ordinate:* mean reduction of $FEV_{1.0}$. See text for discussion. Data from reference 16.

inherent in studies of special groups. It also avoids the problems of selecting random population samples without demonstrable bias. Bias in the selection of the town or area can be overcome by studying more than one town or area, each with its own special features reflected in the composition of its population. Obviously, no group of people represents the general population; any epidemiological survey must deal with a specific group that differs in many ways from other population groups. Thus, conclusions from epidemiological studies are often convincing only if they are based upon independent surveys in different populations, or if they are backed by laboratory data on the effects of exposure.

Size of populations. With industrial exposures, the detailed study of small groups of workers at high risk is often the surest way to establish quickly the existence and severity of a health hazard. Yet, such results may not be representative of the situation throughout the industry; to determine the magnitude of the problem one must also find out the effects of lesser exposure in larger groups of workers under different conditions. The choice of groups, work locations, and factories should obviously be guided by the likelihood of exposure. Usually the most productive approach is to concentrate on work places where the risk occurs. Control groups may be selected among nonrisk groups within the same industry.

In community surveys on obstructive lung disease, one must begin with rather large groups so that when variables are controlled, the remaining subgroups are large enough for meaningful analysis. Consider the 1970 U.S. Census data for 2 small towns, in different states, with a total population of 7215 persons. Let us assume that we want to know the prevalence of obstructive lung disease, and the factors associated with it, among men aged 35–44 years. The census data show 364 men in this age group, which includes smokers and nonsmokers, all ethnic backgrounds, and all occupations. Some men work in the towns, others commute to larger cities nearby. A reasonably homogeneous subgroup might be all white men aged 35–44 years who live and work in the town, who do not smoke, and who work in agriculture. If 50 percent of this age group are nonsmokers, and 33 percent of the total number work in agriculture, the subgroup would include about 30 persons in each of the 2 towns. This number may or may not be large enough for a comparison of, e.g., air-pollution effects, assuming one town has clean air and the other is in a polluted area. With smaller total populations, the numbers of people in such subgroups would certainly be too small for meaningful comparison.

Methods Used in Population Surveys

These methods include specific physical signs, chest x-ray films, lung function tests (Chap. 12), anthropometric data, and questionnaires to record respiratory symptoms.

Questionnaires. These are used to elicit personal data and a history of respiratory symptoms, smoking, occupational exposures, and any other factors relevant to the study. Most questionnaires used by different groups of investigators are derived from the original version developed by Fairbairn, Wood, and Fletcher in Great Britain;[6] many questions still follow the exact phraseology of the original, which was carefully tested in many surveys. Translations in several languages are available. An example of an expanded questionnaire which includes many questions on environmental exposures is given in the Appendix (p. 307). Some of the questions provide semiquantitative information, such as grades of dyspnea. Smoking habits are recorded quantitatively, so that derived values (number of packs smoked in a year, in a lifetime, etc.) can be computed. This is useful when smoking is treated as a continuous variable, for instance, in regression analysis of such dependent variables as lung function values. Age of starting and stopping are important and should, in case of doubt, be elicited by reference to important events in the person's lifetime (leaving school, etc.). Why a person stopped is important; respiratory illness is a common reason.

The importance of a complete occupational history is obvious. Patients should always be asked whether they have ever been exposed to irritant gases, fumes, dusts, or vapors. The complete occupational history should include all jobs after leaving school, including military duties. The name of each job, the nature of the work, and the characteristics of the work place should all be recorded. The history should account for all of the patient's working lifetime. Questions concerning materials handled, procedures, and factory output are often in order. On the part of the interviewer, awareness of potential exposures is crucial. He should know that an electrician may have had silica exposure while working in a foundry, or that two years of work at asbestos lagging in a shipyard during World War II may account for a malignant mesothelioma that developed in the 1960s.

While performing daily chores or in artistic and recreational pursuits, one may be exposed to irritants such as smoke, dust, paints, and solvents. Among primitive populations, exposure to smoke in huts without windows or chimneys may be important. Exposure to noxious agents is not limited to modern industrial societies, since many primitive procedures result in severe lung disease. For instance, grinding of corn between siliceous stones causes silicosis in young girls in Transkei,[23] and batting and hackling of flax or hemp causes byssinosis. In industrial settings, information concerning exposures is often difficult to obtain since complicated technical procedures, trade secrets, and litigation may be involved. Thus, to obtain the necessary information, the physician may need the help of state and federal agencies as well as management and unions.

A listing of residences since birth is important in studies of urban-rural differences in disease prevalence, and it may also provide clues on special exposures or occupations. These data indicate population mobility, which is relevant for follow-up studies. Also, selective mobility may influence disease patterns—for instance, sick or less fit people may move into rural areas in search of clean air, while healthy persons may move to cities in search of jobs.

The administration of questionnaires requires special training of lay interviewers as well as physicians. The questionnaire requires a formalized style of history-taking which some physicians find difficult to accept. With experience, it is possible to ask the questions exactly as listed, while establishing personal rapport with the person interviewed. Self-administration of questionnaires may eliminate observer bias,[12] but most investigators prefer to have trained interviewers administer questionnaires on respiratory symptoms. Self-administered questionnaires may be useful, however, for preliminary data gathering when a large survey is planned. The shortage of trained personnel has led to consideration of computers as interviewing devices, but experience in this field is still minimal. It is feasible to have those interviewed respond to tape-recorded questions and to record the answers with a computer input device. Or, questions can be read by an interviewer guided by computer prompting [2a] (Fig. 13-2), which assures that all relevant questions are asked, and can, with appropriate branching instructions, eliminate or insert questions conditional on other responses. With a teletype or other input/output device, answers can be recorded directly in code, and a hard copy of the interview (Fig. 13-3) can be obtained and data stored in computer-compatible format (e.g., magnetic or paper tape). Additional instructions on the use of questionnaires are available in several papers.[6, 12, 30]

Lung-function tests. The choice of tests is discussed in Chapter 12. When large numbers of subjects are studied, and in particular when follow-up studies are planned, the need for reliable and standardized data is even more important than in a clinical setting. In epidemiological surveys, time for each subject is short and a repeat test to correct technical errors is usually not feasible. Equipment therefore must be simple to operate and repeated calibrations are mandatory. Although the

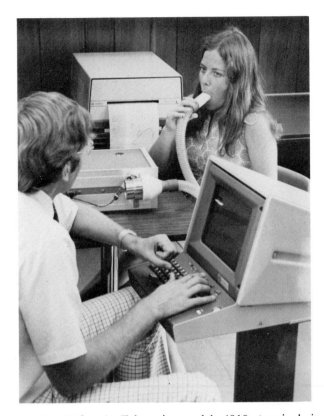

Fig. 13-2. A Tektronix model 4010 terminal is used to record respiratory symptoms and details of environmental exposures, as well as MEFV curves. Expiratory flow data are obtained when the subject performs a forced expiratory maneuver through the breathing tube, which connects to a flowmeter (see Figure 9-7 for hardware configuration). At the end of the interview and function test, all data are displayed on the scope face of the terminal. A hard copy is then obtained (Tektronix model 4610 unit, in background; Figure 13-3 gives an example). At the same time, data are transferred to paper tape for later processing by a digital computer. Examples of MEFV curves recorded with this system are in Figure 9-5 and Figure 18-21.

same instrument should be used whenever possible, when the size of the population precludes this, all instruments should be compared and calibrated to give the same results. Rigorous quality-control procedures must be instituted, so that erroneous results are detected and their cause determined. Unless this is done during the study, technical errors will contribute to the variability of the results. If more than one operator administers tests, the results of different operators must be checked for systematic differences. Every conceivable source of technical and operator error and variability must be considered. If one could standardize methods used in surveys conducted by different investigators, their results could later be

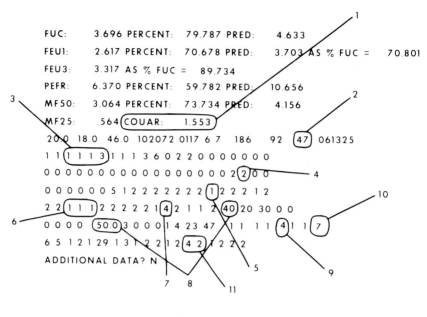

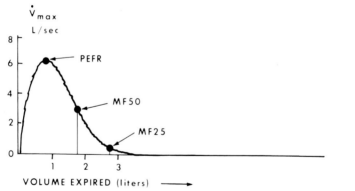

Fig. 13-3. Sample data sheet obtained with terminal and hard copy unit of Figure 13-2. It includes, from the top down, numerical lung-function data (6 lines); subject and test identification (1 line); coded answers to 130 questions on respiratory symptoms, smoking, occupational exposures, and residence (6 lines); and MEFV curve.

Lung function data include forced vital capacity (FVC), forced expiratory volume in 1 and 3 seconds (FEV$_1$, FEV$_3$), peak expiratory flow rate (PEFR), and maximum expiratory flow rate at 50% and 25% of FVC (MF50 and MF25). Data predicted on the basis of subject's sex, age, and height are included and compared with actual test performance. For instance, FVC = 3.696 liters in this subject, which is 79.78% of the predicted value of 4.633 liters.

Identification includes date and time [20.18 hrs (= 8.18 p.m.), Oct. 20, 1972]; subj. no. (0117), age, and anthropometric data. Circled items are as follows: (1) This index shows that the FEV$_{1.0}$ of the best blow in a series of five blows was 1.5% higher than the next best blow. This detects people who produce inconsistent results and introduces an element of data quality control. (2) Age in years. (3) Answers to questions concerning cough. This person usually coughs early in the morning as well as at other times during the day or night. He coughs on most days for as much as 3 months of the year compared or pooled. This would require agreement among investigators on the tests and on the equipment, as well as on operator instructions, calibration procedures, and all other variables. It is already difficult to achieve accuracy and consistency of technical procedures within one laboratory; exact comparability of data from different laboratories is rarely accomplished. However, if suitable control groups are included in each survey, this provides internal validation of procedures in each study.

In the future, performance of lung-function tests under computer control and with on-line data processing can eliminate many sources of error and variability. Test specifications and operator instructions can be built into computer software. The computer can interrupt test sequences and instruct the operator to perform a calibration procedure. The accuracy of calibration procedures can be determined by the computer and appropriate reset procedures instituted. On-line data processing allows immediate comparison of test results with predetermined standards of quality control, so that instructions to repeat the test can be given immediately. Since all test features are accurately determined by computer software, such a system would provide exact reproducibility of test procedures for follow-up studies.

Anthropometric data. In most surveys, anthropometric data are limited to standing height (without shoes) and, sometimes, body weight. When dealing with groups of subjects of different ethnic backgrounds, sitting height should be included since the ratio of sitting-to-standing height differs among the races (large in Japanese, small in blacks). Normal spirometric data obtained in predominantly white populations, based on standing height, are not valid for healthy blacks, Japanese, and other ethnic groups with anthropometric features that differ from those in white people.[3a]

Tests for etiological factors. Reversible airway constriction can be demonstrated by reversal of function loss with isoproterenol. Ideally, all subjects with evidence of reversible airway constriction should receive lung function tests to determine airway reactivity to constrictor drugs quantitatively, prick tests to discover specific allergies, inquiries regarding occupational allergens, and determination of immunoglobulins. Few of these methods have been applied in defined population groups. Tests to discover allergic respiratory disease have been used in a survey of a town in Western Australia (C. A. Mitchell; personal communication), and airway sensitivity to histamine aerosol has been studied in a Dutch population survey.[33] Specific tests for cystic fibrosis and other diseases of known etiology should also be included. It seems likely that the large majority of patients who are placed in the general category of chronic obstructive lung disease have

---

and has had this cough for 5 or more years. (4) No shortness of breath when hurrying on level ground or walking up a slight hill. (5) Subject has had a chest injury in the past (specified on subject identification sheet). (6) Subject is allergic to such drugs as penicillin or sulfa and has frequent (usually at least once a day or night) episodes of sneezing or runny nose. (7) These symptoms are worst in the fall. (8) Subject now smokes 40 cigarettes per day and his total lifetime cigarette consumption is 50 pack-years. (9) Subject worked 1–5 years in a foundry. (10) Subject worked more than 20 years with asbestos. (11) There are 4 people in subject's household, 2 of whom are smokers.

either smoking-induced airway obstruction, allergic airway disease, lung disease
caused by other environmental agents, or a combination of these.

Data Analysis [12]

That epidemiological studies should not be undertaken lightly becomes most
obvious at the time of data analysis. Adequate planning helps to obtain data that
can answer specific questions. However, no plan is complete and one must often
make important decisions concerning selections, choices, and omissions after the
data-gathering phase is already in progress. Such decisions can have a great impact
on the success of the work. The bookkeeping element of the survey work is crucial.
Many studies are never published because of missing, mixed up, or erroneously
recorded data. If several people review data independently, many such errors or
omissions may be discovered while they can still be corrected. The importance of
adequate subject identification, with sufficient redundancy, accurate filing, and
legible handwriting should also be emphasized. An epidemiologist must be a
fussy person who constantly worries about all details.

Transferring data to punch cards or other computer-compatible format introduces the first element of order in the results. By recording interview and lung-
function data directly into a computer-compatible format,[2a] many bookkeeping
errors are eliminated. From punch cards, paper tape, or magnetic tape, suitable
programs can produce tabular output, with checks for errors, inconsistencies, or
incomplete data. Initial sorting can be done if the computer is instructed to group
subjects according to sex, age, and other criteria. Such tables allow preliminary
comparisons between various groups of subjects. Although a complete statistical
analysis is nearly always necessary, this will be most fruitful if guided by an intelli-
gent review of the primary data. The computer can help by allowing the investigator
to sort all data according to many different criteria without the need for data
copying or hand sorting.

Next, simple statistical tests can indicate whether or not differences between
categories are significant. For instance, the χ^2-test may show whether male smokers
aged 25–34 years have significantly more or less dyspnea than male nonsmokers
in the same age group. Or one may compare nonsmokers who work in agriculture
with those in industry. These simple analyses often give clues about environmental
risks. It is frequently also necessary to treat age, sex, smoking, and occupation
as independent variables, while performing a regression analysis on such variables
as lung-function data, which depend upon age (see Fig. 17-9, p. 433). Environmental data also may be used as continuous variables. For instance, one may
study regressions of $FEV_{1.0}$ on the amount smoked, or one may relate lung function to measured pollutant levels. Usually, such analyses require corrections for
additional variables: $FEV_{1.0}$ depends upon body size; if one wants to relate
function to smoking, he should first standardize the $FEV_{1.0}$ data for size.

A frequently used method to facilitate comparisons between groups of people
is to eliminate one variable by calculating an adjusted value. For instance, Figure
13-4 shows regressions of $FEV_{1.0}$ on age in two fictitious population groups with
different but overlapping age distributions. The mean $FEV_{1.0}$ values of the two
groups are similar, but group A is, on the average, younger than group B. A valid
comparison between the groups can be made if one computes the regressions of

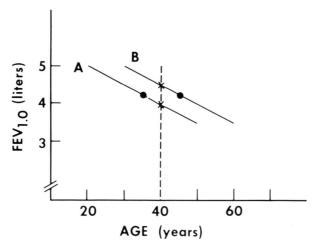

Fig. 13-4. Regression of $FEV_{1.0}$ on age in two fictitious groups of subjects, *A* and *B*. Mean $FEV_{1.0}$ (*dots*) is
the same in both groups, but the age-adjusted mean $FEV_{1.0}$
(*crosses*) is different (see text).

$FEV_{1.0}$ on age for both groups and then determines the value of $FEV_{1.0}$ for a
person of say 40 years of age belonging to either group. This process eliminates
the effect of the different age distributions; the age-adjusted $FEV_{1.0}$ value is clearly
lower in group A than in B, and the difference can be tested for statistical
significance.

Additional problems arise when studying children since the growth of their
lungs and chest cages must be taken into account. Some of these problems are
discussed in connection with the early effects of cigarette smoking (Chap. 14),
and similar considerations apply when one wants to investigate the effect of other
variables on lung function in children and adolescents.

Applications of Epidemiological Methods

Medical surveillance in industry. There is a rapidly increasing need for
regular checks on respiratory symptoms and lung function in workers exposed to
specific inhalants. For instance, the federal standard for asbestos dust exposure
includes provisions for annual health checks of workers, including determination
of vital capacity and $FEV_{1.0}$.[29] The objective of these checks is to detect asbestosis
or other occupational diseases early, in order to prevent disease progression if
possible, and to protect other workers at risk. To promote equitable application
of these standards, it is necessary that the same methods and interpretation be used
in all tests. This uniformity is difficult to attain, given the different spirometric
equipment manufactured by dozens of firms and the multitude of technicians and
nurses performing tests in many different laboratories. Yet, particularly when
one needs to detect relatively small year-to-year deteriorations, as in annual checks
of asbestos workers, it is crucial that exactly the same test be used each time.

Early detection of lung disease. Hospital and clinic patients, often a selected
group of severely ill persons, may represent merely the tip of the iceberg. Many

others, less severely affected or more stoic, are working and do not seek medical care. Population studies outside the hospital or clinic can detect the existence of lung disease in such persons, but whether this represents early detection depends on one's point of view. The patient may be well aware of cough, dyspnea, or other symptoms, even though he has not sought medical aid; he may have had these symptoms for years. The term early detection is more suitable for persons who are unaware of abnormality although objective data indicate disease. Early detection in this sense includes detection of asymptomatic lung cancer or tuberculosis. For chronic bronchitis and emphysema the term early detection may be a misnomer. Even teen-agers who have smoked only a few years have excessive cough, phlegm, and dyspnea [27] in the presence of a demonstrable but slight function loss; the presence of disease is thus apparent without special detection methods.

The value of early detection of chronic bronchitis and emphysema has been questioned because no effective therapy is available. Does the patient benefit from early diagnosis? Cessation of smoking, avoidance of occupational exposures, or a move to a clean-air area may help to halt progression of the disease. Phlegm production decreases in smokers who stop, and other symptoms often improve. The degree of reversibility of the anatomical and functional changes in airways and lungs is not known, but significant symptomatic improvement can often be achieved. However, only medical surveillance programs can provide objective data concerning the value of early detection of lung diseases; at present we do not know enough about their natural history. Until then, early detection programs should probably be undertaken only as a part of studies to obtain objective data on the natural history of disease, with provisions for regular follow-up.

Medical surveillance in communities.   The unsatisfactory state of our knowledge of morbidity from lung diseases and of their natural history can be greatly improved by establishing ongoing lung disease surveillance programs in a few representative towns or geographical areas in the United States. Some programs have already begun as cross-sectional surveys in three communities (Lebanon and Ansonia, Conn.; Winnsboro, S.C.). Given the lack of primary health care in many rural as well as urban areas, such programs should include provisions for medical care and for referrals to specialists. These surveillance systems are feasible, technically as well as economically, now that computerized methods are available. Surveillance should not be limited to older persons. In order to determine the natural history of early lung disease induced by cigarette smoke or other inhalants, it is essential to include children and young adults. Surveillance should also include systematic environmental monitoring. One study of this type has been conducted in Lebanon, Connecticut, a rural town of about 4000 people, where 2450 inhabitants aged 7 years and older were studied, using a mobile laboratory with an on-board computer test system (Fig. 13-2). A second population study has been done in a polluted urban area (Ansonia, Conn.), using the same mobile facility. Initial results of the Lebanon survey are discussed elsewhere in this book (see Tables 16-4, 16-5, 16-6, and 18-1).

Epidemiology of Chronic Bronchitis and Emphysema

This subject merits separate discussion because many epidemiological surveys have been conducted on these diseases. Since the industrial exposures that cause bronchitis and emphysema are discussed in Chapter 15, surveys of community groups only are included here, and the accent is on rural populations. The main problem with studies of urban populations is the ever-changing environment of the city dweller; some studies on urban-rural differences in morbidity are discussed in Chapter 16, and studies mainly concerned with cigarette smoking are in Chapter 14.

Men and women living in a rural area in Wales were surveyed in 1957 by Higgins,[10] who recorded symptoms and ventilatory capacity, and one of the first international comparisons of rural groups was made by Olsen and Gilson,[22] who compared the prevalence of chronic lung disease and ventilatory function in men aged 55–64 years in rural areas in Denmark, Scotland, and Wales. In 1961, Ferris and Anderson [7] did a similar study of men and women over 25 years of age in Berlin, New Hampshire. They confirmed the importance of cigarette smoking as an etiological factor; in Berlin, N.H., smoking proved more important than air pollution from a local paper mill in causing chronic bronchitis.

Comparison of data from population samples in Berlin, N.H., and in Chilliwack, B.C., showed differences not only in the prevalence of respiratory symptoms but also in smoking habits. When smoking was taken into account, the prevalence of symptoms became similar.[1] A cross-sectional survey in 1967 in Berlin, N.H., revealed slightly lower disease prevalence and higher ventilatory capacities than had been found in the same town in 1961.[8] A follow-up study of the subjects seen in 1961 confirmed that this decrease might be related to a reduction in air pollution.[7a] Inevitably, surveys of rural populations include large numbers of cigarette smokers. In Huhti's survey of a rural town in Finland,[14] 81 percent of the men smoked and the group of nonsmokers was too small to study effects of industrial exposures. In Tecumseh, Michigan, only about 12 percent of the men were nonsmokers.[24] Such groups can provide few data on exposures other than cigarette smoking.

To date, studies have focused mostly on older adults, since they have the highest prevalence of disease. However, the seeds of the disease are sown much earlier, and to this end children and young adults should be studied. A large study in Great Britain [13] involved more than 10,000 school children aged 5 to 14 years in 4 geographical areas in Kent. Peak expiratory flow rates (PEF) as well as symptoms of respiratory disease correlated with several factors, in particular, area of residence. Although this might seem to suggest an effect of air pollution, the PEF measurement is insufficiently reliable to permit this conclusion. To a large extent, PEF reflects the subject's effort (Chap. 9, p. 191) and thus may depend on nutritional status and physical development, both of which may be related to social class and residence. Other studies on children are discussed in Chapters 14 and 16.

For practical reasons, many previous studies have been limited to samples of populations. For instance, Ferris et al.'s work in Berlin, New Hampshire, in 1961 included about 1100 subjects from a town of about 15,000,[7] and the survey in Staveley, U.K., dealt with fewer than 800 men and women from a town of

18,000.[11] Since these surveys dealt with people in limited age ranges, the proportion of persons seen in the chosen categories is larger. Even so, the numbers of subjects are suitable for analyzing only a small number of variables. For chronic bronchitis and emphysema, more complete population surveys may detect many as yet unknown or insufficiently recognized environmental factors. In previous surveys only smoking and a few occupational factors (mining, textile industry) have been studied in detail. Studies on nonsmokers in the United States as well as in Great Britain [15, 31] suggest that chronic respiratory symptoms occur in about 5 percent of nonsmokers in rural areas, and this percentage did not increase with age. The causes of chronic respiratory symptoms in nonsmokers in rural areas still need to be established. Bronchial asthma is prevalent in rural areas (Table 18-1). Exposures to dusts and fumes in homes and farms need to be considered. Stebbings [31] has suggested that upper airway disorders, such as sinusitis, may be responsible for chronic cough in nonsmokers.

International comparisons of the prevalence of chronic bronchitis and emphysema pose special problems. In the United Kingdom, death rates from bronchitis are much higher than those in the United States and other European countries. Reid et al.[25] compared men aged 45–64 years in the United States and the United Kingdom; they found more cigarette smokers in the latter, but many more heavy smokers in the former. American city dwellers appeared to have as much bronchitis as people in rural areas in the United Kingdom, and the prevalence of chest illness and dyspnea was much higher in the British towns. People who move from the United Kingdom to the United States have much lower prevalences of chronic respiratory symptoms, similar to those in the United States.[26] The same has been reported for British emigrants to South Africa.[4] Thus, the high death rates from bronchitis in the United Kingdom reflect a high prevalence of disease and not an artifact related to different diagnostic practices or reporting habits.

In international as well as regional comparisons, there may be ethnic differences between population groups. These may affect the risk of lung disease. In a study of a community in Guyana,[17] ethnic origin (African or East Indian) and smoking habits were used as the independent variables. The Indians had more chronic respiratory symptoms than people of African descent, and this was not explained by smoking habits. Indian smokers had 17.3 percent chronic bronchitis, while African smokers had only 2.4 percent. However, many Indian men worked in sugar estates, and occupational exposures were not studied. A greater susceptibility of Indian people also appeared in data from nonsmoking women; 6.1 percent of the Indian women, versus 2.2 percent of the African women, had respiratory symptoms compatible with chronic bronchitis. Such data suggest racial or other genetic differences in sensitivity to environmental exposures. However, careful study of these apparent ethnic differences is necessary. Since cultural or language factors may cause differences in appreciating and reporting of symptoms, objective lung-function tests with adequate anthropometric data are needed.

To facilitate a search for etiological factors in future epidemiological surveys of obstructive lung disease, the following classification (A. Bouhuys, C.A. Mitchell, and R.S.F. Schilling, unpublished material) may be useful:

1. bronchial asthma (Chap. 18), defined as reversible airway obstruction, often of long standing, associated with:

    a. identifiable airborne allergens, such as pollens;
    b. identifiable occupational sensitizers, such as wood dust and flour;
    c. increased sensitivity of airways to exogenous stimuli;
    d. combinations of a, b, and c.
2. chronic bronchitis, associated with:
    a. cigarette smoking;
    b. other identifiable environmental exposures, such as irritant gases and particulates;
    c. genetic factors, e.g., previously undiagnosed cystic fibrosis.
3. emphysema, associated with:
    a. cigarette smoking;
    b. other environmental exposures, such as detergent enzymes or toluene diisocyanate;
    c. genetic factors, e.g., α_1-antitrypsin deficiency.
4. cystic fibrosis in children and young adults;
5. occupational obstructive syndromes, such as byssinosis in textile workers.

This classification can help to establish a baseline on prevalence of different types of obstructive airway disease. Without such a baseline, it is difficult to determine the relative roles of smoking, occupational exposures, and community air pollution. This baseline can be determined by complete cross-sectional surveys of populations of towns with different environmental and population characteristics. The etiological factors involved in obstructive airway disease should be determined in each suspected case, through diagnostic tests as well as environmental measurements. Adequate follow-up is needed to validate the diagnosis of "early" airway disease and to determine progression or improvement as a function of time and of environmental changes. The medical data need to be correlated with environmental data—including climatic and microclimatic data and levels of particulate and gaseous pollutants in the outside atmosphere and in workrooms and homes (Chaps. 12, 15, and 16).

SUMMARY

The prevalence and incidence of lung diseases can be assessed from mortality and morbidity statistics, case registries of patients with specific diseases, and reporting of new cases by physicians. These methods detect primarily illnesses that result in death or significant disability. To obtain closer estimates of true prevalence, including early and preclinical disease states, population surveys are needed. Cross-sectional surveys indicate disease prevalence at one time; longitudinal surveys describe the incidence of new cases and the natural course of diseases. The choice and size of a population or population sample (hospital patients, industrial workers, community groups) depend on goals and available resources. Methods used in population surveys include questionnaires (see Appendix), lung-function tests, anthropometric measurements, and specific diagnostic tests. The principles and techniques of epidemiology should also be applied in programs of medical surveillance in industry or communities for the early detection, prevention, and control of lung disease. Worldwide epidemiological studies have shown a high prevalence of chronic bronchitis and emphysema, with cigarette smoking, occupational exposures, and air pollution as main etiological factors. A classification of obstructive lung disease according to etiological factors and clinical syndromes may allow more detailed diagnostic judgments in future epidemiological surveys.

REFERENCES

1. Anderson DO, Ferris BG Jr, Zickmantel R: The Chilliwack respiratory survey, 1963. Part IV. The effect of tobacco smoking on the prevalence of respiratory disease. Can Med Assoc J 92:1066–1076, 1965

2. Bouhuys A: The forced expiratory volume ($FEV_{0.75}$) in healthy males and in textile workers. Am Rev Respir Dis 87:63–68, 1963

2a. Bouhuys A: A novel computerized method for the study of pulmonary function. Trans NY Acad Sci 35:358–359, 1973

3. Christine B, Flannery JT, Sullivan PD: Cancer in Connecticut, 1966–1968. Conn State Department of Health, 1971

3a. Damon A: Negro-white differences in pulmonary function (vital capacity, timed vital capacity, and expiratory flow rate). Hum Biol 38:380–393, 1966

4. Dean G: The causes of death among South African born and immigrants to South Africa. S Afr Med J (suppl) 39:1–21, 1965

5. Enterline PE: Mortality among asbestos products workers in the United States. Ann NY Acad Sci 132:156–165, 1965

6. Fairbairn AS, Wood CH, Fletcher CM: Variability in answers to a questionnaire on respiratory symptoms. Br J Prev Soc Med 13: 175–193, 1959

7. Ferris BG Jr, Anderson DO: The prevalence of chronic respiratory disease in a New Hampshire town. Am Rev Respir Dis 86:165–177, 1962

7a. Ferris BG Jr, Higgins ITT, Higgins MW, Peters JM: Chronic nonspecific respiratory disease in Berlin, New Hampshire, 1961–1967: A follow-up study. Am Rev Respir Dis 107:110–122, 1973

8. Ferris BG Jr, Higgins ITT, Higgins MW, Peters JM, van Ganse WF, Goldman MD: Chronic nonspecific respiratory disease, Berlin, New Hampshire, 1961–1967: A cross-sectional study. Am Rev Respir Dis 104:232–244, 1971

9. Ferris BG Jr, Speizer FE, Worcester J, Chen HY: Adult mortality in Berlin, New Hampshire, from 1961–1967. Arch Environ Health 23:434–439, 1971

10. Higgins ITT: Tobacco smoking, respiratory symptoms, and ventilatory capacity. Studies in random samples of the population. Br Med J 1:325–329, 1959

11. Higgins ITT, Gilson JC, Ferris BG Jr, Waters ME, Campbell H, Higgins MW: IV. Chronic respiratory disease in an industrial town: A nine-year follow-up study. Preliminary report. Am J Public Health 58:1667–1676, 1968

12. Holland WW (ed): Data Handling in Epidemiology. London, Oxford University Press, 1970

13. Holland WW, Halil T, Bennett AE, Elliott A: Factors influencing the onset of chronic respiratory disease. Br Med J 2:205–208, 1969

14. Huhti E: Prevalence of respiratory symptoms, chronic bronchitis and pulmonary emphysema in a Finnish rural population. Acta Tuberc Pneumol Scand (suppl) 61:1–111, 1965

15. Lowe CR, Khosla T: Chronic bronchitis in ex-coal miners working in the steel industry. Br J Ind Med 29:45–49, 1972

16. Lyons JP, Ryder R, Campbell H, Gough J: Pulmonary disability in coal workers' pneumoconiosis. Br Med J 1:713–716, 1972

17. Miller GJ, Ashcroft MT: A community survey of respiratory disease among East Indian and African adults in Guyana. Thorax 26:331–338, 1971

18. Mitchell RS, Maisel JC, Dart GA, Silvers GW: The accuracy of the death certificate in reporting cause of death in adults. Am Rev Respir Dis 104:844–850, 1971

19. Moss E, Scott TS, Atherley GRC: Mortality of newspaper workers from lung cancer and bronchitis 1952–66. Br J Ind Med 29:1–14, 1972

20. Neumann C: Zur Epidemiologie der Sarkoidose in der Bundesrepublik. Pneumonologie 143:299–330, 1970

21. Occupational Characteristics of Disabled Workers, by Disabling Condition: Disability Insurance Benefit Awards Made in 1959 to 1962 to Men under Age 65. Publication No. 1531, U.S. Dept. of Health, Education and Welfare, PHS, 1967

22. Olsen HC, Gilson JC: Respiratory symptoms, bronchitis, and ventilatory capacity in men. An Anglo-Danish comparison with special reference to differences in smoking habits. Br Med J 1:450–456, 1960

23. Palmer PES, Daynes G: Transkei silicosis. S Afr Med J 41:1182–1188, 1967

24. Payne M, Kjelsberg M: Respiratory symptoms, lung function and smoking habits in an adult population. Am J Public Health 54:261–277, 1969

25. Reid DD, Anderson DO, Ferris BG, Fletcher CM: An Anglo-American comparison of the prevalence of bronchitis. Br Med J 2:1487–1491, 1964

26. Reid DD, Fletcher CM: International studies in chronic respiratory disease. Br Med Bull 27:59–64, 1971

27. Seely JE, Zuskin E, Bouhuys A: Cigarette smoking: Objective evidence for lung damage in teen-agers. Science 172:741–743, 1971

28. Selikoff IJ, Churg J, Hammond EC: The occurrence of asbestosis among insulation workers in the United States. Ann NY Acad Sci 132:139–155, 1965

29. Standard for exposure to asbestos dust. Federal Register, vol 37, no 110, June 7, 1972, pp 11318–11322

30. Standards for epidemiologic surveys in chronic respiratory disease. National Tuberculosis & Respiratory Disease Association, 1969

31. Stebbings JH Jr: Chronic respiratory disease among nonsmokers in Hagerstown, Maryland. I. Design of the study and prevalence of symptoms. Environ Res 4:146–162, 1971

32. Twin Registries in the Study of Chronic Disease. Report of an International Symposium in San Juan, Puerto Rico, 1–4 December 1969. Acta Med Scand [suppl] 523, 1971

33. van der Lende R: Epidemiology of Chronic Non-Specific Lung Disease (Chronic Bronchitis). Assen, The Netherlands, Royal Van Gorcum, 1969

APPENDIX TO CHAPTER 13

Questionnaire on Respiratory Symptoms

and Environmental Exposures

The following questionnaire contains the most important questions used in a survey of residents (7 years and older) of an urban industrialized community (Ansonia, Conn.) from April 1973–July 1973 (Connecticut Lung Survey; Mitchell CA, Schoenberg JB, Schilling RSF, Bouhuys A, et al.). Virtually the same questionnaire was given to 2450 inhabitants of a rural area (Lebanon, Conn.) from October 1972–February 1973. The purpose of these studies is to provide baseline data on prevalence of respiratory disease and on lung function in urban and rural residents, including children, taking into account the variables of age, sex, smoking habits, occupational or domestic pollutant exposures, and urban or rural residence. The questionnaire is administered by a trained interviewer, using the terminal of Figure 13-2. Question numbers are automatically displayed on the screen, in the sequence determined by the subject's responses; e.g., if #30 is answered yes, questions #31 and following are prompted; if #30 is answered no, #31–#53 are skipped. The instruction "specify" requires the interviewer to write the requested information on the subject's master data sheet.

1   Subject number

2   Subject category (coded to classify place of residence)

3   Interviewer number

4 Height (to nearest cm)

5 Weight (to nearest kg)

6 How old are you? (age at last birthday)

7 What is your birthdate?   ( ) ( )   ( ) ( )   ( ) ( )
   (enter 6 digits)   month   day   year

8 Sex   1. male   2. female

9 Race   1. Caucasian
                                                2. Negro
                                                3. other

I SHALL NOW ASK YOU SOME QUESTIONS ABOUT COUGH:

14 Do you *usually* cough first thing in the morning?   1. yes   2. no

15 Do you *usually* cough at other times during the   1. yes   2. no
    day or night?
          (If YES to 14 or 15, ask 16 and 17.)

16 Do you cough on most days for as much as   1. yes   2. no
    3 months of the year?

17 For how many years have you had this cough?   1. less than 2 years
                                                                2. 2–5 years
                                                                3. more than 5 years

I SHALL NOW ASK YOU SOME QUESTIONS ABOUT PHLEGM, SPUTUM, OR
MUCUS THAT COMES FROM YOUR CHEST:

20 Do you *usually* bring up (phlegm), (sputum), or   1. yes   2. no
    (mucus) from your chest first thing in the morning?

21 Do you *usually* bring up (phlegm), (sputum), or   1. yes   2. no
    (mucus) from your chest at other times during
    the day or night?
          (If YES to 20 or 21, ask 22–25.)

22 Do you bring up (phlegm), (sputum), or   1. yes   2. no
    (mucus) from your chest on most days for as
    much as 3 months of the year?

23 For how many years have you raised   1. less than 2 years
    (phlegm), (sputum), or (mucus) from   2. 2–5 years
    your chest?   3. more than 5 years

24 What is the usual color of the (phlegm),   1. don't know
    (sputum), or (mucus) you bring up from   2. clear
    your chest?   3. white
                                                                4. other
                                                                5. yellow
                                                                6. green

          (If 1, 2, 3, or 4 ask 25.)

25 Have you ever had episodes of yellow or green   1. yes   2. no
    (phlegm), (sputum), or (mucus)?

26 Have you ever coughed up blood?   1. yes   2. no
                                                                (specify)

I SHALL NOW ASK YOU SOME QUESTIONS ABOUT WHEEZING, WHISTLING,
AND CHEST TIGHTNESS:

30 Have you ever noticed any wheezing,   1. yes 2. no
    whistling, or tightness in your chest?
          (If YES to 30, ask 31 to 53.)

31 Which of these symptoms have you experienced, wheezing or tightness or both?	1. only wheezing and whistling 2. only chest tightness 3. mainly wheezing and whistling 4. mainly chest tightness 5. both wheezing and whistling and chest tightness
32 At what age did your (wheezing), (whistling), or (chest tightness) first occur?	( ) ( )
33 When did this (wheezing), (whistling), or (chest tightness) last occur?	1. within last 4 weeks 2. within last 12 months 3. more than 1 year ago but less than 5 years ago 4. more than 5 years ago
34 How frequently have you experienced this (wheezing), (whistling), or (chest tightness)?	1. usually at least once a day or night 2. only a few times each week 3. only a few times each month 4. only a few times each year 5. only a few times ever 6. only once

(If answer 5 or 6 to 34, skip to 56.)

35 (Does) or (did) your (wheezing), (whistling), or (chest tightness) occur with colds or sore throats?	1. yes 2. no
36 (Does) or (did) your (wheezing), (whistling), or (chest tightness) occur with episodes of increased phlegm from your chest?	1. yes 2. no
37 (Is) or (was) your (wheezing), (whistling), or (chest tightness) associated with attacks of shortness of breath?	1. yes 2. no

(Is) or (was) your (wheezing), (whistling), or (chest tightness) brought on by, or made worse by exposure to:

38 House dust?	1. yes 2. no
39 Other dusts or fumes in the home?	1. yes 2. no (specify)
40 Contact with animals?	1. yes 2. no (specify)
41 Plants or pollens?	1. yes 2. no (specify)
42 Dusts, gases, or fumes at work?	1. yes 2. no (specify)
43 Tobacco smoke?	1. yes 2. no
44 Other factors?	1. yes 2. no (specify)
45 (Is) or (was) your (wheezing), (whistling), or (chest tightness) worse on any particular day or days of the week? In other words, is there any difference between, say, Friday, Monday, Sunday, or Thursday?	1. yes 2. no

(If YES to 45, ask 46 and 47.)

46 On which day or days is it worse?	1. first day back at work 2. other day(s) at work 3. weekends
47 Did this worsening occur sometimes or always?	1. sometimes 2. always
48 (Is) or (was) your (wheezing), (whistling), or (chest tightness) *better* on any particular day or days of the week or weekend?	1. yes 2. no

(IF YES to 48, ask 49.)

49 When is it better?	1. weekday 2. weekend
50 (Is) or (was) your (wheezing), (whistling), or (chest tightness) better, the same, or worse on vacation?	1. better 2. the same 3. worse
51 (Is) or (was) your (wheezing), (whistling), or (chest tightness) *worse* during a particular season?	1. yes 2. no

(If YES to 51, ask 52 and 53.)

52 Which (is) or (was) the worst season?	1. winter 2. spring 3. summer 4. fall
53 (Do) or (did) these symptoms occur *only* during this season?	1. yes 2. no

I SHALL NOW ASK YOU SOME QUESTIONS ABOUT BREATHLESSNESS:

56 Are you disabled by any condition, other than lung disease, which would interfere with your walking?	1. yes 2. no (specify)

(If YES, go to 60.)

57 Are you troubled by shortness of breath when hurrying on level ground or walking up a slight hill?	1. yes 2. no

(If NO, go to 60.)

58 Do you get short of breath walking with other people of your own age on level ground?	1. yes 2. no

(If NO, go to 60.)

59 Do you get short of breath on walking ¼ mile on level ground in about 15 minutes?	1. yes 2. no

(Dyspnea grades: $0 =$ no to #57
$1 =$ yes to #57; no to #58
$2 =$ yes to #58; no to #59
$3 =$ yes to #59)

NOW SOME QUESTIONS ABOUT CHEST ILLNESS:

60 During the past 3 years, how much trouble have you had with such illnesses as chest colds, bronchitis, or pneumonia?	1. none 2. slight 3. some 4. considerable 5. a great deal

Have you ever had:

70 Bronchial asthma?	1. yes 2. no
71 Bronchitis?	1. yes 2. no
72 Pneumonia?	1. yes 2. no
73 Pleurisy?	1. yes 2. no

74	Pulmonary tuberculosis?	1. yes 2. no
75	A chest injury, such as a fractured rib or spine?	1. yes 2. no (specify)
76	A chest operation?	1. yes 2. no (specify)

NOW SOME QUESTIONS ABOUT SMOKING:

86	Do you *now* smoke cigarettes? (If NO, skip to 93.)	1. yes 2. no
87	Do you smoke cigarettes with or without filters?	1. with filters 2. without filters 3. both with and without filters
88	Do you inhale?	1. yes 2. no
89	How old were you when you began to smoke cigarettes?	_____age
90	How many cigarettes do you usually smoke each day at the present time?	_____number per day
91	At what age did you start smoking this many?	_____age
92	Prior to this, how many did you smoke each day?	_____number per day

(Repeat 91 and 92 until total smoking history has been described.)
(Skip to 102.)

93	Did you *ever* smoke cigarettes? (If NO, skip to 102.)	1. yes 2. no
94	Did you smoke cigarettes with or without filters?	1. with filters 2. without filters 3. both with and without filters
95	Did you inhale?	1. yes 2. no
96	How old were you when you began to smoke cigarettes?	_____age
97	How old were you when you stopped smoking cigarettes regularly?	_____age
98	What was the usual number of cigarettes you smoked per day just before you stopped?	_____number per day
99	At what age did you start smoking this many?	_____age
100	Prior to this how many did you smoke each day?	_____number per day

(Repeat 99 and 100 until total smoking
history has been described.)

101	Were you influenced to stop because you had a cough, wheezing, or shortness of breath?	1. yes 2. no
102	Do you *now* smoke pipes or cigars? (If NO, skip to 106.)	1. yes 2. no
103	How many pipefuls or cigars do you usually smoke each day?	_____number per day
104	Do you usually inhale when you smoke either pipes or cigars?	1. yes 2. no
105	How old were you when you first smoked pipes or cigars? (Skip to 112.)	_____age

106   Did you *ever* smoke pipes or cigars?   1. yes   2. no
          (If NO, skip to 112).

107   How many pipefuls or cigars did you usually   _____number per day
          smoke each day?

108   Did you usually inhale when you smoked either   1. yes   2. no
          pipes or cigars?

109   How old were you when you first smoked   _____age
          pipes or cigars?

110   How old were you when you stopped   _____age
          smoking pipes or cigars?

111   Were you influenced to stop because you had   1. yes   2. no
          a cough, wheezing, or shortness of breath?

NOW SOME QUESTIONS ABOUT SPECIFIC OCCUPATIONS:

Have you ever worked: Answers below apply to
                                                           every question from 112 to 120.

112   At a coal mine?   1. no
113   In any other mine?   2. for less than 3 months
114   In a quarry?   3. for 4 months to 1 year
115   In a foundry?   4. for more than 1–5 years
116   In a pottery?   5. for more than 5–10 years
117   In a cotton, flax, or hemp mill?   6. for more than 10–20 years
118   With asbestos?   7. for more than 20 years
119   On a farm?

          (If YES, specify type of farm.)

120   In any other job with exposure to dust, gas, or fumes?

          (If YES, specify type of exposure.)

I WOULD NOW LIKE TO ASK YOU SOME QUESTIONS ABOUT YOUR HOME
AND HOBBIES:

121   Do you or does any member of your household   1. yes   2. no
          keep animals or pets?   (specify)

122   Have you any hobby that exposes you to dusts,   1. yes   2. no
          gases, or fumes, such as from paints, glues,   (specify)
          or wood dust?

123   Have you ever lived in any town or area other   1. yes   2. no
          than here?

          (If YES, ask 124 and 125.)

124   At what age did you move into this town or area?   (   )   (   )

125   Where did you live previously?   1. mainly country
                                                           2. mainly city
                                                           3. country and city

126   What type of heating system is used in your home?   1. none
                                                           2. forced air heating
                                                           3. circulating hot water
                                                               or steam
                                                           4. electric radiant heating
                                                           5. other (specify)

127   In addition to the above, do you use a fireplace   1. yes   2. no
      in your home?

128   What fuel is used for cooking?   1. electricity
                                                               2. gas
                                                               3. wood
                                                               4. coal

129   Do you have a humidifier?   1. yes   2. no

130   Do you have air-conditioning?   1. yes   2. no

131   Do you have an air-cleaning device in the home?   1. yes   2. no

132   What is the number of people in your household?   (   )   (   )

133   How many are smokers?   (   )   (   )

Chapter 14

Smoking

Cigarette smoking is causally related to lung cancer in men; the magnitude of the effect of cigarette smoking far outweighs all other factors. The data for women, though less extensive, point in the same direction.

The risk of developing lung cancer increases with duration of smoking and the number of cigarettes smoked per day, and is diminished by discontinuing smoking.

For the bulk of the population of the United States, the importance of cigarette smoking as a cause of chronic bronchopulmonary disease is much greater than that of atmospheric pollution or occupational exposures.

—1964 Report of the Advisory Committee to the Surgeon General of the Public Health Service, Smoking and Health [82]

Research summarized in more recent reports [83-87] further strengthens these conclusions from the 1964 Surgeon General's report. Cigarette smoking greatly increases the risk of lung cancer; it is also linked to many noncancerous respiratory and cardiovascular diseases. Even in those population groups where occupational exposures cause more disease than smoking, the smoker may well be at a disadvantage because of interactions between smoking and occupational exposures (Chap. 15).

This chapter concerns recent work on the epidemiology of smoking-induced lung disease, the short- and long-term effects of smoking on the lungs, and the pharmacological agents involved. Early losses in lung function and excesses of respiratory symptoms are described in addition to the more severe disease states. Smoking among teen-agers, the reversibility of the effects of smoking, some considerations for public policies on smoking, and the nature of the habit itself are also discussed.

EPIDEMIOLOGY

Mortality From Lung Disease

One of the most impressive studies on smoking and mortality, conducted among 41,000 British physicians, showed a strong association between smoking and death from lung cancer, chronic bronchitis, and pulmonary tuberculosis.[23]

Table 14-1.
Emphysema Diagnosed at Autopsy (Men Only)

	Grade of Emphysema				
	None (%)	Minimal (%)	Slight (%)	Moderate (%)	Advanced (%)
Nonsmokers (n = 176)	90.0	3.8	3.3	2.9	0
Smokers of 1–9 cigarettes per day (n = 181)	13.1	16.4	33.7	25.1	11.7
Smokers of 20 cigarettes per day (n = 658)	0.3	5.2	42.6	32.7	19.2

Data based on study of whole-lung sections which were graded according to degree of emphysema. Smoking histories were obtained from relatives. The study in lungs of 388 women gave similar results. Data from reference 6.

Among male nonsmokers, the mortality from lung cancer was 7 deaths per 100,000 persons per year; among male smokers of 35 cigarettes per day, the comparable figure was 315 deaths per 100,000 persons. That is, if all 41,000 doctors had been nonsmokers, 34 would have died of lung cancer during the 12-year study period; if all had smoked 35 or more cigarettes per day, about 1550 would have died. Doll and Hill [23] estimated that cigarette smoking accounts for one-third of the total mortality of persons 45 to 64 years old in Great Britain if lung cancer, chronic bronchitis, and coronary thrombosis without hypertension are all attributed to smoking.

Although the excess mortality from lung cancer among smokers is now generally accepted, that from noncancerous lung and airway disease is more difficult to document precisely, because of the problems inherent in mortality data (Chap. 13). A recent study of Auerbach et al.[6] has provided convincing evidence concerning the association of smoking with emphysema (Table 14-1). These authors graded the amount of emphysema in whole-lung sections of large numbers of patients at autopsy. There were very few anatomical lesions of emphysema among nonsmokers, while smokers had a strikingly high prevalence of moderate and advanced lesions. Among continuous smokers, the degree of emphysema increased with age. Thus, this study strongly supports the association between smoking and emphysema, long suspected on the basis of epidemiological and functional data. The strong association between the two makes a cause-effect relationship likely.

Morbidity From Lung Disease

Epidemiological studies in several countries have repeatedly shown associations between smoking, respiratory symptoms, and lung-function loss. Thus, there can be little question about the validity of the Surgeon General's conclusion in 1964: cigarette smoking is indeed a major cause of chronic bronchopulmonary disease, and not just in the United States.

The national morbidity data in the United States probably grossly underestimate the real personal and economical losses. Some of these data are shown in Table 14-2, from the National Health Survey in the United States, which forms the basis for estimates of total morbidity caused by cigarette smoking.[83] This survey, which conducts a yearly interview of 42,000 families representative of the population, includes only self-reported illness, no medical data. Morbidity based on this information yields much lower rates of illness than do medical interviews concerning respiratory symptoms. Table 14-2 includes results from an adult rural population in Finland[40] and from teen-agers in Connecticut.[70] For both cardinal symptoms of bronchitis—cough and phlegm—the interviews show much higher prevalences than do the data from the National Health Survey. This large discrepancy suggests that many people with chronic cough and phlegm do not realize that these symptoms represent illness. For purposes of prevention, the definition of chronic bronchitis should include anyone who admits to regular cough or phlegm or both; a good case could even be made to include everyone who smokes.

Apart from illness, the U.S. National Health Survey also collects annual data on days lost from work, days with restricted activity, and days spent in bed. These were all much higher among smokers, as were the number of chronic illnesses reported by subjects who smoked. Extrapolating from these data, it is estimated that there are about 11 million more cases of chronic illness annually than there would be if all people had the same rate of sickness as persons who never smoked.[83] Chronic bronchitis, emphysema, heart disease, and peptic ulcer account for the majority of this excess. Since chronic bronchitis and emphysema are certainly underestimated (Table 14-2), the figures on chronic illness induced by smoking, impressive as they are, must be far below the true excess. Thus, we do not have a reasonably accurate idea of the total losses in terms of discomfort, illness, and economic loss caused by cigarette smoking. Population surveys have given important baseline information, but further use of this tool is needed to complete the picture.

Population Surveys

Several important population studies, such as those in Berlin, New Hampshire, Tecumseh, Michigan, and Chilliwack, B.C., have been discussed in the previous chapter. These surveys concentrated on associations between smoking and disease; more complete studies in which occupation as well as smoking was carefully considered are available only for special occupational groups. Clearly, the association between smoking and lung disease in itself requires no further evidence. But longitudinal studies of smokers, even over a limited number of years, would provide much-needed information on disease progression and natural history. Also, studies in children and teen-agers are needed to obtain further evidence on the interrelations between smoking, lung growth, and lung damage.

A large study of male nonsmokers in Hagerstown, Maryland, has shown a low prevalence of chronic cough and phlegm. Dyspnea was more common, which Stebbings attributed to an association with coronary disease and hypertension.[74] However, unlike findings among smokers, the prevalence of respiratory symptoms did not increase with age and was unrelated to social class.[75] To counterbalance the many studies on manual workers, one British study investigated respiratory symptoms among 224 executives aged 30–69 years; the relationship between respiratory symptoms and smoking was similar to that in other studies. Although

Table 14-2
Chronic Respiratory Disease and Smoking

Source	Disease/Symptom	Sex, Age	Never Smoked (%) *	Exsmoker (%)	1–10/ day (%)	11–20/ day (%)	21+/ day (%)
National Health Survey, U.S.A.†	Chronic bronchitis and/or emphysema	M, 17+	1.0	2.5	1.1	2.3	3.3
Seely et al.‡	Cough	M, F, 15–19	2.0	—	18.1	27.8	64.7
	Phlegm		3.3	—	19.4	31.9	58.8
					(1–14)	(15–24)	(25+)
Huhti §	Cough	M, 40–64	4.1	8.5	31.5	40.8	42.4
	Phlegm		10.7	17.7	38.0	42.9	42.4

* Percentages in columns 4–8 indicate the number of people with disease or specified symptoms in each smoking category.
† Data reported in reference 83: self-reported disease among adults.
‡ Reference 70—high-school students in Connecticut.
§ Reference 40—rural population in Finland.

chronic bronchitis has sometimes been associated with low social class in the United Kingdom, this study showed that smoking rather than social class determines persistent cough and phlegm.[53] Among women aged 25–54 years, cough, phlegm, and decreased lung function were clearly related to smoking.[96] An ongoing prospective study in Gothenburg, Sweden, concerns the health of the "men of 1913," a sample of men born in that year. In 1963, when they were 50 years old, 46.3 percent of these men were non- or ex-smokers.[94] Of the nonsmokers, 4.8 percent had chronic cough, compared to 52.6 percent of the heavy smokers (> 15 gm/day). For chronic phlegm, these percentages were 1.2 versus 17.1 percent. Function data (VC, $FEV_{1.0}$, PEF, and MMEF; Table 9-1, p. 189) were also lower among the smokers.[94]

Among residents of a rural area in Finland (excluding those with respiratory symptoms), Huhti[41] found significant differences in $FEV_{1.0}$ and PEF between smokers and nonsmokers (420 men and 608 women; aged 40–64 yrs). Non- and ex-smokers (men only) did not differ, suggesting that the effect of smoking is reversible in adults who do not yet have overt symptoms of chronic bronchitis. Yet, in a large population study in The Netherlands, van der Lende[88] found no clear relationship between lung function ($FEV_{1.0}$) and smoking habits. In this survey covering about 5400 men and women in three geographical areas, the smokers had a higher prevalence of respiratory symptoms than the nonsmokers, but the $FEV_{1.0}$ values did not follow the usual pattern (see Fig. 10 in a later paper by van der Lende for a summary of these data[89]). The heavy cigarette smokers (men and women) had an $FEV_{1.0}$ similar to that of nonsmokers, while the light smokers as well as ex-smokers had lower values. The age decrement in $FEV_{1.0}$ (from age 40–60) is similar to that found by other authors.

Such aberrant associations between smoking and lung function can occur when a population is exposed to more than one inhaled agent that causes lung damage. The quantitative relations between the amount smoked and lung function then become complicated by self-selection. We found an example of this process, summarized in Figure 14-1, among older hemp workers in Spain.[10] These men (aged 50–69 yrs) had a high prevalence of chronic respiratory symptoms (Chap. 17). Many (26 percent) were ex-smokers, with an $FEV_{1.0}$ far below that of the active, heavy smokers (> 50 gm/wk). Thus, more smoking appeared to be associated with a higher $FEV_{1.0}$, at least in hemp workers. In contrast, among the control subjects $FEV_{1.0}$ was lower among the moderate to heavy smokers. The likely explanation is that some hemp workers, upon reaching their fifties, find themselves short of breath and decide to quit smoking. Others, less affected by hemp dust, lack this incentive to quit and continue smoking. Through self-selection, then, the smokers are the men with fewer symptoms and a larger $FEV_{1.0}$. We concluded[10] that, whenever the relationship between cigarette smoking and ventilatory capacity does not follow the expected pattern, exposures to agents other than cigarette smoking should be considered.

In fact, occupational exposures may have contributed to van der Lende's data, since the prevalence of symptoms differed significantly among the various occupational groups in the study.[88] The process of self-selection may also be reflected in the large number of pipe and cigar smokers in van der Lende's survey. Although few people in these Dutch groups are lifelong nonsmokers (7.4 percent in the urban group, 6.5 percent in one rural group), the number of ex-smokers

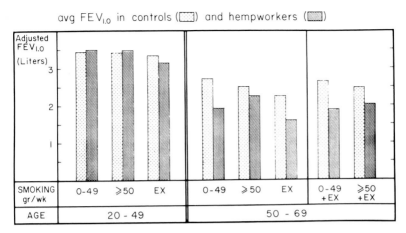

avg FEV$_{1.0}$ in controls (☐) and hempworkers (▓)

Fig. 14-1. Comparison between FEV$_{1.0}$ values of subjects in two age groups, according to present and past smoking habits. *Left-hand panel:* 20–49-year-old hemp workers had FEV$_{1.0}$ values similar to those of control subjects; no significant differences between smoking categories. *Middle panel:* Hemp workers aged 50–69 years, in all smoking categories, have a significantly lower FEV$_{1.0}$ than control subjects. The hemp workers who smoke 50 cigarettes or more per week ($\geq$50 gr/wk) have a significantly *higher* FEV$_{1.0}$ than hemp workers who smoke less (0–49 gr/wk). The exsmokers have the lowest FEV$_{1.0}$ of the three groups. When the exsmokers are added to the groups of active smokers, according to their previous smoking habits (*right-hand panel*), there is no significant difference in FEV$_{1.0}$ between the two groups of hemp workers. These data illustrate the importance of self-selection in population groups (see text). FEV$_{1.0}$ values (*ordinate*) are means adjusted for height and age. Data from reference 10.

is high (15.6 percent in the urban group). About 20 percent of van der Lende's two rural population groups smoked pipes and cigars only, and these men complained more frequently of severe dyspnea than did the cigarette smokers. As among the Spanish hemp workers, those with chronic respiratory symptoms may have selected themselves out of the cigarette-smoker group.

Conclusions from data in such large and heterogeneous population groups are risky. Occupation and social class must be considered in conjunction with smoking habits. Large surveys should focus on relatively homogeneous subgroups, since average data from heterogeneous groups do not provide adequate insight. In fact, the main reason for doing large surveys is the availability of adequately sized, but homogeneous, subgroups for the study of an increased number of variables (Chap. 13, p. 294).

Early Effects of Smoking on the Lungs

The first epidemiological studies on lung function and smoking were directed primarily at men over 40 years of age, a group with a high prevalence of chronic bronchitis and emphysema. In one of the earlier studies, Higgins [37] included men aged 25–34 years and found a decrement of FEV$_{0.75}$ among the smokers almost as large as that in 55–64-year-old smokers. Unfortunately, there were few non-smokers in the sample, a factor that still limits many surveys among men. A later study among U.S. college seniors confirmed clearly that effects of smoking can be demonstrated in people in their twenties. Peters and Ferris [60] found that smoking affected maximum expiratory flow rates in this group, and that the smokers had an excess of respiratory symptoms.

A study of teen-age students in Oklahoma City [1] showed more respiratory symptoms among smokers but no difference in $FEV_{1.0}$ and FVC between non-smokers and smokers. Peters and Ferris [60] had, however, found that flow rates at low lung volumes discriminated clearly between smokers and nonsmokers among their college seniors. We therefore decided to use MEFV curves (Chap. 9) in a study of high school students to determine whether this method, more sensitive to slight airway obstruction than FVC and $FEV_{1.0}$, might show evidence of lung damage after only a few years of smoking.[70]

We asked students not to smoke on the day of the tests, which were done in the morning. A questionnaire on respiratory symptoms was later filled out by a physician-interviewer. The smoking history was recorded separately by the students. Cough, phlegm, and shortness of breath were common among the smokers, with no significant difference between the sexes. This high prevalence of symptoms among the smokers (Table 14-2) confirms results of studies in school children in Great Britain.[38, 39] Smokers and nonsmokers differed also in lung function. We distinguished three types of MEFV curves: concave to the volume axis (A in Fig. 14-2), straight, and convex to the volume axis (B in Fig. 14-2). There was a highly significant difference between the shape of curves in smokers and nonsmokers: many more nonsmokers had type A curves, and many smokers had type B curves.

To analyze the data from the MEFV curves quantitatively is not easy, because adolescent growth alters the relation between lung function and body height, particularly in boys. Age and weight, which reflect these growth changes indirectly, correlate with smoking and flow rates. Consequently, we computed regression equations for the function data ($FEV_{1.0}$, MEF50% and MEF25%) as a function of age, height, and weight for nonsmoking boys as well as non-smoking girls. These equations were then used to test the hypothesis that smokers belong to the same population as the nonsmokers. Figure 14-2 compares the actual values for MEF50% in moderate to heavy smokers with the data predicted by the regression equations. In most smokers, the values are less than the predicted ones, with significant differences in boys who smoked more than 15 and in girls who smoked more than 10 cigarettes per day. These differences in flow rates between smokers and nonsmokers showed up on the MEFV curves but not in the FVC; the $FEV_{1.0}$ data showed a small difference in girls but not in boys. Although smoking affected flow rates among girls who smoked less than 10 cigarettes per day, boys who were light smokers did not differ from the non-smokers. We concluded that 1 to 5 years of regular smoking is sufficient to cause significant lung-function loss in teen-agers and to induce chronic respiratory symptoms and dyspnea. Smoking even a single cigarette affects the MEFV curve. In 17 subjects (teen-age regular smokers) there was a slight but significant decrease of MEF50% but no change of $FEV_{1.0}$ or FVC (Table 9-4). Since these acute effects of smoking disappear in about 1 hour,[54] they cannot explain the differences in function between the nonsmokers and the smokers shown in Figure 14-2.

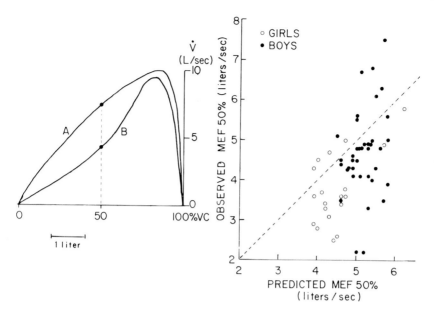

Fig. 14-2. *Left.* Maximum expiratory flow-volume curves in two 18-year-old boys. *A* is a nonsmoker who has no respiratory symptoms. *B* has smoked 16 cigarettes per day since he was 13 and has slight shortness of breath on exertion but no other respiratory symptoms. *Right.* Observed versus predicted values of MEF50% (Table 9-2) in boys smoking more than 15 cigarettes per day and in girls smoking more than 10 cigarettes per day. Line of equality (*dashed*) represents data of the average nonsmoker. Flow rates in smokers are significantly lower than predicted; the majority of points are below the line of equality. The regression equations used for the predicted values (from data in nonsmokers) are:

Boys: MEF50% = −5.75057 + [0.28215 × age (yrs)] + [0.03755 × height(cm)]
                       − [0.00834 × weight (kg)]

Girls: MEF50% = −5.35737 + [0.20808 × age (yrs)] + [0.02828 × height(cm)]
                       + [0.03036 × weight (kg)]

Modified from reference 70.

Low maximum expiratory flow rates reflect partial obstruction in small airways or a decrease of lung static recoil, or both (Chap. 9). The obstruction can result from smooth muscle contraction, mucus secretion, or mucosal edema. These are reversible changes, but since we do not know how reversible the function changes in teen-agers are, the possibility of some degree of developmental arrest remains (discussed in Chap. 1).

The excess respiratory symptoms and the lung-function loss observed in smokers in their teens and twenties [1, 60, 70] contrasts with a lack of demonstrable anatomical changes. Detailed studies at autopsy of the lungs from 11 nonsmokers and 13 smokers (men aged 18 to 46 years) showed no differences in the amounts of smooth muscle and gland tissue in airway walls and no pathological changes indicative of early chronic bronchitis.[73] In detecting early disease, measurements of functional changes are clearly more helpful than pathological studies of the lungs. This is true even when the pathologist attempts to quantitate his findings to the maximum extent feasible. The early signs of airway obstruction, as determined with the MEFV curve and other function tests, indicate small-airway narrowing that could be caused by slight degrees of mucus hypersecretion, slight degrees of smooth muscle contraction, and minor mucosal swelling, or combinations of these. These changes are difficult to quantitate in pathological preparations of airways, even in cases of overt disease. In incipient disease, large portions of the lungs and airways may still be normal. The pathologist's samples can then easily miss the abnormal areas. If we want to emphasize prevention of overt disease and disability, we must accept functional evidence as a sensitive indicator of airway damage in young smokers. In the future, improved methods of studying tissues and cells may indicate the anatomical substrate of these functional changes.

Reactors and Nonreactors

There are probably large differences in the ways individuals respond to smoking.[98] Some may react severely and soon, while others remain normal (as with responses to textile dust, Chap. 17). Similarly, there may be a log-normal distribution of sensitivity to a given dose of smoke (as with other drugs [25]), but this hypothesis cannot be tested in man because of self-selection. Among adults, initial responses to smoking help determine who becomes a smoker and who does not. Persons who are sensitive to the acute effects of smoke on airways probably never become regular smokers. Persons with lung disease also may remain non-smokers. Others, less sensitive, may smoke for some years and then give up. Still others, the so-called nonreactors to the acute effects, are the most likely to remain lifelong smokers. To test a hypothesis concerning the distribution of sensitivity, one would have to measure the effect of cigarette smoke in a large group of children before the age that smoking begins—an inadmissible and impractical experiment. We cannot obtain a clear picture of variations in responses to cigarette smoke merely by measuring effects in a cross section of population groups. The most insensitive nonreactors are obviously those who have normal lung function and few respiratory symptoms even after a lifetime of heavy smoking; such individuals are rare. Most people are neither nonreactors nor highly sensitive; rather, their smoking habits are primarily determined by personal motivation, social custom, and occupational factors (dust inhalation during work; smoking prohibition at work). For instance, when cigars and pipes are a readily available and socially acceptable alternative, many cigarette smokers may switch to these. This practice seems common in The Netherlands (p. 318) and may move those relatively sensitive to cigarette smoke into the category of pipe and cigar smokers. Although sensitivity to the acute effects of cigarette smoke need not correlate with sensitivity to other effects, such as carcinogenicity, it is clearly an important selective factor in determining initial smoking habits. As a result of this pre-selection process, it is not surprising that some studies have not shown convincing dose-response relations for long-term, or chronic, effects of smoking on airways and lungs.

RESPONSES TO CIGARETTE SMOKE

Cigarette smoking elicits acute responses in the body and is associated with chronic diseases and lung cancer. The agents involved in the acute and chronic responses have not been identified with certainty. We shall therefore review the effects and some of the agents in cigarette smoke separately.

Effects on Physiological Functions

Acute responses. Smoking a cigarette induces an increase in airway resistance,[54] a decrease in maximum expiratory flow rates,[60] an increase in carboxyhemoglobin content in blood,[65] an increase in oxygen cost of hyperventilation,[65] and a temporary reduction in clearance of inhaled particles from the airways in man.[59] Several of these effects also occur in long-term smokers and may still be partially reversible during short-term abstinence (days or weeks).

Long-term effects. These include a high prevalence of cough, sputum production, shortness of breath during exercise, and an increased risk of lung cancer as well as heart and peripheral arterial disease. In the following paragraphs we discuss primarily effects on the lungs and airways. The prevalence of respiratory symptoms is discussed in more detail with the epidemiological studies (p. 316); this section deals with effects that can be measured in man or in animals.

Particle deposition and clearance. The physiology and physics of these processes is discussed on pp. 265–267. Smoke from the burning end of a cigarette contains submicronic particles, all less than 0.2 μm in diameter.[22] At the other end of the cigarette, larger particles are present in the smoke, up to about 1 μm diameter. Such particles are deposited in small airways and alveolar spaces and may carry absorbed chemicals to those regions. Particle deposition from smoke decreases at large lung volumes.[9]

Particle deposition does not differ clearly among nonsmokers and smokers, but differences in the clearance of inhaled particles are important. In nonsmokers, clearance begins directly after inhalation of particles; in smokers, this process is delayed for 1 to 4 hours, and clearance takes longer.[49] This is usually attributed to delayed mucociliary transport in smokers. Animal experiments have shown temporary arrest of the ciliary beat and decreased rates of mucociliary transport on the tracheal mucosa.[21] This is a temporary, reversible effect. In intact subjects, particle transport may become slower,[2] faster,[12] or remain unchanged.[29] Albert et al.[2] found impairment of lung particle clearance in donkeys who smoked 90 cigarettes per week during 5–7 months; this improved rapidly after the end of exposure. In the nasal mucosa of these donkeys, particle transport did not change, even after heavy smoke exposure.[29] The clearance of monodisperse particles (inhaled before smoking) increased during intensive smoking in human subjects.[12] Since this result could not be explained by cough, a faster rate of mucociliary transport is likely. If it occurs consistently, this might be an adaptive response. It is conceivable that a given dose of smoking leads to increased mucus production while leaving the ciliary beat unimpaired. This could increase the transport of particles. At a higher dose level, the ciliary beat would slow down or stop, and transport rates would then decrease. In rats, cigarette smoke delays the clearance of silica particles from the airways; but this effect is absent when the smoke is inhaled 1 day before the silica exposure, suggesting that the effect of the smoke lasts no more than 24 hours.[28]

Airway obstruction. Franklin and Lowell found in 1961 that smokers have low maximum expiratory flow rates, particularly at small lung volumes.[30] They suggested that this reflected small-airway obstruction in smokers, which might eventually lead to the development of emphysema. Body plethysmographic measurements of airway resistance also showed evidence of airway obstruction, at least immediately after smoking 1 cigarette.[54] Since this effect results from narrowing of large rather than small airways (Chap. 8), cigarette smoke appears to cause constriction of both. Guyatt et al.[33] studied the acute constrictor response in large numbers of subjects and found that the response (Raw, measured by plethysmography) varied—some subjects had airway dilation rather than constriction. There was a relation between dose and response: heavier smokers constricted more than light smokers and nonsmokers. This acute response to cigarette smoke can be blocked by atropine and isoproterenol,[50] and it can be enhanced by a β-adrenergic blocking drug (see below).

Smokers, even when asymptomatic, have prolonged nitrogen washout curves [18] and an increased airway closing volume.[45] Both findings suggest small-airway obstruction in smokers. Indirectly, arterial blood oxygen tensions also provide evidence for this. Strieder and Kazemi [76] found that arterial P_{O_2} in smokers may be normal in the sitting, but too low in the supine, position. This decrease during the supine posture disappears after a few weeks' abstinence from smoking. Arterial P_{O_2} depends on ventilation-perfusion ratios in the lungs (Chap. 5). Arterial P_{O_2} probably decreased in smokers who were lying down because of increased nonuniformity of ventilation (Chap. 4), a phenomenon associated with partial obstruction of small airways. Thus, several independent findings all point to small-airway obstruction in smokers.

Smoking 2 cigarettes after administration of 40 mg propranolol elicits airway constriction in smokers.[98] Blockade of β-receptors in airway smooth muscle with this drug may render the muscle more sensitive to the action of histamine released by cigarette smoke constituents (p. 326). This explanation fits other observations on interaction between exogenous agents and autonomic stimuli (Chaps. 17 and 18). Regardless of its mechanism, potentiation of the action of smoking by propranolol means that patients treated with this drug should be cautioned against exposure to tobacco smoke.

Diurnal changes of $FEV_{1.0}$ differ in smokers and nonsmokers.[13, 14] The decline during the day (morning versus evening) was larger in smokers (0.07 liters) than in nonsmokers (0.04 liters). These differences are small but not negligible. In comparative studies, a systematic difference of this size can introduce significant errors. They must be taken into account when studying acute effects of dust (as in byssinosis, Chap. 17), in studies of drug effects, and in follow-up studies.

Changes in alveolar macrophage cells. These are important in the clearance of bacteria and other particles in alveolar spaces (Chap. 12). Impairment of their phagocytic function could conceivably increase the risk of lung infections among smokers, but there is no direct evidence for such a sequence of events. Nevertheless, many studies show changes in these cells under the influence of cigarette smoke, and toxic changes in alveolar macrophage cells at least indicate potential damage to clearance mechanisms.

Alveolar macrophage cells are harvested by lavaging the lungs. The yield decreases in acute experiments with cigarette smoke, but after 2 to 4 weeks more cells were obtained.[66] In rabbit alveolar macrophages, the filtered gas phase of cigarette smoke inhibits glyceraldehyde 3-phosphate dehydrogenase,[61] an enzyme of the glycolytic pathway that provides energy for phagocytosis. Alveolar macrophage cells can be obtained in man by bronchial lavage. Cells obtained from smokers and nonsmokers differ in ultrastructure, but not in the capacity to ingest heat-killed yeast cells (Candida albicans [52]). Electronmicrographic studies of the cells show differences in the type and size of inclusion bodies, which may be identical with lysosomes, in nonsmokers and smokers.[62] In another study, fewer nickel monoxide and chromic oxide particles were phagocytosed by hamster macrophage cells under the influence of cigarette smoke.[69] The relation between the ultrastructural changes of the cells and their phagocytic competence is not clear.

Enzyme induction. Components of cigarette smoke may act indirectly by influencing enzyme systems in the body. For instance, smokers have lower plasma phenacetin levels than nonsmokers after oral intake of 900 mg phenacetin.[56] This is attributed to increased activity of enzymes that metabolize phenacetin and could decrease the effect of this analgesic and antipyretic drug in smokers. Other microsomal enzymes, including those that metabolize benzo[a]pyrene, a powerful carcinogenic agent in cigarette smoke, can also be activated. Increased levels of this enzyme activity have been found in rats exposed to smoke and also in the placenta of human smokers.[56, 92] It is not yet clear whether enzyme induction in smokers is useful or dangerous—it might break a carcinogenic agent down to a nontoxic metabolite; it might also convert benzo[a]pyrene to the real carcinogen.[92] It is conceivable that spontaneous or induced variations in benzo[a]pyrene-hydrolase activity levels may be related to the individual differences in sensitivity to the risk of lung cancer.

Pharmacological Agents in Cigarette Smoke

These have recently been reviewed;[87] here we discuss only nicotine and some agents that may act on airways. Carcinogenic substances are discussed later (p. 327).

Nicotine is the most important alkaloid in cigarette smoke.[19] Its metabolism in the body is complex; after a single intravenous injection, about 30–45 percent is recovered in the urine of nonsmokers over a 12-hour period.[7] The nicotine content of tobacco is at least partially responsible for its habit-forming properties. In behavioral experiments with monkeys, nicotine was clearly an incentive for smoking, and oral nicotine could at least partially substitute for smoking.[31] This substitution may also be effective in man but requires high doses of nicotine. In animal studies, Armitage et al.[3] found that small amounts of nicotine "activated the electroencephalogram" of anesthetized cats and made rats press a lever more frequently. The investigators ascribe this to an arousal phenomenon which may find its human counterpart in smokers who state that smoking renders them more alert.

In recent years there has been a tendency to decrease the nicotine and tar content of cigarettes in an effort to decrease their health hazard. Yet, if effects on the lungs were the only consideration, a nicotine-rich cigarette with a low tar content might be the best: one could satisfy one's nicotine requirements by smoking only a few cigarettes, thus minimizing exposure to substances other than nicotine. Unfortunately, nicotine has powerful cardiovascular actions that make this approach undesirable. Other approaches to decreasing smoking risks have been reviewed in a recent report.[97]

Carbon monoxide. The mainstream smoke of a cigarette contains about 4 percent CO in the gas phase, enough to raise the COHb level of the smoker's blood up to 10 percent. Such levels lead to impaired exercise performance.[17] Other effects of CO are discussed in Chapter 16. The exact COHb level at which mental function becomes impaired is still subject to discussion. The production of CO is sufficient reason for prohibiting smoking in enclosed or insufficiently ventilated spaces, in particular those where persons with heart or lung disease may be exposed (e.g., public transport) and those where rapid and accurate judgment is essential (airplane cockpits, air traffic control towers). It is difficult to see how a safe cigarette can be developed: incomplete combustion of any organic material produces CO.

Airway constrictor agents. Cigarette smoke may contain chemical substances that cause airway constriction, but these have not been identified with certainty. Cigarette smoke contains water-soluble agents that cause airway constriction in anesthetized guinea pigs,[32] and these may be identical with agents that release histamine from chopped guinea pig lung.[57] However, other experiments with guinea pig lung have not confirmed the presence of histamine-releasing agents in cigarette smoke.[24] Nicotine and acrolein do not have histamine-releasing activity. Saindelle et al.[67] have proposed that a mixture of aldehydes in cigarette smoke may be responsible for the airway constrictor effect. Alternatively, the airway constriction induced by cigarette smoke in man can be explained on a reflex basis.[54] The fact that the effect is inhibited by atropine[50] is consistent with this view but can also be explained by interaction at the smooth muscle level (p. 465). Immediate, short-lasting effects may be of reflex origin; slowly developing and more persistent effects are better explained by the action of chemicals, perhaps involving release of chemical mediators (Chap. 18, p. 455).

Acetaldehyde is an active ciliostatic agent in cigarette smoke.[26] Most of this soluble vapor may, however, act on the upper respiratory mucosa rather than on the lower airways (Chap. 2).

3-Methylindol. After oral administration, this and related compounds cause interstitial lung edema and emphysema in cattle and goats.[15] They have been identified in cigarette smoke.

Diatomaceous earth, which includes the fibrogenic cristobalite, has been identified in cheap cigars[44] containing up to 40 percent additives. Cristobalite was identified in the mainstream smoke of these cigars.

Types of tobacco. In experiments with rats, the method of curing tobacco appeared to influence the effect of the smoke. Smoke of flue-cured tobacco greatly shortened life span and caused hyperplastic and metaplastic changes in the epithelium of airways; mucous glands were enlarged. Other conditions being equal, smoke of air-cured (cigar type) tobacco had relatively little effect.[58] Compared with cigarette smoking, cigar smoking carries less risk of lung cancer. This may be related to the curing method, as suggested by these experiments; it may also be due to other differences between cigar and cigarette smoking, such as the lower burning temperatures of cigars or the fact that few cigar smokers inhale.

A special kind of tobacco produced in Kentucky and used by East Indian people in Guyana is treated with mineral oil to impart a special flavor to the tobacco. About 20 percent of the long-term smokers of this product, called blackfat tobacco, have lung fibrosis.[53a] Presumably, this is induced by the mineral oil inhalation and is a consequence of lipoid pneumonia.

LUNG CANCER

The epidemic of lung cancer in many Western countries is almost wholly due to cigarette smoking.[82-87] The investigator who tries to decide which agent in cigarette smoke may cause lung cancer has a large choice: [83, 87] aromatic hydrocarbons, phenols, radioactive isotopes, and, perhaps, nitrosamines. There is no conclusive evidence on the relative roles of these substances, but together they form an impressive and persuasive catalog of confirmed or potential carcinogenic substances. Thus, the epidemiological evidence linking smoking with lung cancer is convincingly supported by the presence of such agents in the smoke. For several reasons, further identification of the most important carcinogens is of interest. This might help in the quest for a safe cigarette, useful for those who find it impossible to quit smoking. In addition, the exquisite action of cigarette carcinogens on human airway epithelium may be important for oncological studies. Furthermore, lung cancer provides an impressive example of cocarcinogenesis: asbestos workers who smoke have an 80-fold increased risk of lung cancer, compared to smokers who are not also exposed to asbestos dust (Chap. 15). Cigarette smoke-induced lung cancer is the most prevalent cancer with a known and preventable environmental cause. An understanding of its pathogenesis is almost certainly important for carcinogenesis in general.

Animal Studies

Experimental work on carcinogenesis in animals has been done with cigarette smoke and with smoke condensate. The smoke itself causes cytotoxic effects in the epitheloid cells of lung explants from mice.[47] Induction of the human-type cancer in animals has been tried many times, with negative results. Recently, Auerbach et al. have reported emphysematous lesions as well as granulomatous tumors in the lungs of dogs that smoked cigarettes (3–10 per day for up to 422 days) through a permanent tracheostomy tube, i.e., without benefit of the filter function of nose and upper airways.[4] Later reports from this group dealt with 97 beagles, including 8 nonsmokers and 89 smokers.[5, 34] Among the latter, the 12 that smoked filter cigarettes had less fibrosis and emphysema than those who smoked regular cigarettes. Some of these dogs also had noninvasive bronchoalveolar lung tumors, while 2 animals that smoked nonfilter cigarettes daily for more than 2 years had microscopic squamous cell bronchial carcinomas. The *noninvasive* tumors are not uniquely related to smoking, since they also occurred in 2 of the 8 control dogs. The results relate to effects of smoke inhaled through tracheostomy tubes. Airway temperatures during smoking were not measured and thermal damage to large airways (which can hardly occur during normal smoking) needs to be excluded. Nevertheless, 2 out of 89 smoking dogs had *invasive* tumors, and this finding may be relevant to tumor induction in man. As in these dogs, only a minority of smokers eventually develop lung cancer, even though their risk is much higher than in nonsmokers.

Cocarcinogenesis

The low yield of invasive tumors in dogs may be related to the use of a single carcinogen. In experiments with mice, cigarette smoke condensate could act with cocarcinogens in the induction of skin cancer. The smoke condensate alone was active and caused papillomas, but interaction with a cocarcinogen increased the incidence.[90] An example of cocarcinogenesis in induction of lung cancer has been studied extensively by Kuschner and Laskin (reviewed in reference 36). They showed that neither long-term, low-level SO_2 exposure nor short, daily exposure to low concentrations of benzo[a]pyrene were sufficient to induce lung cancer. However, the combination of the two exposures resulted in a high incidence of lung cancer in their animals.

Radioactive Isotopes

The carcinogenic effect of radioactive isotopes in cigarette smoke is a matter of dispute. Cigarette smoke contains the α-emitting isotope ^{210}Po, which has also been found in lung parenchyma, peribronchial lymph nodes, and bronchial epithelium of smokers. It appears to be absorbed in particular near airway bifurcations, perhaps because of transport by smoke particles which are preferentially deposited in these areas where turbulent airflow patterns are common.[48] The role of this isotope in causing lung cancer is not established, but inhalation of this potential carcinogen is clearly highly undesirable. There is a quantitative argument against the acceptance of ^{210}Po as a principal carcinogen.[63] It is relatively easily removed from cigarette smoke with an ion-exchange resin filter.[11]

Precancerous Lesions

Metaplastic cells occur in the sputum of about 60 percent of heavy smokers, but also frequently (43 percent) in sputum of nonsmokers.[96] Thus, the finding of such preneoplastic cells in sputum does not correlate with the relative lung cancer risks in these two groups. The idea that such precancerous lesions might indicate a high risk of lung cancer was first suggested by Winternitz et al. in 1920.[95] They found preneoplastic lesions in the airways of influenza victims, and they predicted that the survivors of the 1917–1918 pandemic might be susceptible to lung cancer. This prediction has not been fulfilled; Beebe could not confirm an association between influenza in 1918 and the subsequent risk of lung cancer.[8]

Reversibility of the Risk of Lung Cancer

The risk of lung cancer in man decreases considerably when smoking is stopped, but a slight excess risk remains even more than 10 years after stopping. Since no animal or tissue model of this sequence of events is available, one can only speculate on its cellular or subcellular substrate. Most likely, the risk is reduced only in those smokers in whom carcinogenesis has not yet been triggered by some crucial event that requires long-term exposure to cigarette smoke.

REVERSIBILITY OF FUNCTIONAL EFFECTS

Airway Obstruction

Lung-function tests have shown that airway obstruction decreases after one stops smoking. As a result, the oxygen cost of hyperventilation decreases.[65] At the same time, blood carboxyhemoglobin content decreases to less than 2 percent within a few days of abstinence.[65] However, reversibility of effects of smoking has so far been studied only in small numbers of subjects. Krumholz et al.[42] found improved peak flow rates 3 weeks after stopping in 10 adults (25–33 years old). Wilhelmsen[93] showed increased flows at low lung volume (25% VC) about 6 weeks after shopping in 16 adults (average age–44 years), and $FEV_{1.0}$ also increased. Wilhelmsen gave his subjects an anticholinergic drug, which may have contributed to the improved function.

Therefore, at least part of the smoking-induced airway obstruction is reversible within 3–6 weeks. To what extent permanent damage remains is uncertain, and the relationship between degree of reversibility and duration and intensity of smoking is also largely unknown. The graph in Figure 14-3 deals with some of these problems and illustrates different events that may occur when young people stop smoking. We assume that, before age 10, future smokers and nonsmokers are similar with respect to function (an as yet untested assumption). In those who start to smoke, MEF50% continues to increase as they grow older, but less than in nonsmokers.

Three possible courses of events after stopping smoking are shown. Line *C* indicates full reversibility—flow rates increase to the levels found in nonsmokers. Lines *A* and *B* both reflect some degree of permanent function loss. In all three cases, flow rates increase shortly after stopping. Thus, in teen-agers whose lungs still grow, detailed data on flow rates and lung growth (e.g., by measuring TLC; Chap. 1) are needed to determine what happens after a person stops smoking. Complete reversibility (line *C*) would suggest that the airway obstruction of smokers results from events like mucus overproduction, mucosal swelling, or smooth muscle contraction. But if smoking causes damage to alveolar structure during growth (Chap. 1), complete reversibility cannot be expected. The age at which regular smoking began is therefore probably important in determining reversibility of airway obstruction.

It may seem surprising that such simple questions about the damage done by smoking have not yet been answered. However, the answers require controlled studies that are difficult to design and carry out. Accurate follow-up studies on

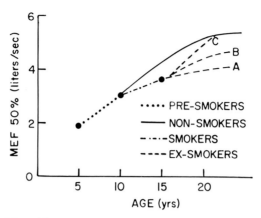

Fig. 14-3. Reversibility of airway obstruction in young smokers. *Ordinate:* maximum expiratory flow rate at 50% VC, as measured on MEFV curves. *A, B,* and *C* indicate three degrees of reversibility; see text for discussion.

lung function are difficult enough to arrange, even without the added problem of inducing people to stop smoking. There is also a need for independent evidence that the smokers have indeed stopped, and we shall briefly review how this can be obtained.

Detection of Smoking

Nicotine and carbon monoxide are at present the most suitable indicators of exposure to cigarette smoke. A noninvasive method, the rebreathing method of Sjöstrand, is available for measuring CO. The subject rebreathes 100 percent oxygen for 2 minutes, after which the CO content of the rebreathing bag or spirometer is determined. This method shows significantly elevated blood COHb content in persons who smoke 10 or more cigarettes per day. Blood COHb should be less than 2 percent during abstinence from smoking.[65] This method is suitable for epidemiological surveys, where blood sampling always greatly decreases subject participation.

The plasma nicotine level may be a very sensitive indicator of current tobacco consumption. Smoking a single cigarette increases it from 1–8 ng/ml to 12–44 ng/ml, with peak levels after 5–10 minutes.[41a] With successive cigarettes smoked, the level continues to increase. The method uses gas chromatographic analysis and requires 20 ml blood. The recovery of intravenous nicotine in urine is limited, and the metabolism of nicotine is complex; determinations of the nicotine level in urine do not offer a suitable substitute for measurements of plasma nicotine levels.[7] Unlike nicotine, the presence of CO (in the blood) may indicate smoking of marijuana as well as tobacco. So far, attempts to devise a breath analysis method to detect cannabis smokers have not resulted in a practical method that can reliably discriminate between cannabis and tobacco.[51]

MARIJUANA AND OPIUM

Surprisingly little is known about the effects of marijuana and opium smoking on the lungs and airways. Recent reviews on the chemistry and pharmacology of marijuana and its main component, the psychopharmacological drug tetrahydro-cannabinol [55a, 71] do not mention effects of the raw product or the pure drug on the lungs. Marijuana and opium induce pronounced psychological changes, including euphoria and alterations of judgment, in the user. Therefore, any respiratory symptoms caused by smoking marijuana or opium are unlikely to be reported accurately. Experiments with objective methods would be needed to study respiratory effects, but legal barriers as well as ethical problems inhibit this kind of research.

Marijuana

Because smoking of marijuana is most common among cigarette smokers (Table 14-3), it is difficult to discern the separate action of the two substances in people who use both. Experiments with naive subjects (nonusers) are difficult to defend on ethical grounds. Experiments with users of marijuana who have stopped smoking tobacco are preferable.[81a] It is, however, very likely that combustion products of plant materials, such as tobacco leaves and marijuana, are similar in several respects. The smoke of marijuana contains CO, particulate matter, and organic chemicals, some of which may well damage lungs and airways. In recent experiments with lung explants of mice,[47] a mixture of cigarette and marijuana smoke caused mitosis and atypism in epitheloid cells, together with increased DNA content. Cigarette smoke alone did not have these effects. Thus,

Table 14-3
Smoking Among Teen-agers

Survey	Total	Never Smoked	1–10/day	11–20/day	20+/day
1969 *					
	n 365	204	72	72	17
	% 100	55.9	19.7	19.7	4.7
1972 †					
	n 256	174	48	28	6
	% 100	68.0	18.8	10.9	2.3
1972 ‡ marijuana					
	n 72	28	24	15	5
	% 28	16.0	50.0	53.5	83.3

* Data from reference 70.

† Unpublished data, Yale University Lung Research Center (Mitchell, Zuskin et al, 1972).

‡ Students who smoked marijuana at least once a month during past 6 months, as a percentage of students in each smoking category.

"Never smoked" = never smoked as much as 1 cigarette regularly per day.

n = number of students in each group.

marijuana smoke may increase the cytological and cytochemical effects of cigarette smoke.

Recent experiments have shown that marijuana induces circulatory changes in man that are blocked by propranolol, suggesting that a β-adrenergic mechanism (Chap. 18) is involved. The authors of this study [6a] recommend caution with vasoactive drugs and anesthetics in marijuana users. In contrast with cigarette smoke, marijuana smoke causes dilatation of small airways.[87a] It increases airway conductance even more than isoproterenol, and this effect is also observed after ingestion of 10–20 mg Δ^9-tetrahydrocannabinol.[81a]

The association between cigarette and marijuana smoking provides an additional reason to intensify programs to prevent teen-agers from becoming cigarette smokers. Cigarettes are the first drug young children are tempted to try. If we could succeed in educating a generation of children unhooked on cigarettes, they would also probably be less likely to smoke marijuana or use other drugs (LSD, heroin). The main message is that drugs, including cigarettes and alcohol, are dangerous to physical and mental health and that the habituated and dependent is not in full control of himself. Since it is a difficult message to get across, it deserves frequent substantiation and repetition.

Opium

Like marijuana smoking, the use of opium is closely associated with cigarette or other tobacco smoking. Opium smokers in Singapore had a high prevalence of productive cough; all smoked cigarettes as well.[41b] There was no excess in airway obstruction that could clearly be attributed to opium smoking. Yet, opium smoking is considered likely to cause chronic airway obstruction, since opium smokers often have severe airway obstruction and overinflation of the lungs.[20]

THE SMOKING HABIT

Psychologists have described smoking as a chain of conditioned behavioral events, starting with the procurement of cigarettes, and with positive and negative reinforcers.[16] Among the positive reinforcers are the pharmacological effects of smoking, at least in part due to nicotine (e.g., relaxation, increased awareness, alertness), peer approval in teen-agers, and the avoidance of situational anxieties and tension. Negative reinforcers may include cough, shortness of breath, information on health effects, observation of one's own decreased performance, or the observation that smoking has impaired the health of one's friends or relatives.

The relation between smoking habits and personality factors is controversial. Eysenck believes that smokers as well as overeaters are extroverts who have a stimulus hunger.[27] This need for exogenous stimuli may explain why many people who stop smoking tend to overeat. A recent review covering about 30 studies showed a close link between smoking and low social status.[46] Thus, smoking would be associated with other aspects of low social status, and the relative roles of social and personality factors would be difficult to separate.

Why do people begin to smoke, continue to smoke, and have difficulty quitting? The powerful motivational factors involved must be taken into account by physicians who want their patients to stop smoking and also by private and public bodies that need to design rational policies on smoking.

Beginning to Smoke

For teen-agers, smoking habits of friends and older siblings are the most important factor in initiating smoking, which suggests that efforts to change smoking behavior should be directed primarily at smokers who serve as models within peer groups.[43] These may in turn carry the message to others in their group, with perhaps more chance of success than repeated lectures by adults. Apart from peer group pressure, smoking is associated with poor academic performance in high school as well as in college. Tamerin,[77] who reviews these data, points out that many values of today's youth—risk-taking, immediate experience rather than delayed gratification, and decreased interest in academic achievement—reinforce smoking.

Antismoking propaganda in schools has had no perceptible effect on smoking habits in Great Britain.[38] An approach focused on 10–14-year-olds, perhaps even on younger children, is necessary, since smoking habits are already much more established in older children.[68] In many western countries, one-third of all children are regular smokers by the age of 15. In high schools in the New Haven, Connecticut, area, about 50 percent of the boys and 37 percent of the girls in 1969 were regular smokers at the age of 15 to 19 years. A recent study in one of these schools (1972) showed a decrease in the number of moderate and heavy smokers (Table 14-3). This encouraging result in one school contrasts with national figures, which suggest that teen-age smoking is increasing or at least not decreasing.[77, 87] Perhaps the health information conveyed through our surveys had some impact, but more systematic and more frequent evaluation of these methods is necessary. The association between cigarette and marijuana smoking has already been discussed (p. 331; Table 14-3). Many students first smoke cigarettes in their pre-teens and become regular smokers by the age of 12 to 14. It then may seem only a small step to replace one kind of plant material in the cigarette with another.

Programs to reduce smoking among teen-agers are urgently needed. They must objectively present the health risks, especially the immediate ones—accumulation of CO, decreased lung function, and impaired athletic performance. These effects can be demonstrated with objective methods of measurement. If presented to suitable groups of nonsmokers and smokers, interaction between students may reinforce the need to change smoking behavior. One should ask teen-agers to talk to one another about the risks of smoking,[77] with adults available to answer questions regarding objective health information or to offer psychological support when needed. Unfortunately, few programs implement and evaluate behavioral methods along these lines. Yet, it is likely that intensive and repeated exposure to the health risks of smoking is at least one factor in convincing teen-agers not to smoke.[79]

Risk-taking Behavior

Smoking is a form of risk-taking behavior.[16, 81] Tamerin and Resnik contrast creative or constructive risk-taking, characterized by positive aims, rational decision, and adequate preparation, with the impulsive and irrational features of destructive risk-taking.[81] As in other forms of neurotic risk-taking, the real risks of smoking far outweigh the real benefits. The fact that smoking is so prevalent indicates that many of us are prone to this kind of irrational risk-taking.

A quantitative assessment of the degree of risk involved in smoking, in terms of the individual, may help to highlight the need for changing smoking behavior. The presentation of national statistics (in terms of excess mortality and morbidity) is not sufficiently visible to the individual, who often likes to believe that statistics apply only to others. In fact, these statistics greatly underestimate the total risk. They do not assess the discomfort and the social and economical losses caused by chronic respiratory symptoms and disability. They also take no account of the demand for medical services created by these diseases. The loss to society caused by premature death of smokers is likewise ignored. A quantitative assessment of these effects of smoking needs to be made. A similar assessment of the risk of community air pollution and of such acknowledged high-risk activities as car racing would help to place the risk of smoking in proper perspective. Although such assessments probably add nothing to our understanding of smoking-induced disease in medical terms, from the social and political viewpoint they may be essential in designing policies and assigning priorities.

A rough computation of losses and gains from smoking, including only those losses ascribed to lung cancer and coronary infarction, has been made in Norway.[91] The total national loss for Norway, in 1964, amounted to about $40,000,000, in a country of 3.7 million people. If losses due to chronic bronchitis and emphysema as well as other social and economic losses (see above) were added, this figure would be much higher. The Norwegian smoker paid about $60,000,000 in tax revenues for tobacco in 1964. Thus, it appears that in Norway the smoker approximately "pays his own way" through taxation. A more precise assessment of losses would probably negate this statement and show that losses are much greater than tax revenues.

Giving up Smoking

The study of risk-taking behavior is of recent vintage, and the scientific basis for methods to change such behavior is weak. Methods and approaches to stop smoking are widely discussed (as in this chapter), but objective evaluations of these methods are lacking.[16, 55, 91] A few studies provide some tentative insights. Among 1527 exsmokers in Norway,[91] 39 percent cited symptoms as the principal reason for stopping smoking. A study of Hammond and Percy [35] indicated that 62 percent of 333 exsmokers quit because of symptoms; less than 10 percent of them were influenced by information about smoking and lung cancer. Since these studies were completed (in the 1950's), the impact of health information has probably increased. In any case, evidence concerning a person's present state of health appeared to be more persuasive than the risk of cancer. Even middle-aged people may consider the cancer threat to be far-off.

Studies of physicians also show how important the individual's personal experience is. Although US psychiatrists and internists have both tried hard to give up smoking, the internists have been far more successful in quitting. Tamerin and Eisinger [79] believe that the daily exposure of internists to smoking-induced disease helps them to stop; psychiatrists and pediatricians, who are equally unsuccessful, miss the exposure. Psychiatrists may also be too preoccupied with the difficulties in changing irrational human behavior. In 1968, only 22 percent of the internists in a random national sample of 5000 American physicians were current smokers; 50 percent were ex-smokers. Among psychiatrists, 42 percent were current smokers. Tamerin and Eisinger [79] outline the following factors as important in determining success with giving up smoking: "1) the extent of difficulty the individual anticipates in changing, 2) the individual's concern with setting an example for others, and particularly 3) the identification with the health consequences of smoking (i.e., damage to himself) as a result of direct, repeated exposure to this damage in others." Thus, the physician should not overemphasize the difficulty involved when he discusses a stop-smoking program with patients.

Smoking clinics, which have been organized in many U.S. and Canadian cities, use a variety of tactics to get the participants to quit, including group support. They may attract chiefly those who have already decided that they want to stop. Most smoking clinics have had only marginal success; only a minority of those attending become permanent exsmokers.[64] An intensive 2-week program guided by a psychiatrist resulted after 3 months in 5 exsmokers, from a group of 16 middle-aged, heavy-smoking suburban housewives.[78] Thus, a 30 percent success rate was achieved in a group that was strongly motivated toward smoking and whose members had been smoking, on the average, for more than 20 years. A well-designed program directed at younger people should be able to do at least as well, and probably better. The antismoking clinic may be too negative in its approach, and no-smoking advocates, in particular reformed smokers, are often untactful in their attitudes toward smokers. Attempts to quit among neurotic persons who are suddenly deprived of cigarettes by others, or who stop during a time of other stress, are usually unsuccessful and may, in fact, be harmful.[80]

Health education programs. A more positive approach would be to include information on health effects of smoking in comprehensive health education programs. Rode and Shephard [64] advocate a change of emphasis in antismoking programs, away from the more remote hazard of lung cancer, to the immediate health effects. The same idea motivated our studies among teen-agers in the New Haven area (p. 320). A comprehensive program should include preventive health surveillance as well as objective information on smoking, diet, physical fitness, and exercise. The approach should emphasize "health, well-being and mastery of self." [80] Adequate resources for preventive care in this sense (a task for Health Maintenance Organizations in the United States) would eliminate the need for special antismoking clinics. Positive policies and funding for such programs could sharply decrease the demand for medical care for lung and heart disease within the next 10 to 20 years. Objective methods to demonstrate health effects of smoking should be used in health education programs, as outlined above (p. 333). Scare tactics have no success and may be counterproductive.

Within the past ten years or so, millions of adults in the United States have stopped smoking, and the social acceptability of smoking has declined. Since the steady repetition of health information has almost certainly contributed to these changes in attitude and behavior, the information process should be reinforced and amplified. Information on the health hazards of smoking is widely available in the United States: on every pack of cigarettes, in brochures and on posters, and in messages in the mass media. The US government compiles and publishes periodic reviews on smoking and health.[82-87] Objective information on smoking and health should remain the principal basis for programs to reduce smoking.

Smoking Policies

Since the smoking habit is unlikely to be eliminated in the foreseeable future, a number of organizations need policies on smoking. Public policy should include a prohibition of smoking in all areas where this is warranted on the basis of (1) fire hazards, (2) accumulation of CO, (3) irritant effects upon nonsmokers, and (4) other health, hygienic, or safety considerations. Smoking at meetings is becoming a policy issue in many societies and organizations; as more people stop smoking, the habit is becoming socially less acceptable. Safety considerations (CO accumulation) apply in airplanes and buses. Prohibition of smoking by automobile drivers has been proposed.

Schools and hospitals are in a special position because of their social function as exemplary institutions. Smoking policies are debated in high schools throughout the country. Although teachers are aware of their importance as models, many of them smoke. Punitive measures against children for behavior that is condoned in adults are hard to defend. It is unjust to allow teachers to smoke on campus while expelling students who do the same. Apart from its unfairness, this places smoking in the position of desirable adult behavior. Every teen-ager wants to be considered mature, and if only adults may smoke, smoking becomes a logical way of achieving that aim. Some schools allow student smoking in approved areas and request teachers to limit or give up smoking on campus. Other school boards consider that the health risks of smoking make any official stamp of approval on smoking unethical, e.g., by designating smoking areas. That these issues are so actively discussed in our schools is highly encouraging. As a result of concerted efforts by schools and professionals, smoking among teen-agers and young adults will undoubtedly decrease over the next 5 years.

For hospitals, rational smoking policies should be easier to develop. Institutions charged with health care should be among the first to help educate the public concerning the health risks of smoking. A British organization, Action on Smoking and Health, Ltd., chaired by Dr. Charles Fletcher, has issued recommendations for smoking policies in hospitals,[72a] some of which follow here in abridged form.

"Hospital Staff: Workers in a Service for Health should not smoke. Those who do should not smoke in the presence of patients, nor while wearing white coats or hospital uniform. Smoking by doctors and nurses is particularly inappropriate and should only take place in their private rooms, if at all.

"Hospital Boards and Committees should not smoke. They should set an example to others and help them to comply with the rules they will be making.

"The hospital should become a place where cigarette smoking is only accepted for patients in exceptional circumstances. More than half the population are non-smokers and non-smoking in hospitals must be considered the normal. Notices should be placed in all wards such as 'In view of the health hazard and the discomfort to others, Please Do Not Smoke' or 'This is a Smoke-free Area.'

"Visitors and out-patients should not smoke and this policy should be enforced. Occasional exceptions may have to be made for relatives or patients in distress.

"Cigarettes should not be sold in hospital shops or on ward trolleys. Several hospitals have already stopped the sale of tobacco and this policy should be the rule. To discourage smoking and then to profit by the sale of cigarettes cannot be justified.

"Doctors and nurses should encourage patients to stop smoking while in hospital whatever the reason for their admission. Many patients have shown that they can do so.

"Teaching Hospitals and Medical Schools have a particular responsibility on smoking. They should give a lead on the control of smoking in the hospital and the education of students about its effects, and should devote more resources to research into the problem of smoking withdrawal."

SUMMARY

This chapter reviews the mortality and morbidity of smoking-induced lung disease, from official statistics and from surveys in diverse population groups. The early effects of smoking on lung function in young people are described, as is the individual variability of responses to smoke. Smoke and its constituents have both a short- and long-term effect on lung and airways; several mechanisms that can account for some of these effects are discussed. Cigarette smoke-induced lung cancer is highly prevalent, and several potential carcinogens in cigarette smoke have been identified.

We do not know to what extent early effects of smoking are reversible. Little is known about effects of marijuana smoking on the lungs. The smoking habit is discussed as a form of risk-taking behavior. Requirements and difficulties of programs to help people give up smoking are described, and recommendations concerning public policies, especially in schools and hospitals, are detailed.

REFERENCES

1. Addington WW, Carpenter RL, McCoy JF, Duncan KA, Mogg K: The association of cigarette smoking with respiratory symptoms and pulmonary function in a group of high school students. J Okla State Med Assoc, pp 525–529, Nov 1970

2. Albert RE, Alessandro D, Lippmann M, Berger J: Long-term smoking in the donkey. Arch Environ Health 22:12–19, 1971

3. Armitage AK, Hall GH, Morrison CF: Pharmacological basis for the tobacco smoking habit. Nature 217:331–334, 1968

4. Auerbach O, Hammond EC, Kirman D, Garfinkel L: Emphysema produced in dogs by cigarette smoking. JAMA 199:241–246, 1967

5. Auerbach O, Hammond EC, Kirman D, Garfinkel L: Effects of cigarette smoking on dogs. II. Pulmonary neoplasms. Arch Environ Health 21:754–768, 1970

6. Auerbach O, Hammond EC, Garfinkel L, Benante C: Relation of smoking and age to emphysema. Whole-lung section study. N Eng J Med 286:853–857, 1972

6a. Beaconsfield P, Ginsburg J, Rainsbury R: Marihuana smoking. Cardiovascular effects in man and possible mechanisms. N Eng J Med 287:209–212, 1972

7. Beckett AH, Gorrod JW, Jenner P: The effect of smoking on nicotine metabolism in vivo in man. J Pharm Pharmacol (suppl) 23:62S–67S, 1971

8. Beebe GW: Lung cancer in World War I veterans. Possible relation to mustard gas injury and 1918 influenza epidemic. J Natl Cancer Inst 25:1231–1252, 1960

9. Beeckmans JM: The deposition of aero-

sols in the respiratory tract. II. Deposition in cigarette smoking. Can J Physiol Pharmacol 43:707–714, 1965

10. Bouhuys A, Schilling RSF, van de Woestijne KP: Cigarette smoking, occupational dust exposure and ventilatory capacity. Arch Environ Health 19:793–797, 1969

11. Bretthauer EW, Black SC: Polonium–210: Removal from smoke by resin filters. Science 156:1375–1376, 1967

12. Camner P, Philipson K, Arvidsson T: Cigarette smoking in man. Short-term effect on mucociliary transport. Arch Environ Health 23:421–426, 1971

13. Carey GCR, Dawson TAJ, Merrett JD: Daily changes in ventilatory capacity in smokers and in non-smokers. Br J Prev Soc Med 21: 86–89, 1967

14. Carey GCR, Dawson TAJ, Merrett JD: Addendum to daily changes in ventilatory capacity in smokers and non-smokers. Br J Prev Soc Med 22:59, 1968

15. Carlson JR, Yokoyama MT, Dickinson EO: Induction of pulmonary edema and emphysema in cattle and goats with 3-methylindole. Science 176:298–299, 1972

16. Carney RE (ed): Risk-Taking Behavior. Springfield, Charles C Thomas, 1971

17. Chevalier RB, Krumholz RA, Ross JC: Reaction of nonsmokers to carbon monoxide inhalation. Cardiopulmonary responses at rest and during exercise. JAMA 198:1061–1064, 1966

18. Chiang ST, Wang BC: Acute effects of cigarette smoking on pulmonary function. Am Rev Respir Dis 101:860–868, 1970

19. Clark MSG, Rand MJ, Vanov S: Comparison of pharmacological activity of nicotine and related alkaloids occurring in cigarette smoke. Arch Int Pharmacodyn Ther 156:363–379, 1965

20. DaCosta JL, Tock EPC, Boey HK: Lung disease with chronic obstruction in opium smokers in Singapore. Clinical, electrocardiographic, radiological, functional, and pathological features. Thorax 26: 555–571, 1971

21. Dalhamn T, Rylander R: Ciliastatic action of smoke from filter-tipped and non-tipped cigarettes. Nature 201:401–402, 1963

22. Dautrebande L, Walkenhorst W: New studies on aerosols XXIV. Deposition rate of various microaerosols in human

lung with special reference to the hygroscopicity of the material inhaled and to cigarette smoke. Arch Int Pharmacodyn Ther 162:194–218, 1966

23. Doll R, Hill AB: Mortality in relation to smoking: Ten years' observations of British doctors. Br Med J 1:1399–1410 and 1460–1467, 1964

24. Douglas JS, Ridgway P, Dennis MW: Histamine release by air pollutants. Arch Environ Health 18:627–630, 1969

25. Douglas JS, Dennis MW, Ridgway P, Bouhuys A: Airway constriction in guinea pigs: Interaction of histamine and autonomic drugs. J Pharmacol Exp Ther 184:169–179, 1973

26. Egle JL Jr: Single-breath retention of acetaldehyde in man. Arch Environ Health 23:427–433, 1971

27. Eysenck HJ: Personality and cigarette smoking. Life Sci 3:777–792, 1964

28. Ferin J, Urbánková G, Vlčková A: Influence of tobacco smoke on the elimination of particles from the lungs. Nature 206:515–516, 1965

29. Frances R, Alessandro D, Lippmann M, Proctor DF, Albert RE: Effect of cigarette smoke on particle transport on nasociliary mucosa of donkeys. Arch Environ Health 21:25–31, 1970

30. Franklin W, Lowell FC: Unrecognized airway obstruction associated with smoking: A probable forerunner of obstructive pulmonary emphysema. Ann Intern Med 54:379–386, 1961

31. Glick SD, Zimmerberg B, Jarvik ME: Titration of oral nicotine intake with smoking behaviour in monkeys. Nature 233:207–208, 1971

32. Guillerm R, Saindelle A, Faltot P, Hée J: Étude chez le Cobaye des effets bronchomoteurs de la fumée de cigarette et de quelques-uns de ses constituants. J Physiol (Paris) 57:619–620, 1965

33. Guyatt AR, Berry G, Alpers JH, Bramley AC, Fletcher CM: Relationship of airway conductance and its immediate change on smoking to smoking habits and symptoms of chronic bronchitis. Am Rev Respir Dis 101:44–54, 1970

34. Hammond EC, Auerbach O, Kirman D, Garfinkel L: Effects of cigarette smoking on dogs. I. Design of experiment, mortality, and findings in lung parenchyma. Arch Environ Health 21:740–753, 1970

35. Hammond EC, Percy C: Ex-smokers. NY State J Med 58:2956–2959, 1958

36. Hanna MG Jr, Nettesheim P, Gilbert JR (eds): Inhalation Carcinogenesis. US Atomic Energy Commission, Division of Technical Information, 1970

37. Higgins ITT: Tobacco smoking, respiratory symptoms, and ventilatory capacity. Studies in random samples of the population. Br Med J 1:325–329, 1959

38. Holland WW, Elliott A: Cigarette smoking, respiratory symptoms and anti-smoking propaganda. Lancet 1:41–43, 1968

39. Holland WW, Halil T, Bennett AE, Elliott A: Factors influencing the onset of chronic respiratory disease. Br Med J 2:205–208, 1969

40. Huhti E: Prevalence of respiratory symptoms, chronic bronchitis and pulmonary emphysema in a Finnish rural population. Field survey of age 40–64 in the Harjavalta area. Acta Tuberc Pneumol Scand suppl 61:1–111, 1965

41. Huhti E: Ventilatory function in healthy non-smokers and smokers. Scand J Respir Dis 48:149–155, 1967

41a. Isaac PF, Rand MJ: Cigarette smoking and plasma levels of nicotine. Nature 236:308–310, 1972

41b. Koon LH, Chuan PS, Gandevia B: Ventilatory capacity in a group of opium smokers. Singapore Med J 11:75–79, 1970

42. Krumholz RA, Chevalier RB, Ross JC: Changes in cardiopulmonary functions related to abstinence from smoking. Ann Intern Med 62:197–207, 1965

43. Lanese RR, Banks FR, Keller MD: Smoking behavior in a teenage population: A multivariate conceptual approach. Am J Public Health 62:807–813, 1972

44. Langer AM, Mackler AD, Rubin I, Hammond EC, Selikoff IJ: Inorganic particles in cigars and cigar smoke. Science 174:585–587, 1971

45. LeBlanc P, Ruff F, Milic-Emili J: Effects of age and body position on "airway closure" in man. J Appl Physiol 28:448–451, 1970

46. Lebovits B, Ostfeld A: Smoking and personality: a methological analysis. J Chronic Dis 23:813–821, 1971

47. Leuchtenberger C, Leuchtenberger R: Morphological and cytochemical effects of marijuana cigarette smoke on epithelioid cells of lung explants from mice. Nature 234:227–229, 1971

48. Little JB, Radford EP Jr, McCombs HL, Hunt VR: Distribution of polonium[210] in pulmonary tissue of cigarette smokers. N Engl J Med 273:1343–1351, 1965

49. Lourenço RV, Klimek MF, Borowski CJ: Deposition and clearance of 2μ particles in the tracheobronchial tree of normal subjects—smokers and non-smokers. J Clin Invest 50:1411–1420, 1971

50. Lovejoy FW Jr, Dautrebande L: New studies on aerosols, XX. Effects of cigarette smoke on the airway conductance in smokers and non-smokers. Arch Int Pharmacodyn Ther 143:258–267, 1963

51. McCarthy TJ, van Zyl JD: Breath analysis of cannabis smokers. J Pharm Pharmacol 24:489, 1972

52. Mann PEG, Cohen AB, Finley TN, Ladman AJ: Alveolar macrophages. Structural and functional differences between nonsmokers and smokers of marijuana and tobacco. Lab Invest 25:111–120, 1971

53. Meadows SH, Wood CH, Schilling RSF: Respiratory symptoms and smoking habits of senior industrial staff. Br J Ind Med 22:149–153, 1965

53a. Miller GJ, Ashcroft MT, Beadnell HMSG, Wagner JC, Pepys J: The lipoid pneumonia of blackfat tobacco smokers in Guyana. Q J Med 40:457–470, 1971

54. Nadel JA, Comroe JH Jr: Acute effects of inhalation of cigarette smoke on airway conductance. J Appl Physiol 16:713–716, 1961

55. National Conference on Smoking and Health. A Summary of Proceedings. National Interagency Council on Smoking and Health, New York, 1970

55a. Neumeyer JL, Shagoury RA: Chemistry and pharmacology of marijuana. J Pharm Sci 60:1433–1457, 1971

56. Pantuck EJ, Kuntzman R, Conney AH: Decreased concentration of phenacetin in plasma of cigarette smokers. Science 175:1248–1250, 1972

57. Parrot J-L, Guillerm R, Ruff F, Saindelle A: Libération d'histamine par la fumée de cigarette et par quelques-uns de ses constituants. J Physiol (Paris) 58:580, 1966

58. Passey RD, Blackmore M, Warbrick-Smith D, Jones R: Smoking risks of different tobaccos. Br Med J 4:198–201, 1971

59. Pavia D, Thomson ML, Pocock SJ:

Evidence for temporary slowing of muco-ciliary clearance in the lung caused by tobacco smoking. Nature 231:325–326, 1971

60. Peters JM, Ferris BG Jr: Smoking, pulmonary function, and respiratory symptoms in a college age group. Am Rev Respir Dis 95:774–782, 1967

61. Powell GM, Green GM: Cigarette smoke—a proposed metabolic lesion in alveolar macrophages. Biochem Pharmacol 21:1785–1798, 1972

62. Pratt SA, Smith MH, Ladman AJ, Finley TN: The ultrastructure of alveolar macrophages from human cigarette smokers and nonsmokers. Lab Invest 24:331–338, 1971

63. Rajewsky B, Stahlhofen W: Polonium-210 activity in the lungs of cigarette smokers. Nature 209:1312–1313, 1966

64. Rode A, Ross R, Shephard RJ; Smoking withdrawal programme. Personality and cardiorespiratory fitness. Arch Environ Health 24:27–36, 1972

65. Rode A, Shephard RJ: The influence of cigarette smoking upon the oxygen cost of breathing in near-maximal exercise. Med Sci Sports 3:51–55, 1971

66. Rylander R: Free lung cell studies in cigarette smoke inhalation experiments. Scand J Respir Dis 52:121–128, 1971

67. Saindelle A, Flavian N, Guillerm R, Hée J: Libération d'histamine par la fumée de cigarette et ses constituants. CR Acad Sci [D] (Paris) 264:2926–2928, 1967

68. Salber EJ: Smoking among teen-agers. Bull NY Acad Med 44:1521–1525, 1968

69. Sanders CL, Jackson TA, Adee RR, Powers GJ, Wehner AP: Distribution of inhaled metal oxide particles in pulmonary alveoli. Arch Intern Med 127:1085–1089, 1971

70. Seely JE, Zuskin E, Bouhuys A: Cigarette smoking: Objective evidence for lung damage in teen-agers. Science 172:741–743, 1971

71. Singer AJ (ed): Marijuana: Chemistry, pharmacology, and patterns of social use. Ann NY Acad Sci 191:1–269, 1971

72. Sjöstrand T: Endogenous formation of carbon monoxide in man under normal and pathological conditions. Scand J Clin Lab Invest 1:201–214, 1949

72a. Smoking and the Hospital, A Conference jointly sponsored by ASH and the King's Fund Hospital Centre. Mimeographed transcript available from Action on

Smoking and Health, Ltd., 11 St. Andrew's Place, London, England

73. Sobonya RE, Kleinerman J: Morphometric studies of bronchi in young smokers. Am Rev Respir Dis 105:768–775, 1972

74. Stebbings JH Jr: Chronic respiratory disease among nonsmokers in Hagerstown, Maryland. I. Design of the study and prevalence of symptoms. Environ Res 4:146–162, 1971.

75. Stebbings, JH Jr: Chronic respiratory disease among nonsmokers in Hagerstown, Maryland. III. Social class and chronic respiratory disease. Environ Res 4:213–232, 1971

76. Strieder DJ, Kazemi H: Hypoxemia in young asymptomatic cigarette smokers. Ann Thorac Surg 4:523–531, 1967

77. Tamerin JS: The recent increase in adolescent cigarette smoking: A disquieting phenomenon examined. Arch Gen Psychiatry 28:116–119, 1973

78. Tamerin JS: The psychodynamics of quitting smoking in a group. Am J Psychiatry 129:589–594, 1972

79. Tamerin JS, Eisinger RA: Cigarette smoking and the psychiatrist. Am J Psychiatry 128:1224–1229, 1972

80. Tamerin JS, Neumann CP: Casualties of the antismoking campaign. Compr Psychiatry 14:35–40, 1973

81. Tamerin JS, Resnik HLP: Risk-taking by individual option. Case study: Cigarette smoking. Perspectives on benefit-risk decision making; the report of the colloquium of the National Academy of Engineering, Washington, pp 73–84, 1972

81a. Tashkin DP, Shapiro BJ, Frank IM: Acute pulmonary physiologic effects of smoked marijuana and oral Δ^9-tetrahydrocannibinol in young men. N Engl J Med 289:336–341, 1973

82. US Public Health Service: Smoking and Health. Report of the Advisory Committee to the Surgeon General of the Public Health Service. Washington, US Dept of Health, Education and Welfare, PHS publication no 1103, 1964

83. US Public Health Service: The Health Consequences of Smoking. A Public Health Service Review: 1967. Washington, US Dept of Health, Education and Welfare, PHS publication no 1696, January 1968

84. US Public Health Service: The Health Consequences of Smoking, 1968 Supple-

ment to the 1967 Public Health Service Review. Washington, US Dept of Health, Education and Welfare, PHS publication no 1696, 1968

85. US Public Health Service: The Health Consequences of Smoking, 1969 Supplement to the 1967 Public Health Service Review. Washington, US Dept of Health, Education and Welfare, PHS publication no 1696-2, 1969

86. US Public Health Service: The Health Consequences of Smoking, A Report of the Surgeon General: 1971. Washington, US Dept of Health, Education and Welfare, DHEW no (HSM) 71-7513, 1971

87. US Public Health Service: The Health Consequences of Smoking, A Report of the Surgeon General: 1972. Washington, US Dept of Health, Education and Welfare, DHEW no (HSM) 72-7516, 1972

87a. Vachon L, FitzGerald MX, Solliday NH, Gould IA, Gaensler EA: Single-dose effect of marijuana smoke: Bronchial dynamics and respiratory-center sensitivity in normal subjects. N Eng J Med 288: 985–989, 1973

88. van der Lende R: Epidemiology of Chronic Non-Specific Lung Disease (Chronic Bronchitis). Springfield, Charles C Thomas, 1969

89. van der Lende R, deKroon JPM, van der Meulen GG, Tammeling GJ, Visser BF, deVries K, Orie NGM: Possible indicators of endogenous factors in the development of CNSLD, in Orie NGM, van der Lende R (eds): Bronchitis III. Assen, The Netherlands, Royal Van Gorcum, 1970, pp 52–70

90. van Duuren BL, Sivak A, Katz C, Melchionne S: Cigarette smoke carcinogenesis: Importance of tumor promoters. J Natl Cancer Inst 47:235–240, 1971

91. Wakefield J (ed): Influencing Smoking Behaviour. UICC Technical Report Series, vol 3. Geneva, International Union against Cancer, 1969

92. Welch RM, Loh A, Conney AH: Cigarette smoke: Stimulatory effect on metabolism of 3,4-benzpyrene by enzymes in rat lung. Life Sci [I] 10:215–221, 1971

93. Wilhelmsen L: Effects on bronchopulmonary symptoms, ventilation, and lung mechanics of abstinence from tobacco smoking. Scand J Respir Dis 48:407–414, 1967

94. Wilhelmsen L, Tibblin G: Tobacco smoking in fifty-year-old men. I. Respiratory symptoms and ventilatory function tests. Scand J Respir Dis 47:121–130, 1966

95. Winternitz MC, Wason IM, McNamara FP: The Pathology of Influenza. New Haven, Yale University Press, 1920

96. Woolf CR, Suero JT: The respiratory effects of regular cigarette smoking in women. Am Rev Respir Dis 103:26–37, 1971

97. Wynder EL, Hoffmann D, Ashwanden P (eds): Less Harmful Ways of Smoking. A Workshop of the Second World Conference on Smoking and Health, held in London, England, Sept. 20–24, 1971. J Natl Cancer Inst 48:1739–1891, 1972

98. Zuskin E, Mitchell CA, Bouhuys A: Interaction between effects of beta blockade and cigarette smoke on airways. J Appl Physiol (In press)

Chapter 15

Occupational Lung Disease

Occupational lung diseases are caused by environmental exposures that occur during one's work. Thus, the circumstances of exposure rather than the nature of the inhalant or of its effects on the lungs determine whether a disease is included among the occupational lung diseases. For example, smokers (Chap. 16, p. 395), and possibly city dwellers (Chap. 16, p. 403), are exposed to potentially injurious levels of NO_2. However, only silage workers, welders, and others whose work leads to NO_2 exposures can, by definition, develop an occupational lung disease. Similarly, while many environmental inhalants, such as grass pollens, can induce asthma, only pollen exposure resulting from one's job, e.g., as a professional gardener, causes occupational asthma.

Occupational lung diseases are grouped together because they share certain legal and social implications and because they can be prevented by changing the work environment—that is, by removing either the inhalant from the atmosphere or the worker from the noxious environment. Occupational exposures occur in industry as well as in agriculture and may lead to acute disease after brief, heavy exposures, or to chronic disease after lesser but prolonged exposures. In addition, repeated exposures may cause repeated acute lung damage. Three main classes of agents can cause occupational lung disease: (1) gases, vapors, and fumes (pp. 344–351); (2) mineral dusts (pp. 351–371); and (3) organic dusts (pp. 371–374).

Gases, vapors, and fumes usually cause mainly acute responses, including chemical bronchitis, lung edema, chemical pneumonitis, and, in some cases, asthma (Table 15-1). Mineral dusts may or may not cause acute responses (cough, sputum production), but the main risks are the chronic tissue responses resulting from long-term exposure: lung fibrosis, granuloma formation, pneumonitis (Table 15-2). Organic dusts lead to pharmacological and immunologic responses (Table 15-2), which may be acute, recurrent, or chronic, depending primarily on the level and frequency of exposure.

Since the mechanisms of lung disease have already been discussed in general terms (Chap. 12), this chapter focuses on the specific exposures and their effects, classified according to agent. Occupational causes of lung cancer are discussed in a separate section, because a variety of agents may lead to this disease. Before discussing specific agents and diseases, however, a general approach to the detection and prevention of occupational lung disease will be presented.

DETECTION AND PREVENTION

Risks of lung disease caused by dust produced during tool grinding, textile processing, coal mining, quarrying, and pottery making are as old as the activities themselves. Ramazzini [153] described these and many other occupational hazards in the early 18th century. But new materials and procedures discovered since then continue to increase the list of hazardous inhaled substances. Concentration of workers in factories and the faster production rates of the 19th and 20th centuries have increased the amounts of inhalants as well as the number of people exposed for a substantial portion of their lives.

The systematic study of occupational lung diseases is about 100 years old. In the United States, Dr. Alice Hamilton (1869–1970) did pioneering work early in this century. In Great Britain, J.S. Haldane undertook physiological studies in miners as early as 1890. However, only in the past 20 years have laboratory studies led to a broader understanding of the pathogenesis of several occupational lung diseases. Most progress has been made from epidemiological studies of disease prevalence (Chap. 13) combined with environmental measurements to quantitate the exposures, and with laboratory research to elucidate the action of the inhaled agents. Detailed epidemiological studies that include control groups are necessary for reasons discussed in Chapter 13 and illustrated in Table 13–2. Environmental measurements help to pinpoint the sources and describe the distribution of inhalants in workrooms, an essential step in determining who is at risk and how to prevent exposure.

Prevention of occupational lung disease is the employer's responsibility, described in detail in the US Williams-Steiger Occupational Safety and Health Act of 1970. The Act states that: "The Congress declares it to be its purpose and policy . . . to assure as far as possible every working man and woman in the Nation safe and healthful working conditions. . . ." The Act provides for the setting and enforcement of exposure standards, for assistance to the states in their occupational health and safety programs, and for research, education, and training.

In providing for uniform standards, the OSH Act has already improved US occupational health. In the past, management and labor unions alike were often either unaware of health risks, confused by conflicting or unconvincing data, or unwilling to accept evidence that risks existed and should be eliminated. Although working conditions in risk industries have been much improved in the past 20 years, these improvements depended largely on chance—the persistence of individual hygienists or physicians rather than a concerted effort to develop safe conditions throughout industry. Given the increasing number and variety of hazardous industrial exposures, a legal framework to protect workers became essential.

Now that a national policy on occupational health has been established, the OSH Act's ultimate effectiveness will depend on its enforcement. This requires consistent interpretation of the Act's scope and intent,[175] along with the setting of standards for programs to prevent specific hazards.[179] These standards should include not only appropriate threshold limit values (TLV's) but also mandatory medical examinations of workers, environmental measurements to obtain baseline data for prevention programs, and appropriate environmental control measures. The US Department of Labor has designated five target health hazards as priority items, including three important pulmonary hazards: asbestos, cotton, and silica.[187] In some industries, occupational health programs are beginning to be a subject of management-union negotiations, and much can be achieved by programs under their joint sponsorship.[186a] Unfortunately, the resources to operate prevention and control programs in industry are still quite limited, and the most basic deficiency is in the supply of physicians and other personnel trained in occupational health. One hopeful sign is a recent textbook [165] which provides much-needed guidance for students in this field.

The task of the individual industrial physician responsible for the health of employees is complex. He must assess the risks of the many possible exposures within industry, and he is up against ever-changing industrial procedures as well as changes in the worker population. For instance, since his experience usually is limited to the active work force exposed in a factory, he often loses track of retired workers; thus, his population is biased in favor of healthy individuals. He must deal with many health problems and usually does not have adequate resources to investigate each fully. The industrial physician often requires support resources from regional or national groups with expertise in epidemiology, occupational diseases, and environmental hygiene.

Compensation laws, which provide financial recompense to workers disabled by conditions arising from their employment, differ among the various states and countries with respect to compensable diseases, the degree of disability required for an award, and the level of compensation provided. These laws can provide incentives for prevention and control; for example, if the awards are financed from contributions of industry, or if the law includes provisions for early reassignment of affected workers to nonrisk jobs. Usually, however, the laws offer only solace to individual victims and add little impetus to disease prevention.

Previous chapters provide more detailed discussions of methods in environmental hygiene (Chap. 12, pp. 280–282), epidemiology (Chap. 13), and medical surveillance (Chap. 13, pp. 301–302). In the sections which follow, these methods will be applied to discussions of specific exposures.

EFFECTS OF GASES, VAPORS, AND FUMES

Gaseous pollutants and fumes may cause illnesses by their own actions or they may, by displacing oxygen, result in hypoxia (asphyxiant atmospheres). Table 15-1 lists some agents that cause lung or airways responses in animals and in man, notes some circumstances under which human exposure may occur, indicates the approximate nature of the effects observed, and shows the pollutant levels presently considered relatively safe for workrooms. These data are derived from several sources [4, 139] and other references quoted in this section. The description of the responses comes largely from observations of gross and microscopic pathology in animals and from qualitative clinical observations in man. Since quantitative data on the time course of responses and the effects of minor exposures are rare, Table 15-1 is based primarily on older studies, which probably overestimate some threshold limit values (Chap. 12, p. 281). The lack of objective laboratory data on many agents in humans results largely from difficulties in studying their effects under controlled conditions. The responses are often brief and may go undetected; in other instances they are severe and require intensive emergency treatment, which does not allow time for detailed and controlled laboratory studies of lung function. Since control data on the patient before exposure are usually not available, it is difficult to determine if his recovery is complete. A person whose vital capacity is 85 percent of the predicted value some weeks after an acute response to chlorine exposure may be fully recovered (since his VC might have been 85 percent before exposure), or he may have a significant lung volume decrement (since his VC might also have been 120 percent of that predicted before exposure).

In the following sections, a few agents for which more data are available are discussed in greater detail; these illustrate the main responses to their respective class of pollutants. Only exposures to single substances will be discussed, since information on interactions occurring with mixed exposures is minimal. While many workers are exposed to mixtures of pollutants, the contribution of each component to the overall response is often difficult to evaluate. For instance, silver brazers are exposed to cadmium (from the solder), nitrogen dioxide (formed by the torch), and fluorides (from the flux);[115] arc welders are exposed to an even more complex mixture.[180] Some cumulative hazard probably results from these combined exposures.

Cadmium

Acute exposures to cadmium oxide fume occur during welding and silver brazing.[19] Small amounts of Cd are normally ingested with food (shellfish in particular). Cigarette smoke contains about 0.7 μg Cd per cigarette. Cadmium accumulates in the kidneys, pancreas, liver, and hair, and it damages the kidneys.[132, 133] Tissues of smokers contain more Cd than those of nonsmokers.[108] Acute exposure to high concentrations of cadmium oxide fume causes acute pneumonitis, often resembling a viral infection.[18] Early recognition of the exposure is important; steroids rather than antibiotics may arrest the inflammatory process. Airway obstruction and emphysema may occur after prolonged Cd exposure.[20] Recent function studies in 11 men exposed to 1.21–2.70 mg Cd/cu m during 7 to 11 years did not show emphysema or airway obstruction; 5 of these workers had unexplained grade 3 dyspnea on exertion.[188]

Chlorine

Agents such as acids and ammonia cause immediate responses (tearing eyes, sore throat, severe cough), alerting the worker to withdraw quickly from exposure. Chlorine has fewer immediate effects but causes severe responses after several hours. Exposure is often prolonged because of insufficient warning from the immediate responses. Inflammation of small airways and lung edema with cough,

Table 15-1

Gases, Vapors, and Fumes With Effects on Lower Airways and Lungs

Compound	Principal Effect on Airways and Lungs	TLV (1973) ppm	Examples of Usage and Exposures
Acetaldehyde	B	100	Chemical synthesis
Acetic acid	B *	10	
Acetic anhydride	B	C 5	Cellulose production
Acrolein	B, E	0.1	Coating of paper
Ammonia	B *, E *	25	
Boron trifluoride	P	C 1	Catalyst
Bromine	E *	0.1	
Cadmium oxide fume	P *	C 0.1 (0.05) mg Cd/cu m	Electroplating, alloys, welding
Chlorine	B *, E *	1	Bleaching
Chlorine dioxide	B *	0.1	Bleaching; cellulose manufacturing
Chlorine trifluoride	B, E	C 0.1	Oxidant; high-energy fuel
α-chloroacetophenone	E *	0.05	Tear gas (riot-control agent)
Diazomethane	A, P *	0.2	Chemical laboratories
Diborane	E	0.1	High-energy fuel
Dimethylamine	B, E, P	10	Chemical synthesis
Diphenyl	B	0.2	Coolant
Formaldehyde	B	C 2	
Formic acid	B	5	
Hydrogen chloride	B *	C 5	
Hydrogen fluoride	E *	3	Etching
Hydrogen sulfide	E, P *, RP	10	
Indium sesquioxide	E *	0.1 mg In/cu m	Welding transistor parts
Iodine	B *, E	C 0.1	
Isopropylamine	E	5	
Ketene	E	0.5	Oxidant; chemical industry
Lithium hydride	B	0.025 mg/cu m	Isotope extraction
Mercury vapor	E *, P *	0.05 mg/cu m	Power plants; laboratories
Methylacetate	B *	200	Solvent
Methylamine	B *	10	Chemical synthesis
Methylformate	E *	100	Solvent
Methylmercaptan	E, RP	0.5	
Methylene bisphenyl isocyanate (MDI)	A	C 0.02	Spraying of polyurethane foam
Nickel carbonyl	C *	0.007 mg/cu m	Nickel refineries (Mond process)
Nitric acid	B, P *	2	
Nitrogen dioxide	P *	C 5	Welding; component of photochemical smog
Osmium tetroxide	B *, E	0.002 mg/cu m	Metal refining; electron microscopy
Oxygendifluoride	E	0.05	Oxidant

Table 15-1   (Continued)

Gases, Vapors, and Fumes With Effects on Lower Airways and Lungs

Compound	Principal Effect on Airways and Lungs	TLV (1973) ppm	Examples of Usage and Exposures
Ozone	E *	0.1	Welding; component of photochemical smog
Perchloryl fluoride	E, P	3	
Phosgene	E *, P *	0.1	Organic synthesis; product of combustion of chlorinated solvents
Phosphine	E *	0.3	Generation of acetylene
Phthalic anhydride	B *	2	Manufacture of plasticizers, resins, and dyes
Selenium compounds	A *, B *, P *	0.2 mg Se/ cu m	Metal refining
Sulfur dioxide	B *	5	Product of fossil fuel combustion; oil refining; paper industry
Sulfuric acid	B *	1 mg/cu m	Battery manufacture; air pollutant
Sulfur monochloride	B	1	Rubber curing
Sulfur pentafluoride	E	0.025	
Sulfuryl fluoride	E	5	Fumigant
Tellurium hexafluoride	E	0.02	
Terphenyls	B *, E	C 1	Coolants
Tetranitromethane	E *, P *	1	Explosives industry
Toluene -2, 4-diisocyanate (TDI)	A *	C 0.02	Polyurethane manufacture
Trimethylbenzene	A *	25	Solvent
Vanadium pentoxide	B *, E *, P *	0.5 mg V/cu m for dust C 0.05 mg V/ cu m for fumes	Mining and milling of V; cleaning oil burners
Vinylacetate	B *	10	
Yttrium	F	1 mg/cu m	Metal industry
Zinc chloride fume	B *, P *, F *	1 mg/cu m	Smoke generators
Zinc oxide fume	M	5 mg/cu m	Galvanizing

This table lists selected compounds with effects on the respiratory system. Many of these have other toxic effects as well. Agents for which these other effects are the principal determinant of toxicity have not been listed. Asphyxiant gases also have been omitted.

Effects on airways and lungs: A=asthma, B=chemical bronchitis, C=lung cancer, E=lung edema, F=lung fibrosis, M=metal fume fever, P=chemical pneumonitis, RP= respiratory paralysis.

* Indicates that the description of effects is at least in part based on human exposures.

TLV=threshold limit values according to reference 5, reproduced with permission of the American Conference of Governmental Industrial Hygienists. TLV values are listed as parts per million except where shown otherwise. TLV values are time-weighted averages for an 8-hour exposure except when preceded by C, which indicates a ceiling value which should never be exceeded. Values in parentheses are intended changes of TLV (see reference 5). Examples of usage have not been listed for compounds used in many chemical and other industries. Sources: see text and references 4 and 139.

sputum production, chest tightness, dyspnea, and cyanosis may take up to 24 hours to develop. Blood gas determinations show arterial hypoxemia. Treatment is empirical and usually requires oxygen to abolish hypoxemia, antibiotics to prevent infection, and steroids to reduce inflammation.[21] Recovery is the rule in hospital-treated patients; nevertheless, residual function loss (reduced lung volumes, compliance, and diffusing capacity) persisted several years after a severe acute exposure in one group of 17 men.[98]

Isocyanates

Exposures to toluene diisocyanate (TDI) and to methylene-bisphenylisocyanate (MDI) occur in the manufacture and spraying of polyurethane.[143] These polymer compounds, widely used as insulation material, also emit TDI and MDI when heated, although the compounds are not combustible in the strict sense. Thus, isocyanate exposure occurs during fires in polyurethane factories [121] and may contribute to passenger deaths during fires in airplane wrecks. Recently, US space officials became concerned about TDI exposure when the interior of Skylab was severely overheated and toxic vapors including isocyanates were released from the insulation material (New York Times, May 31, 1973). Exposed persons may develop chest tightness, wheezing, and shortness of breath immediately or after several years of exposure without symptoms, suggesting that sensitization takes place.[9] Delayed effects may also follow a single intensive exposure, as in some firemen where sputum production and decreased lung function appeared only several months after exposure.[121] Low levels of TDI exposure lead to less dramatic but nevertheless significant effects on lung function, often without accompanying symptoms. Frequently $FEV_{1.0}$ decreases during a single work shift, especially in the beginning of the work week.[64, 143] In addition, $FEV_{1.0}$ decreases more rapidly over the longer term than can be expected from the normal effect of aging. In workers exposed to less than 0.02 ppm TDI, a presumably safe level (Table 15-1), the long-term decrement of $FEV_{1.0}$ (over 2.5 years) was several times increased and correlated with the acute $FEV_{1.0}$ changes observed initially.[144] Airway constriction may contribute to the decreased flow rates after TDI exposures,[104] but an effect of TDI on lung elastic recoil has not been ruled out. A recent code of practice provides detailed descriptions of precautionary measures and medical surveillance.[191]

Another isocyanate, 2-chlorethylisocyanate, used in the pharmaceutical industry, causes bronchitis and pneumonia in rats. Its inhalation toxicology resembles that of MDI; a TLV of 0.02 ppm has been suggested.[88]

Mercury Vapor

Accidental inhalation of mercury vapor may cause severe acute interstitial pneumonitis leading to permanent lung damage.[78]

Nickel Carbonyl

See lung cancer (p. 375).

Nitrogen Dioxide

Effects of low levels of nitrogen oxides on the lungs are discussed in Chapter 16. Acute high exposures occur, for instance, in insufficiently ventilated grain silos (silo-filler's disease [113]) and in welders who work in closed spaces.[134] Such exposures may cause acute chemical pneumonitis, usually after a latent period. Thus, clinical observation for 48 hours in exposed persons is recommended.[193] The main symptom is shortness of breath. The effects on the lungs may be in two stages—first, an acute phase with pulmonary edema, and second, a more slowly developing phase with small-airway obstruction (bronchiolitis). The acute stage may remain subclinical, with no symptoms of dyspnea and nonproductive cough until 2 to 6 weeks after exposure.[93] Severe restrictive function loss with arterial hypoxemia, hyperventilation and reduced diffusing capacity occurs in both phases of the disease.[93] Treatment with corticosteroids is probably effective, although no controlled studies have been made. Functional recovery is not always complete.

Ozone

See Chapter 16.

Phosgene

Phosgene ($COCl_2$) inhalation occurred on a large scale during World War I when it was used as a war gas, but inhalation is rare today. The damaging effects of this highly irritant gas probably result from its release of HCl and chlorine in the lungs. This hydrolysis takes time, and the gas does not irritate upper airways but exerts its effects only on the small airways and lung parenchyma. Acute severe exposure leads to lung edema and destruction of the epithelium of small airways. Low exposure levels cause proliferative changes in the alveoli and bronchioles.[75] In dogs, low-level exposure (24–40 ppm) produced pulmonary emphysema, probably at least in part as a result of widespread small-airway obstruction.[26]

Sulfur Dioxide

A single severe exposure to this gas can cause lung edema, followed by progressive loss of lung function and irreversible damage to the airways (case report in reference 12). Long-term industrial exposure (pulp mill workers) to 2–36 ppm SO_2 was associated with an increased prevalence of cough, sputum, and dyspnea.[176] Although, in experimental exposures (see Chap. 16), 1 ppm SO_2 in air for less than 5 minutes can cause significant decreases in maximum flow rates, the TLV for SO_2 in workroom air (for an 8-hour exposure) is five times higher than this level (Table 15-1). Workers continuously exposed to high levels of SO_2 in industry may be a selected group of individuals insensitive to this gas, but unfortunately no objective data are available to support the validity of the 5 ppm TLV. The two surveys quoted in documenting this TLV[4] did not include objective function data which reflect airway obstruction; the peak flow rate used in one of them[176] does not qualify as such (see p. 191, Chap. 9). The effects of low levels of SO_2 are further discussed in Chapter 16.

Other Exposures With Acute Effects on Lungs and Airways

This group includes some imprecisely defined exposures, agents for which no TLV has been set, and one agent that causes lung damage after ingestion.

Metal fumes. Various metal fumes, including zinc oxide (Table 15-1), cadmium, manganese, and nickel may cause an ill-documented syndrome consisting of fever, chills, and malaise, often occurring on first working days after absence from work. It lasts 24–48 hours and is not accompanied by x-ray changes. No function tests appear to have been done in workers at risk.

Polymer fumes. Heat-degradation products of polytetrafluorethylene (Teflon®) can cause short-lasting attacks of chest tightness, cough, and fever easily mistaken for a cold.[149] In one instance, a worker exposed herself with contaminated cigarettes; nonsmokers in the same workplace were unaffected.[200]

CS. Orthochloro-benzylidene malonitrile, dispersed as an aerosol, is used as a riot-control agent because of its immediate irritating effects on the eyes and airways. In use for at least 10 years, it is considered safe, since exposed persons withdraw quickly from exposure and the effects then cease in minutes. Gradual exposure leads to some degree of habituation.[17] Vital capacity and peak flow remained unchanged during exposures to higher levels than those encountered in actual use,[17] and diffusing capacity measurements showed small and transient changes.[32] However, no measurements of flows at low lung volumes, which reflect small-airway obstruction, have been reported. Since the immediate effects of CS aerosol include chest tightness and difficulty in breathing,[17] these measurements might be more relevant than those reported (see Chap. 9).

Tear gas (Table 15-1), a riot-control agent of longer standing, is known to have caused lethal pulmonary edema and permanent eye damage.[4] The populations exposed to these agents are likely to include persons with asthma or other chronic lung diseases, who may be more sensitive to them than others. Because there is probably a wide dispersion of sensitivities to any kind of toxicological agent used for riot control, development of a safe agent may be an illusory goal.

Asphyxiant atmospheres. These commonly develop during fires in which persons are trapped in closed spaces where burning depletes oxygen, while carbon monoxide and other toxic gases accumulate. Although these exposures cause what is often described as smoke inhalation effects, several agents and mechanisms may be involved. Hypoxia and CO exposure caused coronary infarction in 2 out of 6 people trapped in an elevator during a fire.[102] Smoke from burning wood and cotton may cause lung edema because of its aldehyde content.[203] Fatalities have also occurred in the absence of fire, for instance, in the holds of cutters landing trash fish for use in fish-meal plants in Denmark. The air in some of these holds contained less than 7 percent oxygen, up to 40 percent CO_2, from 25 to over 2000 ppm H_2S (TLV = 10 ppm), and high concentrations of various amines. Three fatal exposures occurred in such holds and several crew members were removed unconscious. Among workers in confined spaces, even instances of minor fainting should lead to air sampling and assessment of atmospheric conditions in the work area.[35]

Paraquat. Ingestion of this herbicide causes extensive tissue damage, and may result in death from renal or respiratory failure. Lung lesions—including lung edema, cellular proliferation in the alveoli, and bronchiolitis—are usually irreversible and may lead to death from respiratory failure at a later stage. However, clinical recovery is possible.[65] Lung function tests showed restriction of lung volumes and a decreased diffusing capacity during the first 2 days after ingestion, with partial recovery 3 weeks later. In rats, paraquat causes infiltration of the lungs with macrophage cells.[59]

CHRONIC OCCUPATIONAL DISEASES
CAUSED BY MINERAL DUSTS

Table 15-2 lists chronic occupational lung diseases under two main headings—those caused by inhalation of mineral dusts and those caused by inhalation of organic dusts. The former are often referred to as the pneumoconioses, but there is no general agreement on the definition of this term (p. 267). Its use is often reserved for diseases that cause changes on chest x-ray films due to dust accumulation or tissue response to dust, or both. However, chest x-ray changes usually do not correlate well with the degree of functional impairment. Extensive shadows on the chest x-ray film may occur without much functional impairment; disabling function loss may occur while the chest x-ray film remains normal or nearly so. Lung-function tests are often more sensitive than x-ray films for purposes of early detection and offer a better guide to a person's ability to perform manual work. In the following paragraphs, individual exposures are discussed in the order of their appearance in Table 15-2.

Aluminum

Aluminum and aluminum oxide dust are usually considered inert substances. However, several cases of lung fibrosis in workers exposed to these dusts have been documented, in part from lung-function studies showing restrictive and obstructive function loss.[12, 178] No prevalence studies appear to have been performed.

Asbestos

Many industries (Table 15-2) use asbestos for its thermal and electrical insulation properties, its tensile strength, and its immunity to attack by chemicals. Table 15-3 describes the various forms of hydrated silicates which are the most common commercial forms of asbestos. Virtually indestructible, the fibers persist indefinitely when inhaled into the lungs. Three main health risks are associated with inhalation of asbestos fibers: asbestosis, lung cancer, and mesothelioma. Pleural plaques, the most frequent sign of asbestos exposure, are a benign process.

Asbestosis. Asbestos fibers cause widespread increase of connective tissue throughout the lung parenchyma. This diffuse interstitial lung fibrosis usually results from prolonged and heavy asbestos exposure. It is often accompanied by pleural plaques (see below). In animal experiments, injection of chrysotile or

Table 15-2
Summary of Chronic Occupational Lung Diseases

Agent	Industries	Diseases	Pathology	TLV (1973)
Mineral dusts				
Aluminum and aluminum oxide	Bauxite mining; corundum smelting; abrasives; explosives; paints; fireworks	Aluminosis, bauxite lung	F	10 mg Al_2O_3/cu m *
Asbestos	Insulation; brake linings; lagging; construction; shipyards	Asbestosis; mesothelioma; lung cancer	See text	5 fibers/ml †
Barium sulfate	Barite mining	Baritosis	D	0.5 mg Ba/cu m
Beryllium compounds	Aircraft manufacturing; metallurgy; rocket fuels	Beryllium disease	F,G,P	0.002 mg Be/cu m
Coal dust	Coal mining; transport of coal	Coal workers' pneumoconiosis (CWP)	B,F	2 mg/cu m ‡
Cobalt	Cutting-tool industry	Hard metal disease	F	0.1 mg/cu m
Iron oxide	Welding; foundries	Siderosis	D	5 mg/cu m
Kaolin	Porcelain	Kaolin pneumoconiosis	F	10 mg/cu m *
Magnesium silicates (talc)	Rubber industry; lubricants	Talcosis	F+	6.7 mg/cu m
Platinum salts	Refineries; chemicals; electronics	Platinum asthma	A	0.002 mg Pt/cu m
Silica (SiO_2)	Mining (gold, tin, copper, graphite, coal); pottery; sand blasting; foundries; quarries (granite, slate, sandstone)	Silicosis	F	See legend
Tin oxide	Tin foundries	Stannosis	D	10 mg/cu m *

Organic dusts

Allergens (partial listing)				
Castor bean	Castor oil manufacture			
Flour	Bakeries			
Grain weevil	Grain handling			
Guinea pig hair	Laboratories	Asthma	A	—
Gum acacia	Printing			
Tamarind seed	Yarn finishing			
Bagasse	Sugar cane waste processing	Bagassosis	P, F	—
Cotton, flax, and hemp dust	Textiles	Byssinosis	A, B	1 (0.2) mg/cu m §
Enzyme detergents	Laundry products	Asthma	A	0.06 µg/cu m ‖
Moldy hay	Farming	Farmer's lung	P, F	—
Pigeon and other bird droppings	Pigeon breeders; bird fanciers	Pigeon breeder's lung Bird fancier's lung	P, F	—

Modified and expanded from reference 21.

Pathology: A=reversible airway obstruction (chronic effects, see text); B=bronchitis; D=dust deposits without marked tissue response; F=fibrosis; G=granulomas; P=pneumonitis; +=fibrous forms of talc behave like asbestos.

Threshold limit values (TLV):

For silica derive TLV from equation: $TLV = \dfrac{300}{\%\ \text{quartz} + 10} \times 35.3$ particles/ml, where % quartz=concentration in airborne dust. For example, for dust with 25% quartz, TLV=302 particles/ml. [*Note:* Recent reports on dust exposure, lung function and roentgenographic changes in Vermont granite workers (Theriault GP et al, Arch Environ Health 28:12–27, 1974) favor the setting of a TLV in terms of respirable quartz; we (A. Bouhuys and J. B. Schoenberg) have concluded from their data that this TLV might be set at 35 µg/m³ respirable quartz.]

* Nuisance particulate (see text).   † Fibers > 5 µm long.   ‡ If respirable dust fraction contains less than 5% quartz.   § Present TLV 1 mg/cu m total dust; intended change to 0.2 mg/cu m lintfree dust measured with vertical elutriator (see Chap. 17).   ‖ As 100 percent pure crystalline enzyme. —: no TLV established.

For references see text; TLV data from reference 5, with permission of the American Conference of Governmental Industrial Hygienists.

Table 15-3
Varieties of Asbestos

Variety	Formula	Principal sites of origin
Serpentine		
Chrysotile	$Mg_3Si_2O_5(OH_4)$	Canada
Amphibole		
Anthophyllite	$(Mg\ Fe)_7Si_8O_{22}(OH)$	South Africa
Amosite	$Ca_2MgFe_2Na_3Si_8O_{22}(OH)$	South Africa
Crocidolite	$Na_3Fe_3Fe_2Si_8O_{23}(OH)$	South Africa

Reproduced from reference 202.

crocidolite asbestos into the pleural cavity causes formation of granulomas followed by fibrosis.[36] Intratracheal injection of a suspension of chrysotile in rats causes extensive lesions of small airways and fibrosis.[22] Phagocytosis of fibers by alveolar macrophage cells and subsequent death of the macrophage may influence the initiation of this process (see p. 268).

In lung tissue, peculiar reaction products, or asbestos bodies, form around asbestos fibers. These bodies, which often occur in the sputum of exposed persons, are coated asbestos fibers. Once coated, the fibers may lose their effect on lung tissue.[89] Their coating contains iron, probably in ferritin or hemosiderin.[37] Since the bodies can also be induced by other fibers (e.g., fine glass fibers or ceramic aluminum silicate [37]), some prefer the name ferruginous bodies to asbestos bodies. Electronmicroscopic studies can distinguish asbestos fibers from these other fibers.[74, 150] The origin of the coating of the fibers in asbestos bodies is uncertain. Since the coating contains acid mucopolysaccharides, it may be derived from intercellular matter rather than from cells.[71]

Asbestos exposure can be demonstrated by finding asbestos bodies in sputum and, recently, by mapping the magnetic field around the chest with a magnetometer.[29] The diagnosis of asbestosis requires a history of exposure (usually more than 10 years in risk jobs) and certain clinical findings—bilateral rales over the lung bases; clubbing of the fingers; increased and irregular, linear, nodular markings evident on the chest x-ray film; and restrictive lung-function loss (Fig. 9-6). The diffusing capacity is usually decreased, and the patient complains of dyspnea on exertion. Obstructive lung disease is equally common among asbestos workers and control subjects;[125] the prevalence of bronchitic symptoms in asbestos workers is related to smoking and not to dust exposure, while dyspnea correlates with age and dust exposure and not with smoking.[119] Hence, cough is not a symptom of asbestosis, while dyspnea is.

Epidemiological surveys of asbestos workers require standardization of history taking (by questionnaire, Chap. 13), chest x-ray film reading (Chap. 12), and lung-function testing. A recent survey in a large asbestos-processing factory underlined the importance of standardization: a radiologist had read all chest x-ray films as within normal limits (C. A. Mitchell et al., unpublished data). Yet, when an experienced reader later read a sample of these films using the UICC-Cincinnati classification (p. 276), 24 out of 80 films were graded 1/0 or more (Table 15-4). Thus, although abnormal films were in fact frequent, they were not detected when

Table 15-4

Results of Survey of Asbestos Workers and Control Subjects

Method	Asbestos Workers	Controls	χ^2
Basal rales (n = 101)			
Score < 4	54	21	5.27
Score ⩾ 4	25	1	(p<0.025)
Chest x-ray film (n = 80)			
Score < 1/0	44	12	0.39
Score ⩾ 1/0	21	3	NS
FVC (n = 101)			
> 80% predicted	69	22	1.83
⩽ 80% predicted	10	0	NS
$FEV_{1.0}$ (n = 101)			
> 80% predicted	69	22	1.83
⩽ 80% predicted	10	0	NS

Basal rales at 4 points on the lower chest scored as follows: a few transient rales=1; many transient=2; a few persistent rales=4; many persistent=8; score at all points added to obtain total score, thus giving a range of 0 to 32. Chest x-ray film (only available in 80 subjects): profusion of small irregular opacities scored according to UICC-Cincinnati classification (Chap. 12, p. 276). Asbestos workers and control subjects worked in the same factory (manufacturing friction materials); control subjects did not work in areas with asbestos exposure risk. (Data from Mitchell CA et al., unpublished material, Yale University Lung Research Center.)

viewed individually because of the wide range of normal variability. Since basal rales are an early sign of asbestosis, auscultation is important; semiquantitative grading of the results can introduce an element of objectivity into this observer-error-prone method (Table 15-4; see also reference 127a).

Asbestosis, once established, progresses even after exposure is terminated. No treatment for asbestosis exists and only supportive measures can be taken for the individual patient with asbestosis. Therefore, early detection of the disease is mainly important as a method of biological monitoring of the workroom atmosphere. The finding of asbestosis cases indicates the need for controlling workroom dust in order to protect those not yet affected. Sensitive methods are needed to detect early asbestosis in the interest of the total work force at risk. Basal rales may be among the earliest positive findings [126] (Table 15-4); other early changes include decreases in vital capacity or single-breath diffusing capacity, or both,[126] even in persons with normal x-ray films. The arterial P_{O_2} may be low at rest or during exercise, with an increased A-a P_{O_2} difference (Chap. 5) in the presence of a normal FVC and TLC.[117] Lung compliance is usually reduced, and static recoil pressure at TLC may be increased.[92]

The functional findings in early asbestosis are consistent with the pathological finding of extensive fibrosis of the lung parenchyma, leading to increased lung stiffness and decreased gas exchange (Figs. 15-1, 15-5A). Hence, it is important to diagnose early asbestosis even in the presence of a normal chest x-ray film, if the functional findings as well as the history support the diagnosis. In-plant surveys

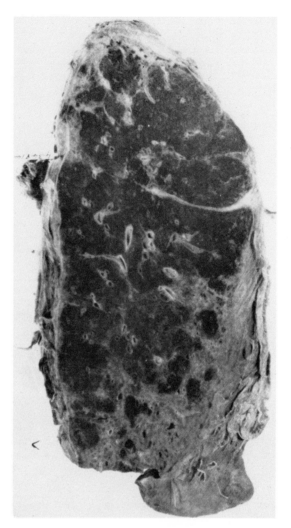

Fig. 15-1. Section of a lung with asbestosis. Extensive pleural adhesions around the lower lobe. Approx. ×
½. From reference 178, with permission from the author
and Pergamon Press, Ltd (copyright 1968).

may detect few if any severe cases of asbestosis, since affected workers often retire
because of disability.

The prevalence of asbestosis varies with the degree and length of exposure
and with the criteria used for diagnosis. In different surveys, the prevalence of
chest x-ray changes varied from 26 to 90 percent in heavily exposed men working
more than 30 years (Table 15-5). Selection factors may in part account for the
differences in prevalence. A policy of early transfer to nondusty jobs for affected
workers in one of the Canadian mining areas could explain why prevalence appeared lower there.[162] In the United States and Canada, most cases of asbestosis
are caused by chrysotile asbestos, but all commercially used forms of asbestos can
induce the disease (e.g., amosite [170]). There is good evidence that asbestosis can

Table 15-5

Prevalence of Lung Tissue Changes on Chest X-ray Films of Asbestos Workers

Population	Exposure	No. Workers	Years worked with asbestos.	
			10–30 yrs (%)	30 + yrs (%)
(1) US insulation workers	Probably heavy	1,117	49	90
(2) UK dockyard workers	Heavy	369	17	60
(3) Canadian chrysotile production workers (age 36–65)	Heavy	466	18	26
Total Population	(All exposure levels)	6,127	5	18

Figures indicate prevalence of asbestosis grade 1 or more (1) and for radiological category 1+(2 and 3; UICC-Cincinnati classification). Thus, they include all films in which the lung parenchyma was judged to be definitely abnormal, to varying degrees. From Rossiter et al.[162]

be induced by long-term exposures to dust levels previously considered safe. Among pipe coverers with 20 years' exposure in new ship construction, 38 percent had asbestosis, using standardized diagnostic criteria. These men had been exposed to dust levels near the previously recommended TLV (5 million particles per cu ft, which equals 17.6 fibers/ml if the dust contained 10 percent asbestos fibers). In a 4-year follow-up of these men, it was found that both FVC and diffusing capacity decreased significantly.[125]

Lung cancer. Asbestos workers have an increased risk of lung cancer that is closely linked to smoking habits. Nonsmoking asbestos workers rarely get lung cancer, while smoking asbestos workers are at much greater risk than other smokers.[16, 79, 169] In one study, the excess of lung cancer was greater among female than among male asbestos workers.[130] A large excess of lung cancer deaths occurred among workers exclusively exposed to amosite;[170] chrysotile and amosite may have similar carcinogenic properties.[171] Death from lung cancer may occur after 10–14 years of asbestos exposure.[171] As a cause of death among asbestos workers, lung cancer is more important than asbestosis. Among a group of insulation workers, 7.1 percent died of lung cancer over a 20-year period (a sevenfold excess), while 1.9 percent died of asbestosis. Many workers with asbestosis eventually die of lung cancer (see also p. 360).

The nature of the carcinogenic effect of asbestos is not clear. In rodents, chrysotile and amosite cause fibrosis but not cancer. The carcinogenic effect may be inherent to the fibers themselves or it may depend on other substances intimately associated with asbestos.[156] Trace metals and oils are probably not a factor.[160]

Mesothelioma (Fig. 15-2). This rare and fatal tumor of the pleural and peritoneal cavities is almost exclusively associated with asbestos exposure either in industry, in residential areas near asbestos factories, or in the neighborhood of

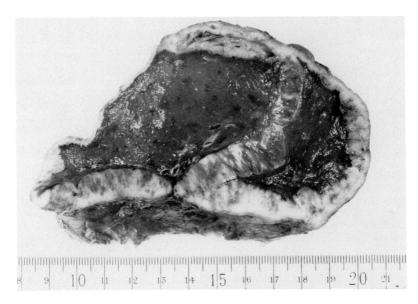

Fig. 15-2.   Mesothelioma, showing masses of tumor tissue surrounding the lung. Figure
reproduced by courtesy of Dr. D. O'B. Hourihane.

other sources of asbestos dust. In some groups of patients, contact with asbestos
was demonstrated in nearly all cases (Table 15-6). In one case, laundering of
asbestos-contaminated overalls was the source of exposure.[120] The duration of
asbestos exposure is frequently short or of low intensity. Cases have been reported
in persons who worked only a few years in a risk area.[186] There is usually a long
interval (20–50 years) between exposure and tumor development. In the United
States, mesotheliomas were diagnosed in the 1960s among persons who had worked
for short periods in shipyards during World War II. In Germany, an 84-year-old
man died in 1964 of mesothelioma; his exposure had been in a shipyard from
1895–1914.[97a] Age at death in patients with mesothelioma differs little from that
in the general population,[97a] so mesothelioma is not a frequent cause of premature
death. No excess of mesotheliomas has been found among persons living near
chrysotile or amosite mines; with these fibers the risk appears to be greater in
manufacturing.[160] One case of mesothelioma has been reported among installers
of asbestos floor tiles, with exposures in the order of 1.2 fibers/ml.[127] This suggests
that the present TLV's (2 fibers/ml in the UK and 5 fibers/ml in the US) are
insufficient to prevent development of this tumor.

The long latency between exposure and the clinical appearance of mesotheliomas is surprising since pleural tissue responds rapidly to contact with asbestos
fibers. In rats, intratracheal injection of chrysotile labeled with radioactive thymi-
dine led to labeling of mesothelial cells in 14 days or less, suggesting that DNA
formation was increased.[22] Human pleural tissue proliferates within 8 days when
brought in contact with crocidolite in tissue culture.[152] Although the risk of mesothelioma in man is much higher with exposure to crocidolite than to chrysotile,
intrapleural injection of all types of asbestos in rats leads to mesothelioma.[190] The
danger of crocidolite inhalation in man probably arises from the straightness of
these fibers, which facilitates penetration of small airways and greater retention

Table 15-6
Asbestos Exposure and Mesothelioma

Location	n	Direct Exposure	Casual Exposure	Environmental or Domestic	None
London, UK	76	31	0	20	25
Belfast, UK	42	8	24	— *	10
Liverpool, UK	17	7	6	— *	4
South Africa †	148	93	0	31	24
Walcheren, Netherlands ‡	25	23 §	0	0	2
Harrisburg, Pa	42	10	0	11	21
Newcastle, UK	22	13	0	7	2
Melbourne, Australia	15	12	0	1	2
Total	387	197 (51%)	30 (8%)	70 (18%)	90 (23%)

n = number of persons in each group.
* Domestic and environmental exposures not investigated.
† From Webster I, in Shapiro HA (ed): Pneumoconiosis; Proceedings of the International Conference, Johannesburg, 1969. Cape Town, Oxford University Press, 1970, pp 209–212.
‡ From reference 186. All other data from Elmes PC, Postgrad Med J 42:623–635, 1966, and Rubino GF et al., Br J Ind Med 29:436–442, 1972, which supply references to the original papers.
§ 9 of these shipyard workers worked in jobs with no or negligible asbestos; 1 worked for 1 month in the yard.

than occurs with the coiled fibers of chrysotile.[190] The same property probably enables more crocidolite than chrysotile to penetrate the pleural space. Fiber shape also is important after it has reached the pleural space. In rats, 40 mg crocidolite implanted in the pleura caused mesotheliomas in 61 percent in 2 years; when the fibers were first pulverized, the incidence was greatly reduced. Glass fibers produced no tumors under similar conditions, except when the fibers were first split into thin fibrous fragments.[181] Fiber length also influences in vitro responses of pleural tissue: long fibers (larger than 40 μm) induce fibroblast growth; short fibers cause monocyte accumulation.[116]

These laboratory observations correspond to epidemiological observations. In South Africa, Cape Province crocidolite (with thin, short fibers) causes more mesothelioma than Transvaal crocidolite, which has longer and thicker fibers.[190] The prevalence of mesothelioma in Canada, where only chrysotile is mined, has not increased in recent years.[118] The increased risk of mesothelioma during manufacturing of chrysotile products may be related to the separation of thick bundles into individual thin fibers which better penetrate the lungs and pleura.

Pleural plaques. In surveys of asbestos workers, the majority of lesions seen on x-ray films are pleural plaques, or zones of pleural thickening which result from localized fibrosis. These plaques are often calcified and show particularly well on 45° oblique films.[82] Their prevalence correlates with the extent and duration of dust exposure.[162] While not all plaques are caused by asbestos exposure,[160] the association is strong enough to serve as a monitor for asbestos exposure. Although plaques must be extensive to produce symptoms and restrictive function loss,[82] their presence indicates that asbestos fibers have penetrated the pleural space; in one study, mortality from mesothelioma and lung cancer was higher among shipyard workers with pleural plaques than among those without.[58]

Other effects of asbestos. Asbestos workers have an excess of deaths from gastrointestinal cancer; an earlier suspicion of increased risk of ovarian cancer among women has not been confirmed.[160] Ingested asbestos fibers can penetrate through the wall of the digestive tract in rats,[148] a disturbing fact in view of the presence of asbestos in drinking water of towns near sources of asbestos. Asbestos exposure was frequent (31 percent) in one series of patients with cancer of the larynx, with an average duration of 27 years' exposure.[182a]

Asbestos air pollution. Small numbers of asbestos bodies occur in the lungs of city dwellers, and at least some of these are caused by chrysotile exposure.[173] The finding of asbestos bodies by itself does not prove exposure to asbestos;[73] identification of the fibers by electron microscopy is required.[103] The amounts of asbestos involved are minimal, and there is at present no evidence that the general public in cities is exposed to increased risk of asbestos-related diseases.[160] Exceptions to this rule are people who live near asbestos factories or mines or in areas where asbestos-containing rock is used for building purposes.[173] Small numbers of asbestos fibers are found in the air in many cities, including those without asbestos factories.[89] In New York City, chrysotile levels up to 6×10^{-5} mg/cu m have been found;[173] however, quantitating these levels is difficult.[89, 161] Thus, although present risks to the public appear negligible, asbestos emission into community air, such as spraying of asbestos for fireproofing of buildings, should be forbidden.[158] In New York City, all asbestos spraying has been prohibited since 1972.

Overall mortality from asbestos-related diseases. The mortality of heavily exposed asbestos workers over a 25-year period is about three times the expected rate, with lung cancer the major cause of death, asbestosis the second, and mesothelioma and gastrointestinal cancer accounting for additional excess mortality.[48, 52] A large proportion of such workers (about 40 percent) die of asbestos-related diseases. Early death from asbestosis may be less frequent now than in the past, since high exposure levels are less common;[68] instead, asbestos workers die in increasing numbers from lung cancer and mesothelioma. The increased risks should be judged in relation to the lower prevalence of lung cancer and the virtual absence of mesothelioma in the general population. Thus, the overall excess mortality of asbestos workers, from all causes, is similar to the excess mortality among male smokers of 20 or more cigarettes per day.[67] "Confusion sometimes occurs between the proportion of individuals exposed who develop a disease and the excess risk of a particular disease in exposed individuals compared with the general public. The first may be relatively small and the second extremely high."[67] This statement concerning the absolute and relative risks of asbestos may be useful in counseling persons with light or moderate past asbestos exposure who are concerned about their future health.

Prevention and control.   A recent review on behalf of the National Academy of Sciences[30] stresses the need for further data on dose-response relations in asbestos-induced diseases. However, better protection of exposed persons is urgently needed on the basis of present, admittedly incomplete, knowledge. Present protective measures should include frequent monitoring of fiber levels in work-rooms, better housekeeping practices in industry,[8] scheduling and segregation of work to keep the number of persons exposed at a minimum, respirator use in risk areas, and improved dust control. Since dust control is costly and its effects may be offset by increased production rates,[66] many asbestos users are switching to substitutes (see below). Medical surveillance is now mandatory in the United States for all persons exposed to asbestos. A yearly examination— including measurement of at least FVC and $FEV_{1.0}$—is prescribed by the Federal Standard for Asbestos.[179] Unfortunately, the standard includes no provisions for test quality control and does not explicitly require auscultation for basal rales. In order to provide the early detection of asbestosis essential for biological monitoring (p. 355), the standard should require both auscultation for basal rales and standardized chest x-ray film reading according to the UICC-Cincinnati classification (Chap. 12, p. 276).[166] Workers with early asbestosis must be urged to stop smoking. Termination of their jobs in risk areas after many years' employment is often unwarranted, since present dust levels in many operations add little to their total asbestos load, and asbestosis progresses in spite of cessation of exposure.

There is little cause for optimism about the future morbidity and mortality trends among asbestos workers. The TLV for asbestos in the United States has been set at 5 fibers/ml until July 1, 1976, and at 2 fibers/ml thereafter.[179] These are time-weighted average values for 8-hour working days, and higher exposures (up to 10 fibers/ml) are allowed as long as the average is below the TLV. At present, many asbestos-processing factories do not comply with the standard (Fig. 15-3). In a recent survey of the Connecticut asbestos industry, 8 out of 15 factories reported levels of 5 or more fibers/ml in workrooms. In addition, 4 of these factories reported measurements above the ceiling limit of 10 fibers/ml.[166] Some of these companies may switch to substitutes; others will hopefully decrease their fiber levels. In any case, even the lower standard (2 fibers/ml) now applicable in the United Kingdom probably will not prevent all significant asbestos-related disease, in particular mesothelioma.[127]

Asbestos substitutes.   For many industries, replacing asbestos with a substitute appears to be the best way to reduce risks of lung disease among workers. However, the introduction of new materials, equally as stable and chemically resistant as asbestos, should be closely monitored with biological methods. Glass fibers are frequently used as an asbestos substitute. Although there are at present no data to indicate that they pose risks on inhalation,[87] a healthy suspicion seems warranted on the basis of several in vitro studies. Thin glass fiber fragments can induce mesothelioma in rats.[181] In cultures of macrophage cells, glass fibers as well as chrysotile increased the permeability of the cell membrane, leading to release of intracellular enzymes into the medium. Both types of fibers may penetrate more than one cell, and the microscopic appearance of cells attached to each type of fiber is remarkably similar.[14] Thus, the mechanical effects of

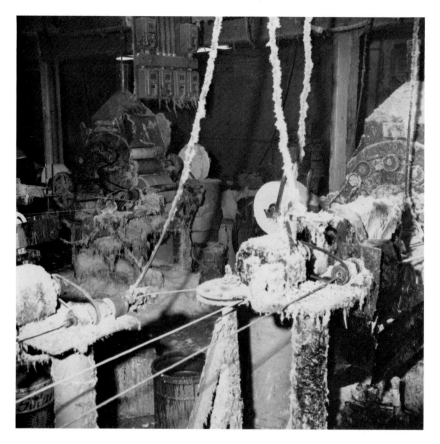

Fig. 15-3. Interior of a small factory producing asbestos-coated wire. Photograph taken in January 1973. Since this factory is operated by a partnership, without employees, it does not fall within the scope of the OSHA 1970. Asbestos carding machine in background. As far as could be ascertained, the settled dust visible in the picture is nearly pure asbestos. Photo: Yale University Lung Research Center.

the fibers, rather than any special physicochemical property, may initiate tissue lesions by damaging macrophage cells. Another asbestos substitute, vermiculite (a silicate that occurs in flakes rather than fibers), caused no mesotheliomas in rats under conditions where chrysotile caused tumors in about 50 percent. Instead, the vermiculite-injected rats had pleural granulomas,[90] which may encapsulate the material so that its potential carcinogenicity remains latent.

With the asbestos experience at hand, there seems to be every reason to practice equally stringent dust control when using these substitute fibers until acceptable evidence of their lack of fibrogenicity and carcinogenicity is available. Asbestos was introduced into industry about 100 years ago, when infectious diseases still caused most people to die at an age before they could develop asbestos-induced disease. Future generations should not be able to reproach us for having replaced one dangerous fiber with another; we now know better than that.

Barium

Inhalation of barium sulfate occurs in workers in barite mines. The inhaled barium causes radiopaque dust deposits, with dense shadows on the chest x-ray film but little functional impairment.[12, 178]

Beryllium

An estimated 8000 US workplaces involved exposure to Be in 1969,[114] in mining and processing of Be ores and in manufacturing alloys and propellants for spacecraft.[192] Beryllium is emitted when new mantle-type gas lanterns are first lit.[72a] Beryllium is no longer used in fluorescent lamp manufacturing, which was formerly a chief risk of exposure.

In body tissues, Be is bound to proteins and affects enzyme actions; it may concentrate in lysosomes and react with nucleic acids. It also inhibits DNA synthesis and causes liver necrosis in rats.[70] In the lungs, severe Be exposures can cause widespread acute pneumonitis leading to death. Chronic, lower-level exposures cause granulomatous disease of the lungs, liver, and spleen.[81, 185] Although the diffuse nodular x-ray changes may be confused with those of sarcoidosis, other signs of this disease (hypercalcemia, eye involvement, and lymph node enlargement) are absent. In patients with sarcoidosis, certain antigens transform the lymphocytes into precursor forms; this lymphocyte transformation test is negative in Be lung disease.[194] Lung-function changes usually include restrictive function loss and arterial hypoxemia in Be lung disease; the diffusing capacity is often decreased.[63] However, airway obstruction has also been observed, even in nonsmoking Be workers.[6] While Be usage increased from 100–500 metric tons in 1947–1950 to over 1200 tons in 1966, the number of new cases of Be disease reported to the beryllium registry has steadily declined since 1947.[154] The decrease in new cases may be real, but a recent in-plant survey found 26 (14 percent) workers with x-ray changes suggesting mild interstitial lung disease.[184] Since Be usage is still increasing (a sixfold increase was predicted in 1968 [192]), further epidemiological studies are needed to establish disease prevalence and to investigate risks of neighborhood exposures among people living near Be factories.

Whether industries effectively implement the TLV of 2 μg/cu m is unknown. The documentation of the TLV [4] quotes the occurrence of cases during exposure near this level. Thus, adequate medical surveillance of workers at risk of Be exposure as well as documentation of Be levels in the workroom atmosphere is needed; it is likely that Be disease has been underreported in recent years.

Coal Dust

Lung disease among coal miners has long been attributed to silica exposure and tuberculosis; coal dust was thought to be innocuous. Haldane [77] noted that the lungs of city dwellers are "more or less blackened by smoke particles, but remain perfectly healthy"; he thought this also applied to coal miners. At present there is little doubt that coal dust without silica can cause lung lesions (coal workers' pneumoconiosis—CWP), since the disease occurs in mines with rocks low in silica, in workers exposed to nearly pure carbon (synthetic graphite [109]), in workers loading processed coal without silica, and in carbon-electrode workers. Cases in which no silica was found in the lungs at autopsy have been documented. The main debate at the present time, however, is to what extent the lesions induced by coal dust on the one hand, and chronic bronchitis on the other hand, are responsible for symptoms and for disability.[96, 172]

CWP LESIONS

Pathology. The three main anatomical features of CWP are the coal macula, fibrosis, and emphysema. Initially, coal dust accumulates around respiratory bronchioles and local fibrosis ensues. The contracting fibrous tissue widens the bronchiole and exerts traction on the surrounding lung tissue. As a result, dust accumulations and emphysematous lesions appear in the center of the lung lobules (Fig. 15-4). More extensive dust deposits cause fibrotic nodules, which differ from those in silicosis (Fig. 15-5*B*). Later, extensive centrilobular emphysema may occur throughout the lungs. Because this form of emphysema infrequently affects the general population,[83] its high prevalence in patients with CWP is probably due to the initial lesions around the respiratory bronchioles. The term simple pneumoconiosis is used to describe the x-ray changes induced by widespread but discrete fibrous changes (Fig. 15-6). As the disease progresses, solid, confluent tissue masses may develop (progressive massive fibrosis, PMF, or complicated pneumoconiosis). Formerly, PMF was thought to be caused by tuberculous infection, but this is not true for many cases of PMF seen at present. After dust exposure ceases, PMF continues to progress—more rapidly in younger than in older persons [28, 69]—while simple pneumoconiosis does not.

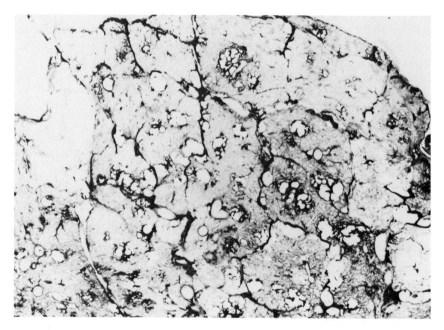

Fig. 15-4. Coal-workers' pneumoconiosis. Twelve or more secondary lobules are outlined by the coal dust deposited in their periphery. Widened respiratory bronchioles, surrounded by dust deposits, are in the center of the lobules. Portion of a whole-lung paper section. $\times$ 8.2. From reference 202.

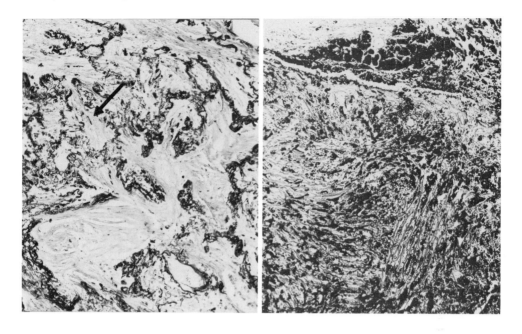

A   B

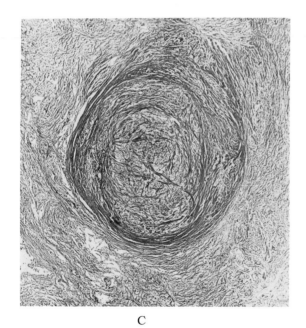

C

Fig. 15-5. *A*. Asbestosis (× 140). Generalized fibrosis and obliteration of alveolar spaces, with intact alveolar elastic network. Arrow indicates an asbestos particle. Modified Sheridan's stain and hematoxylin. *B*. Coal dust nodule (× 140). Collagen and reticulin fibers run in all directions, with coal dust particles between them. Modified Foot's stain. *C*. Silicotic nodule (× 40). Note concentric arrangement of collagen fibers. Foot's reticulin stain. From reference 178, with permission from the author and Pergamon Press, Ltd (copyright 1968).

The prevalence of CWP among US coal miners varies widely, in part as a function of the type of coal mined.[96, 172] Among 300,000 British coal miners seen during 1964–1968, 9.7 percent had simple CWP, and 1 percent progressive massive fibrosis.[151] Using periodic records of dust exposure in the mines over a 15-year period, it could be shown that the progression of x-ray changes correlated with the mass of dust inhaled. The risk of contracting CWP during a 35-year

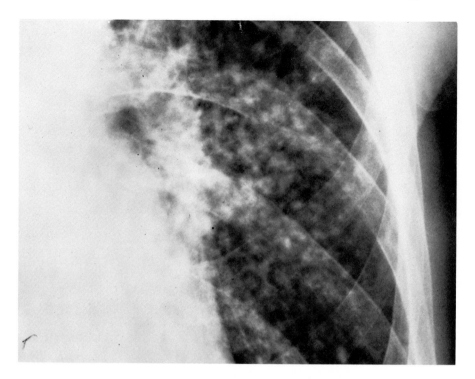

Fig. 15-6.   Portion of a chest x-ray film of a patient with coal workers' pneumo-coniosis.   There are small rounded opacities as well as some irregular opacities in the lung.   From E.P. Pendergrass et al., in reference 96.

working life at the coal face increased from about 3 percent at a dust level of 4 mg/cu m to about 18 percent at 8 mg/cu m.   Thus, doubling the dust level caused a sixfold increase in lesions apparent on x-ray films in 35 years.   The human lungs appear to act as an excellent filter for coal dust; their coal dust content after death correlates with the amount of dust inhaled during life (see Table 12-1, p. 277).

Lung function.   Centrilobular emphysema involves widening of the respiratory bronchioles—air spaces in series with the alveoli.   This widening can impair gas exchange through series ventilation (Chap. 4, p. 64), resulting in ventilation-perfusion maldistribution.   The fibrotic parenchymal lesions also impair local ventilation-perfusion relations.   These two causes of maldistribution probably account for the increased A-a P_{O_2} difference even in miners with no significant chest x-ray changes and no bronchitis (Chap. 5, p. 89).[128]   Small disseminated lesions (pinhead nodules) appear to affect gas exchange more than larger nodules, leading to a larger dead space, a smaller diffusing capacity, and a lower arterial P_{O_2}.[33, 168]   These gas-exchange abnormalities also occur in nonsmoking miners but contribute little to disability or symptoms.[124]

BRONCHITIS IN COAL MINERS

Chronic cough and sputum production (chronic bronchitis) are common symptoms among coal miners, and their prevalence is greatly influenced by smoking habits. In one study of men aged 45–54 years, smoking control subjects had more bronchitis than nonsmoking men with past exposures to coal dust; the latter had more bronchitis than nonsmoking control subjects.[112] Thus, mine dust exposure causes an excess of bronchitis among nonsmokers, but smoking nonminers have an even greater excess, while smoking miners have the highest bronchitis prevalence. The symptoms of bronchitis (cough and sputum production) are accompanied by functional evidence of airway obstruction.[167] Reduction of $FEV_{1.0}$ may occur at an early age (25–34 years [23]) and may not progress much with continued exposure to coal dust.[86]

Since most miners smoke, the contributions of coal dust and cigarette smoke to their obstructive function loss are difficult to separate, although smoking is probably more important than coal dust. In nonsmoking miners, coal dust alone, or concomitant exposures to gases and fumes in mines, may be responsible. While the lesions in terminal lung units (simple pneumoconiosis) must be due to inhalation of small particles that can penetrate deeply into the lungs, airway obstruction may be caused by larger particles which settle in the bronchi.[124] During a work shift underground in coal mines, many workers develop wheezing on auscultation [201] and their flow rates at low lung volumes on MEFV curves (Chap. 9) decrease.[105] Consequently, exposure in coal mines can lead to acute airway obstruction. Although the responsible agent has not been isolated, it may be relevant that pure carbon dust can cause airway obstruction in laboratory experiments with healthy subjects.[43]

IMPLICATIONS FOR PREVENTION AND CONTROL

The respiratory symptoms of many coal miners appear to result from a combination of smoking and coal dust exposure, with the latter perhaps the minor contributor. In contrast, the lesions of pneumoconiosis apparent on x-ray films as well as the gas-exchange abnormalities, appear to result primarily from coal dust deposition in the lungs. The roentgenographic changes are not closely correlated with disabling function loss.[124] Although lung volumes are reduced in many coal miners, gross mechanical changes suggesting extensive fibrosis occur mostly in miners with PMF.[167] Thus, among the lesions primarily induced by coal dust, PMF may be the only one that leads to significant disability. On the other hand, bronchitis is a common cause of disability among miners without PMF, particularly among smokers.

Confusion of the effects of smoking and coal dust exposure in coal miners has led to widespread disagreement over the criteria to be used for disability evaluation. In the United States, rejection rates of applications for disability benefits vary from 33 percent in one state to 78 percent in another.[146] These discrepancies could be largely eliminated if appropriate standardized tests and interpretations were used. Lung-function tests and exercise performance, not roentgenographic changes, should be the primary standard for evaluating ability to work. However, chest x-ray films that show lesions induced by coal dust should be used to help prevent and control pneumoconiosis. Since the risk of PMF increases as the severity of simple pneumoconiosis progresses, workers whose lesions of simple pneumoconiosis exceed an arbitrary limit should be assigned to nondusty jobs; unlike asbestosis, simple CWP then does not progress further. According to the British experience,[151] consistent reduction of coal dust loads to the present TLV (3 mg/cu m in both the United States and Britain [7, 97]) should reduce the increase of CWP over a 35-year working lifetime to less than 3 percent. Coupled with adequate medical surveillance, including periodic chest x-ray films interpreted with a standardized method, enforcement of this TLV should eliminate PMF if workers with simple CWP are transferred to nondusty jobs in time. The medical surveillance program should include continued attempts to induce miners to stop smoking in order to reduce the prevalence of airway obstruction and chronic bronchitis.

Hard Metals

Exposure to hard metal (mainly tungsten carbide) in the manufacture and repair of cutting tools for rock drilling can induce interstitial fibrosis. The lung tissue lesions include mononuclear infiltrates with varying amounts of fibrosis. In one series of 12 patients there were 8 deaths. Nine patients were from one plant with 1500 employees. Although these data may suggest a low prevalence, it is uncertain whether all workers were equally exposed. Since tungsten carbide is milled with 3 to 25 percent cobalt, and the latter is toxic in animals while the former is not, the disease is attributed to cobalt inhalation.[13, 27]

Iron Oxide

Inhalation of iron oxide causes dust deposits visible on the chest x-ray film (siderosis), but these are considered innocuous. However, there is often exposure to other substances as well. In one series, there was exposure to iron, nickel, and chromium oxides; 4 out of 14 workers had pneumoconiosis (roentgenographic category 2 or 3), with 2 also having function loss.[94] In foundry workers, simple pneumoconiosis is about equally prevalent among those exposed to iron, aluminum, or magnesium; progressive massive fibrosis is absent or infrequent. The prevalence of pneumoconiosis in these workers appears to be related to the silica content of the inhaled dust rather than to the metals themselves.[95] Lung compliance was somewhat reduced in arc welders with siderosis. This could, however, be due to other agents, since arc welders are exposed to an impressive number of inhalants— iron, ozone, nitrogen dioxide, cadmium, chromium, manganese, zinc, silica, and asbestos.[180]

Kaolin

Reports of cases of severe lung fibrosis following exposure to kaolin (china clay; $Al_2O_3 \cdot 2SiO_2 \cdot 2H_2O$) have been published.[178] No prevalence studies appear to have been done.

Talc

Excessive usage of cosmetic talcum powder may lead to acute airway obstruction in infants or to diffuse lung fibrosis (case description in reference 12). More commonly, interstitial fibrosis due to talc occurs in workers manufacturing or using talc.[178] Talc may contain up to 50 percent free silica,[34] and some fibrous types of talc appear to behave like asbestos.[57] Hence, "talcosis" is probably not a uniform entity.

Platinum

Inhalation of dust containing platinum salts, in the refining industry or in the manufacture of chloroplatinates, causes asthma. A prevalence of 70 percent was observed in one refining factory. Sodium chloroplatinate causes delayed-onset asthma in guinea pigs, but has no direct effect on the guinea pig ileum. It probably acts through the release of histamine in lung tissue.[138]

Silica

The Occupational Safety and Health Administration estimates that more than 1.1 million Americans are exposed to free silica (SiO_2) in their jobs.[187] Free silica occurs in several crystalline forms, of which quartz is the most important. Exposure occurs not only in jobs classically linked with a silicosis-risk (Table 15-2), but also in work where the primary exposure is to other agents, with silica as an admixture. Home exposures have occurred in people laundering overalls of pottery workers.[53] Silicosis, a disease known to the ancients, still occurs among people in primitive trades. For instance, in Transkei (southern Africa), girls who grind mealies with stones containing quartz often contract silicosis in their twenties.[136] In one hospital, 132 such patients were seen per year.[38]

Acute silicosis, leading to death within a few years after heavy exposure, is now rare.[12, 159] Ashing of lung tissue and x-ray diffraction or electron microprobe analysis may establish the diagnosis.[137, 159] The histological findings vary and include cellular infiltration around blood vessels, interstitial granulomas, and thickening of the alveolocapillary membrane.[12]

More commonly, symptoms—including gradually increasing dyspnea and decreased exercise performance—occur after 10 or more years of exposure. The characteristic chest x-ray film shows diffuse nodular lesions, predominantly in the upper lobes, and sometimes "eggshells," calcifications of the cortex of lymph nodes near the large bronchi. Fibrotic nodules are disseminated throughout the lungs (Fig. 15-5C). Lung-function findings usually include restrictive function loss (Chap. 9), with decreases in VC and TLC paralleling the extent of the roentgenographic changes.[61] Nonuniform inspired gas distribution (Chap. 4) and a decreased arterial P_{O_2}, suggesting ventilation-perfusion maldistribution (Chap. 5), have been found in a group of workers whose mean VC was normal.[157] Nonsmoking silica-exposed workers may have restrictive function loss in the presence of minimal chest changes apparent on x-ray film.[24]

An early theory of the pathogenesis of silicosis attributed the lung lesions to the release of silicic acid from quartz in lung tissue. Phagocytes ingest silica more slowly than carbon,[54] but, once ingested, silica particles render the membrane of the intracellular lysosomes in macrophages permeable, an effect probably mediated by silicic acid. The lysosomes release enzymes into the cell, leading to its death. Quartz particles coated with polyvinylpyridine-N-oxide (PVPNO) do not kill the macrophage cell, perhaps because PVPNO binds silicic acid.[3] How macrophage death leads to fibrosis is not clear; in vitro, macrophages and SiO_2 together stimulate collagen formation in fibroblast cultures.[85] In animal exposures with SiO_2, biochemical changes in lung tissue occur within 48 hours, including an increase in lung phospholipids, in particular dipalmityllecithin, the main component of lung surfactant [76, 84] (Chap. 1). In some experiments with rats, quartz led to alveolar lipoproteinosis rather than to silicosis;[84] in another series, typical silicosis developed 4 months after injection of 50 mg quartz into the trachea.[99]

As with coal workers' pneumoconiosis, cigarette smoking probably contributes significantly to the respiratory symptoms. In a survey of foundrymen,[111] dyspnea and episodes of acute chest illness were more related to smoking habits than to occupational exposure. Thus, the combination of silica exposure, cigarette smoking, and concomitant occupational exposures can result in a variable clinical picture, depending on the extent and the time course of each exposure. Formerly, complicating tuberculosis was a leading cause of death among silicotics.

Recent US reports include cases of silicosis among bentonite workers in Wyoming [145] and among slate workers in Pennsylvania.[163] In Sweden, the incidence of new cases of silicosis (average age at diagnosis, 54 years) is about 67 per 1000 workers exposed more than 10 years.[2] In West Germany, a decreasing trend in new case reports (1955–1960) did not continue over 1964–1968, and silicotuberculosis actually increased.[129] Amorphous silica rather than quartz causes pneumoconiosis in workers with diatomaceous earth (the siliceous skeletons of diatoms, unicellular plants). Among 251 workers with 5 or more years' exposure, 25 percent had lesions apparent on x-ray films.[31]

The lack of detailed epidemiological studies on silicosis leaves unanswered many questions concerning its natural history. It is not clear whether the disease progresses after exposure ceases, nor whether the prognosis is better now that complicating tuberculosis is less common.[69]

Tin

Exposure to tin oxide in mining and processing of tin and tin ore causes dense shadows (stannosis) visible on x-ray film, but the dust deposits do not elicit significant tissue reactions.[178]

Other Mineral Dusts

Among 14,076 US metal miners, 3.3 percent had roentgenographic lesions of pneumoconiosis; the type of metals was not specified.[101] Although chromite miners in South Africa had fine nodulations on chest x-ray films (10 out of 1500 workers), this was considered a benign deposit of chromite dust (Cr_2O_3FeO).[177] Lung-function data were not reported in these studies. Inhalation of dust from an arc-lamp electrode can lead to accumulation of rare earth elements (cerium, lanthanum, and others) in the lungs of reproduction photographers.[183]

Nuisance Particulates

The US TLV Committee states that all types of dust exposure should be limited, if only for hygienic reasons. Therefore, an arbitrary TLV of 10 mg/cu m is assigned to dusts containing less than 1 percent quartz, for which no positive evidence in favor of a lower TLV is available. Among these nuisance particulates listed in Table 15-2 are aluminum, aluminum oxide, kaolin, and tin oxide. Others are calcium carbonate, cellulose, Portland cement, and synthetic graphite.[5] Since the lack of evidence concerning risks in most cases reflects lack of data rather than convincing negative evidence, some of these dusts will probably be assigned lower TLVs as more data become available.

CHRONIC OCCUPATIONAL LUNG DISEASES CAUSED BY ORGANIC DUSTS

Most exposures to dust containing vegetable or animal matter occur on farms and in industries where farm products are processed into consumer goods. These dusts contain large numbers of organic substances, and in most instances the exact nature of the agent that causes the lung disease is not known. Organic dusts cause two main types of lung disease. Some agents affect the airways by acting as allergens (e.g., enzymes; occupational asthma) or through direct toxic effects (byssinosis, Chap. 17). Other organic dusts cause parenchymal lung disease (pneumonitis or alveolitis, as in farmer's lung). Occupational asthma is discussed in Chapter 18. In industry, patients with nonoccupational asthma may need protection from irritants at exposure levels that do not affect persons without asthma. Job placement of asthmatic but otherwise healthy persons needs to take into account their probable susceptibility to any kind of irritant exposure.

The remaining group of organic dusts are chiefly those that contain antigenic material that induces other than reaginic antibodies in exposed persons. After a period of sensitization, further exposure may lead to parenchymal lung disease, mediated through an antigen-antibody reaction. The most common exposures are listed in Table 15-2.

Bagasse

Bagasse, the residue after extracting sugar from sugar cane, consists mainly of cellulose and is used in the manufacture of paper and board. Bagassosis is clinically similar to farmer's lung (see below), but while bagasse contains many fungal spores, especially when stored wet, no definite causal organism has been identified. Although many patients appear to recover from bagassosis,[196] reduced lung volumes and decreased diffusing capacity may occur 7 to 10 years after exposure.[122] A single acute episode of bagassosis can lead to permanent lung damage.[147]

Cotton and Other Textile Dusts

The most important disease associated with exposure to cotton dust in cardroom and other cotton textile workers is byssinosis. This disease also occurs among preparers and spinners of flax and soft hemp fibers (see Chap. 17).

Enzymes in Laundry Products

Concentrated autolyzates of *Bacillus subtilis,* which have an enzymatic (proteolytic) action that helps clean laundry, are widely used in various washing powders. One preparation contains 35 percent organic material, 5–10 percent of which is enzyme.[131] These products have been marketed since 1963; the first instances of lung disease among workers exposed to concentrated enzyme powder in industry were reported in 1969.[60] The syndrome resembles bronchial asthma (dyspnea, wheezing, and cough). Sensitization to one or more components of the enzyme powder may be responsible. Skin tests showed hypersensitivity in many workers, and sensitization was more common among those with a history of allergic disease.[131, 197] Obstructive function loss, reversed by isoproterenol, is common among sensitized workers, whose $FEV_{1.0}$ often decreases over the working day.[131] The asthmatic response to exposure appears to include an early and a delayed phase.[141] The risk of disease is much higher among workers handling the concentrated enzyme powder than among those processing a more diluted preparation.[197] In a high-risk plant, symptoms usually appeared several hours after the affected employees left work (delayed response). Employees in this plant had significantly more airway obstruction than those in a low-risk factory, as shown by measurement of maximum flow rates at low lung volumes (Chap. 9). Early responses usually occur on first exposure; delayed responses do not appear until several months later.[133] Positive skin tests correlate better with nasal symptoms than with lower-airway responses.[123] Hence, medical surveillance should not be based on skin tests alone.

The enzymes may also have direct toxic effects independent of sensitization. A few long-term workers had decreased lung elastic recoil,[123] which is not surprising considering the ease with which another proteolytic enzyme, papain, induces reduced lung recoil and emphysema in animals (see Chap. 7, p. 139). Direct toxic effects of these enzyme preparations—including weight loss, hemolysis, and hemagglutination—have been observed in mice; as little as 2 μg increased the mortality from lung infection induced by *Klebsiella pneumoniae.*[42] One study reported lasting decreases of diffusing capacity in enzyme workers and evidence of airway obstruction in some, but no control subjects were included.[174]

The TLV for proteolytic enzyme (in terms of 100 percent pure crystalline enzyme) is 0.06 μg/cu m. Continuing improvement of atmospheric conditions in one factory reduced levels considerably, but only to levels of about 0.25–1.10 μg/cu m.[62] The risk to consumers using the final product, which contains much less enzyme than the concentrated material handled in factories, is probably minimal under conditions of normal use, although eye and respiratory symptoms as well as evidence of sensitization have been reported in 3 Swedish consumers.[15]

Moldy Hay

Exposure to dust of moldy hay, which contains fungi and fungal spores, causes farmer's lung, an acute lung disease with shortness of breath, fever, and cough. In the early stage of disease, the chest x-ray film shows diffuse infiltration, especially in the lower lung zones. The initial tissue lesion includes lung edema, followed by cellular infiltration of the alveoli and alveolar walls. This results in granulomatous lesions, resembling those of sarcoidosis, and interstitial fibrosis. The disease has variously been called a fibrosing alveolitis, an interstitial pneumonitis, or an extrinsic allergic alveolitis.[55, 182] Although clinical recovery is the rule, permanent lung damage may occur, especially if repeated acute attacks follow renewed exposures to moldy hay. Lung-function loss in farmer's lung is usually restrictive and accompanied by arterial hypoxemia. Chronic lung damage is often apparent from a decrease in diffusing capacity.[11]

The prevalence of the disease varies with climate and farm practices. Prevalence data from Scotland show a high prevalence (86 per 1000 persons) in two areas with much rainfall. In a third area with modern farms and less rain, the prevalence was only 27 per 1000.[72] Many cases of farmer's lung have been reported in the United States, but no prevalence data are available since most observations were hospital based. Farmer's lung can be prevented by improved farm techniques: drying of hay, ventilation of farm buildings, and mechanical feeding of cattle.[72]

Although farmer's lung is probably caused by inhalation of spores of fungi of the class of thermophylic actinomycetes,[50, 140, 142] the precise immunological mechanism is not known. Serum of patients often contains precipitating antibodies against extracts of spores of Micropolyspora faeni and other fungi.[91, 142] However, the sera of 50 percent of nonfarmers and other healthy persons also contain such precipitins, if sensitive methods are used.[91] Immunoglobulins and a polysaccharide antigen have been found in airway epithelium as well as in granulomas from patients with farmer's lung.[199] While the serum precipitins suggest exposure to antigens from thermophylic actinomycetes, the lung lesions may represent a cytotoxic response caused by antigen binding on cells.[199] Among the cases diagnosed during the farm survey in Scotland (criteria: history of exposure to moldy hay and acute bouts of chest illness after exposure), 57 percent had no serum precipitins.[72] However, purified antigens have only recently become available,[45] and their use may help clarify the immunological mechanisms.

Other Organic Antigens

Several clinical syndromes similar to farmer's lung have been described in persons exposed to organic dusts—pigeon breeders, bird fanciers, malt workers, mushroom workers, cork workers in Portugal, paprika splitters in Hungary, and sequoia workers in California.[10, 164, 178, 204]

Pigeon breeder's lung. Among members of a Swedish pigeon breeders' club, 8 percent had a history of pigeon breeder's lung;[47] however, affected persons may have left the club, and thus the true prevalence may be higher. The breeders usually become ill after exposure to dust of bird droppings. The antigenic activity of the droppings is greater than that of bird serum.[46] While most breeders (60 percent) have serum precipitins against bird antigen, control subjects do not. But precipitins occurred equally among breeders with and without disease.[47] The disease of bird fanciers (caused by exposure to budgerigars) develops more slowly than that of pigeon breeders and is often detected in a stage of marked fibrosis.[140]

Maple bark disease. Inhalation of spores from *Cryptostroma corticale,* a fungus growing in maple logs, causes maple bark disease, a disease similar to farmer's lung in persons exposed to maple bark dust in paper mills.[49] Among 37 men exposed to this dust in the same room, 14 had active or minor disease, and 4 others had a positive serum-precipitin test.[198] The disease usually lasts from 2–4 months; function tests show restrictive function loss and arterial hypoxemia.[51] Inhalation of the spores in guinea pigs causes granulomatous lung disease similar to the human disease.[189]

Yet another fungus, *Aspergillus clavatus,* may contaminate germinating barley on the maltfloor in distilleries.[25] Inhalation of the spores can reproduce the acute phase of the disease, which is the same as that of farmer's lung. While many workers have spores of the fungus in their sputum, only a few become diseased.

Chronic respiratory symptoms and airway obstruction are common among workers exposed to grain dust. These workers experience increased symptoms during dust exposure. Few workers have serum precipitins against grain dust, and the presence of these precipitins does not correlate with disease severity. Therefore, the pathogenesis of this syndrome may be similar to that of byssinosis (Chap. 17), involving direct toxic actions of the dust rather than a hypersensitivity reaction.[192a]

LUNG CANCER

The most common lung cancer develops from cells in the bronchial epithelium (bronchogenic carcinoma). Its malignancy in terms of local invasive growth and of metastasis varies with the type of tumor cells. Tumors with undifferentiated cells (oat-cell tumors) are highly malignant, while tumors with more differentiated cells (squamous cell carcinoma) often grow slower and develop metastases later. However, the prognosis of bronchogenic carcinoma in any form is poor. In the upper respiratory tract, cancer of the larynx is the most frequent tumor. Since it leads to hoarseness while still localized, it is often detected in the stage of local growth and can then be removed successfully, though often at the cost of a total laryngectomy.

Mortality due to lung cancer has risen steadily during the past 30 years, largely because of the carcinogenic effects of cigarette smoke (Chap. 14). However, detailed studies of certain occupational groups have detected other agents that can cause lung cancer. The classic example of environmentally induced lung cancer is that of uranium miners,[195] first discovered among miners in Schneeberg, Germany, in 1899. Asbestos exposure, which potentiates the effects of smoking, has already been discussed (p. 357). Other examples are discussed in this section. Whether community air pollution plays a role in causing lung cancer is discussed in Chapter 16.

Lung cancer mortality is much higher among workers exposed to products of the carbonization of coal in gas works[41] or in workers involved in producing coke from bituminous coal in steel works[110, 155] than it is among the general population. These workers are exposed to coal tar and volatile substances released from coal tar, including 3,4-benzo[a]pyrene, a potent carcinogen. The risks of skin, bladder, and scrotal cancer are also increased in these workers, again most likely as a result of exposure to coal tar products. The excess of lung cancer is especially high for men subject to severe exposures, with some categories having a sevenfold excess risk.[155]

Among iron ore (haematite) miners in Great Britain, lung cancer deaths occurred at about twice the expected rate. The excess cancer mortality may be related to radioactivity in the air of these mines, or perhaps to a carcinogenic effect of iron oxide.[21a] Bis(chloromethyl)ether (BCME) causes squamous cell carcinoma of the lung in rats when inhaled in as little as 0.1 ppm concentration.[107] This agent also caused tumors of the olfactory epithelium in the nose in rats. The substance is formed from a parent compound (chloromethyl methylether, CMME) which is widely used as an ion-exchange resin, in polymer manufacture, and in organic synthesis. Workers exposed to CMME in a chemical factory had at least an eightfold excess of lung cancer, and the majority of these cancers were of the highly malignant oat-cell type.[56]

Excess lung cancer occurs in workers exposed to nickel carbonyl in the early stages of nickel refining, in workers exposed to dust of chrome ore and chromates, and in workers manufacturing mustard gas (reviewed in reference 40). Under several conditions, arsenic exposure has been suspected of causing lung cancer.[40] For instance, gold miners in Rhodesia have a high incidence of lung cancer, related to exposure to arsenopyrites in these mines, and excess cancer also occurs in nonsmokers who work underground in arsenic mines.[135] A possible interaction between cigarette smoking and arsenic exposure, as with asbestos, was noted in this study.[135]

Other agents that may lead to increased cancer risks are wood dust in the furniture industry (associated with a high prevalence of adenocarcinoma in the nasal cavity [1]) and polyurethane foam dust, which induces squamous cell bronchial cancer in rats.[106]

Basic studies of carcinogenesis may lead to early recognition of substances likely to induce cancer.[80] An early cellular change induced by benzo[a]pyrene in airway epithelium is the transformation of mucous cells into keratinizing cells, which contain less glycoproteins.[39] A similar change is induced by vitamin A deficiency, and administration of this vitamin can convert keratinizing cells back into goblet cells. In several instances, the experimental induction of cancer appears to involve two agents (cocarcinogenesis), one that initiates an essential step in the process of cancer formation (initiating agent), followed by development of cancer when a second agent (tumor-promoting agent) is administered. The tumor-promoting agent by itself has only weak carcinogenetic properties. Although there are no examples of experimental lung cancer resulting from successive administration of two agents, the induction of lung cancer in mice exposed to benzo[a]pyrene and SO_2, neither of which caused cancer in the doses used,[100] and the potentiation of the effect of cigarette smoking by asbestos exposure may be related to this process.

Even when bronchial carcinoma is detected before symptoms appear, the patient's prognosis is usually poor, with only a 4 percent 5-year survival rate in the United States and the United Kingdom.[44] In one series of cases detected through annual chest roentgenograms in an industrial population, the 5-year survival rate was 18 percent. Of those who were diagnosed when symptom-free, 26 percent survived 5 years or more after surgery.[44] However, their longer survival time includes the period between early detection and the point at which they would have developed symptoms. Thus, the increased survival time in part reflects the fact that these patients were operated on earlier than if their tumor had been diagnosed after they developed symptoms. The dubious advantages of early lung cancer detection programs have to be weighed against their low yield of positive findings and their high cost. However, in industries with demonstrated or suspected cancer risks, semiannual chest x-ray films (including a lateral film) should be made and a history of respiratory symptoms recorded. The experience with asbestos strongly suggests that workers in such risk industries should be discouraged from smoking through an active health-education program. In addition, every effort must be made to prevent exposure to occupational carcinogenic agents.

SUMMARY

Occupational lung diseases are a major cause of acute illness, recurrent symptoms, chronic disability, and premature death among workers in agriculture and industry. The effects of gases, vapors, and fumes on airways and lungs are summarized in Table 15-1, those of mineral and organic dusts in Table 15-2. These effects range from acute bronchitis or lung edema to severe, irreversible obstructive or restrictive function loss caused by airway obstruction or lung fibrosis, respectively. In addition, many cases of bronchial carcinoma are related to exposures at work. Special emphasis has been placed on asbestos and coal dust exposures, which have been studied intensively in recent years. Many other exposures may be no less important but have received less attention, partly because of insufficient resources in the occupational health field. The Occupational Safety and Health Act of 1970 provides a basis for improving prevention and control programs in the United States. Some approaches toward implementing goals of the act have been outlined.

REFERENCES

1. Acheson ED, Cowdell RH, Rang E: Adenocarcinoma of the nasal cavity and sinuses in England and Wales. Br J Ind Med 29:21–30, 1972
2. Ahlmark A: Silicosis, dust conditions and dust control in Sweden. Staub-Reinhalt. Luft 29:1–6, 1969
3. Allison AC: Lysosomes and the toxicity of particulate pollutants. Arch Intern Med 128:131–139, 1971
4. American Conference of Governmental Industrial Hygienists: Documentation of the threshold limit values for substances in workroom air, ed 3, 1971. Direct requests for copies to the Chairman, TLV Committee, Cincinnati
5. American Conference of Governmental Industrial Hygienists: TLVs: Threshold limit values for chemical substances in workroom air. Cincinnati, 1973
6. Andrews JL, Kazemi H, Hardy HL: Patterns of lung dysfunction in chronic beryllium disease. Am Rev Respir Dis 100:791–800, 1969
7. Annotation: Dust sampling in coalmines. Lancet 2:306, 1971
8. Asbestos Research Council: The cleaning of premises and plant in accordance with the asbestos regulations. Control and Safety Guide, No. 9. London, Thomas Jenkins (Printers) Ltd, 1972
9. Avery SB, Stetson DM, Pan PM, Mathews KP: Immunological investigation of individuals with toluene diisocyanate asthma. Clin Exp Immunol 4:585–596, 1969

10. Avila R, Villar TG: Suberosis: Respiratory disease in cork workers. Lancet 1:620–621, 1968

11. Barbee RA, Callies Q, Dickie HA, Rankin J: The long-term prognosis in farmer's lung. Am Rev Respir Dis 97:223–231, 1968

12. Bates DV, Macklem PT, Christie RV: Respiratory function in disease, ed 2. Philadelphia, WB Saunders Company, 1971

13. Bech AO, Kipling MD, Heather JC: Hard metal disease. Br J Ind Med 19:239–252, 1962

14. Beck EG, Holt PF, Manojlovic N: Comparison of effects on macrophage cultures of glass fibre, glass powder, and chrysotile asbestos. Br J Ind Med 29:280–286, 1972

15. Belin L, Falsen E, Hoborn J, André J: Enzyme sensitisation in consumers of enzyme-containing washing powder. Lancet 2:1153–1157, 1970

16. Berry G, Newhouse ML, Turok M: Combined effect of asbestos exposure and smoking on mortality from lung cancer in factory workers. Lancet 2:476–479, 1972

17. Beswick FW, Holland P, Hemp KH: Acute effects of exposure to orthochlorobenzylidene malononitrile (CS) and the development of tolerance. Br J Ind Med 29:298–306, 1972

18. Beton DC, Andrews GS, Davies HJ, Howells L, Smith GF: Acute cadmium fume poisoning. Five cases with one death from renal necrosis. Br J Ind Med 23:292–301, 1966

19. Blejer HP, Caplan PE (eds): Occupational Health Aspects of Cadmium Inhalation Poisoning with Special Reference to Welding and Silver Brazing, ed 2, 1972. Available free of charge from: Bureau of Occupational Health and Environmental Epidemiology, State of California, Dept of Public Health, 2151 Berkeley Way, Berkeley, Calif, 94704

20. Bonnell JA: Emphysema and proteinuria in men casting copper-cadmium alloys. Br J Ind Med 12:181–197, 1955

21. Bouhuys A, Gee JBL: Environmental lung disease, in: Harrison's Principles of Internal Medicine, ed 7. New York, McGraw-Hill, 1974

21a. Boyd JT, Doll R, Faulds JS, Leiper J: Cancer of the lung in iron ore (haematite) miners. Br J Ind Med 27:97–105, 1970

22. Bryks S, Bertalanffy FD: Cytodynamic reactivity of the mesothelium. Pleural reaction to chrysotile asbestos. Arch Environ Health 23:469–472, 1971

23. Carpenter RG, Cochrane AL, Gilson JC, Higgins ITT: The relationship between ventilatory capacity and simple pneumoconiosis in coalworkers. Br J Ind Med 13:166–176, 1956

24. Carnow BW, Abrams HK, Carnow V: Pulmonary function for detection of incipient disease in foundry workers. Proceedings of the XIV International Congress on Occupational Health, Madrid, 1963. Excerpta Medica, International Congress Series, No. 62:1046–1050, 1963

25. Channell S, Blyth W, Lloyd M, Weir DM, Amos WMG, Littlewood AP, Riddle HFV, Grant IWB: Allergic alveolitis in maltworkers. A clinical, mycological, and immunological study. Q J Med 38:351–376, 1969

26. Clay JR, Rossing RG: Histopathology of exposure to phosgene. Arch Pathol 78:544–551, 1964

27. Coates EO, Watson JHL: Diffuse interstitial lung disease in tungsten carbide workers. Ann Intern Med 75:709–716, 1971

28. Cochrane AL, Carpenter RG: Factors influencing the radiological progression rate of progressive massive fibrosis. Br J Ind Med 13:177–183, 1956

29. Cohen D: Ferromagnetic contamination in the lungs and other organs of the human body. Science 180:745–748, 1973

30. Committee on Biologic Effects of Atmospheric Pollutants: Asbestos: The Need for and Feasibility of Air Pollution Controls. Division of Medical Sciences, National Research Council, National Academy of Sciences, Washington, D.C., 1971

31. Cooper WD, Cralley LJ: Pneumoconiosis in diatomite mining and processing. Public Health Service Publication No. 601, US Government Printing Office, Washington, D.C., 1958

32. Cotes JE, Dabbs JM, Evans MR, Holland P: Effect of CS aerosol upon lung gas transfer and alveolar volume in healthy men. Q J Exp Physiol 57:199–206, 1972

33. Cotes JE, Field GB: Lung gas exchange in simple pneumoconiosis of coal workers. Br J Ind Med 29:268–273, 1972

34. Cralley LJ, Key MM, Groth DH, Lainhart WS, Ligo RM: Fibrous and mineral content of cosmetic talcum products. Am Ind Hyg Assoc J 29:350–354, 1968

35. Dalgaard JB, Dencker F, Fallentin B, Hansen P, Kaempe B, Steensberg J, Wilhardt P: Fatal poisoning and other health hazards connected with industrial fishing. Br J Ind Med 29:307–316, 1972

36. Davis JMG: The long term fibrogenic effects of chrysotile and crocidolite asbestos dust injected into the pleural cavity of experimental animals. Br J Exp Pathol 51:617–627, 1970

37. Davis JMG, Gross P, DeTreville RTP: "Ferruginous Bodies" in guinea pigs. Arch Pathol 89:364–373, 1970

38. Daynes WG: The prevention of Transkei silicosis. S Afr Med J 47:352–353, 1973

39. DeLuca L, Anderson GH, Wolf G: The in vivo and in vitro biosynthesis of lung tissue glycopeptides. Arch Intern Med 127:853–857, 1971

40. Doll R: Practical steps towards the prevention of bronchial carcinoma. Scott Med J 15:433–447, 1970

41. Doll R, Vessey MP, Beasley RWR, Buckley AR, Fear EC, Fisher REW, Gammon EJ, Gunn W, Hughes GO, Lee K, Norman-Smith B: Mortality of gasworkers—final report of a prospective study. Br J Ind Med 29:394–406, 1972

42. Dubos R: Toxic factors in enzymes used in laundry products. Science 173:259–260, 1971

43. DuBois AB, Dautrebande ·L: Acute effects of breathing inert dust particles and of carbachol aerosol on the mechanical characteristics of the lungs in man. Changes in response after inhaling sympathomimetic aerosols. J Clin Invest 37:1746–1755, 1958

44. Duncan KP, Howell RW: Detection of lung cancer in a male industrial population. Br J Prev Soc Med 21:30–34, 1967

45. Edwards JH: The double dialysis method of producing farmer's lung antigens. J Lab Clin Med 79:683–688, 1972

46. Edwards JH, Barboriak JJ, Fink JN: Antigens in pigeon breeders' disease. Immunology 19:729–734, 1970

47. Elgefors B, Belin L, Hanson LA: Pigeon breeder's lung. Clinical and immunological observations. Scand J Respir Dis 52:167–176, 1971

48. Elmes PC, Simpson MJC: Insulation workers in Belfast. 3. Mortality 1940–66. Br J Ind Med 28:226–236, 1971

49. Emanuel DA, Lawton BR, Wenzel FJ: Maple-bark disease. Pneumonitis due to Coniosporum corticale. N Engl J Med 266:333–337, 1962

50. Emanuel DA, Wenzel FJ, Bowerman CI, Lawton BR: Farmer's lung. Clinical, pathologic, and immunologic study of twenty-four patients. Am J Med 37:392–401, 1964

51. Emanuel DA, Wenzel FJ, Lawton BR: Pneumonitis due to cryptostroma corticale (maple-bark disease). N Engl J Med 274:1413–1418, 1966

52. Enterline P, de Coufle P, Henderson V: Respiratory cancer in relation to occupational exposures among retired asbestos workers. Br J Ind Med 30:162–166, 1973

53. Evans DJ, Posner E: Pneumoconiosis in laundry workers. Environ Res 4:121–128, 1971

54. Fenn WO: The phagocytosis of solid particles. III. Carbon and quartz. J Gen Physiol 3:575–593, 1921

55. Fibrosing alveolitis (editorial). Lancet 1:999–1000, 1971

56. Figueroa WF, Raszkowski R, Weiss W: Lung cancer in chloromethyl methyl ether workers. N Engl J Med 288:1096–1097, 1973

57. FitzGerald MX, Carrington CB, Gaensler EA: Environmental lung disease, in: Symposium on Chronic Respiratory Disease, The Medical Clinics of North America, 57:593–622, Philadelphia, WB Saunders Company, 1973

58. Fletcher DE: A mortality study of shipyard workers with pleural plaques. Br J Ind Med 29:142–145, 1972

59. Fletcher K, Wyatt I: The composition of lung lipids after poisoning with paraquat. Br J Exp Pathol 51:604–610, 1970

60. Flindt MLH: Pulmonary disease due to inhalation of derivatives of Bacillus

subtilis containing proteolytic enzyme. Lancet 1:1177–1181, 1969

61. Frost J, Georg J: The clinical evaluation of disability in silicosis. Acta Med Scand 147:349–357, 1953

62. Fulwiler RD, Abbott JC, Darcy FJ: Evaluation of detergent enzymes in air. Am Ind Hyg Assoc J 33:231–236, 1972

63. Gaensler EA, Verstraeten JM, Weil WB, Cugell DW, Marks A, Cadigan JB, Jones RH, Ellicott MF: Respiratory pathophysiology in chronic beryllium disease. AMA Arch Ind Health 19: 132–145, 1959

64. Gandevia B: Studies of ventilatory capacity and histamine response during exposure to isocyanate vapour in polyurethane foam manufacture. Br J Ind Med 20:204–209, 1963

65. Gardiner AJS: Pulmonary oedema in paraquat poisoning. Thorax 27:132–135, 1972

66. Gibbs GW, Lachance M: Dust exposure in the chrysotile asbestos mines and mills of Quebec. Arch Environ Health 24:189–197, 1972

67. Gilson JC: Health hazards of asbestos. Composites 3:57–59, 1972

68. Gilson JC: Problems and perspectives: The changing hazards of exposure to asbestos, in: Biological effects of asbestos. Ann NY Acad Sci 132:696–705, 1965

69. Gilson JC: The first Wade lecture: The changing pattern of pneumoconiosis, in: Health Conditions in the Ceramic Industry. International Symposium, Stoke-on-Trent. Oxford, Pergamon Press, 1969, pp 11–28

70. Goldblatt PJ, Lieberman MW, Witschi H: Beryllium-induced ultrastructural changes in intact and regenerating liver. Arch Environ Health 26:48–56, 1973

71. Governa M, Rosanda C: A histochemical study of the asbestos body coating. Br J Ind Med 29:154–159, 1972

72. Grant IWB, Blyth W, Wardrop VE, Gordon RM, Pearson JCG, Mair A: Prevalence of farmer's lung in Scotland: A pilot survey. Br Med J 1:530–534, 1972

72a. Griggs K: Toxic metal fumes from mantle-type camp lanterns. Science 181: 842–843, 1973

73. Gross P, deTreville RTP, Haller MN: Pulmonary ferruginous bodies in city dwellers. Arch Environ Health 19: 186–188, 1969

74. Gross P, deTreville RTP, Haller MN: Asbestos versus nonasbestos fibers. Arch Environ Health 20:571–578, 1970

75. Gross P, Rinehart WE, deTreville RTP: The pulmonary reactions to toxic gases. Am Ind Hyg Assoc J 28:315–321, 1967

76. Grünspan M, Antweiler H, Dehnen W: Effect of silica on phospholipids in the rat lung. Br J Ind Med 30:74–77, 1973

77. Haldane JS, Priestley JG: Respiration. London, Oxford University Press, 1935

78. Hallee TJ: Diffuse lung disease caused by inhalation of mercury vapor. Am Rev Respir Dis 99:430–436, 1969

79. Hammond EC, Selikoff IJ: Relation of cigarette smoking to risk of death of asbestos-associated disease among insulation workers in the United States. Environmental Cancer Research Project, presented at meeting of the Working Group to Assess Biological Effects of Asbestos, Lyon, International Agency for Research on Cancer, 1972

80. Hanna MG Jr, Nettesheim P, Gilbert JR (eds): Inhalation Carcinogenesis. US Atomic Energy Commission, Division of Technical Information, 1970

81. Hardy HL, Chamberlin RI: Beryllium, Alloys, Compounds. Encyclopaedia of Occupational Health and Safety. vol I, A–K. Geneva, International Labour Office, 1971, pp 170–175

82. Harries PG, MacKenzie FAF, Sheers G, Kemp JH, Oliver TP, Wright DS: Radiological survey of men exposed to asbestos in naval dockyards. Br J Ind Med 29:274–279, 1972

83. Hasleton PS: Incidence of emphysema at necropsy as assessed by point-counting. Thorax 27:552–556, 1972

84. Heppleston AG, Fletcher K, Wyatt I: Abnormalities of lung lipids following inhalation of quartz. Experientia 28: 938–939, 1972

85. Heppleston AG, Styles JA: Activity of a macrophage factor in collagen formation by silica. Nature 214:521–522, 1967

86. Higgins ITT, Oldham PD: Ventilatory capacity in miners. A five-year follow-up study. Br J Ind Med 19:65–76, 1962

87. Hill JW, Whitehead WS, Cameron JD, Hedgecock GA: Glass fibres: absence of pulmonary hazard in production

workers. Br J Ind Med 30:174–179, 1973

88. Hofmann A, Neufelder M: Tierexperimentelle Untersuchungen zur gewerbetoxikologischen Beurteilung von 2-Chloräthylisocyanat. Arch Toxikol 29:73–84, 1972

89. Holt PF, Young DK: Asbestos fibres in the air of towns. Atmos Environ 7:481–483, 1973

90. Hunter B, Thomson C: Evaluation of the tumorigenic potential of vermiculite by intrapleural injection in rats. Br J Ind Med 30:167–173, 1973

91. Jameson JE: Precipitins with relevance to farmer's lung and aspergillosis in normal and other sera. J Clin Pathol 22:519–526, 1969

92. Jodoin G, Gibbs GW, Macklem PT, McDonald JC, Becklake MR: Early effects of asbestos exposure on lung function. Am Rev Respir Dis 104:525–535, 1971

93. Jones GR, Proudfoot AT, Hall JI: Pulmonary effects of acute exposure to nitrous fumes. Thorax 28:61–65, 1973

94. Jones JG, Warner CG: Chronic exposure to iron oxide, chromium oxide, and nickel oxide fumes of metal dressers in a steelworks. Br J Ind Med 29:169–177, 1972

95. Jones WW: The newer pneumoconioses (with special regard to foundry risks). Ann Occup Hyg 10:241–248, 1967

96. Key MM, Kerr LE, Bundy M: Pulmonary Reactions to Coal Dust: A Review of U.S. Experience. New York, Academic Press, 1971

97. Key MM: Health standards and standard setting in the United States. Ann NY Acad Sci 200: 707–711, 1972

97a. Knappmann J: Beobachtungen an 251 obduzierten Mesotheliom-Fällen in Hamburg (1958–1968). Pneumonologie 148:60–65, 1972

98. Kowitz TA, Reba RC, Parker RT. Spicer WS Jr: Effects of chlorine gas upon respiratory function. Arch Environ Health 14:545–558, 1967

99. Kuncová M, Havránková J, Holusa R, Palecek F: Experimental silicosis of the rat. Correlation of functional, biochemical, and histological changes. Arch Environ Health 23:365–372, 1971

100. Kuschner M: The J. Burns Amberson Lecture. The causes of lung cancer. Am Rev Respir Dis 98:573–590, 1968

101. Lainhart WS, Felson B, Jacobson G, Pendergrass EP: Pneumoconiotic lesions in bituminous coal miners and metal miners. Arch Environ Health 16:207–210, 1968

102. Landa J, Avery WG, Sackner MA: Some physiologic observations in smoke inhalation. Chest 61:62–64, 1972

103. Langer AM, Selikoff IJ, Sastre A: Chrysotile asbestos in the lungs of persons in New York City. Arch Environ Health 22:348–361, 1971

104. Lapp NL: Physiological changes as diagnostic aids in isocyanate exposure. Am Ind Hyg Assoc J 32:378–382, 1971

105. Lapp NL, Hankinson JL, Burgess DB, O'Brien R: Changes in ventilatory function in coal miners after a work shift. Arch Environ Health 24:204–208, 1972

106. Laskin S, Drew RT, Cappiello VP, Kuschner M: Inhalation studies with freshly generated polyurethane foam dust, in Mercer TT, Morrow PE, Stöber W (eds): Assessment of Airborne Particles. Springfield, Charles C Thomas, 1972, pp 382–404

107. Laskin S, Kuschner M, Drew RT, Cappiello VP, Nelson N: Tumors of the respiratory tract induced by inhalation of bis(chloromethyl)ether. Arch Environ Health 23:135–136, 1971

108. Lewis GP, Jusko WJ, Coughlin LL, Hartz S: Contribution of cigarette smoking to cadmium accumulation in man. Lancet 1:291–292, 1972

109. Lister WB, Wimborne D: Carbon pneumoconiosis in a synthetic graphite worker. Br J Ind Med 29:108–110, 1972

110. Lloyd JW: Long-term mortality study of steelworkers. V. Respiratory cancer in coke plant workers. J Occup Med 13:53–68, 1971

111. Lloyd-Davies TA: Respiratory Disease in Foundrymen, Report of a Survey. London, HMSO, 1971

112. Lowe CR, Khosla T: Chronic bronchitis in ex-coal miners working in the steel industry. Br J Ind Med 29:45–49, 1972

113. Lowry T, Schuman LM: "Silo-filler's disease"—a syndrome caused by nitrogen dioxide. JAMA 162:153–160, 1956

114. Mancuso TF: Relation of duration of employment and prior respiratory illness to respiratory cancer among beryllium workers. Environ Res 3:251–275, 1970

115. Mangold CA, Beckett RR: Combined occupational exposure of silver brazers to cadmium oxide, nitrogen dioxide and fluorides at a naval shipyard. Am Ind Hyg Assoc J 32:115–118, 1971

116. Maroudas NG, O'Neill CH, Stanton MF: Fibroblast anchorage in carcinogenesis by fibres. Lancet 1:807–809, 1973

117. Mattson S-B, Ringquist T: Pleural plaques and exposure to asbestos. Scand J Respir Dis (suppl 75), 1970

118. McDonald AD, Harper A, El Attar OA, McDonald JC: Epidemiology of primary malignant mesothelial tumors in Canada. Cancer 26:914–919, 1970

119. McDonald JC, Becklake MR, Fournier-Massey G, Rossiter CE: Respiratory symptoms in chrysotile asbestos mine and mill workers of Quebec. Arch Environ Health 24:358–363, 1972

120. McEwen J, Finlayson A, Mair A: Asbestos and mesothelioma in Scotland. An epidemiological study. Int Arch Arbeitsmed 28:301–311, 1971

121. McKerrow CB, Davies HJ, Jones AP: Symptoms and lung function following acute and chronic exposure to tolyene diisocyanate. Proc R Soc Med 63:376–378, 1970

122. Miller GJ, Hearn CED, Edwards RHT: Pulmonary function at rest and during exercise following bagassosis. Br J Ind Med 28:152–158, 1971

123. Mitchell CA, Gandevia B: Respiratory symptoms and skin reactivity in workers exposed to proteolytic enzymes in the detergent industry. Am Rev Respir Dis 104:1–12, 1971

124. Morgan WKC, Lapp NL, Seaton A: Respiratory impairment in simple coal workers' pneumoconiosis. J Occup Med 14:839–844, 1972

125. Murphy RLH, Ferris BG Jr, Burgess WA, Worcester J, Gaensler EA: Effects of low concentrations of asbestos. N Engl J Med 285:1271–1278, 1971

126. Murphy RLH Jr, Gaensler EA, Redding RA, Belleau R, Keelan PJ, Smith AA, Goff AM, Ferris BG Jr: Low exposure to asbestos: gas exchange in ship pipe coverers and controls. Arch Environ Health 25:253–264, 1972

127. Murphy RL, Levine BW, Al Bazzaz FJ, Lynch JJ, Burgess WA: Floor tile installation as a source of asbestos exposure. Am Rev Respir Dis 104:576–580, 1971

127a. Murphy, RLH Jr, Dorensen K: Chest auscultation in the diagnosis of pulmonary asbestosis. J Occup Med 15:272–276, 1973

128. Muysers K, Siehoff F, Worth G, Gasthaus L: Die Lungenfunktion bei der Bronchitis unter Berücksichtigung beruflich bedingter Exposition gegenüber Luftverunreinigungen. Med Thorac 23:265–282, 1966

129. Neubert H: Zur Silicose in der gewerblichen Wirtschaft: Ein statistischer Ueberblick. Zentralbl Arbeitsmed 21:252–256, 1971

130. Newhouse ML, Berry G, Wagner JC, Turok ME: A study of the mortality of female asbestos workers. Br J Ind Med 29:134–141, 1972

131. Newhouse ML, Tagg B, Pocock SJ, McEwan AC: An epidemiological study of workers producing enzyme washing powders. Lancet 1:689–693, 1970

132. Nishizumi M: Electron microscopic study of cadmium nephrotoxicity in the rat. Arch Environ Health 24:215–225, 1972

133. Norberg GF, Nishiyama K: Whole-body and hair retention of cadmium in mice. Arch Environ Health 24:209–214, 1972

134. Norwood WD, Wisehart DE, Earl CA, Adley FE, Anderson DE: Nitrogen dioxide poisoning due to metal-cutting with oxyacetylene torch. J Occup Med 8:301–306, 1966

135. Osburn HS: Lung cancer in a mining district in Rhodesia. S Afr Med J 43:1307–1312, 1969

136. Palmer PES, Daynes G: Transkei silicosis. S Afr Med J 41:1182–1188, 1967

137. Pariente R, Berry JP, Galle P, Cayrol E, Brouet G: A study of pulmonary dust deposits using the electron microscope in conjunction with the electron sound analyser. Thorax 27:80–82, 1972

138. Parrot JL, Hébert R, Saindelle A, Ruff F: Platinum and platinosis. Allergy and histamine release due to some platinum salts. Arch Environ Health 19:685–691, 1969

139. Patty FA (ed): Industrial hygiene and toxicology, (ed 2) vol II, Toxicology, Fassett DW, Irish DD (eds). New York, Interscience Publishers, 1963

140. Pepys J: Pulmonary hypersensitivity disease due to inhaled organic antigens. Ann Intern Med 64:943–948, 1966

141. Pepys J, Hargreave FE, Longbottom JL, Faux J: Allergic reactions of the lungs to enzymes of Bacillus subtilis. Lancet 1:1181–1184, 1969

142. Pepys J, Jenkins PA: Precipitin (F.L. H.) test in farmer's lung. Thorax 20: 21–35, 1965

143. Peters JM, Murphy RLH, Pagnotto LD, van Ganse WF: Acute respiratory effects in workers exposed to low levels of toluene diisocyanate (TDI). Arch Environ Health 16:642–647, 1968

144. Peters JM, Murphy RLH, Pagnotto LD, Whittenberger JL: Respiratory impairment in workers exposed to "safe" levels of toluene diisocyanate (TDI). Arch Environ Health 20:364–367, 1970

145. Phibbs BP, Sundin RE, Mitchell RS: Silicosis in Wyoming bentonite workers. Am Rev Respir Dis 103:1–17, 1971

146. Pichirallo J: Black lung: Dispute about diagnosis of miners' ailment. Science 174:132–134, 1971

147. Pierce AK, Nicholson DP, Miller JM, Johnson RL Jr: Pulmonary function in bagasse worker's lung disease: Am Rev Respir Dis 97:561–570, 1968

148. Pontefract RD, Cunningham HM: Penetration of asbestos through the digestive tract of rats. Nature 243:352–353, 1973

149. Polymer-fume fever (editorial). Lancet 2:27–28, 1972

150. Pooley FD: Electron microscope characteristics of inhaled chrysotile asbestos fibre. Br J Ind Med 29:146–153, 1972

151. Rae S: Pneumoconiosis and coal dust exposure. Br Med Bull 27:53–58, 1971

152. Rajan KT, Wagner JC, Evans PH: The response of human pleura in organ culture to asbestos. Nature 238:346–347, 1972

153. Ramazzini B: De Morbis Artificum Diatriba. Wright WC (ed). Chicago, University of Chicago Press, 1940

154. Redding RA, Hardy HL, Gaensler EA: Beryllium disease: a 16-year follow-up case study. Respiration 25:263–278, 1968

155. Redmond CK, Ciocco A, Lloyd JW, Rush HW: Long-term mortality study of steelworkers; VI—Mortality from malignant neoplasms among coke oven workers. J Occup Med 14:621–629, 1972

156. Reeves AL, Puro HE, Smith RG, Vorwald AJ: Experimental asbestos carcinogenesis. Environ Res 4:496–511, 1971

157. Refsum HE: Pulmonary gas exchange during and after exercise of short duration in silicosis. Scand J Clin Lab Invest 29 (suppl 121): 1–45, 1972

158. Reitze WB, Nicholson WJ, Holaday DA, Selikoff IJ: Application of sprayed inorganic fiber containing asbestos: occupational health hazards. Am Ind Hyg Assoc J 33:178–191, 1972

159. Renie O, Cavigneaux A, Le Bouffant L, Martin J-C, Durif S, Krespine C: Silicose aigüe. A propos d'un cas. Arch Mal Prof 33:298–300, 1972

160. Report of the Advisory Committee on Asbestos Cancers to the Director of the International Agency for Research on Cancer. Br J Ind Med 30:180–186, 1973

161. Rickards AL, Badami DV: Chrysotile asbestos in urban air. Nature 234:93–94, 1971

162. Rossiter CE, Bristol LJ, Cartier PH, Gilson JC, Grainger TR, Sluis-Cremer GK, McDonald JC: Radiographic changes in chrysotile asbestos mine and millworkers of Quebec. Arch Environ Health 24:388–400, 1972

163. Sacharov KM, Knauss KG, Kubala PJ: Reductions of dust exposures in the slate industry. Am Ind Hyg Assoc J 32:119–122, 1971

164. Sakula A: Mushroom-worker's lung. Br Med J 3:708–710, 1967

165. Schilling RSF (ed): Occupational Health Practice. London, Butterworths, 1973

166. Schoenberg JB: The OSHA asbestos standard and its medical surveillance requirement: purposes, implementation and implications. MPH Thesis, Yale University, 1973

167. Seaton A, Lapp NL, Morgan WKC: Lung mechanics and frequency dependence of compliance in coal miners. J Clin Invest 51:1203–1211, 1972

168. Seaton A, Lapp NL, Morgan WKC: Relationship of pulmonary impairment in simple coal workers' pneumoconiosis to type of radiographic opacity. Br J Ind Med 29:50–55, 1972

169. Selikoff IJ, Churg J, Hammond EC: Asbestos exposure and neoplasia. JAMA 188:22–26, 1964

170. Selikoff IJ, Hammond EC, Churg J:

Carcinogenicity of amosite asbestos. Arch Environ Health 25:183–186, 1972

171. Selikoff IJ, Hammond EC, Seidman H: Cancer risk of insulation workers in the United States. Environmental Cancer Research Project, presented at meeting of Working Group to Assess Biological Effects of Asbestos, Lyon, International Agency for Research on Cancer, 1972

172. Selikoff IJ, Key MM, Lee DHK (eds): Coal workers' pneumoconiosis. Ann NY Acad Sci 200:1–861, 1972

173. Selikoff IJ, Nicholson WJ, Langer AM: Asbestos air pollution. Arch Environ Health 25:1–13, 1972

174. Shore NS, Greene R, Kazemi H: Lung dysfunction in workers exposed to Bacillus subtilis enzyme. Environ Res 4: 512–519, 1971

175. Showalter DR: How to Make the OSHA-1970 Work For You. Handbook of the Williams-Steiger Occupational Safety and Health Administration. Ann Arbor, Ann Arbor Science Publishers, Inc, 1972

176. Skalpe IO: Long-term effects of sulphur dioxide exposure in pulp mills. Br J Ind Med 21:69–73, 1964

177. Sluis-Cremer GK, DuToit RSJ: Pneumoconiosis in chromite miners in South Africa. Br J Ind Med 25:63–67, 1968

178. Spencer H: Pathology of the Lung, ed 2. Oxford, Pergamon Press, 1968

179. Standard for exposure to asbestos dust. Title 29: Labor, Part 1910, Occupational Safety and Health Standards. Fed Regis 37:11318–11322, June 7, 1972

180. Stănescu DC, Pilat L, Gavrilescu N, Teculescu DB, Cristescu I: Aspects of pulmonary mechanics in arc welders' siderosis. Br J Ind Med 24:143–147, 1967

181. Stanton MF, Wrench C: Mechanisms of mesothelioma induction with asbestos and fibrous glass. J Natl Cancer Inst 48:797–821, 1972

182. Stack BHR: The clinical manifestations and diagnosis of fibrosing alveolitis. BTTA Rev 1:15–22, 1971

182a. Stell PM, McGill T: Asbestos and laryngeal carcinoma. Lancet 2:416–417, 1973

183. Sticher H, Spycher MA, Ruettner JR: Crystallization in vivo of rhabdophane in human lungs. Nature 241:49, 1973

184. Stoeckle JD, Kazemi H, Chamberlin R: Exposure, complaints, chest film abnormalities and lung function tests among beryllium workers: Preliminary report. J Occup Med 15:301, 1973

185. Stokinger HE (ed): Beryllium, Its Industrial Hygiene Aspects. New York, Academic Press, 1966

186. Stumphius J: Epidemiology of mesothelioma on Walcheren Island. Br J Ind Med 28:59–66, 1971

186a. Tabershaw IR, Cooper WC, Balzer JL: A labor-management occupational health service in a construction industry. Arch Environ Health 21:784–788, 1970

187. Target health hazards. Washington, D.C., US Dept of Labor, Occupational Safety and Health Administration, 1972

188. Teculescu DB, Stănescu DC: Pulmonary function in workers with chronic exposure to cadmium oxide fumes. Int Arch Arbeitsmed 26:335–345, 1970

189. Tewksbury DA, Wenzel FJ, Emanuel DA: An immunological study of maple bark disease. Clin Exp Immunol 3:857–863, 1968

190. Timbrell V: Inhalation and biological effects of asbestos, in Mercer TT, Morrow PE, Stöber W (eds): Assessment of Airborne Particles. Springfield, Charles C Thomas, 1972, pp 429–445

191. Toluene di-isocyanate in industry. Operating and Medical Codes of Practice. A Report of the Isocyanate Sub-Committee of the British Manufacturers' Association, Ltd. Health Advisory Committee, BRMA, Health Research Unit, Scala House, Birmingham, 1971

192. Trends in usage of beryllium and beryllium oxide. Committee on Technical Aspects of Critical and Strategic Materials. Materials Advisory Board. National Research Council Publication, MAB-238, 1968

192a. Tse KS, Warren P, Janusz M, McCarthy DS, Cherniack RM: Respiratory abnormalities in workers exposed to grain dust. Arch Environ Health 27:74–77, 1973

193. Tse RL, Bockman AA: Nitrogen dioxide toxicity: report of four cases in firemen. JAMA 212:1341–1344, 1970

194. van Ganse WF, Oleffe J, van Hove W, Groetenbriel C: Lymphocyte transformation in chronic pulmonary berylliosis. Lancet 1:1023, 1972

195. Wagoner JK, Archer VE, Lundin FE Jr, Holaday DA, Lloyd JW: Radiation

as the cause of lung cancer among uranium miners. N Engl J Med 273:181–188, 1965

196. Weill H, Buechner HA, Gonzalez E, Herbert SJ, Aucoin E, Ziskind MM: Bagassosis: A study of pulmonary function in 20 cases. Ann Intern Med 64:737–747, 1966

197. Weill H, Waddell LC, Ziskind M: A study of workers exposed to detergent enzymes. JAMA 217:425–433, 1971

198. Wenzel FJ, Emanuel DA: The epidemiology of maple bark disease. Arch Environ Health 14:385–389, 1967

199. Wenzel FJ, Emanuel DA, Gray RL: Immunofluorescent studies in patients with farmer's lung. J Aller Clin Immunol 48:224–229, 1971

200. Williams N, Smith FK: Polymer-fume fever. An elusive diagnosis. JAMA 219:1587–1589, 1972

201. Worth G, Valentin H, Venrath H, Gasthaus L, Hoffmann H: Weitere klinische und spirographische Untersuchungen bei Bergleuten vor, während und nach der Untertagearbeit. Arch Gewerbepath Gewerbehyg 14:269–290, 1956

202. Wyatt JP: Occupational lung diseases and inferential relationships to general population hazards. Am J Pathol 64:197–208, 1971

203. Zikria BA, Ferrer JM, Floch HF: The chemical factors contributing to pulmonary damage in "smoke poisoning." Surgery 71:704–709, 1972

204. Hargreave FE: Extrinsic allergic alveolitis. Can Med Assoc J 108:1150–1154, 1973

Chapter 16

Air Pollution

Unlike smoking and industrial exposures, air pollution concerns us all. Newspaper photographs of Tokyo residents and Venetian gondoliers wearing gas masks have dramatized this concern. Dead orange trees and damaged crops in southern California and elsewhere are silent witnesses that air pollutants can kill at least some forms of life. Yet, while air pollution is a legitimate public concern, the actual risks to human health are ill-documented and thus a source of confusion and debate.

Does air pollution in fact endanger human health, or are its risks less tangible, including discomfort, lack of visibility, and a decreased quality of life? If there is a risk to health, are the effects of pollution mainly immediate or delayed? Are these effects primarily on the lungs, or also on other organs and functions, as on the body's ability to fight infection? Finally, what constitutes a safe exposure to air pollution—the lowest level which affects the most sensitive individual, or the highest level consistent with minimal effects in the majority of people?

These questions are more than academic. Present US law and proposed pollution-abatement programs are based on the assumption that air pollution poses a grave threat to health, and most evidence quoted to support this assumption relates to lung diseases. However, this evidence is inadequate and the assumption is therefore unwarranted. For instance, the primary standards for ambient air quality which arise from the Clean Air Act of 1970 are supposedly those "requisite to protect the public health." [31] Based on these standards, the Environmental Protection Agency (EPA) recently called for measures of far-reaching social and economic impact—measures which, most notably, might require an 80 percent reduction in automobile traffic in Los Angeles County by 1975. [47, 105] Yet, the primary standards are based largely on weak and in some instances even misleading data from epidemiological studies that lack sufficient controls.

Better-controlled, short-term toxicological studies have generally shown pollutant effects only in concentrations that exceed those in heavily polluted cities. An increased death rate, mainly affecting people with preexisting lung or heart disease, has been documented during often-quoted but infrequent pollution disasters (e.g., in the Meuse Valley, Belgium, 1930; in Donora, Pa., 1948; and in London, UK, 1952). But the evidence for major health damage from lesser degrees of air pollution is much more tenuous. In fact, the bulk of the reliable data available seems to point the other way. Statements to the effect that "man is very close to suffocating himself" [80] are clearly unwarranted and misinformed.

On the other hand, the absence of reliable data does not prove that polluted air is harmless. It may merely mean that the methods used to assess the effects have been inappropriate or too insensitive. Furthermore, most of the better studies have related only to acute effects of pure pollutants. Until long-term toxicological studies are performed that test the effects of low-level, mixed exposures to pollutants commonly found in urban air, harmful effects to the lungs from realistic pollutant levels cannot be positively excluded.

In addition to the primary standards for air quality, secondary standards, or those "requisite to protect the public welfare from any known or anticipated adverse effects" of air pollution, such as those on vegetation and materials, arose from the Clean Air Act of 1970. But it is the primary, or health, standards which, by the law's definition, necessarily shape plans to improve air quality in cities. Since health effects are quoted as the only factor to be considered in setting primary standards for air quality under present law,[31] a critical review of the known dangers of air pollutants to human lungs appears to be in order.

The first two sections of this chapter will review the characteristics of polluted air masses and the methods used to study their effects on man's lungs. Subsequent sections will review the toxic effects of individual pollutants, based on observations in man and in animals. Next, the epidemiological evidence linking polluted air and specific pollutants with lung diseases is discussed. Finally, the implications of toxicological as well as epidemiological evidence for control programs will be critically reviewed.

CHARACTERISTICS OF POLLUTED AIR MASSES

Atmospheric air commonly contains small amounts of gases other than its normal constituents (O_2, N_2, CO_2, inert gases, and water vapor) as well as liquid droplets and solid particles. The term pollutant is usually applied to objectionable air additives. Standardized methods and instruments for quantitative determinations of many pollutants in ambient air are available.[5, 55] The types and amounts of pollutants found in community air depend on (1) the sources of pollutants, (2) geographical and meteorological factors, and (3) chemical reactions in the atmosphere which alter pollutant levels.[102]

Sources of pollutants. The main sources of pollutants include industrial operations, automobiles, incinerators and home-heating fuel burners, in addition to natural sources (e.g., volcanoes, forest fires, swamps). Factories sometimes emit gases, fumes, and dusts formed during industrial processes (see Tables 15-1 and 15-2) into the surrounding community. Incinerators, power plants, and home-heating burners release products of complete and incomplete combustion into the air unless provided with emission-control systems. Automobiles, primarily through exhaust fumes, emit a complex pollutant mixture. Some pollutants emitted by man-made sources are also formed in nature (e.g., carbon monoxide); other pollutants rarely occur naturally (e.g., sulfur dioxide). Geographical factors, such as mountain ranges and river valleys, affect the dispersion of pollutants in a more or less confined area. On a smaller scale, elevation above ground level in or outside buildings or emission of pollutants in confined areas (tunnels) determine local variations in pollutant levels. Climatic influences on air pollution include wind speed and direction, rain and snow, sunlight and temperature. Lack of wind prevents dispersion and dilution of pollutants, and prevailing wind directions determine where pollutants spread. Rain and snow decrease air-pollutant levels by dissolving gases and by precipitating suspended particulate matter. Sunlight is a main ingredient in the formation of photochemical smog (see below). Temperature influences the dispersion of pollutants by affecting airflow patterns, a particularly important effect where masses of cooler air may be trapped under a layer of warmer air, as often occurs in the Los Angeles basin. When such temperature inversions occur, polluted masses of air build up below the layer of warm air and cannot be dispersed until wind speeds increase sufficiently. Physical and chemical reactions in the atmosphere alter many pollutants. Thus, sulfur dioxide is converted to sulfuric acid in mists, gases may be adsorbed on particle surfaces, and intricate chemical reactions occur in photochemical smog. These reactions may increase the irritating potential of the pollutants in several ways. On the other hand, chemical reactions may also neutralize pollutant effects, as when sulfur dioxide is bound by ammonia. In addition many pollutants are absorbed and converted into other compounds in the soil [1] and in building materials.[7] Thus, naturally occurring reactions may help to increase or decrease air-pollutant levels.

Two main classes of pollution account for the majority of air-quality problems in our cities: (1) sulfur oxides and particulate pollution, and (2) photochemical smog. The former results mainly from burning coal and other types of fossil fuel containing sulfur. This type of pollution occurs in cities and industrialized areas, and it is often worst in cold and moist weather. Photochemical smog, on the other hand, results from complex chemical reactions in the atmosphere, with automobile exhaust gases as its main substrate, and requires sunlight to form its irritating components. Thus, it is worst in areas with heavy automobile traffic and a sunny climate.

EPIDEMIOLOGICAL VERSUS TOXICOLOGICAL STUDIES

The World Health Organization, the US Environmental Protection Agency, and national organizations in other countries base standards for pollution control on epidemiological as well as toxicological studies. These two types of studies differ in particular in the degree of certainty that can be attached to their findings. Epidemiological studies are extremely difficult to design and to control, since both the population and pollution levels vary in time and in place. Hence, these studies usually do not meet a prime requirement of scientific work, i.e., that the results be subject to verification by other investigators studying the same phenomenon with the same methods. Short-term toxicological studies, on the other hand, are relatively easy to control and repeat, and, if verified, carry considerable scientific weight.

Unfortunately, verifying the results of long-term toxicological studies, designed to test effects of chronic low-level exposures, will require many years of costly work. Thus, while it is tempting to propose control measures on the basis of short-term toxicological or epidemiological studies, the evidence from these is insufficient for this purpose.

In the following sections, results of both kinds of studies will be reviewed.

TOXIC EFFECTS OF AIR POLLUTANTS

In experiments with controlled exposures, most single pollutants exert toxic effects on human and animal airways or lungs only in concentrations that exceed those actually found in urban polluted air (Table 16-1). Experiments with pollutant mixtures resembling actual polluted air and with long-term exposures are few. Consequently, the assessment of pollutant toxicology which follows is necessarily tentative and incomplete.

To determine which ambient pollutant levels are safe for prolonged exposure in the general population and in sensitive individuals, controlled experiments in suitable inhalation facilities, with exposure lasting several weeks, are needed. The experiments would require a facility perhaps somewhat similar to Skylab in the US space program. Some suggestions for exposure levels for such studies are inserted in the last column of Table 16-1. More use could also be made of lung-function measurements in persons exposed to urban air. For instance, no one appears to have determined whether or not the short-lasting oxidant peaks in Los Angeles are accompanied by fluctuations in lung function, using sensitive methods of assessment.

Sulfur Compounds [79]

The most important pollutants in this group are sulfur dioxide (SO_2) and sulfuric acid and its salts. High concentrations of SO_2 cause chemical bronchitis (Chap. 15), with increased mucus production and inflammation of the mucosa. Low-grade SO_2-induced (7–20 ppm) inflammation promotes experimental virus pneumonia in mice.[34] Concentrations in the order of 50–100 mg/cu m (17.5–35 ppm) are associated with increased chronic respiratory symptoms during prolonged exposure in industry (Chap. 15). In healthy persons, maximum flow rates at low lung volumes decrease after brief exposures to SO_2 in concentrations of 2.86 mg/cu m (1 ppm).[100] No effect occurred after exposure to 0.5 ppm (1.43 mg/cu m) up to 5 minutes (unpublished observation from our laboratory by CA Mitchell et al). These experiments were done during mouth breathing and thus demonstrate the effect of SO_2 in the absence of the nose's scrubbing function (Chap. 2). Since healthy persons normally breathe through their mouths during exercise, and sometimes even at rest, the effect of SO_2 during experiments with mouth breathing is relevant to air-pollution health effects. When breathing through the nose, only a fraction of the inhaled SO_2 reaches lower airways, so that the response would be less.

Changes in maximum flow rates suggest that 1 ppm SO_2 can cause narrowing of small airways in man (Chap. 9). Whether continued exposure leads to chronic

Table 16-1

Summary of Selected Air Pollutants, Exposure Standards,
and Respiratory Health Effects

Pollutant	TLV (mg/ cu m)	AQS Primary (mg/ cu m)	Typical US High Urban Level (mg/ cu m)	Acute Effects in Man (mg/ cu m)	Chronic Exposure Levels to Be Studied (mg/cu m)
SO_2 [79]	13.0	0.365 [a]	0.860 [h]	2.86 [100]	0.08–1.80
Particulates [77]	10.0 [b]	0.260 [a]	0.180 [i]	> 10.0 [77]	Note A
Carbon mono- xide [75]	55.0	10.0 [c]	20.0 [f]	58.0 [m 75]	Note B
Oxidants (ozone) [78]	0.2	0.160 [d]	0.500 [k]	0.74 [45a]	0.10–0.80
Nitrogen dioxide [3]	9.0	0.100 [g]	0.480 [l]	7.5 [3]	0.10–1.00
Hydrocarbons [76]	—	0.160 [e]	2.60 [j]	—	Note C

[a] 24-hour average, ne (=not to be exceeded more than once per year).

[b] Nuisance dusts, see Table 15-2.

[c] 8-hour average, ne.

[d] 1-hour average, ne.

[e] 3-hour average, 6–9 a.m., ne.

[f] In heavy traffic zones, e.g., midtown Manhattan.[75]

[g] Annual arithmetic mean.

[h] 90 percent of samples in Chicago, 1962–1967, were below this level; other cities had lower levels.[79]

[i] Highest level among 60 urban areas, 1961–1965.[77]

[j] 4 ppm (carbon) average total hydrocarbon concentration, a near-maximum level observed in several cities.[76]

[k] Highest 1-hour average oxidant level, downtown Los Angeles, 1965.[78]

[l] 90th percentile level in highest NO_2 area around a TNT factory.[97]

[m] Impaired auditory discrimination after 90 minutes, not confirmed by others.[75]

The table lists pollutants for which air criteria documents have been published (references indicated in *column 1*). TLV=threshold limit values for industrial exposures (see Chap. 15, Tables 15-1, 15-2). AQS=primary ambient air-quality standards in the United States.[31] *Column 4:* typical high urban levels chosen from sources indicated in footnotes. "Acute effects in man" (*column 5*): levels at which health effects (respiratory, except for CO) have been shown in controlled exposures lasting minutes or hours; from sources referenced in superscripts. No relevant human data are available for hydrocarbon mixtures; for effects of individual hydrocarbons (aldehydes, acrolein) see chapter 15, Table 15-1. *Column 6:* suggested exposure levels of interest in long-term human exposures. With sensitive and frequent lung-function monitoring, exposures at these levels should entail minimal risks for healthy humans.

Note A: data on effect of long-term exposures to specific particulates can be obtained from industrial exposures (Chap. 15). Note B: Toxic effects of CO depend on COHb levels and have been studied extensively during exposures of adequate duration (up to 16 hours); longer-term exposures at constant elevations of COHb levels are needed to evaluate functional changes that might result from minor tissue hypoxia. Note C: Longer-term effects of hydrocarbons are probably determined chiefly by secondary irritant products including oxidants formed in photochemical smog (see text).

lung disease is not known but may be suspected by analogy with other exposures that cause similar acute effects on maximum flows (e.g., textile dusts, Chap. 17; TDI, Chap. 15). The mechanism that causes airway constriction is not certain. SO_2 can act directly on the airway mucosa, but results of exposures in vagotomized animals suggest that reflexes from receptors in the nose and upper airways may also be involved.[30, 73] However, the effect of vagotomy might also be explained by interaction between the inhaled agent and cholinergic stimuli at the cellular level (see Chap. 17, p. 431 and Chap. 18, p. 465). Earlier studies using airway-resistance measurements showed that a second exposure to 5 and 13 ppm SO_2 (14.3–37.2 mg/cu m) in man causes less effect than the first exposure.[36, 37] Increased mucus formation, which increases SO_2 binding in mucus and thus protects the mucosa, might account for the decreased response on second exposure. As an adaptive mechanism, however, this would be of questionable value, since increased mucus production itself promotes airway obstruction.

J. S. Haldane suspected that the choking effect of dense fog in man resulted mainly from sulfate rather than from SO_2.[43] In guinea pigs, sulfuric acid and particulate sulfates cause more airway obstruction than equivalent amounts of SO_2.[4] In these experiments, the effect of SO_2 was potentiated when a liquid-droplet aerosol was administered simultaneously with SO_2. The explanation may be that SO_2 is concentrated in the droplets and converted to the more irritant sulfuric acid. Although two independent studies in man have failed to confirm a potentiating effect of NaCl liquid-droplet aerosols on the effects of SO_2 in man,[16, 36] other aerosols may be more effective in converting SO_2 to irritating salts such as zinc-ammonium sulfate. Also, a high relative humidity appears to be required for SO_2-aerosol potentiation.[67]

Since 1.0 ppm SO_2 (2.86 mg/cu m) causes acute effects in minutes, lower concentrations may well damage airways when inhaled over the long term; controlled experiments are therefore needed to detect the effects of chronic exposures. Until we know more about the long-term effects of SO_2 itself, it will be difficult to assess the additional risks posed by secondary products formed by SO_2.

Particulates [77]

As a group, particles suspended in the air range from the potentially harmful to the relatively innocuous and include organic substances, pollens, viruses, metals, bacteria, and droplets. The composition of the particulate matter in air depends largely on the nature of the nearby sources, ranging from plants, which emit pollens, to industrial processes. Measurements of total particulate matter in the air express in quantitative terms the dirtiness responsible for such physical effects of pollution as limitation of visibility and soiling of buildings. However, no clear relation between the air's total particulate matter and health effects is to be expected, since (1) only particles in a limited size range are inhaled and deposited in the respiratory tract (Chap. 12, p. 265), and (2) the health effects of particles, once deposited, depend on their nature. Thus, persons with asthma develop symptoms in relatively clean air if it contains pollens to which they are sensitive, while dirty air may be innocuous to health if most of the suspended particles are inert. Some health risks posed by specific particles (asbestos, beryllium) in persons living near emission sources have been discussed in Chapter 15. Knowledge of health effects of separate chemical components of particulate pollution is still too limited to warrant a more detailed classification on this basis. In addition to having their own actions, particles may serve as vehicles for substances adsorbed in their surfaces, and gaseous pollutants may dissolve in liquid droplets. In experiments with humans, even inert particles in sufficiently large amounts can cause airway constriction (see Chap. 12, p. 271). Both coal and textile dusts have been shown to have acute effects on lung function (Chap. 15, p. 367 and Chap. 17). However, the amounts required (1–10 or more mg/per cu m total dust) exceed the amount of particulate matter currently found in highly polluted city air (up to 0.2 mg/cu m), and these effects are therefore rarely relevant to community air exposures.

The particle size distribution of aerosols in ambient air varies with the sources, the dispersion by air motion, and the time available for sedimentation of large particles. Thus, in relatively still air indoors, large particles settle out, and the remaining suspended matter consists chiefly of small particles (up to 91 percent ≤ 1 μm [63]). Outdoors, particles ≤ 1 μm in diameter account for 50–75 percent of the total aerosol mass.[63] Such aerosols are deposited largely in small airways and alveoli. However, their effect depends on their nature, and the chemical composition of aerosols in ambient air is complex, including carbon compounds from auto exhaust, polymers from tire dust, and salts from sea water, soil dust and fly ash.[37a] In the London Underground, airborne particles (0.3–5.5 μm size range) contained 10 percent (by weight) skin particles, presumably mostly of human origin.[17a] The effects of coal dust (Chap. 15, p. 367) are among the few for which dose-related responses to acute exposure are available. To prevent disease, efforts to control particulate matter should focus on particles with specific damage effects (such as asbestos), rather than on the total particulate matter. Exposures near asbestos sources, for instance, may well be significant even when total particulate levels are low.

Carbon Monoxide [75]

CO is inhaled via the lungs and binds with Hb to form a blood pigment (COHb) that is inactive in oxygen transport (Chap. 6). Heavy exposures lead to rapid death because of tissue hypoxia, at blood COHb levels of about 50 percent or more. Lesser exposures, leading to blood COHb levels between 20 and 50 percent, decrease tissue oxygenation, which affects physical and psychomotor performance. In community air pollution, even CO levels which lead to lower blood COHb levels (less than 20 percent) are of concern. Such exposures occur in heavy traffic and in tunnels. Although there is some evidence that such low-level exposures interfere with performance in physiological and visual function tests, the effects of COHb levels less than 5 percent are controversial.[75] Vision disturbances, particularly when light is dim, may occur with blood COHb levels as low as 5 percent.[45] According to one study, 1 to 2½ hours exposure to about 120 mg/cu m (111 ppm) CO, with final COHb levels averaging 6.6 percent, may reduce vigilance.[52] Others found no performance deficit after 9 hours at 83.3 or 166.7 mg/cu m (75 or 150 ppm), with COHb levels up to 12.9 percent.[57] Still higher levels (250 mg/cu m CO) decrease exercise performance (maximum oxygen uptake) in healthy persons, at COHb levels of about 20 percent; [106] similar effects occurred in another study at 25–33 percent COHb.[83]

Since the sidestream smoke of a single cigarette generates about 75 ml CO,[48] smoking is a major source of indoor CO exposure. Indoor exposure to CO also occurs during cooking on charcoal fires. CO exposure used to be common among cooks; hence the old French term *folie des cuisiniers* for the effects of CO on mental function. Outdoors, in heavy traffic areas, CO levels fluctuate during the day, with hourly averages of at most 25 mg/cu m (23 ppm), and short-lasting peaks of about 110 mg/cu m (102 ppm).[107] Even 4 hours' exposure to this peak level raises blood COHb to only about 10 percent;[35] the actual increase during short peaks is much less. Furthermore, there is little reason to believe that CO air pollution outdoors is increasing as a health risk. The CO levels of 110 mg/cu m (102 ppm) measured in New York City in 1922 by Henderson and Haggard[46] occurred in congested areas where traffic could not further increase. In London, CO levels were about 110 mg/cu m during dense fogs in the early 1900s, through partial combustion of coal in train engines and home fireplaces.[43] Nevertheless, even on the short term, the highest ambient CO levels today may endanger persons who are at special risk because of lung or heart (especially coronary heart) disease.[40] For healthy persons, however, exposure to CO levels in heavy traffic is a negligible health risk. In nonsmokers exposed under actual traffic conditions, blood CO levels increase (Table 16-2) but remain far below CO levels found in smokers not exposed to traffic.[91] In smokers exposed to traffic while not smoking, blood CO levels decrease while smoking increases their blood CO (Table 16-2). Hence, for the smoking driver, CO from cigarette smoke poses a greater risk than CO from car exhaust.

The effects of long-term, low-level CO exposures (beyond 16 hours) have not been studied experimentally in man.[75] Two-year exposures of monkeys to atmospheres containing CO (with blood COHb levels up to 8.3 percent) caused no chronic tissue damage demonstrable with extensive biochemical and pathological studies.[29] The subtle effects of low levels of CO (blood COHb levels of 5 percent

Table 16-2

Comparison of Acute Effects of Air Pollution and Smoking in Healthy Persons

Exposure	ΔP_{O_2} (mm Hg)	ΔRaw (%)	CO (vol %) before	after	ΔCO (%)
Nonsmokers, 3 hr at busy intersection (n = 16)	+1.6	+12 (10/16)	0.210	0.308	+47 (15/16)
Smokers, 3 hr at busy intersection without smoking (n = 14)	+2.3	+18 (8/14)	0.830	0.556	−33 (13/14)
Smokers indoors (2 cigars or 3 cigarettes) (n = 9; for Raw, n = 8)	−3.2	+24 (5/8)	0.823	1.030	+25 (8/9)

ΔP_{O_2}=change in arterial P_{O_2}; ΔRaw=change in airway resistance. Blood CO content measured with infrared analyzer after vacuum extraction of gases from blood. Numbers in parentheses in columns for ΔRaw and ΔCO indicate proportion of subjects showing a change in the direction of the average change. The changes of P_{O_2} and airway resistance are not significant. Averages calculated from Tables 1 and 2 of Reichel et al.[91]

and higher) may be important in persons whose tasks depend on accurate psycho-motor performance (car drivers, airline pilots, traffic controllers). It seems likely, however, that the best way to reduce these low levels is to control pollution in the immediate environment (chiefly by prohibiting smoking) rather than to attempt to decrease short-lasting peaks of CO levels in ambient air.[70] As long as smoking is permitted in public transportation, reducing other sources of CO is unlikely to reduce its passengers' blood COHb levels significantly.

Oxidants [78]

When ultraviolet light acts on the mixture of hydrocarbons and nitrogen oxides emitted in automobile exhaust, ozone and other oxidants are formed. In areas prone to oxidant or photochemical smog, such as Los Angeles, peak measurements of primary pollutants (hydrocarbons and nitrogen oxides) cor-respond with maximum traffic hours in the morning and late afternoon. Since the action of sunlight requires time, oxidant peaks occur around noontime. No oxidant peak follows the evening rush hour, since sunlight is reduced. Oxidant smog, which irritates the eyes and damages vegetation, is undesirable for these reasons alone. Its effect on respiratory health, however, is questionable.

Under the influence of sunlight, NO_2 in the atmosphere splits into NO and O. The free oxygen atom is highly reactive and, if hydrocarbons also are present, causes the formation of both hydrocarbon free radicals and ozone. The presence of hydrocarbons also increases the formation of ozone and NO_2. The hydrocarbon free radical is probably used, together with NO_2, to form another oxidant, per-oxyacetylnitrate (PAN). However, the major component of oxidant smog is ozone; contributions of PAN and other oxidants are minor. One-hour average concentrations of ozone frequently reach values of 0.2–0.3 ppm (0.4–0.6 mg/cu m) in Los Angeles and less commonly in other cities.[78] Concentrations of PAN are in the order of 0.06 ppm (0.3 mg/cu m) when the ozone level is 0.20 ppm (0.4 mg/cu m). Peak oxidant levels up to 0.67 ppm have been measured in the Los Angeles area,[78] and higher levels may have occurred at other sites and at other times (SK Friedlander, personal communication, 1973). The level of 0.67 ppm is close to that at which Bates et al.[11, 112] observed acute lung function changes after 2-hour exposures. However, ambient ozone exposures are not continuous since the peak concentrations occur only around noon on days that the climatic factors are favorable to photochemical smog formation. Thus, exposure is dis-continuous, and year-round and 24-hour average values of ozone and oxidant levels are much lower than the peak values. Ozone is formed not only in photo-chemical smog but also by electrical discharge in the atmosphere. In some rural areas, concentrations up to 0.05 ppm (0.1 mg/cu m) have been measured.[78]

Ozone, the main harmful component of oxidant smog, is a highly toxic gas [56] with effects on the lungs in concentrations near those prevailing, under adverse conditions, in ambient air of communities with photochemical smog. In intact animals, the main effect of ozone is to produce lung edema.[95] After the first exposure, tolerance develops [26] and the mortality during subsequent exposures decreases. Ozone causes lung edema in rats (1 ppm=2 mg/cu m, 2 hours), mice (3 ppm=6 mg/cu m, 4 hours), and guinea pigs (3 ppm, 2 hours) (un-published data from this laboratory [84]). Although chemical mediators (histamine,

5-hydroxytryptamine) have been suspected of contributing to edema, significant edema develops in the absence of demonstrable changes in the content of these mediators in lung tissue.[84] Hence, it is more likely that edema develops as a consequence of an effect of ozone on vascular epithelium. In rabbits, 0.4 ppm O_3 causes lesions of small pulmonary blood vessels.[86]

In addition to its direct effects, ozone can damage the lungs via interference with defense mechanisms against infection. For instance, ozone inhibits lysozyme, a bacteriostatic enzyme in bronchial mucus.[51] More importantly, ozone interferes with the phagocytic function of alveolar macrophage cells, probably by damaging their cell membranes,[53] an effect observed with concentrations as low as 0.25 ppm (0.5 mg/cu m) after a 3-hour exposure.[54] The damaged macrophages and perhaps other cells release lysosomal enzymes into the culture medium in vitro,[53] and this release in vivo is probably an early sign of an inflammatory response.[25] A third component of the impaired defense mechanism is probably a decrease in the available number of macrophage cells.[18] These effects of ozone on alveolar macrophage cells and on lysozyme in bronchial mucus can account for the fact that 0.62 ppm O_3 (1.22 mg/cu m) impairs the killing of bacteria in the lungs of mice.[42]

It should be stressed, however, that on inhalation ozone is largely removed in the nose (see Chap. 2 and reference 13). Furthermore, its effects on the lungs are probably mediated via free oxygen radicals. Inhalation of compounds that bind free radicals (with SH or SS groups) protect against O_3 toxicity in mice.[33] Since free radicals are unlikely to penetrate into the tissues, they probably induce the formation of other compounds with potentially harmful biological actions. For instance, ozone can induce aldehyde formation by oxidizing fatty acids; aldehydes can cross-link protein molecules and oxidize hyaluronic acid, thus profoundly affecting the ground substance of lung tissue.[15] The formation of lipid peroxides by ozone may be of particular importance. One of these peroxides (linoleic acid hydroperoxide) impairs phagocytosis by rabbit alveolar macrophages in vitro, via an effect on the cell membrane.[61] Thus, this peroxide mimics some of the effects of ozone on macrophage cells. Another argument in favor of lipid peroxidation as an intermediary mechanism in ozone toxicity is that antioxidants (vitamin E, para-aminobenzoic acid) protect animals against the toxic effects of ozone.[41, 69, 92]

Ozone tolerance develops with respect to edema formation but not with respect to the inflammatory response nor its toxic effects on macrophages.[38] In rabbits, 0.75 ppm (1.47 mg/cu m) and higher concentrations of ozone inhibit the activity of the enzyme that breaks down benzo[a]pyrene (benzpyrene hydrolase).[85] Consequently, benzo[a]pyrene might be a more active carcinogen when ozone exposure occurs simultaneously.

In man, 1- to-2 hours' exposure to 0.6–0.8 ppm (1.18–1.57 mg/cu m) ozone increases airway resistance, reduces vital capacity and diffusing capacity, and decreases flow rates on MEFV curves.[11, 112] Significant decreases of $FEV_{1.0}$ and MEF50% (Chap. 9, p. 189) also occur after 2 hours at 0.37 ppm O_3 (0.74 mg/cu m).[45a] Large as well as small airways appear to be affected by concentrations similar to the high levels observed in Los Angeles (see Table 16-1). Higher concentrations (1–3 ppm during 30 minutes or less) cause chest tightness, dyspnea, and cough, with a 20 percent drop in $FEV_{1.0}$ and a reduction of vital capacity and diffusing capacity.[44] Thus, ambient ozone levels should be controlled to less than about 0.4 ppm (0.80 mg/cu m), but research on lower-level exposures is still needed to establish a level that causes no detectable responses.

Nitrogen Dioxide [3]

Nitrogen dioxide, a toxic gas in high concentrations (see Chap. 15, p. 349), is an essential ingredient of photochemical smog (p. 393). Another important source of NO_2 is cigarette smoke. The NO_2 concentrations inhaled by smokers may perhaps account for their increased prevalence of emphysema, which can be induced experimentally with NO_2 in rats (see also Chap. 14). Toxic effects in man and animals have been observed at concentrations considerably higher (at least 4–5 times) than those observed in ambient air, which may reach up to about 0.25 ppm (0.5 mg/cu m). Fifteen ppm NO_2 (28.5 mg/cu m) suppresses the phagocytic activity of rabbit alveolar macrophage cells and renders the animals more sensitive to some virus infections.[2] This is related to failure of the cells to produce interferon when exposed to NO_2.[109] Seventeen ppm NO_2 (32.3 mg/cu m) injures the alveolar epithelium, leads to loss of cilia in terminal bronchioles, and causes increased cell division in rat lung after 2 to 3 days' exposure. In 24–48 hours a repair process with cuboid cells, which are resistant to NO_2, begins. A lower concentration (2 ppm=3.8 mg/cu m) caused similar changes, but these reversed to normal when exposure was terminated.[32, 101] Other effects of NO_2 include increased mucociliary clearance in rats (6 ppm=11.4 mg/cu m over several months,[39] reduced surfactant activity of lung wash fluid, and decreased lung lipid content in rats (2.9 ppm=5.5 mg/cu m over 9 months).[9] NO_2 does not affect benzpyrene hydrolase activity (5–50 ppm=9.5–95 mg/cu m).[85]

In man, 5–8 ppm NO_2 (9.5–15.2 mg/cu m) in air increases airway resistance. This effect, which can be prevented with an antihistamine drug, may thus result from histamine release.[82] Histamine release may also explain the delayed action (maximal after 30 minutes) of NO_2 in other short-term exposures (2.5 ppm=4.8 mg/cu m) in man.[3]

Hydrocarbons [76]

Sensitive chemical analysis can detect dozens of organic compounds in the atmosphere. Among these, the aliphatic hydrocarbons (e.g., methane) are biologically inert; some unsaturated members of this group have anesthetic properties (e.g., acetylene). Aldehydes, another group of hydrocarbons, are irritants (Table 15-1, p. 346). Formaldehyde and acrolein, an unsaturated aldehyde, primarily irritate the eyes and nose in man. They are formed photochemically by irradiation of automobile exhaust and may account for a significant portion of the response of guinea pigs (increased airway resistance) to irradiated auto exhaust.[72] The response of guinea pigs to 1.2–1.5 ppm (3.3–4.1 mg/cu m) acrolein is blocked by atropine, aminophylline and isoproterenol, but not by antihistamine drugs.[71] Since autonomic drugs can modulate sensitivity to acrolein (see also Chap. 17, p. 431 and Chap. 18, p. 465), human responses may vary as a function of autonomic responses. These irritating hydrocarbons in ambient air may contribute to eye irritation in photochemical smog at ambient air levels that probably do not significantly affect the lungs and airways. Since hydrocarbons participate in the photochemical reactions that lead to oxidant production (p. 393), reducing hydrocarbon emissions can help control photo-oxidant smog. Nevertheless, since the direct health effects of hydrocarbons are slight, controlling their emissions is unlikely to improve air quality significantly in areas with less sunshine than Los Angeles and hence only incidental and minimal photochemical smog formation. The effects of polycyclic hydrocarbons are discussed later (p. 406).

Lead

Possible toxic effects of lead, when inhaled from car exhaust fumes in traffic, have aroused much public concern. In a study of London taxi drivers, however, inhaled lead played only a minor role in elevating blood lead levels.[57] Most of our lead intake appears to come from foods [23] and, in children, from paint that contains lead. Although increases in ambient lead levels have been observed in heavy traffic, they were considered well within safe limits.[107] For a comprehensive review of the possible risks of airborne lead exposure, see reference 23.

EPIDEMIOLOGICAL STUDIES OF AIR POLLUTION AND LUNG DISEASE

The prevalence of lung diseases in populations and the mortality associated with the diseases depend on large numbers of variables (Chap. 13)—age and sex distribution, social status, educational level, occupation, housing conditions, smoking habits, and availability of health care. Efforts to conduct population surveys are further complicated by differences in people's subjective appreciation of respiratory symptoms and in their understanding of questions posed by investigators. Also, since mortality for specific diseases depends on reporting practices that may vary widely, variations in reported deaths in different geographical areas cannot be interpreted with any degree of confidence. Chronic respiratory disease is probably markedly underreported as a cause of death (Chap. 13). In morbidity studies, objective measurements of lung function are needed in addition to data on symptoms and medical history. Even when such objective data show differences that might be related to air pollution, their correlation with ambient air measurements presents serious problems. Since, for practical reasons, the number of sampling stations is usually small, it is risky to relate the data obtained to a wide area around the sampling point. In the surrounding area, pollution levels may be either higher or lower than those at the air-monitoring station. In addition, pollutant levels vary over the day and the year, causing uncertainty as to which level is relevant to disease. For chronic disease developing over many years, annual average levels may be relevant. For short-term exacerbations of disease, acute mortality, or acute respiratory effects, daily or hourly averages are the ones to consider. In studies showing chronic disease prevalence at one point in time, present pollutant levels may not adequately reflect the pollutant load during years past. Longitudinal studies in which changes in prevalence or severity of disease are related to changes in pollutant levels in time may allow more definite conclusions about the association between pollution and lung disease.

Mortality Studies

Increased mortality, primarily of older people with preexisting lung or heart disease, has occurred during severe air-pollution disasters.[79] For instance, about 4000 excess deaths were attributed to smog in London during December 1952. In New York City, lesser mortality peaks have been related to levels of SO_2 and smoke,[66] but no other episodic increase in mortality has reached the level obtained in London in 1952. The association between pollutant levels and mortality does not prove a causal effect of pollution. In fact, when Dublin, Ireland, residents switched to peat from coal for home-heating during World War II, pollution levels decreased, but mortality continued to be much higher in January than in June (Fig. 16-1).[64] Any effect of continuous lower level pollutant exposures on mortality has not been clearly established. In Los Angeles County, mortality rates among people aged 65 years and older in nursing homes show peaks related to heat waves rather than to air pollution.[78] Two studies in other US cities (Buffalo, N.Y., and Nashville, Tenn.; reviewed in reference 77) have suggested that particulate levels above 0.08 mg/cu m, together with increased SO_2 levels, may be associated with increased mortality in persons over 50 years of age. However, smoking habits were not taken into account, and mortality and pollution were not measured over the same period of time (e.g., mortality rates in 1959–1961 were related to pollution in 1961–1963).

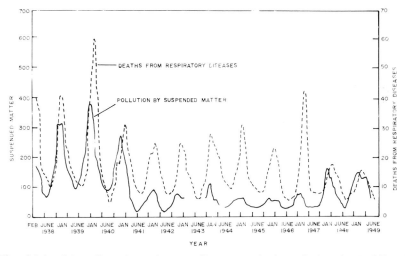

Fig. 16-1. Mortality of respiratory diseases and air pollution in Dublin, 1938–1949 (curves of moving averages). Total suspended matter per week was obtained by summing hourly values (100 = 32 mg/cu m). Monthly SO_2 values (lead peroxide method) showed trends similar to the curve for suspended matter. From 1941 to 1947, particulate levels decreased as a result of a change in the main fuel (coal until 1941, peat from 1941 to 1947). The high winter peaks of particulate matter from January 1939 through January 1941 were accompanied by increased deaths from respiratory diseases. During the years 1942 to 1947, these mortality peaks persisted while particulate levels were much lower. Adapted from reference 64.

Comparisons of Respiratory Disease Morbidity in Communities

To compare disease prevalence in communities with contrasting air-pollutant levels would seem to be a straightforward way to assess effects of air pollution on health. However, when the populations are scrutinized, additional variables that are difficult to control often become apparent. For instance, a comparison of lung function in about 800 persons living in a polluted town (Seward, Pa.) and a nearby cleaner town (New Florence, Pa.) showed differences related only to age, height, and sex. Many coal miners lived in the polluted town, and smoking habits differed in the two towns, but only about 20 percent of the persons studied were nonsmokers.[89] Thus, despite a marked difference in pollutant levels (SO_2 nine times higher in Seward than in New Florence; particulates 40 percent higher), no clear effect of pollution on respiratory health could be demonstrated. A comparison of urban and rural residents (Berlin, N.H., versus Chilliwack, B.C.) has been discussed elsewhere (Chap. 13, p. 303). The air-pollution contrast was greater than that between Seward and New Florence, and the data show that the higher pollutant levels in Berlin, N.H., are associated with a higher prevalence of respiratory symptoms and a lower $FEV_{1.0}$ among its population if suitable subgroups in both towns are compared.[8] However, the differences are small, and smoking was a much more important variable related to lung disease. A large-scale study in urban residents (Duisburg), small-town residents (Bocholt), and nearby rural residents (Borken) has been undertaken in Germany.[90] The main finding was a high prevalence of airway obstruction in all groups, including women and rural residents. No significant differences between urban and rural residents emerged from the data. Rather, the study shows the importance of distinguishing occupational groups within community populations. For instance, the high disease prevalence in the small town was at least in part related to the fact that 23 percent of the men and 12.5 percent of the women worked in textile mills (Chap. 17). When urban and rural population groups are studied in detail with personal interviews and lung-function testing, variables become apparent which remain unknown in studies confined to mortality data or gross indicators of morbidity, such as hospital admissions and clinic visits.

Studies in Occupational Groups

These offer an opportunity to compare people of similar educational and social status in communities with contrasting pollutant levels. An example of such a study is a survey of telephone workers in four geographical areas in the United States and Britain (Table 16-3). The average results show no effects of SO_2 levels on the $FEV_{1.0}$ of nonsmokers and on the percentage of subjects who produced sputum. The respiratory findings correlate better with the particulate levels, but the results might also be related to differences in housing conditions, recreational pursuits, or other social differences between British and American telephone workers.[50] As in other studies, smoking was a major variable affecting symptoms and lung function.

Nonsmoking housewives, aged 65 years and older, were studied as a relatively homogeneous occupational group in Genoa, Italy [87] (Table 16-4). Persons with histories of occupational exposures were excluded. The prevalence of chronic

Table 16-3

Telephone Workers in the US and UK

	SO$_2$ (ppm)	Particu-lates (μg/ cu m)	Males 40–49 yr		Males 50–59 yr	
			FEV$_{1.0}$ * (liters)	Spu-tum † (%)	FEV$_{1.0}$ * (liters)	Spu-tum † (%)
San Francisco	0.01	120	3.7	9	3.3	14
Rural UK	0.02	200	3.0	22	2.8	24
US east coast ‡	0.04	120	3.5	7	3.1	10
London	0.10	220	2.8	29	2.6	43

* FEV$_{1.0}$ data for nonsmokers only.
† % with sputum production > 2 ml (smokers and nonsmokers).
‡ Baltimore, Md., Washington, D.C., and Westchester County, N.Y.
Data quoted from reference 77 (p. 163).

cough and dyspnea was much greater among residents of a highly polluted industrial zone than among suburban residents. Women living in an area with intermediate pollutant levels also had a high prevalence of respiratory symptoms. In the suburban area, where SO$_2$ and particulate levels were lower but were still higher than the US primary air quality standards,[31] symptom prevalence was similar to that among older rural women in Connecticut, where pollutant levels are much lower. If the differences may be attributed to air pollution, the data of Table 16-4 suggest that lowering the SO$_2$ and particulate levels below those prevailing in the suburban area of Genoa may not lead to perceptible improvement in respiratory health among older women.

It is often suspected that urban air pollution aggravates the effects of cigarette smoking. Figure 16-2 shows that mailmen in London had a lower FEV$_{1.0}$ than rural UK mailmen in each smoking category. The smallest difference is between

Table 16-4

Respiratory Symptoms in Women 65 Years and Older

	n	Cough Winter (%)	Summer (%)	Dyspnea (%)	Particu-lates (mg/ cu m)	SO$_2$ (mg/ cu m)
Genoa, Italy						
Suburban	81	13.5	6.2	19.8	0.09	0.086
Intermediate	70	30.0	15.7	37.1	0.22	0.114
Industrial	162	44.4	19.8	43.8	0.35	0.315
Lebanon, Connecticut						
Rural	50	12.0	—	22.0	0.03	0.025

Data for Genoa residents from reference 87. n=number of persons.
Data for Lebanon, Connecticut, from Connecticut Lung Survey (Yale University Lung Research Center, unpublished material).

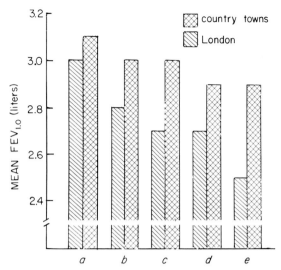

Fig. 16-2. Mean $FEV_{1.0}$ of mailmen in country towns and in London, U.K., standardized to age 40. *a:* Non-smokers; *b:* ex-smokers; *c:* smokers, 1–14 gram/day; *d:* smokers, 15–24 gram/day; *e:* smokers, 25 gram or more/day. In each smoking category, the urban men have a lower $FEV_{1.0}$ than the rural men; the difference is smallest for non-smokers and largest in the heaviest smokers. From reference 49.

urban and rural nonsmokers. Air pollution is the most likely cause of the differences; climatic and social variables were thought to be of minor importance.[49]

Studies in Children

Since such variables as smoking and occupational hazards are absent or minor, children are good subjects for air-pollution studies. In addition, pollutants might have more serious effects on developing individuals than on adults; they might, for instance, interfere with lung growth (Chap. 1) or induce lasting changes leading to severe disease later in life. Studies of school children in relation to SO_2 and particulates, the most common form of urban pollution, are discussed below; studies of the effects of oxidants and NO_2 on children are discussed in the sections dealing with these specific pollutants.

An association between pollution and lower respiratory tract infections in children has been suspected in Great Britain.[28] However, childhood bronchitis in polluted areas was increased only among children of semiskilled and unskilled workers. Also, the higher rates in Wales were unrelated to air pollution.[22] Since air-pollution levels and social class are associated in Great Britain, their separate effects on disease prevalence are not known.[21] Higher indoor pollutant levels in the homes of the poor (e.g., from kerosene heaters) may contribute to class differences in prevalence of respiratory illness. In Sheffield, UK, respiratory symptoms and a history of chest illness were more common in 5-year-old children living in polluted zones than among those in clean areas. However, although pollutant loads differed markedly between the zones (e.g., SO_2 up to 0.30 mg/cu m=0.1 ppm in the polluted areas, versus 0.10 mg/cu m=0.03 ppm in the clean zone, in 1964), the differences in symptom prevalences are small (e.g., 35.2 percent persistent cough in the polluted areas, versus 22.4 percent in the clean zone). Moreover, no significant differences in $FEV_{1.0}$ or FVC were found between children living in the different areas.[60] Four years after the initial study (1963–1965), about 500 of the same children were studied again. There had been considerable improvement in air quality, particularly in smoke levels. SO_2 levels were still high in the polluted zones (up to 0.25 mg/cu m=0.09 ppm); nevertheless, differences in symptom or chest illness prevalence between the zones were no longer demonstrable. Again, the lung-function tests did not reveal any difference between the groups.[60] In Czechoslovakia, children (10–11 years old) living in a severely polluted city (SO_2 up to 0.675 mg/cu m=0.24 ppm; dust levels up to 0.525 mg/cu m) showed no excess respiratory symptoms nor increased chest illness; lung function test data were mainly within normal limits.[113] Thus, there are indications that high SO_2 and particulate levels were associated with increased chest illness among children in Sheffield some years ago. Partial pollution abatement has eliminated this risk in Sheffield, while in Czechoslovakia no excess disease was shown in spite of very high SO_2 and particulate levels. Infection and allergy are important causes of respiratory disease among children; it seems likely that any additional effect of air pollution is minimal and difficult to demonstrate against the background of other causes of lung disease.

Studies of Effects of Specific Pollutants

SO$_2$ and particulate pollution. The epidemiological studies discussed in the preceding paragraphs all concern the effects of the SO_2 and particulate type of smog prevalent in many industrial areas. In most studies, SO_2 and particulate levels are closely associated so that the effects of the two cannot be evaluated separately.[110] Both SO_2 and particulate levels rise in winter when sulfur-containing fuel is burnt. In summer, SO_2 levels are lower and particulates vary independently. The World Health Organization has concluded that adverse health effects (respiratory symptoms) can be expected at SO_2 and smoke levels of 0.1 mg/cu m each (annual means).[110] Bates summarized several studies by stating that annual average levels of SO_2 higher than 0.08 ppm (0.23 mg/cu m), especially if combined with particulate levels higher than 0.15 mg/cu m lead to increased bronchitis morbidity among adult urban populations.[10] These conclusions are based on the studies summarized earlier, particularly the Genoa survey (Table 16-4), as well as on studies in Great Britain showing increased symptoms in bronchitic patients when ambient pollutant levels were high. The latter data are based on surveys using mailed questionnaires or diaries kept by the patients.[58, 62] Although such studies may provide valuable pointers for detailed objective studies, no reliance should be placed on such data in setting air-quality standards of broad economic impact. Similar remarks can be made about other studies using the patient's own subjective assessment of his degree of illness, often without provisions to account for differences in smoking habits or social status.[79] Furthermore, there is no need to rely on such evidence, since portable pollution-sampling equipment* makes it feasible to correlate variations in a patient's lung function and symptoms with changes in pollutant levels in his environment. Well-controlled studies of this nature in small numbers of patients would provide more convincing evidence on the relations between pollution and bronchitis symptoms than statistical analysis of large bodies of data with many hidden variables.

Recent US epidemiological studies, not yet published in detail, suggest that suspended sulfates pose a greater risk than sulfur dioxide (see p. 390).[99] Sulfate pollution may increase if and when automobiles are provided with new exhaust control systems (catalytic converters) to reduce hydrocarbon and CO emission. These devices produce sulfuric acid mist, leading to sulfate formation in the atmosphere. Some calculations suggest that roadside sulfate levels might reach 35 to 150 μg/cu m, compared to current US levels in the order of 7 to 13 μg/cu m, if all cars were equipped with catalytic converters.[96a] The health effects of these sulfate levels still need to be assessed. In the meantime, it seems highly undesirable to equip our cars (as will be required for all new 1976 cars under present law) with devices that, while perhaps improving photooxidant pollution in some cities, might lead to a nationwide increase in sulfate pollution.

Oxidant pollution. In spite of the demonstrated toxic properties of oxidants at levels close to those in ambient air under adverse conditions (p. 394), there is no convincing epidemiological evidence linking oxidant smog with increased prevalence or severity of respiratory disease. The lack of evidence may largely be due to the uncontrolled nature and the lack of objective methods in several surveys (reviewed in reference 78). Nevertheless, one careful study of nonsmokers in an area with high oxidant levels (San Gabriel Valley; 45 percent of all days with 0.15 ppm or higher maximum hourly average) and in an area with lower oxidant levels (San Diego; 6 percent of days with similar high levels) showed no difference in lung function and in respiratory symptom prevalence.[20] In Los Angeles, peak flows were higher rather than lower among school children living in a high-oxidant area (up to 0.34 ppm).[68] On the other hand, studies of patients with obstructive lung disease have suggested some improvement in lung function during a stay in a controlled environment free of oxidant smog. Smoking, however, was an uncontrolled variable in most of these individuals.[78]

An increased incidence of asthmatic attacks among patients with asthma has been reported in Pasadena when the oxidant level rose to about 0.25 ppm. However, of all reported attacks, only 5 percent were attributed to smog and none of these was severe.[96] No lung function or other clinical data were reported. Thus, while a small number of asthma patients may have increased symptoms due to smog, no confirming objective evidence has been reported since this study was performed in 1956. Asthma is a common disease even among rural nonsmokers in an area with minimal air pollution (Table 16-6), and factors other than oxidant pollution clearly predominate in its pathogenesis (Chap. 18). Yet, the Pasadena report [96] has been quoted as a principal reason for setting the oxidant air-quality standard

---

* Portable sampling equipment, built in a small suitcase, has been designed for assessment of NO$_2$, CO, total hydrocarbons, respirable particles, lead and sulfur dioxide (Burgess W et al, Arch Environ Health, 26:325–329, 1973; Hosein HR et al, Yale University Lung Research Center). Since these instruments sample air beyond the subject's breathing zone (flow rate approx. 250 liters/min), they differ from personal samplers (Chap. 12, p 282).

at 0.160 mg/cu m (0.08 ppm).[31] However, since many other inhalants (including allergens, Chap. 18) cause asthma, it is very unlikely that implementing this standard will result in any measurable improvement in the condition of asthma patients, even in the Los Angeles area.

Another uncontrolled study quoted in favor of low oxidant standards concerns decreased track performance among high school students in the Los Angeles area.[108] Data on running times were collected by a coach, during each of the years from 1959 to 1964. The boys were not examined by the investigators. Running times were correlated with oxidant levels measured 2 miles away from the track. It was noted that on high oxidant days, a high percentage of team members did not improve their performance in comparison with the previous meet. This percentage correlated significantly with the oxidant level during the hour preceding each meet. However, the extent of the performance deficit was not reported, and no explanation of the decreased performance was offered other than that it might be related to discomfort, e.g., eye irritation. Another explanation is discussed in Chapter 12, p. 264. In fact, for the teams as a whole, performance improved consistently from 1959 to 1964, but there is no evidence that pollution decreased over this period. In spite of the obvious deficiencies of this work, which has not received supporting evidence from other studies, the Air Quality Criteria document for Photochemical Oxidants concludes that these data ". . . . provide convincing evidence that some component of the air which was measured as oxidant had a causal effect on team performances." (See pp. 9–12 in reference 78.)

Nitrogen dioxide. Since NO_2 interferes with biochemical mechanisms that protect the lung against viral infections (p. 395), the report that acute respiratory illnesses are more prevalent among people living in an area with relatively high NO_2 levels is of interest.[98] However, NO_2 levels in this population study were much lower than those used in the experimental work (average 24-hour level— 0.109 ppm in the highest NO_2 area, versus 15 or 25 ppm in the virus studies [2, 109]). Within each of the four study areas (a high NO_2 and a high particulate area as well as two control areas), the incidence of acute illness varied from about 25 percent to about 7 percent over the 12-week study period. One high-incidence peak was related to an outbreak of influenza, when incidence increases were similar in the high NO_2 and the control areas. Over the total period there was an 18.8 percent excess incidence among people in the high NO_2 area, which might be due to pollution. Even if this excess is confirmed, the effect of pollution is clearly secondary in comparison with the large temporal variations in incidence caused by epidemics of illness induced by respiratory viruses.

In the same study area, ventilatory function in 987 second grade elementary school children was measured. According to an analysis of variance, children in the high NO_2 area, as a group, had a slightly lower $FEV_{0.75}$ than children in the two control areas. However, the difference was very small (e.g., 1.19 liters among boys in the high NO_2 area in March 1969, versus 1.23 and 1.18 in the two control areas), and some details of the testing procedure (e.g., number of blows; use of single or average values, p. 436) were not reported.[97] In addition, the NO_2 levels were different for three schools in the high NO_2 area, but the $FEV_{0.75}$ did not differ among children in these schools. Thus, these data offer no convincing evidence that exposures up to mean daily values of 0.109 ppm cause a physiologically meaningful decrement in ventilatory function among young children.

Studies of Chronic Respiratory Disease

Asthma. An increased prevalence or severity of asthma related to air pollution has been reported in some geographical areas. In New Orleans, this observation was based on the number of emergency clinic visits for asthma.[65] A clinical description of Tokyo-Yokohama asthma among US personnel in Japan [88] did not include adequate epidemiological data, and its seasonal prevalence does not coincide with the highest dust and SO_2 levels in that area.[104] In New Cumberland, West Virginia, pollutant levels (SO_2, particulates, sulfates, and nitrates) did correlate with the number of attacks reported by patients with asthma. However, there was an even stronger correlation between ambient temperature and the attack rate. In addition, the study did not include asthma patients in a control area without pollution, and 9 out of 29 patients who reported no attacks were omitted from the analysis.[19] Although some pollutants may well initiate or aggravate asthma, no convincing epidemiological evidence concerning this relationship is available. Detailed and frequent monitoring of lung function in individual patients, together with the use of portable samplers (p. 402), may offer a more suitable approach to such studies. Seasonal variations in prevalence must be taken into account.[12]

Prevalence of respiratory disease in a rural community. Since all US air-quality standards except that for CO are primarily based upon respiratory health effects, one wonders how much the prevalence of respiratory disease would decrease if these standards were implemented in our cities. Data from a survey in a rural community (Lebanon, Conn.; see Chap. 13, p. 302) where SO_2 and particulate levels are consistently below the primary standard, and where NO_2 levels only infrequently exceed the standard (Table 16-5), may be relevant to

Table 16-5
Air Pollution in Lebanon, Connecticut

Pollutant	Primary Air-Quality Standard (See Table 16–1)	Mean 24-hr Average	Range of 24-hr Averages	Times > Standard (%)
SO_2 (μg/cu m)	365	30	10–65	0
Particulates (μg/cu m)	260	19	4–47	0
NO_2 (μg/cu m)	100	45	18–138	9
Oxidants (μg/cu m)	160	40	30–61	0

Measurements of pollutants (with methods recommended by the Environmental Protection Agency) during the period November 1972 through April 1973. The last column indicates the number of times a 24-hour average exceeded the primary air-quality standard. Data from Connecticut Lung Survey, Yale University Lung Research Center, unpublished material.

Table 16-6
Prevalence of Respiratory Symptoms and Illness Among Nonsmoking
Lifetime Rural Residents (Lebanon, Connecticut)

| | Age Group (yrs) | | | | | | | |
| | 15–24 | | 25–44 | | 45–64 | | Total | |
Symptom/Illness	M	F	M	F	M	F	M	F
n	68	74	48	66	38	41	154	181
% chronic cough (16)	4	1	4	3	11	15	6	5
% chronic phlegm (22)	3	1	10	2	8	2	6	2
% dyspnea (57–59)	0	11	0	15	16	22	4	15
% frequent chest illness (60, 3–5)	12	7	6	9	5	10	8	8
% bronchitis (71)	7	12	6	9	13	12	8	11
% pneumonia (72)	13	16	40	18	24	10	24	15
% frequent wheezing (34, 1–3)	7	4	4	0	5	15	6	5
% asthma (70)	7	0	8	2	5	0	7	<1

Results from answers to standardized questions in all nonsmokers, seen in a total community survey, who had always lived in a rural area. The percentages on each line refer to the number of positive answers to questions listed by their number in the questionnaire (see p. 307 for text of questions and coding of answers). Source: See Table 16–5.

this question. Chronic cough, dyspnea, and histories of bronchitis, pneumonia, and asthma are common in several categories of subjects (Table 16-6). There is a high prevalence of dyspnea and frequent wheezing among older women. Asthma is particularly common among younger men. In several symptom categories, particularly chronic cough, chronic phlegm, dyspnea, and frequent wheezing (see also Table 18-1, p. 445), prevalences were higher among smokers. Occupational exposures, for instance on farms, may account for some symptoms and illnesses. In any case, respiratory disease clearly remains a common cause of symptoms and illness even in nonsmokers living in clean ambient air. Hence, it is difficult to reconcile suggestions that air-pollution abatement may be the "single most effective way of improving the health of middle-class families" (recent statistical analysis of US mortality data)[59] with the data on morbidity in the nonsmokers of rural Lebanon, Conn. Air pollution seems relatively insignificant as a health factor, particularly if one takes into account the considerable excess morbidity and mortality due to smoking among a large additional segment of the US population.

Air Pollution and Cancer

Unlike smoking and certain occupational exposures, which are known to increase risks of lung cancer significantly (Chap. 14, p. 327 and Chap. 15, p. 374), an additional carcinogenic role of other air pollutants is exceedingly difficult to detect. Concern about a possible relation between community air pollution and cancer has arisen for two main reasons.[24] First, epidemiological studies suggest that smoking habits cannot fully explain the excess cancer mortality in urban residents. Second, known carcinogenic agents such as benzo[a]pyrene have been identified in urban air. In Zürich, Switzerland, the amount of benzo[a]pyrene inhaled per year may correspond roughly to the amount inhaled by a smoker of 5–6 cigarettes per day. In rural areas, the amount may be about 20–40 percent of that inhaled by the urban dweller, depending on the season and traffic density.[94] However, the excess cancer risk among those who smoke 5–6 cigarettes per day is small. At present, there is no convincing evidence that benzo[a]pyrene and other polycyclic hydrocarbons in urban air contribute significantly to lung cancer mortality. Even in workers exposed to benzo[a]pyrene levels about 10,000 times higher than those in London air, the excess lung cancer risk was only 38 percent.[27] Thus, an increased risk to the city dweller is hardly likely. Nevertheless, benzo[a]pyrene might merely be an indicator of cancer-causing pollution; the true carcinogen might be another substance prevalent in polluted urban air. Also, cocarcinogenesis (p. 328) might lead to increased cancer risks for smokers exposed to urban air, and decreased breakdown of benzo[a]pyrene in the body due to concomitant other exposures (e.g., ozone, p. 394) might increase the carcinogenetic effects of low-level benzo[a]pyrene exposures. These largely theoretical suggestions can be verified only in prospective epidemiological studies in which cancer mortality can be related to exposure data over the long term. At present, prevention and control programs should focus on smoking and occupational exposures as well-established causes of excess cancer deaths. If cocarcinogenetic effects of smoking and urban air pollution in fact exist, there are presently more facts to support prevention through efforts to reduce smoking than through air-pollution control.

Effects of Indoor Air Pollution

Few systematic studies have dealt with health risks of pollutants in domestic and other indoor environments, even though many of us spend most of our time there. The risk of accidental carbon monoxide poisoning in homes has greatly diminished as electric power replaced gas for home illumination, and natural gas without CO replaced manufactured gas for use in appliances. However, even natural gas appliances may produce CO when combustion is incomplete, a danger inherent in insufficiently vented gas-fired water heaters.[46] In most homes, tobacco smoke is the main source of carbon monoxide and other pollutants. However, this is not a significant hazard for nonsmokers, even though sidestream smoke contains more CO than mainstream smoke.[14] In an experiment with considerably worse than usual conditions, large amounts of cigarette smoke were generated in a small, unventilated room, and CO levels averaged 38 ppm (=42 mg/cu m). Blood COHb of nonsmokers rose by 1 percent in 1 hour, while that of smokers, who smoked during the experiment, increased more (from average 5.9 to average 9.6 percent).[93] Since some performance deficit can be expected in smokers with these blood COHb levels (see p. 391), adverse indoor conditions that aggravate COHb accumulation appear to pose some risk to smokers. Accumulation of suspended particulates as a result of smoking is significant [14, 48] and well known to housewives. Indoor particulate aerosols consist predominantly of particles less than 1 μm in diameter,[63] which are able to reach and sediment in small airways and alveoli. Indoor particulate pollution can be reduced by air-cleaning devices (electrostatic precipitators), often installed in home-heating systems in the United States. The health benefits of such devices have not been evaluated critically, but some patients with asthma appear to benefit from eliminating suspended particulates, in particular pollens, from their homes. Levels of sulfur dioxide are often lower indoors than outdoors; the difference is determined in part by absorption of SO_2 in building materials.[7] The use of aerosolized household and cosmetic products merits attention as a source of indoor pollution in modern homes. Commercial hairspray preparations cause airway constriction (measured with flow-volume curves, Chap. 9) in the user who breathes quietly while applying the spray to the hair during 20 seconds [114] (see also page 447 and Fig. 18-3). The component(s) responsible for this effect have not been identified. Other aerosolized products may also cause airway constriction, sometimes accompanied by wheezing and chest tightness.[115] In hospitals, particularly in intensive care units, piped air supplies may pose risks of oil mist inhalation from compressors in the system. This risk needs to be prevented, since inhaled oil particles may cause chemical pneumonitis.[17]

IMPLICATIONS FOR POLLUTION-CONTROL PROGRAMS

Observations on Air-Quality Standards

Evidence for present standards. In accordance with the Clean Air Act of 1970, primary air-quality standards, and hence, pollution-control plans, are based on health considerations alone [31] (see also p. 385). The background data used to determine these standards are set forth in air-quality criteria documents.[3, 75–79] However, considering the limited, sometimes questionable nature of the data available on health effects of pollutants, the plight of those assembling the criteria documents is clear. In several cases, evidence of toxic effects was available only for pollutant concentrations much higher than those in highly polluted ambient air, and lower standards were set solely on epidemiological evidence. One critique of the criteria documents concludes: "The respiratory system of healthy persons has not been demonstrated to react to any of these agents at the concentrations thus far reported in community air. Some evidence suggests that oxidants may aggravate symptoms of persons with pre-existing lung disease, but this cannot account for the fluctuations of mortality in the general population. There are no data upon which to base a judgment of whether or not oxidants, nitrogen dioxide, or hydrocarbons at levels now existing in community air play any role in causation of respiratory disease." [111] On the basis of present data, the only exception required to this statement is that ozone has demonstrable toxic effects on the lungs of healthy persons at levels similar to those occurring under adverse conditions in Los Angeles (p. 393).

With respect to particulates and SO_2, the use of epidemiological surveys to set air-quality criteria is misleading, since these studies do not assess responses to single pollutants, but only to the complex mixtures in ambient air.[62] In fact, the epidemiological evidence quoted in the air-quality document for particulates [77] concerns much the same material as that quoted in the similar document for SO_2.[79]

The World Health Organization has suggested a combined guideline level for SO_2 and particulates.[110] The standard for total particulates does not take into account either particle size distribution or health effects of specific particles. Given the difficulties in determining these health effects, it may be more logical to base control of particulate matter primarily on its effect in reducing visibility and in soiling of materials, with health effects as an additional guide when specific toxic substances (e.g., asbestos, beryllium, cotton) may be involved.

Differences between industrial and community air standards. The standards for acceptable concentrations of pollutants in atmospheric air differ markedly for industrial and community exposures.[103] For instance, the TLV for sulfur dioxide in the United States is 5 ppm (13 mg/cu m) for industrial exposures, while the primary air-quality standard, based on health effects in man, is 0.08 mg/cu m as an annual arithmetic average; a 24–hour maximum of 0.365 mg/cu m should not be exceeded more than once per year (Table 16-1). The rationale given for these different standards includes: (1) industrial workers represent a selected, healthy group in the population; (2) industrial exposures last only 40 hours per week; (3) in contrast to urban residents, who can do little about the air they breathe, industry has better means of localizing pollution and protecting against its effects; and (4) since the general population includes many sick individuals who may be more than usually sensitive to pollutants, air-quality standards should aim to protect these individuals. However, no controlled studies show that industrial workers as a group are less sensitive to pollutants, or that persons with lung disease as a group are more sensitive to all pollutants. The only exception to this statement is that patients with asthma (Chap. 18) are more than usually sensitive to many substances, perhaps including gaseous pollutants. Many industrial workers have chronic bronchitis due to cigarette smoking, and they are probably equally as sensitive to pollutants as other cigarette smokers.

The argument is largely fallacious that community air standards must be more stringent than industrial-exposure standards in order to provide continuous protection over 24 hours, rather than just during working hours. Actually, the average urban housewife might maximally spend about 32 hours per week outdoors, and the average man working indoors perhaps about 17 hours per week (estimate of Dr. C. A. Mitchell and myself). Even people working outdoors are unlikely to spend more than 80 hours outdoors per week. Thus, it seems unrealistic to base air-quality standards on the expectation of continuous exposure. In summer, open windows promote uniform pollutant concentrations indoors and outdoors; in winter, indoor pollution may be high and different from that outdoors (see p. 406).

The large discrepancies between industrial and community air standards reflect two different philosophical approaches to similar data. Industrial TLV's are not meant to provide complete protection to all persons exposed, but only to set a limit below which major health effects are believed not to occur frequently.[6] On the other hand, community air standards have been set at levels thought to be low enough to prevent any health effect in any person who might be exposed. Therefore, the question raised when setting a TLV for industrial exposure is roughly: What is the highest pollutant level consistent with minimal health effects in most people? In contrast, the US ambient air-quality standards try to answer the question: What is the lowest pollutant level at which health effects can be anticipated in the most sensitive persons? Since responses to biological agents vary greatly among individuals, it is not surprising that widely different standards have emerged from these quite different philosophies. In addition, however, elements of uncertainty, related to the uncontrolled nature of many studies on community air pollution and to the limitations of air-quality monitoring, have led to setting air-quality standards at very low (i.e., stringent) levels, in hopes of providing an adequate safety margin.[31]

There is some justification for more stringent community-air standards than industrial-exposure standards, principally because it is generally easier for a sensitive individual to change jobs than to move from a polluted urban area to a rural clean air area lacking in job opportunities. However, the different philosophies used in standard setting have led to unrealistic differences between the two sets of standards. For instance, under the prevailing standards (Table 16-1), an industrial worker might inhale nearly 10 gm SO_2 per year if he is continuously exposed, 40 hours per week, to air containing SO_2 at the TLV. In contrast, the urban dweller is thought to be liable to health risks if the total amount of SO_2 per year inhaled exceeds about 60 mg.* Even if the urban dweller were exposed to 0.08 mg SO_2/cu m (0.028 ppm) during 24 hours per day, the yearly SO_2 load would be only about 250 mg. I believe that this difference is unjustifiably large. The evidence reviewed in this chapter suggests that the TLV for industrial exposure should be lowered to 0.5 ppm [1 ppm (1.43 mg/cu m) is the lowest level at which acute respiratory effects have been observed]. In order to provide an adequate safety margin for the general population, an ambient air-quality standard five times below the suggested industrial TLV (i.e., 0.1 ppm = 0.286 mg/cu m) might be reasonable. In support of this level, no significant differences in respiratory symptoms and lung function were found between groups of British children living in areas with SO_2 levels varying from 0.094–0.253 mg/cu m (1968–1969[60]).

Provisions for variations in regional conditions and individual sensitivity. The present air-quality standards are too rigid; that is, they do not allow sufficiently for the local, regional, climatic, and other variations that affect pollution. Although the current legislation correctly aims to prevent promoters in rural areas from attracting industry with promises that no undue fuss will be made over air pollution,[81] its present provisions lead to grossly uneconomical control programs. For instance, it makes little sense to have home owners and industries burn expensive low-fuel oil in areas where SO_2 levels are far below the present standards for SO_2. Similarly, little or no gain in terms of respiratory health can be expected from curbing automobile traffic in areas where photo-oxidant pollution occurs incidentally and at low levels. Reducing hydrocarbon and NO_2 emissions in such areas accomplishes little, since these pollutants themselves are not highly toxic and require two other factors—sunlight and air stagnation—to produce irritant photochemical smog. In the approach to standard setting, the aim to protect even the most sensitive individual against lung or airway irritants is also unrealistic. A small number

* Assume minute ventilation = 6 liters/min = 14.4 cu m during a 40-hour workweek = 720 cu m per year of 50 workweeks. TLV = 13 mg/cu m; total amount of SO_2 inhaled per year = 720 × 13 = 9360 mg. Urban dweller exposed to ambient air during same time period: total amount of SO_2 inhaled = 720 × 0.08 = 57.6 mg.

of people is probably highly sensitive to minute amounts of pollutants. But efforts to protect these people should focus on research and treatment to modify their individual sensitivities, not on the imposition of unrealistic air-quality standards that impose undue costs on everybody.

If the air-quality standards are to be based on stronger data on health effects, research on the long-term health effects of pollutants should be expanded. Well-designed exposure and epidemiological studies using objective, quality-controlled methods should provide better data than we now have. However, if this research is to help in designing pollution-control measures, it should not be delayed.

Recommendations for Air-Pollution Control

Even though there is no evidence that present pollutant levels in US cities pose grave dangers to health, it is necessary to limit pollutant emissions as much as is feasible. Further increases in pollutant levels in our cities must be prevented, since many pollutants do cause toxic effects at higher levels than those now prevailing. Also, the discomfort, public nuisance and crop damage associated with high pollutant levels in several areas must be reduced. Mass transit systems should be greatly improved in our cities to reduce dependence on the automobile for urban and suburban transport. Improved urban housing, adequate planning of residential and industrial zones, and control of industrial pollutant emissions are also needed to improve air quality or at least prevent further deterioration.

It is, however, counterproductive to defend these measures on our present knowledge of human health effects of air pollution. The evidence for respiratory health effects most often quoted in favor of the present air-quality standards is tenuous and unconvincing on many points. Indeed, until better-controlled studies are performed, there is more evidence to support an upward revision of the standards than their maintenance at present levels. Also, it should be made clear that control of man-made ambient air pollution can never eliminate asthma, bronchitis, emphysema, and other lung diseases, certainly not as long as people continue to smoke. It is therefore misleading to impress the public with a sense of impending disaster because of air pollution, and to suggest that pollution control will prevent most respiratory disease.

Among certain high-risk groups where pollution does pose an immediate health risk, additional protective measures are needed. Stopping of smoking, controlling the indoor domestic environment, or moving to a low-pollution area are measures within reach of many citizens. In addition, adequate pollution warning systems, which exist in most states of the U.S., can alert persons who must continue to live in risk areas and who need protection against effects of episodic high pollutant levels. Clinics for symptomatic treatment, hospital wards provided with clean air, and advice on protective measures should be available to these groups.

The decision expressed in the Clean Air Act of 1970 to base air pollution-control measures on anticipated health effects was intended to protect the public. Present evidence, however, suggests that while there are many compelling reasons to reduce pollution, ill health is not foremost among them. Thus, the less specific secondary standards for ambient air quality—those "requisite to protect the general welfare"—may turn out to offer the strongest grounds for pollution control.

SUMMARY

The health effects of air pollution are poorly documented and ill understood. Although many pollutants have potentially toxic effects on the lungs and airways, and some on other physiological systems, these effects require dose levels much higher than those now present in urban air even under adverse conditions.

The physical and chemical characteristics of polluted air masses are determined by the nature of pollutant emissions, by climatic and geographic factors, and by complex chemical reactions in the polluted atmosphere. The two main types of pollution are (1) sulfur and particulate pollution and (2) photochemical smog. Air pollutants with potential health effects include sulfur dioxide, sulfates, particulates, carbon monoxide, oxidants (including ozone), nitrogen dioxide, and hydrocarbons. The last two participate in chemical reactions, promoted by sunlight, which form photochemical (oxidant) smog.

The health effects of pollutants can be studied in the laboratory, with experiments involving controlled exposures (toxicology), and in the community, with studies which compare mortality and morbidity in populations exposed to pollutants with similar indices in nonexposed populations (epidemiology). Unfortunately, most toxicological studies have been limited to short-term exposures (minutes or hours); studies of long-term exposures (days or weeks) in humans are urgently needed. Epidemiological studies have suffered from insufficient controls and from failure to include some toxicological elements: few if any studies in polluted areas, such as Los Angeles, have used sensitive tests to measure pollutant effects on human lung function. Thus, while some epidemiological studies have suggested associations between SO_2 and particulate pollution and the prevalence of respiratory symptoms, these studies cannot substitute for well-designed, well-executed toxicological studies. Unless, and until, such studies confirm the health risks posed by air pollutants, the scientific basis for air-pollution control to promote public health will be tenuous indeed.

REFERENCES

1. Abeles FB, Craker LE, Forrence LE, Leather GR: Fate of air pollutants: removal of ethylene, sulfur dioxide, and nitrogen dioxide by soil. Science 173:914–916, 1971
2. Acton JD, Myrvik QN: Nitrogen dioxide effects on alveolar macrophages. Arch Environ Health 24:48–52, 1972
3. Air Pollution Control Office: Air quality criteria for nitrogen oxides. Washington, D.C., Environmental Protection Agency, 1971
4. Amdur MO: Aerosols formed by oxidation of sulfur dioxide. Arch Environ Health 23:459–468, 1971
5. American Conference of Governmental Industrial Hygienists: Air Sampling Instruments, ed 4. Cincinnati, 1972
6. American Conference of Governmental Industrial Hygienists: TLV's: Threshold limit values for chemical substances and physical agents in the workroom environment with intended changes for 1973. Cincinnati, 1973
7. Andersen I: Relationships between outdoor and indoor air pollution. Atmos Environ 6:275–278, 1972
8. Anderson DO, Ferris BG Jr: Community studies of the health effects of air pollution—a critique. J Air Pollut Control Assoc 15:587–593, 1965
9. Arner EC, Rhoades RA: Long-term

nitrogen dioxide exposure. Arch Environ Health 26:156–160, 1973

10. Bates DV: Air pollutants and the human lung. Am Rev Respir Dis 105:1–13, 1972

11. Bates DV, Bell GM, Burnham CD, Hazucha M, Mantha J, Pengelly LD, Silverman F: Short-term effects of ozone on the lung. J Appl Physiol 32:176–181, 1972

12. Booth S, DeGroot I, Markush R, Horton RJM: Detection of asthma epidemics in seven cities. Arch Environ Health 10:152–155, 1965

13. Brain JD: The uptake of inhaled gases by the nose. Ann Otol Rhinol Laryngol 79:529–539, 1970

14. Bridge DP, Corn M: Contribution to the assessment of exposure of nonsmokers to air pollution from cigarette and cigar smoke in occupied spaces. Environ Res 5:192–209, 1972

15. Buell GC, Tokiwa Y, Mueller PK: Potential crosslinking agents in lung tissue. Arch Environ Health 10:213–219, 1965

16. Burton GG, Corn M, Gee JBL, Vasallo C, Thomas AP: Response of healthy men to inhaled low concentrations of gas-aerosol mixtures. Arch Environ Health 18:681–692, 1969

17. Bushman JA, Clark PA: Oil mist hazard and piped air supplies. Br Med J 3:588–590, 1967

17a. Clark RP, Shirley SG: Identification of skin in airborne particulate matter. Nature 246:39–40, 1973

18. Coffin DL, Gardner DE, Holzman RS, Wolock FJ: Influence of ozone on pulmonary cells. Arch Environ Health 16:633–636, 1968

19. Cohen AA, Bromberg S, Buechley RW, Heiderscheit LT, Shy CM: Asthma and air pollution from a coal-fueled power plant. Am J Public Health 62:1181–1188, 1972

20. Cohen CA, Hudson AR, Clausen JL, Knelson JH: Respiratory symptoms, spirometry, and oxidant air pollution in nonsmoking adults. Am Rev Respir Dis 105:251–261, 1972

21. Colley JRT: Respiratory disease in childhood. Br Med Bull 27:9–14, 1971

22. Colley JRT, Reid DD: Urban and social origins of childhood bronchitis in England and Wales. Br Med J 2:213–217, 1970

23. Committee on Biologic Effects of At-

mospheric Pollutants: Airborne lead in perspective. Washington, D.C., Division of Medical Sciences, National Research Council, National Academy of Sciences, 1971

24. Committee on Biologic Effects of Atmospheric Pollutants: Particulate polycyclic organic matter. Washington, D.C., Division of Medical Sciences, National Research Council, National Academy of Sciences, 1972

25. Dillard CJ, Urribarri N, Reddy K, Fletcher B, Taylor S, deLumen B, Langberg S, Tappel AL: Increased lysosomal enzymes in lungs of ozone-exposed rats. Arch Environ Health 25:426–431, 1972

26. Dixon JR, Mountain JT: Role of histamine and related substances in development of tolerance to edemagenic gases. Toxicol Appl Pharmacol 7:756–766, 1965

27. Doll R: Practical steps towards the prevention of bronchial carcinoma. Scott Med J 15:433–447, 1970

28. Douglas JWB, Waller RE: Air pollution and respiratory infection in children. Br J Prev Soc Med 20:1–8, 1966

29. Eckhardt RE, MacFarland HN, Alarie YCE, Busey WM: The biologic effect from long-term exposure of primates to carbon monoxide. Arch Environ Health 25:381–387, 1972

30. Einthoven W: Ueber die Wirkung der Bronchialmuskeln, nach einer neuen Methode untersucht, und über Asthma nervosum. Arch ges Physiol 51:367–444, 1892

31. Environmental Protection Agency: National primary and secondary ambient air quality standards. Fed Regis 36:8186–8201, 1971

32. Evans MJ, Stephens RJ, Cabral LJ, Freeman G: Cell renewal in the lungs of rats exposed to low levels of NO_2. Arch Environ Health 24:180–188, 1972

33. Fairchild EJ, Murphy SD, Stokinger HE: Protection by sulfur compounds against the air pollutants ozone and nitrogen dioxide. Science 130:861–862, 1959

34. Fairchild GA, Roan J, McCarroll J: Atmospheric pollutants and the pathogenesis of viral respiratory infection. Arch Environ Health 25:174–182, 1972

35. Forbes WH: Carbon monoxide uptake

via the lungs. Ann NY Acad Sci 174: 72–75, 1970

36. Frank NR: Studies on the effects of acute exposure to sulfur dioxide in human subjects. Proc R Soc Med 57:1029–1033, 1964

37. Frank NR, Amdur MO, Worcester J, Whittenberger JL: Effects of acute controlled exposure to SO₂ on respiratory mechanics in healthy male adults. J Appl Physiol 17:252–258, 1962

37a. Friedlander SK: Chemical element balances and identification of air pollution sources. Environ Sci Tech: 7:235–240, 1973

38. Gardner DE, Lewis TR, Alpert SM, Hurst DJ, Coffin DL: The role of tolerance in pulmonary defense mechanisms. Arch Environ Health 25:432–438, 1972

39. Giordano AM Jr, Morrow PE: Chronic low-level nitrogen dioxide exposure and mucociliary clearance. Arch Environ Health 25:443–449, 1972

40. Goldsmith JR, Cohen SI: Epidemiological bases for possible air quality criteria for carbon monoxide. J Air Pollut Control Assoc 19:704–713, 1969

41. Goldstein BD, Levine MR, Cuzzi-Spada R, Cardenas R, Buckley RD, Balchum OJ: P-aminobenzoic acid as a protective agent in ozone toxicity. Arch Environ Health 24:243–247, 1972

42. Goldstein E, Tyler WS, Hoeprich PD, Eagle C: Adverse influence of ozone on pulmonary bactericidal activity of murine lung. Nature 229:262–263, 1971

43. Haldane JS, Priestley JG: Respiration. London, Oxford University Press, 1935

44. Hallett WY: Effect of ozone and cigarette smoke on lung function. Arch Environ Health 10:295–302, 1965

45. Halperin MH, McFarland RA, Niven JI, Roughton FJW: The time course of the effects of carbon monoxide on visual thresholds. J Physiol (London) 146:583–593, 1959

45a. Hazucha M, Silverman F, Parent C, Field S, Bates DV: Pulmonary function in man after short-term exposure to ozone. Arch Environ Health 27:183–188, 1973

46. Henderson Y, Haggard HW: Noxious Gases, ed 2. New York, Reinhold Publishing Corporation, 1943

47. Hill G: "Los Angeles faces strict auto curbs." NY Times, p 1, Jan 14, 1973

48. Hoegg UR: Cigarette smoke in closed spaces. Environ Health Perspect 2, 117–128, 1972

49. Holland WW, Reid DD: The urban factor in chronic bronchitis. Lancet 1:445–448, 1965

50. Holland WW, Reid DD, Seltser R, Stone RW: Respiratory disease in England and the United States. Arch Environ Health 10:338–345, 1965

51. Holzman RS, Gardner DE, Coffin DL: In vivo inactivation of lysozyme by ozone. J Bacteriol 96:1562–1566, 1968

52. Horvath SM, Dahms TE, O'Hanlon JF: Carbon monoxide and human vigilance. A deleterious effect of present urban concentrations. Arch Environ Health 23:343–347, 1971

53. Hurst DJ, Coffin DL: Ozone effect on lysosomal hydrolases of alveolar macrophages in vitro. Arch Intern Med 127:1059–1063, 1971

54. Hurst DJ, Gardner DE, Coffin DL: Effect of ozone on acid hydrolases of the pulmonary alveolar macrophage. J Reticuloendothel Soc 8:288–301, 1970

55. Intersociety Committee: Methods of air sampling and analysis. Washington, D.C., American Public Health Association, 1972

56. Jaffe LS: The biological effects of ozone on man and animals. Am Ind Hyg Assoc J 28:267–277, 1967

57. Jones RD, Commins BT, Cernik AA: Blood lead and carboxyhemoglobin levels in London taxi drivers. Lancet 2:302–303, 1972

58. Lambert PM, Reid DD: Smoking, air pollution and bronchitis in Britain. Lancet 1:853–857, 1970

59. Lave LB, Seskin EP: Air pollution, climate and home heating: their effects on U.S. mortality rates. Am J Public Health 62:909–916, 1972

60. Lunn JE, Knowelden J, Roe JW: Patterns of respiratory illness in Sheffield junior school children: A follow-up study. Br J Prev Soc Med 24:223–228, 1970

61. Khandwala A, Gee JBL: Linoleic acid hydroperoxide: Impaired bacterial uptake by alveolar macrophages, a mechanism of oxidant lung injury. Science 182:1364–1365, 1973

62. Lawther PJ, Waller RE, Henderson M: Air pollution and exacerbations of bronchitis. Thorax 25:525–539, 1970

63. Lee RE Jr: The size of suspended

particulate matter in air. Science 178: 567–575, 1972

64. Leonard AGG, Crowley D, Belton J: Atmospheric pollution in Dublin during the years 1944 to 1950. Sci Proc Royal Dublin Soc 25:166–167, 1950

65. Lewis R, Gilkeson MM, McCaldin RO: Air pollution and New Orleans asthma. Pub Health Reps 77:947–954, 1962

66. McCarroll J, Bradley W: Excess mortality as an indicator of health effects of air pollution. Am J Public Health 56:1933–1942, 1966

67. McJilton C, Frank R, Charlson R: Role of relative humidity in the synergistic effect of a sulfur dioxide-aerosol mixture on the lung. Science 182:503–504, 1973

68. McMillan RS, Wiseman DH, Hanes B, Wehrle PF: Effects of oxidant air pollution on peak expiratory flow rates in Los Angeles school children. Arch Environ Health 18:941–949, 1969

69. Menzel DB: Toxicity of ozone, oxygen and radiation. Ann Rev Pharmacol 10:379–394, 1970

70. Motley HL: Environmental air pollution effect on pulmonary function. Aerosp Med 42:1108–1110, 1971

71. Murphy SD, Klingshirn DA, Ulrich CE: Respiratory response of guinea pigs during acrolein inhalation and its modification by drugs. J Pharmacol Exp Ther 141:79–83, 1963

72. Murphy SD, Leng JK, Ulrich CE, Davis HV: Effects on animals of exposure to auto exhaust. Arch Environ Health 7: 60–70, 1963

73. Nadel JA, Salem H, Tamplin B, Tokiwa Y: Mechanism of bronchoconstriction. Arch Environ Health 10:175–178, 1965

74. Nadel JA, Salem H, Tamplin B, Tokiwa Y: Mechanism of bronchoconstriction during inhalation of sulfur dioxide. J Appl Physiol 20:164–167, 1965

75. National Air Pollution Control Administration: Air quality criteria for carbon monoxide. Washington, D.C., Environmental Health Service, PHS, US Dept of Health, Education, and Welfare, 1970

76. National Air Pollution Control Administration: Air quality criteria for hydrocarbons. Washington, D.C., Environmental Health Service, PHS, US Dept of Health, Education, and Welfare, 1970

77. National Air Pollution Control Admin-istration: Air quality criteria for particulate matter. Washington, D.C., Environmental Health Service, PHS, US Dept of Health, Education and Welfare, 1969

78. National Air Pollution Control Administration: Air quality criteria for photochemical oxidants. Washington, D.C., Environmental Health Service, PHS, US Dept of Health, Education and Welfare, 1970

79. National Air Pollution Control Administration: Air quality criteria for sulfur oxides. Washington, D.C., Environmental Health Service, PHS, US Dept of Health, Education, and Welfare, 1970

80. National Tuberculosis and Respiratory Disease Association: Air Pollution Primer, New York, 1969

81. de Nevers N: Enforcing the Clean Air Act of 1970. Sci Am 228:14–21, 1973

82. Nieding G von, Krekeler H: Pharma-kologische Beeinflussung der akuten NO_2-Wirkung auf die Lungenfunktion von Gesunden und Kranken mit einer chronischen Bronchitis. Int Arch Arbeitsmed 29:55–63, 1971

83. Nielsen B: Thermoregulation during work in carbon monoxide poisoning. Acta Physiol Scand 82:98–106, 1971

84. Okulicz WC: Lung biogenic amines and pulmonary edema in ozone exposed rats, mice, and guinea pigs. MPH Thesis, Yale University, 1971

85. Palmer MS, Exley RW, Coffin DL: Influence of pollutant gases on benz-pyrene hydroxylase activity. Arch Environ Health 25:439–442, 1972

86. P'an AYS, Béland J, Jegier Z: Ozone-induced arterial lesions. Arch Environ Health 24:229–232, 1972

87. Petrilli FL, Agnese G, Kanitz S: Epidemiologic studies of air pollution effects in Genoa, Italy. Arch Environ Health 12:733–740, 1966

88. Phelps HW, Koike S: "Tokyo-Yokohama asthma." The rapid development of respiratory distress presumably due to air pollution. Am Rev Respir Dis 86:55–63, 1962

89. Prindle RA, Wright GW, McCaldin RO, Marcus SC, Lloyd TC, Bye WE: Comparison of pulmonary function and other parameters in two communities with widely different air pollution levels. Am J Public Health 53:200–217, 1963

90. Reichel G, Ulmer WT (eds): Luft-verschmutzung und unspezifische Atem-

wegserkrankungen. Berlin, Springer-Verlag, 1970

91. Reichel G, Wobith F, Ulmer WT: Akute und chronische Wirkung von Strassenluft an verkehrsreicher Kreuzung auf die Lungenfunktion des Menschen, den CO- Hb- und Bleigehalt des Blutes, in: Reichel G, Ulmer WT, (eds): Luftverschmutzung und Unspezifische Atemwegserkrankungen. Berlin, Springer-Verlag, 1970

92. Roehm JN, Hadley JG, Menzel DB: Antioxidants vs. lung disease. Arch Intern Med 128:88–93, 1971

93. Russell MAH, Cole PV, Brown E: Absorption by non-smokers of carbon monoxide from room air polluted by tobacco smoke. Lancet 1:576–579, 1973

94. Schaad R, Gilgen A: 3,4-Benzpyren im Staubsediment von Zürich. Z Präventivmedizin 15:87–96, 1970

95. Scheel LD, Dobrogorski OJ, Mountain JT, Svirbely JL, Stokinger HE: Physiologic, biochemical, immunologic and pathologic changes following ozone exposure. J Appl Physiol 14:67–80, 1959

96. Schoettlin CE, Landau E: Air pollution and asthmatic attacks in the Los Angeles area. Pub. Health Reps 76: 545–548, 1961

96a. Shapley D: Auto pollution: EPA worrying that the catalyst may backfire. Science 182:368–371, 1973

97. Shy CM, Creason JP, Pearlman ME, McClain KE, Benson FB, Young MM: The Chattanooga school children study: Effects of community exposure to nitrogen dioxide. I. Methods, description of pollutant exposure, and results of ventilatory function testing. J Air Pollut Control Assoc 20:539–545, 1970

98. Shy CM, Creason JP, Pearlman ME, McClain KE, Benson FB, Young MM: The Chattanooga school children study: Effects of community exposure to nitrogen dioxide. II. Incidence of acute respiratory illness. J Air Pollut Control Assoc 20:582–588, 1970

99. Shy CM, Finklea JF: Air pollution affects community health. Environ Sci Tech 7:204–208, 1973

100. Snell RE, Luchsinger PC: Effects of sulfur dioxide on expiratory flow rates and total respiratory resistance in normal human subjects. Arch Environ Health 18:693–698, 1969

101. Stephens RJ, Freeman G, Evans MJ: Early response of lungs to low levels of nitrogen dioxide. Arch Environ Health 24:160–179, 1972

102. Stern A (ed): Air Pollution, vol I (2 ed): Air Pollution and Its Effects. New York, Academic Press, 1968

103. Stokinger HE: Toxicity of airborne chemicals: Air quality standards—A national and international view. Ann Rev Pharmacol 12:407–422, 1972

104. Toyama T: Air pollution and its health effects in Japan. Arch Environ Health 8:153–173, 1964

105. "U.S. accepts traffic plan to cut air pollution here." NY Times, p 1, June 16, 1973

106. Vogel JA, Gleser MA, Wheeler RC, Whitten BK: Carbon monoxide and physical work capacity. Arch Environ Health 24:198–203, 1972

107. Waller RE, Commins BT, Lawther PJ: Air pollution in a city street. Br J Ind Med 22:128–138, 1965

108. Wayne WS, Wehrle PF, Carroll RE: Oxidant air pollution and athletic performance. JAMA 199:901–904, 1967

109. Williams RD, Acton JD, Myrvik QN: Influence of nitrogen dioxide on the uptake of parainfluenza-3 virus by alveolar macrophages. J Reticuloendothel Soc 11:627–636, 1972

110. World Health Organization: Health hazards of the human environment. Geneva, 1972

111. Wright GW: An appraisal of epidemiologic data concerning the effect of oxidants, nitrogen dioxide, and hydrocarbons upon human populations. J Air Pollut Control Assoc 19:679–682, 1969

112. Young WA, Shaw DB, Bates DV: Effect of low concentrations of ozone on pulmonary function in man. J Appl Physiol 19:765–768, 1964

113. Zapletal A, Jech J, Paul T, Samánek M: Pulmonary function studies in children living in an air-polluted area. Am Rev Respir Dis 107:400–409, 1973

114. Zuskin E, Bouhuys A: Acute airway responses to hairspray preparations. N Engl J Med (in press)

115. Zuskin E: Exposure to inhalants in the home. Mexico City, Symposium on Environmental Health in the Americas, July 3–4, 1973

Chapter 17

Byssinosis*

> But after all these profound reasonings on breeches, I should like to know what is the best material to make them of. I am now wearing a kind of black stuff. . . . It is composed of linen and silk, but it is extremely thin and does not wear well. I have worn breeches made of this stuff only three or four weeks, and they are already miserably torn. I am much ashamed of them. . . .
>
> I undertake to be Mademoiselle's knight-errant if she will kindly mend my breeches with her own fair hand. I have the honour to say that it is not the first time I have asked and obtained such a favour. My breeches have been mended by ladies before now. They have been mended by the most famous beauty in the north of Scotland, and even when I had them on. I must admit, however, that it was only in one of the knees.
>
> James Boswell, November 1763 [46]

Before the Industrial Revolution made cheap and high-quality cotton goods widely available, even well-to-do men like Boswell had difficulty keeping their clothes in good repair. Boswell made the most of that problem, but few of us would like to trade pants with him. The Lancashire mills began to increase their production of cotton yarn and cloth within a few years after Eli Whitney, of New Haven, invented the cotton gin in 1793. Concomitantly, their machines began to pollute the air in the mills with dust, an unfortunate consequence of the increase in cotton production. In the 1820s, Lancashire physicians reported an excess of respiratory disease in cotton mill workers. Even earlier, Ramazzini [47] had recognized that flax dust causes an asthma-like disease, and Morgagni [41] had described pathological changes in the lungs of hemp workers. Byssinosis due to flax dust probably occurred in colonial America.[18a] Despite this early recognition of undesirable side-effects on human health, the problem of byssinosis in the cotton textile industry remains. There is certainly no lack of medical literature on the subject. In addition to many studies in the 19th and first half of the 20th century,

---

* Based in part on the MacArthur Postgraduate Lecture given at the University of Edinburgh, October 28, 1970.

research in the past 20 years has provided the knowledge to prevent and control the disease. That it still exists, therefore, reflects not so much a shortage of facts, but rather a failure to apply the knowledge to practical control measures. Hopefully, the post-industrial revolution of our times, which should emphasize timely prevention of harmful side-effects of new technology, will eliminate a health hazard introduced by the "new" technology of the 18th century.

Clinical Syndrome

The early literature on byssinosis has been admirably reviewed by Schilling.[49] The cardinal acute symptoms, dyspnea and shortness of breath on Mondays after a weekend off work, were first described by two Belgian physicians—Mareska and Heyman[34]—who, in 1845, interviewed 1000 men and 1000 women in the mills of Ghent. "All workers declared that the dust troubled them much less on the last days of the week than on Monday and Tuesday. The masters find the reason of this greater sensitivity in the excesses of the Sunday; but the workers never fail to attribute it to the interruption of work which makes them lose, they say, part of their habituation to dust."[34] Our present knowledge confirms the workers' view.

The acute symptoms that develop on Mondays differ primarily in degree and in duration from the chronic symptoms (Table 17-1). The former are reversible;

Table 17-1
Main Features of Byssinosis

At risk:	Cotton, flax, and soft-hemp workers in carding, spinning, and other dusty operations.
Symptoms:	Chest tightness, shortness of breath, cough, and wheezing.
Symptoms appear:	*Initially* *— on Mondays or other first workdays after absence from work;
	Later *— also on Tuesdays and subsequent weekdays during work;
	Eventually *— chronic shortness of breath and other respiratory symptoms, even in absence of dust exposure, and continuing after retirement from work.

Clinical grades [12, 49–51]:

$\frac{1}{2}$—occasional chest tightness or cough, or both, on first day of the working week;

1—chest tightness on every first day of the working week;

2—chest tightness on the first and other days of the working week;

3—grade 2 symptoms accompanied by evidence of permanent incapacity from reduced ventilatory capacity.

* Initially=on starting employment in risk area; later=usually after more than 2–5 years' exposure to dust in a risk area; eventually=as a rule, after more than 10 years' exposure. Aggravation of symptoms on Monday continues, also in the later stages, if the worker remains at work in risk areas.

the latter are not. Although the symptoms of byssinosis are clear-cut and not easily misinterpreted, the absence of characteristic anatomical changes visible in chest x-ray films has delayed the recognition of the disease as an occupational hazard. The clinical syndrome of byssinosis differs in many aspects from diseases caused by organic antigens, such as farmer's lung and occupational asthma. In byssinosis, chest x-ray films are not diagnostic and show, if anything, changes similar to those in patients with chronic bronchitis or emphysema.[49] However, objective evidence about the lung's response to dust exposure can be obtained with lung-function measurements. Byssinosis is a lung disease in which accurate function studies are essential for diagnosis, as well as for prevention and control measures.

Prevalence of Byssinosis

The epidemiology of byssinosis shows why it is important to study a disease in its natural setting. The prevalence of byssinosis in the textile industry not only indicates its importance as a public health problem, but also provides clues about its pathogenesis. A full discussion of the epidemiology of byssinosis is beyond the scope of this book. The examples chosen for discussion deal principally with conditions in the United States. Most studies of byssinosis include (1) a question-naire interview (Chap. 13), (2) measurement of lung function, and (3) measure-ment of airborne dust. A standard questionnaire is available in English, Spanish, and other languages.[8, 32, 51] Lung-function measurements should detect irreversible, long-term changes as well as acute effects of dust exposure. Airborne dust concen-trations should be measured to quantitate the degree of dust exposure and to provide baseline data for control measures.

Most data on byssinosis prevalence are based on responses to standard ques-tions concerning chest tightness and dyspnea on Monday. These reflect the subjec-tive experience of the workers and underestimate the prevalence of airway responses as measured with objective methods, especially when the interview is conducted at a time that the symptoms are absent or minimal, such as on Fridays.[8] Recent recommendations, therefore, emphasize the need to determine the worker's objective response to dust exposure.[12, 50]

Prevalence studies in US cotton mills have shown that about 20–30 percent of cardroom workers, and a similar or lower percentage of spinning room workers, have acute symptoms of byssinosis (all grades; Table 17-2). Age and duration of employment in the mill do not clearly affect the prevalence of acute symptoms.[4, 21, 60] In one of these mills (mill F in Table 17-2), many workers had been employed less than 1 year, but were just as often affected by chest tightness on Monday as the long-term workers.[21] If these prevalence rates, found in a small number of mills, are valid for the US cotton textile industry as a whole, some 8000 cardroom workers and 9000 spinning room workers may have byssinosis.[60] Since this estimate is based on studies of people at work in the industry, it does not include retired workers. This omission is important because those who are disabled by byssinosis (clinical grade 3; Table 17-1) often retire prematurely;[14] the problem of chronic disease in this group is discussed later (p. 431).

The results of prevalence studies in US mills [21, 21a, 52, 60] agree with those in cotton textile mills in other countries and are probably reasonably representative

Table 17-2
Prevalence of Byssinosis in US Cotton Mills

	Workers (no.)	Mean Age (yrs)	Average Duration of Employment in Cotton Mills (yrs)	Byssinosis * (% of Workers)
Mill A				
Carders	25	36	16	32 }
Spinners	84	43	18	12 } <0.05
Total	109	40	17	17
Mill B				
Carders	34	48	17	21 }
Spinners	15	43	12	13 } NS †
Total	49	46	15	18
Mill F				
Carders	47	38	3	26 }
Spinners	167	41	4	29 } NS †
Total	214	40	4	29

* Positive history of byssinosis (all grades).
† Not significant (χ^2 test).
Data from Bouhuys et al. (mill F[21]) and from Zuskin et al. (mills *A and B*[60]).

for the industry as a whole. There is no question, however, that the prevalence of byssinosis may vary among mills for several reasons. The risk is highest among people exposed to dust in initial processing stages (e.g., carding—for description of cotton processing, see references 21, 39, and 49) and to dust of low-quality cotton. In such groups, 70 percent or more of the workers may be affected. They inhale large amounts of dust containing toxic contaminants (see below). Some other textile dusts (rayon dust or dust of chemically treated cotton waste—which consist of nearly pure cellulose—or dust of chemically degummed flax) do not cause byssinosis. Workers exposed to these apparently nontoxic dusts have no symptoms, and byssinotic workers transferred from risk areas to such workrooms stop complaining of acute symptoms.[3, 13, 56] Thus, epidemiological data indicate that byssinosis is probably caused by some contaminant of cotton, since pure cellulose dust, derived from cotton with relatively simple chemical procedures, is nontoxic.

Dust Exposure and Lung Function

The first objective evidence that textile dust exposure affects the lungs came from lung-function studies by McKerrow et al.[37] They showed that forced expiratory volume ($FEV_{0.75}$) decreases during dust exposure in cotton cardroom workers, and more so on Monday than on other weekdays. They suggested that cotton dust contains a pharmacological agent that causes airway constriction. At that time, however, the use of spirometric tests to measure changes in airway caliber was not generally accepted. At the University of Lund, the late Gunnar Lundin and I were sufficiently skeptical of the idea that cotton dust contains a constrictor agent that we served as subjects in experiments with aerosols of cotton dust extract. We began these studies (with S.-E. Lindell) because we thought that a few controlled laboratory experiments might dismiss the idea. We were wrong: both of us became short of breath and felt tight in the chest after inhaling the extract aerosol for 10 minutes. Our N_2 washout curves (Chap. 4, p. 71) showed objective evidence of function changes, which we interpreted as reflecting reversible small-airway obstruction.[18] Later, we obtained the same changes of N_2 washout curves in cotton cardroom workers exposed to dust on Monday[1] (Fig. 17-1) and also in flax workers.[11] Several more recent studies have confirmed these results with a variety of function tests. A few hours' exposure to cotton, flax, or hemp dust causes the typical symptoms, decreased maximum expiratory flow rates,[4, 8, 11, 18a, 20, 21, 58, 60] and increased airway resistance.[37, 38] Decreases in arterial oxygen tensions have also been recorded in hemp workers,[33] while static lung recoil pressures are unchanged.[20] In addition, laboratory exposures to dust clouds or dust-extract aerosols have resulted in chest tightness and dyspnea, and in decreases of expiratory flow[14, 15] and dynamic lung compliance.[19, 36] These changes are compatible with narrowing

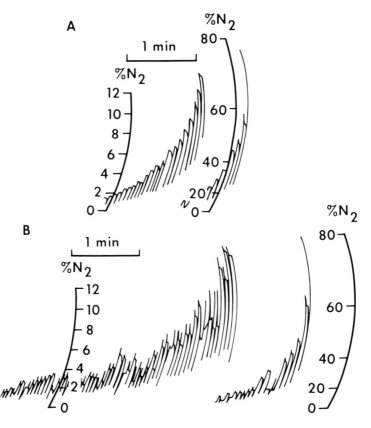

Fig. 17-1. Nitrogen clearance before work (*A*) and at the end of 6 hours' work in the cardroom (*B*). Read from right to left. Records made during quiet breathing at rest. See also discussion of N_2 clearance in Chapter 4. Lung clearance index: 6.9 (*A*) and 9.1 (*B*). Reproduced from Arnoldsson et al.[1]

of small airways as the principal effect of acute dust exposure. Increases in airway resistance [36] and pulmonary resistance have also been reported,[19, 36] suggesting that larger airways may also be involved (Chap. 8).

Effect of Dust on Airways

The preceding section summarized the evidence that cotton dust exposure may result in small-airway narrowing; this section discusses how that effect occurs. The first clue was that β-adrenergic drugs (isoproterenol, orciprenaline, epinephrine [11, 20, 37]) can prevent or abolish the dust effect. After the end of a work shift, inhalation of a small dose of isoproterenol often reverses most of the functional deficit within 30 minutes. Most workers, or healthy subjects, do not produce any mucus secretions from their airways either during exposure or while its effect wears off. Therefore, airway smooth muscle contraction is probably the major factor in obstructing the airways.

Another important clue was the time course of the effect of dust extract (Fig. 17-2). The symptoms and function changes developed about 20 minutes after the end of a 10-minute exposure period and lasted several hours. The acute effect of dust in industry, too, lasts hours rather than minutes. Histamine aerosol induces qualitatively similar function changes, but with a shorter time course. The slowly

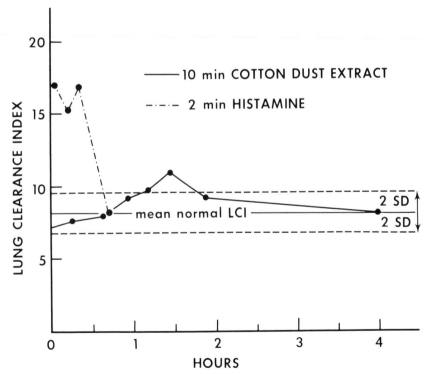

Fig. 17-2. Time course of the effects of inhalation of histamine aerosol and of cotton dust extract aerosol in a healthy man, as estimated from changes in lung N_2 clearance during oxygen breathing. Exposures were performed before first data point on each curve. After Bouhuys A, Ned Tijdschr Geneeskd 103:2356, 1959.

developing and prolonged effect of the dust and of its extract suggested an indirect action of the dust, such as through release of histamine.

The following experimental data provide clues on the mechanism of dust action: (1) the response can be elicited not only by cotton dust but also by aerosol inhalation of an aqueous dust extract;[18, 19, 23] (2) the large majority of people at risk are affected when toxic dust concentrations are high;[4, 8] (3) healthy people exposed for the first time to dust or dust extract respond as severely as long-term workers;[8, 18, 38] (4) after a single exposure to dust extract, repeat exposure 24 hours later has no effect.[18, 19] These findings indicate that the response is mediated by one or more water-soluble agents in the dust, that no special sensitization is required for the dust to take effect, that most people are sensitive to the dust action, and that the response exhibits marked tachyphylaxis.

Our experiments in 1958 suggested that the actions of dust extract in healthy subjects, and some of the acute symptoms of byssinosis, might result from a non-antigenic histamine-releasing agent in the dust.[18] This could explain why most people are sensitive to the dust action, and the depletion and replenishment of histamine stores in lung tissue could explain the tachyphylaxis observed. In the industrial worker with grade 1 byssinosis, exposure to dust on Monday would deplete the histamine stores, so that repeated exposure on Tuesday and subsequent workdays has less or no effect. Absence from exposure over a weekend would allow the histamine stores to be refilled, and dust exposure on Monday would again cause symptoms and lung-function changes. This hypothesis explains the acute effects of dust in the initial stages of byssinosis. In later stages, chronic changes in airways and lungs complicate the situation, and this may account for the more prolonged symptomatology in grade 2 byssinosis.

Other researchers have suggested that an antigen-antibody reaction is involved in the pathogenesis of byssinosis.[55] The proposed antigen, however, has aspecific protein-precipitating properties,[25] and this action is difficult to distinguish from specific binding processes between antigen and antibodies. Popa and his associates have demonstrated that the serum of byssinotic textile workers contains several types of antibodies;[45] they conclude that none of these is likely to be of pathogenetic importance. Thus, there is no convincing evidence on the role of antigen-antibody reactions in byssinosis. The histamine-releasing agent in textile dusts probably acts directly on target cells in lung tissue and airways. It has been suggested that proteolytic enzymes in cotton dust might cause histamine release.[57] However, there is no direct evidence supporting this view: the acute actions of cotton dust differ from those of proteolytic enzymes (Chap. 15, p. 372).

Histamine Release by Textile Dust

Experiments with chopped human lung tissue have shown that cotton-, flax-, and hemp-dust extracts release histamine from human lung, during about one-half hour incubation at 37°C.[17] Data from early experiments are shown in Figure 17-3. This result, confirmed by Nicholls et al.,[43] focuses attention on the origin of the histamine-releasing agent. It had sometimes been thought that active agents in cotton dust might be formed during the prolonged storage of tightly packed cotton in bales, and it seemed worthwhile to investigate whether fresh plant

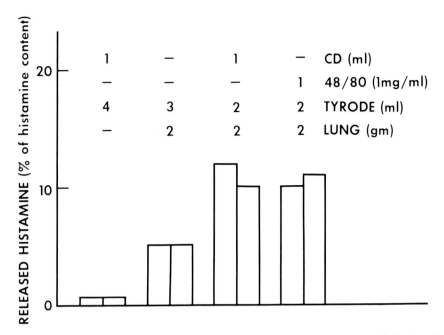

1	—	1	—	CD (ml)
—	—	—	1	48/80 (1mg/ml)
4	3	2	2	TYRODE (ml)
—	2	2	2	LUNG (gm)

Fig. 17-3. Each bar represents one incubation flask; contents of flasks above columns. Cotton dust extract (CD) contains traces of histamine (*left-hand bars*). Chopped human lung tissue alone releases about 5% of its total histamine content (*second set of bars*). With CD, twice as much histamine is released (*3rd set*), and a well-known histamine releaser (Compound 48/80) has a similar action (*4th set*). Data from Bouhuys and Lindell.[17]

components would have any activity in the in vitro system. A suitable animal model would have greatly facilitated experiments on this problem. Unfortunately, in vitro histamine-release experiments had consistently negative results with non-human lung tissues, including guinea pig, rat, cat, sheep, cow, and horse lung.[23, 43] Monkey lung gave small but consistent releases,[23] but not enough to serve for assay purposes. More recently, Nicholls (personal communication) found that an agent in cotton dust releases histamine from pig lung tissue, and Douglas confirmed this with cotton bract extract (unpublished data, 1972). We now use histamine from chopped pig lung as an initial assay system, with human lung available to confirm whether or not the actions on human and on pig lung are similar.

The cotton boll (Fig. 17-4) consists of pericarps (fruit capsules), bracts, and fibers that surround the seeds. The seeds and pericarps are removed during ginning. The bracts are friable; their particles cling to the fibers and are found in baled cotton. Among the parts of the plant tested, only bract extract showed consistent histamine-releasing properties.[43] This has since been confirmed in our laboratory in different series of experiments.[23, 28] The agent in bracts is stable during storage of the leaves; samples collected in 1963 have produced histamine release in experiments done in 1968 and 1969. Other plant components, including fibers and pericarps, have given negative results.[23, 28, 43]

Until recently, we used resection specimens of human lung tissue, obtained during thoracic surgery,[17, 43] which limited the number of samples and the amount

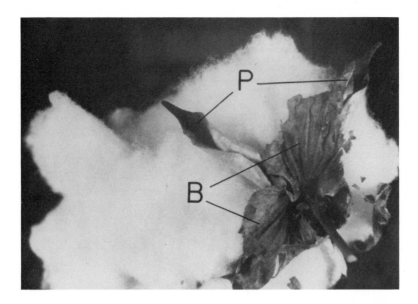

Fig. 17-4. Cotton boll with pericarps (*P*) and bracts (*B*). The stem of the boll points to the lower right-hand corner of the photograph. Reproduced from Nicholls et al.[43]

of tissue available. Fortunately, autopsy lung can also be used, provided the lungs are removed within 16 hours after death.[23, 28] Some samples show excessive histamine release in control flasks, due to tissue breakdown, and results from such samples must be discarded. In one series of experiments, distillation of the bract extract (under vacuum at 40°C) resulted in a distillate which proved to be more active than the original bract extract, while there was no activity in the residue.[28] This result suggests that the histamine-releasing agent in cotton bracts may be steam volatile.

Identification of the agent(s) in bracts. Vegetable matter contains many organic substances that can be isolated by chemical extraction and separation procedures and then identified by analysis of the fractions. Many of these substances probably have some type of biological activity. However, to identify one or more chemical compounds in cotton bracts as the, or one of the, agents that cause airway constriction in cotton workers, the following two criteria must be fulfilled:

1. The agent(s) must have a biological activity that is likely to lead to airway constriction in man (e.g., histamine release in human lung tissue; contraction of isolated human airway muscle; reversible airway constriction in man in vivo). A substance that does not have such an activity is unlikely to be the causal agent in byssinosis, even though it may have many other biological actions.

2. Since the inhaled bracts particles are unlikely to pass through the intact airway mucosa, the agent(s) must be released from the particles under conditions similar to those in the airways. For example, an agent which

can only be separated from bracts particles with strong acid or alkali would probably not be released in the mucous layer of the airways.

To date, no agents that fulfill both criteria have been identified. Methyl-piperonylate, a heat-stable, volatile compound of a class that occurs naturally in several plants, including Cannabis sativa (soft hemp),[22, 31, 44] has been proposed as a likely candidate.[28] Methylpiperonylate, in very low concentrations (as little as 5×10^{-9} final molar concentration), releases histamine from human lung tissue.[28] However, more recent chromatographic work in our laboratory (Dutka et al, unpublished material, 1973) indicates that the histamine-releasing agent in cotton bracts distillate is not identical with methylpiperonylate.

Thus, more complete chemical analysis of bract extracts, together with assessment of the biological activity of different fractions on the lungs, is necessary before one or more substances can be positively identified as agents causing airway constriction in cotton textile workers. Largely because of the decreasing economical importance of flax and hemp, few if any attempts have been made to identify the agent(s) in these plants that cause byssinosis.

Further Experiments in Man

If textile dusts indeed cause airway constriction through release of histamine, one would expect histamine release also in vivo. To demonstrate this, histamine determinations in blood are of no value since they reflect largely the number of basophil cells. Although determinations of histamine levels in blood plasma might be informative, these require stringent conditions for blood sampling that are difficult to meet in field studies. In a study of hemp workers on a histidine-poor diet we collected 10-hour urine samples during dust exposure and several hours thereafter. Determinations of a major histamine metabolite [1,4-methylimidazolacetic acid (MeIAA)][27] in urine suggested that increased amounts of histamine were released and metabolized on Monday in persons who responded to dust exposure with symptoms and function changes.[8] This result has been confirmed by Edwards et al.,[26] who exposed their subjects to cotton dust clouds produced in an exposure chamber. Both studies include small numbers of subjects, and they provide only partial information on histamine metabolism. Although the results are therefore tentative, they are consistent with histamine release during dust exposure in textile workers as well as in healthy subjects.

Aerosolized bract extract causes lung function changes in vivo as well as histamine release in lung tissue. Measurements of lung mechanics in 4 healthy subjects showed significant responses in the sense of small-airway obstruction; tachyphylaxis was also observed, as in the earlier experiments with cotton dust extract.[19] At the time we wrote: "Formal proof of the identity of the agent in bracts which releases histamine with the agent which causes pulmonary function changes in man would require isolation of the active agent from bracts by chemical procedures."[19] This has not yet been accomplished. Yet, it is very likely that the histamine-releasing and the airway-constrictor agents in cotton bracts are identical. Both are water-soluble, heat-stable agents that are active in human but not in guinea pig lung. The time course of the constrictor effect in vivo is similar to the time course of histamine release in vitro. Lastly, the tachyphylaxis observed with the constrictor agent in vivo is characteristic for the action of nonantigenic hista-mine-releasing agents.

Reactors and nonreactors. Even in dusty workrooms where most people ex-perience serious chest tightness and acute lung-function loss, a few workers have no symptoms at all. In several surveys we have encountered long-term workers who have never felt chest tightness on Monday and whose flow rates do not decrease in dust, while others who work in the same room are severely affected. This differ-ence in response was pronounced among a small group of Spanish hemp workers whom we could study under relatively well-controlled conditions in a field survey in 1965 [8] (Fig. 17-5). Most of the men reacted to dust exposure on Monday with severe chest tightness and large decreases of $FEV_{1.0}$. One of the investigators who inhaled the dust for the first time responded similarly. In contrast, 4 men who worked in the same factory had few symptoms and no decrease of $FEV_{1.0}$. The 4 nonreactors as well as the 9 reactors were long-term hemp workers, with at least 15 years in the industry. One explanation for the difference between reactors and nonreactors may be that the former release more histamine in their lungs, after

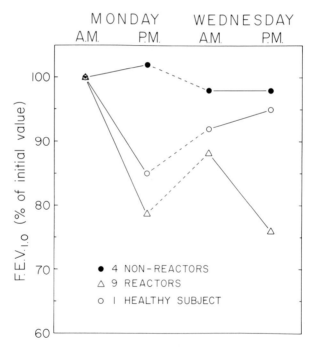

Fig. 17-5. Change in $FEV_{1.0}$ (as a percentage of initial value on Monday AM, before work = 100) during workshifts in a Spanish hemp factory. The healthy subject was exposed to dust only on Monday; his Wednesday data indicate incomplete recovery from the response on Mon-day. The reactors had a significant drop in $FEV_{1.0}$ on Monday and Wednesday: 4/9 of these had byssinosis grade 2 (Table 17-1). Data from Bouhuys et al.[8]

similar exposures, than the nonreactors. Human lung tissue samples indeed release varying amounts of histamine with dust or bract extract; some samples do not release any.[43]

The difference between reactors and nonreactors was explored in greater detail when we installed a body plethysmograph in our field laboratory in Spain in 1967.[20] We used it to measure lung volumes, including total lung capacity, as well as airway conductance (during panting) and MEFV curves (Chap. 9) in 25 men, before and after exposure to dust in a hemp fiber factory. Six of these subjects felt no chest tightness and had no other symptoms during and after exposure. The only significant function change in these men was a decrease in airway conductance (C in Fig. 17-6). In contrast, the function changes in the 19 men who had chest tightness included (1) decreases in flow rates on MEFV curves, (2) decreases in vital capacity, and (3) increases in residual volume (Fig. 17-6). Total lung capacity did not change, and airway conductance decreased only in those who felt the dust effect more severely.

Thus, it appeared that hemp dust exposure may cause two distinct responses: (1) a flow rate response, accompanied by chest tightness and dyspnea in the symptomatic reactors, and (2) a conductance response without symptoms, found in nonreactors. From other studies (p. 420) we know that chest tightness is also associated with prolonged N_2 washout and decreased dynamic compliance. These changes and the decreases in maximum flow reflect obstruction in small airways (see Chap. 9, p. 197). Histamine can elicit the same changes when administered by aerosol.[15, 16] Thus, there is strong presumptive evidence that the flow rate response is caused by small-airway obstruction due to histamine release in lung tissue. There is less evidence concerning the nature of the conductance response. It probably involves narrowing of large intrathoracic airways, which are the major site of resistance to airflow (Chap. 8), and whose caliber has little direct effect on gas distribution, flow-volume curves, and dynamic lung compliance. The conductance response, like the flow rate response, is abolished by isoproterenol inhalation. Therefore, it is unlikely that it occurs in the larynx or in supraglottal airways not controlled by smooth muscle. The conductance response may be similar to inert dust responses of reflex origin.[24]

Since textile dusts contain particles of different sizes, deposition probably occurs throughout the bronchial tree.[42] If all airways receive dust particles, why does the site of smooth muscle contraction appear to vary individually? Since airway smooth muscle is functionally not homogeneous,[54] local variations in responses to histamine may be a factor. Also, the distribution of sympathetic or vagal nerve fibers to airway smooth muscle may vary among individuals. For instance, persons with a flow rate response might have few sympathetic fibers in small airways; the norepinephrine output of these fibers might be insufficient to protect these airways from constriction by locally released histamine. In persons with a conductance response, on the other hand, adrenergic fibers might be predominant in small airways, and the large ones might be relatively unprotected. Interaction between histamine and autonomic-mediating substances may thus also be involved in determining the site of the dust response in the airways. Recent experiments with autonomic drugs have shown that such an interaction may play a role in determining the effect of textile dusts on the airways (see next section).

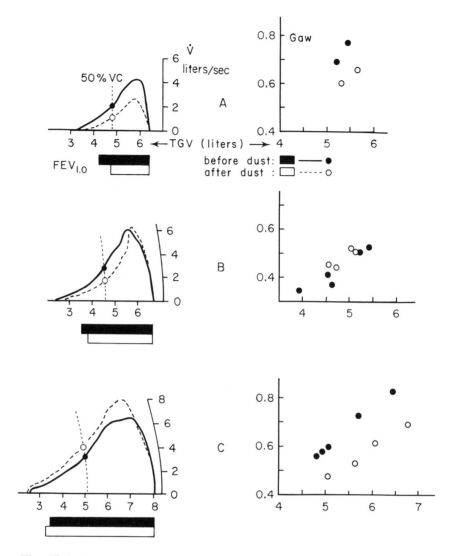

Fig. 17-6. MEFV curves and Gaw-TGV graphs before and after dust in 3 soft-hemp workers, *A, B,* and *C. Right-hand graphs,* airway conductance (Gaw) (liters per second per cm H_2O) versus thoracic gas volume (TGV). The curved flow ordinates in the MEFV curves of *B* and *C* reflect the curvilinear pen excursions of the flow-volume spirometer. MEFV curves in *A* were made with the body plethysmograph. Bars under MEFV curves indicate $FEV_{1.0}$ before and after dust; refer to TGV scale for volume calibration. Dashed vertical lines indicate volume level for measurements of MEF 50%. These flow values are indicated by a dot and a circle on the MEFV curves. In all instances, 5 $FEV_{1.0}$ values were obtained and the changes (decreases in *A* and *B;* increase in *C*) were significant at the 0.1% level.

Experiment *B* shows a typical flow rate response, experiment *C* a typical conductance response. In the subject of experiment *A,* a pronounced flow rate response was associated with decreased airway conductance.

Reproduced from Bouhuys and van de Woestijne.[20]

Modulation of Dust Responses by Autonomic Drugs (See also Chap. 18)

Prior administration of β-adrenergic stimulants [20] or of an antihistamine drug [7] can prevent the constrictor response to textile dust exposure. This is consistent with the histamine-releasing action of the dust, and subsequent histamine-induced smooth muscle contraction. In a recent field study in hemp workers [10] we used two other drugs, atropine and propranolol, in an attempt to modify responses to hemp dust exposure as well as to histamine. To assess the responses we used partial expiratory flow-volume (PEFV) curves (Chap. 9). Figures 17-7 and 17-8

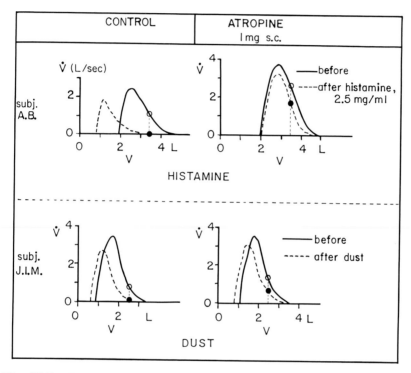

Fig. 17-7. Partial expiratory flow-volume (*PEFV*) curves before and after exposure to histamine aerosol or hemp dust. Lung volume scales are in liters, with the point of maximum inspiration (total lung capacity, TLC; on the left in each graph) as zero. This procedure was used because no absolute volume measurements were made in this study. Dust and histamine aerosol do not affect TLC significantly.[20]

Each curve begins at a lung volume less than total lung capacity; for instance, at TLC minus about 2 liters in the control experiment before histamine in subject A.B. After completing the maximum expiration (*right-hand side of each graph*), the subject inspired maximally to establish the TLC point (*left-hand side*). After histamine exposure, flow rates decrease, and, in most instances, more air remains in the lungs after the maximum expiration is completed (increased residual volume). Maximum flow rates at a fixed degree of lung inflation (TLC − 75% of control VC) are indicated (*circles and dots*); these flow rates can be used to quantitate the drug or dust effect. After prior administration of atropine, equal doses of histamine aerosols have much less effect. A similar protection occurs when hemp dust exposure is preceded by administration of atropine. After atropine administration alone, maximum flow rates were increased compared with the control. Data of Bouhuys et al.[10]

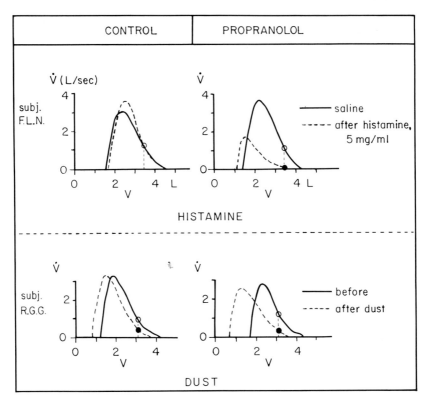

Fig. 17-8. Similar to Figure 17-7, to demonstrate the potentiation of the effects of histamine aerosol and of hemp dust exposure by prior administration of propranolol (40 mg orally). About 90 minutes was allowed for absorption of propranolol, before exposures were repeated. Continued β-block existed in all subjects throughout the experimental period, as shown by decreased heart rates. Data of Bouhuys et al.[10]

illustrate the results. Qualitatively, the responses to histamine and to dust were similar. Effective exposures to both agents caused chest tightness, shortness of breath, and decreases in maximum expiratory flow rates. This is not surprising if the dust acts via release of histamine. Atropine (1 mg subcutaneously) inhibits the responses to both agents (Fig. 17-7). One explanation of the atropine effect is that histamine (exogenous, or endogenously released) elicits a reflex with its efferent path in the vagal nerve, thereby reinforcing the airway constriction. Atropine prevents the vagal efferent impulses from acting on airway smooth muscle; hence, atropine inhibits the action of the dust and of histamine. This view is consistent with several experiments of Widdicombe and his co-workers.[40]

   The opposite effect was obtained with administration of a small dose of propranolol (40 mg orally). This drug alone did not alter flow rates, but it potentiated the effects of both inhaled histamine and hemp dust (Fig. 17-8). Propranolol blocks β-adrenergic receptors, and the potentiation of airway constriction could be explained by assuming a bronchodilator reflex as proposed by McCulloch et al.[35] Thus, some of the data (with atropine) could be explained if histamine elicits a reflex that reinforces its constrictor action. Another part of the data (with propranolol) could be explained if histamine elicits a reflex that inhibits its direct constrictor action. Thus, operation of different reflexes with opposing effects on the target organ could explain the data, but this implies the assumption of a complex central control system. A simpler concept, which could explain the actions of both drugs, is discussed in the next section.

Interaction between dust effect and autonomic mediators. The effects of acetylcholine, isoproterenol, and histamine on airway smooth muscle are inhibited, with relatively high specificity, by different antagonists (atropine, β-adrenergic blockers, and antihistamine drugs, respectively). Therefore, these drugs are believed to act on separate and distinct receptor sites on the cell membrane. This makes it difficult to understand their interaction, unless there is partial overlap of receptor sites or other reasons for action of a drug on more than one receptor. The interaction of different drugs on airway smooth muscle in vitro is discussed in Chapter 18. The concept of interaction is based on experiments with isolated smooth muscle and with drug responses in animals, and it may also be relevant to the action of textile dusts in man. The inhibition of the dust effect by atropine and its potentiation by propranolol would be consistent with modulation of airway constrictor responses by vagal or sympathetic impulses. Increased vagal tone appears to render airway smooth muscle more susceptible to the constrictor effect of histamine, while an increase in sympathetic tone makes them less sensitive. This interaction between autonomic mediating substances and exogenous agents, such as histamine or dust, may occur within the smooth muscle cells. Many intracellular events occur between receptor activation and smooth muscle fiber contraction, and any one of several could be a site of interaction (see Fig. 18-6).

The concept of interaction does not conflict with other experiments that have demonstrated reflex bronchoconstriction under a variety of conditions.[24, 40, 53] The time course of these reflex events differs considerably from those that occur in byssinosis. Reflex bronchoconstriction may start within seconds after an appropriate stimulus (e.g., cough) and may last only 1–3 minutes.[53] In contrast, the action of textile dust on the airways takes at least 15–30 minutes to develop and may last for several hours. One may think of bronchoconstrictor reflexes as short-term events that either help clear the airways of foreign material or serve as a warning signal for the presence of irritating gases in the inspired air. Thus, these reflexes may protect the individual against noxious matter in the airways, whereas the response to textile dust is harmful on both the short and the long term.

Chronic Lung Disease in Textile Workers

Early studies on byssinosis suggested that textile workers had more chronic lung disease than people not exposed to dust.[49] Lung-function measurements in cotton and flax workers in The Netherlands[6] showed that these men had lower ventilatory capacities than control subjects. In a survey of Swedish cotton workers, the prevalence of chronic respiratory symptoms was higher than expected.[4] Since disabled workers usually retire prematurely, a higher than expected prevalence of chronic symptoms and of function loss among active workers suggested that retired workers might be even more affected.

Several conditions for a population study that includes retired workers were fulfilled in Callosa de Segura, a town in Spain where people have processed soft hemp fiber (*Cannabis sativa*) for centuries.[9] A list of persons who had worked in the hemp industry during the past 15 years was available, and a random sample of men from this list was studied. Most of the men over 50 years of age no longer worked in hemp, some because of disability, others because of contraction of the trade. Suitable control groups were studied in the same geographical area: men in agriculture, marble cutting, and shoe manufacturing. The difference between the older hemp workers and control subjects was large, both in terms of symptom prevalence and function loss. Seventy percent of the older hemp workers had chronic cough (26 percent in the controls), and 37 percent of them had severe shortness of breath (dyspnea grades 4 and 5). Only 11 percent of the controls had such severe dyspnea. Measurement of the $FEV_{1.0}$, in the absence of acute dust exposure, showed large differences between older hemp workers and controls, and this difference persisted when moderate and heavy cigarette smokers were excluded from the analysis (Fig. 17-9). We concluded that 27 out of 146 older men (50–69 years of age) were completely disabled, with an $FEV_{1.0}$ of 1 liter or less, and 31 percent of this group had an $FEV_{1.0}$ less than 50 percent of the value expected for their age and height (controls: 4 percent). Thus, the long-term hemp workers were severely disabled men, and there is little doubt that hemp dust exposure caused their disability.[9] When we returned to Callosa 3 years later, 6 of the 27 men with an $FEV_{1.0}$ of 1 liter or less had died, and among the surviving group of older men there was a continuing decrease in the $FEV_{1.0}$ (See Table 13-1, p. 290). None of them improved while out of the dust, as would be expected if a significant portion of the dust effect were reversible. Isoproterenol and other bronchodilator drugs gave a degree of subjective relief in some, but no one had any significant improvement in lung function. The irreversibly decreased maximum expiratory flows in the older hemp workers are at least partially related to loss of lung elastic recoil.[27a] Thus, many of these workers may have parenchymal lung damage similar to that of emphysema (Chap. 7, p. 139).

The hemp workers in Spain have worked for many years under detrimental conditions.[2, 8, 9] In Callosa de Segura, only a few of the disabled men received a disability award. In Great Britain, disabled cotton workers are eligible for pensions under the Byssinosis Act, but there are probably many who never receive a pension. In the United States, a survey along the lines of the study in Callosa de Segura has been performed in a defined population of older cotton workers (March 1973; Yale University Lung Research Center, in preparation).

Relation between acute and chronic effects of textile dust. Textile workers with irreversible lung function loss have usually worked in the industry for 10 or more years. Such a slowly-developing decrement in function is very hard to trace without access to long-term follow-up medical records, and no such data are available. The pathogenesis of the chronic lung disease in byssinosis is also difficult to study in the laboratory; as discussed above (p. 423), we have no suitable animal model for byssinosis. Thus, we do not know how the acute stages of byssinosis progress to the chronic and irreversible clinical grade 3 (Table 17-1). A 3-year follow-up study in England produced no conclusive data.[5] However, there are a few clues that indicate a relationship between the acute and chronic phases.

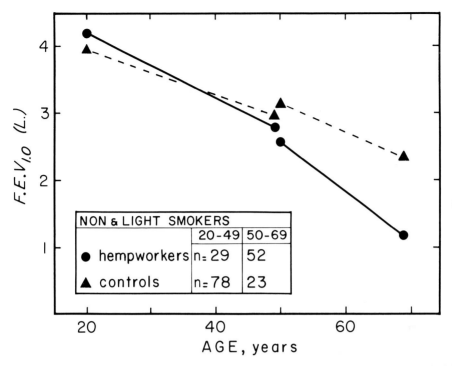

Fig. 17-9. Regression of $FEV_{1.0}$ on age (for height 165 cm) in non- and light smokers aged 20–49 and 50–69 years. *Dashed lines:* controls; *solid lines:* hemp workers. The slopes of the equations within each group do not differ significantly. The mean adjusted $FEV_{1.0}$ for men aged 20–49 years is similar for controls and hemp workers ($F = 0.10$; $p > 0.25$); for men aged 50–69 years, the adjusted $FEV_{1.0}$ values differ significantly ($F = 17.33$; $p < 0.005$), with the hemp workers having the lower values. Reproduced from Bouhuys et al.[9]

Among older hemp workers, irreversible lung-function loss was moderate or severe ($FEV_{1.0} < 65$ percent of expected) only among men who had acute Monday symptoms when they worked in the industry. Thirteen men never had such symptoms, and their $FEV_{1.0}$ was 65 percent of that predicted or higher. Thus, people who regularly experienced the acute symptoms of byssinosis were at much higher risk of developing chronic disease than those who never had these symptoms.[9] The Monday symptoms of byssinosis are associated with the flow-rate response (see p. 427). Among the 25 hemp workers who were studied in detail with the body plethysmograph,[20] irreversible function loss was found only among those with a flow rate response to acute dust exposure.

As a working hypothesis, one may assume that the repeated microinsults to the lungs that occur each time a worker is exposed to toxic dust, especially on Monday, have a cumulative damaging effect. The damage mechanism is not known. If the histamine release from mast cells during acute exposure involves damage to cell walls, this process might represent such a microinsult. Chronic lung damage might result from these and possibly other microinsults on the cellular elements, if regularly repeated during many years.

Dust Exposure Measurements

There is no agreement on standard procedures for dust sampling in the cotton industry, and data from different surveys are therefore not strictly comparable. Yet, if the prevalence of byssinosis is related to the amounts of dust found in different mills, a definite pattern emerges (Fig. 17-10). This graph includes the majority of studies where data on total dust (all sizes of particles) as well as on fine dust (all particles <7 μm diameter or less) were obtained. These experiences show that byssinosis risk is low (< 10 percent prevalence of acute symptoms) when the workrooms contain less dust than about 1.5 mg/cu m, as long as most of this dust consists of larger particles. In workrooms where much of the dust (> 20 percent) consists of particles less than 7 μm in diameter, the risk of byssinosis increases considerably, for the same amount of total dust. Lines A and B approximate the upper limits of the byssinosis risk under these different sets of conditions. When similar prevalence data are plotted against concentrations of fine dust (Fig. 17-11), it is clear that even small amounts of respirable particles are sufficient to cause a significant byssinosis hazard. At higher levels of fine dust, the relations between amount of dust and disease prevalence are variable. This probably is due to differences in the toxicity of dusts, and the amounts of dust serve mainly as a guide to the maximum risk of byssinosis when the dust is highly toxic.

Emission of textile dust into workrooms must be prevented not only for health reasons, but also because of technical and general hygienic considerations.

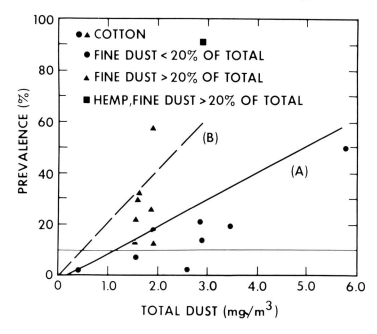

Fig. 17-10. Byssinosis prevalence (defined by symptoms) as a function of total dust concentration in workrooms. Line A indicates approximate upper limit for risk of byssinosis when fine dust is < 20% of total dust. Line B is the similar limit for work places with more fine dust (> 20% of total).

Data from references 8, 21, 29, 32, 39, 59, and 60.

Until recently, a value of 1 mg/cu m airborne cotton dust was thought to pose a minimal risk of byssinosis.[48] Although many cotton mills have installed air-treatment plants that remove coarse dust and lint from the air, such installations do not remove fine dust adequately, and much respirable dust remains in the air of the mills. It is, therefore, no longer enough to specify a safe limit in terms of total dust. Rather, a limit must be established in terms of the dust that is likely to be deposited in the worker's lungs when inhaled. For fine dust less than 7 μm in diameter, even concentrations as low as 0.2 mg/cu m (respirable dust), if used as threshold limit values (Chap. 12, p. 280; Chap. 15, p. 353) do not offer complete protection (Fig. 17-11); additional medical surveillance is needed.

Prevention and Control

Recommendations for programs to prevent and control byssinosis among cotton and other textile workers [12, 50, 51] include technical measures to prevent dust emission from machines and to remove dust from the air, and medical programs to protect workers from health risks. Steaming of raw cotton is under study as a possible means of removing the toxic agents from cotton before it is processed in the mills.[30] The medical surveillance of textile workers should include pre-employment examinations; people with preexisting lung disease should not be employed in risk areas. New entrants should be checked soon for evidence of reactor status, using the $FEV_{1.0}$ test before and after a shift on Monday to detect their acute responses to dust exposure. People who are consistent and pronounced reactors should be removed from risk areas before they become disabled and while they can still be retrained for other jobs.

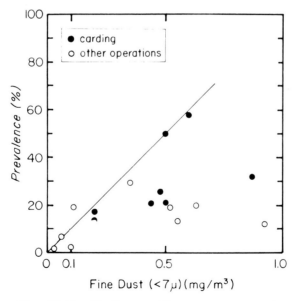

Fig. 17-11. Similar to Figure 17-10. Byssinosis prevalence as a function of respirable cotton dust concentration in workrooms. Data from references 21, 29, 32, 39, 59, and 60.

It is now clear that lung-function tests are indispensable for an adequate prevention and control program in textile workers, and a functional grading system has been proposed for this purpose (Table 17-3 [12, 50]). The system is based on the use of the $FEV_{1.0}$ test, since it has provided most of the existing industrial data and has proved simple as well as reliable. That the $FEV_{1.0}$ test is not as sensitive as some other tests (Chap. 9) is not necessarily a disadvantage here: one needs to screen out obvious reactors rather than persons who only experience minimal effects of the dust. The test should be performed according to standard specifications.[50] The functional grading system, which incorporates an assessment of both the acute and the chronic effects of textile dusts on ventilatory capacity, should significantly improve the amount and quality of objective data concerning the respiratory health of textile workers. Use of this system, coupled with appropriate action as outlined here, should prevent most if not all new cases of disabling byssinosis. The letter F (for function) is used to distinguish the present grades from the previously recommended clinical grades 0–3 (Table 17-1). The practical significance of the functional grades (see Table 17-3) is as follows:

F 0: no demonstrable acute effect of the dust on ventilatory capacity; no evidence of chronic ventilatory impairment.

F ½: slight acute effect of dust on ventilatory capacity; no evidence of chronic ventilatory impairment.

F 1: definite acute effect of dust on ventilatory capacity; no evidence of chronic ventilatory impairment.

F 2: evidence of slight to moderate irreversible impairment of ventilatory capacity.

F 3: evidence of moderate to severe irreversible impairment of ventilatory capacity.

Increasing grades indicate increasing severity of functional impairment. F ½ and F 1 indicate acute dust effects. Workers in grade F 1 should, if at all possible, be removed to jobs in nonrisk areas. If this is not feasible, they ought to be

Table 17-3
Recommended Functional Grades in Byssinosis

Grade *	$\Delta FEV_{1.0}$ † (liters)	$FEV_{1.0}$ ‡ (% of predicted)
F 0	−0.05–0; or +	> 80
F ½	−0.06– −0.20	> 80
F 1	>– −0.20	> 80
F 2	—	60–79
F 3	—	< 60

* If the grades based on $\Delta FEV_{1.0}$ and $FEV_{1.0}$ differ, assign the highest of the two grades.
† Difference between $FEV_{1.0}$ before and after work shift on a first working day of the week.
‡ $FEV_{1.0}$ in the absence of dust exposure (2 days or longer); use value postisoproterenol whenever this drug can be used.

followed regularly so that any worsening of their condition can be detected in time. For workers in grade F 2, removal to nonrisk jobs is highly desirable; they should also be followed regularly, with an $FEV_{1.0}$ test at least every year. Such workers may improve slightly in ventilatory capacity after termination of dust exposure, but others may progress to chronic lung disease even if they leave their jobs. Immediate removal to nondusty jobs is necessary for workers in grade F 3. These persons should be followed to determine whether they improve after cessation; more detailed function studies and other diagnostic work may be required.

SUMMARY

Chest tightness and dyspnea on Monday—the cardinal symptoms of byssinosis in cotton, flax, and hemp workers—are particularly prevalent among cardroom workers in mills spinning coarse grades of cotton. Some 17,000 US cotton workers may be affected, and the number of disabled retired workers is unknown. The symptoms are accompanied by lung-function changes that reflect obstruction of small airways. Inhalation of dust results in airway constriction, probably as a result of histamine release by an agent in the dust. Cotton dust and the bracts of the cotton boll contain a heat-stable substance that releases histamine in human lung tissue. The airway-constrictor agent and the histamine-releasing agent in cotton bracts are probably identical, but their chemical nature has not yet been established.

Some persons react to dust exposure with symptoms and decreases in maximum flow rates (flow rate response). Others have no symptoms, but their airway conductance decreases (conductance response). The flow rate response is inhibited by atropine and potentiated by propranolol. The opposite effects of these autonomic drugs may be explained by interaction of released histamine with autonomic mediators on the smooth muscle cell.

Long-term exposure to textile dust may lead to irreversible lung-function loss and chronic respiratory symptoms. Disabling obstructive lung disease is highly prevalent among older hemp workers, affecting only those who had acute Monday symptoms earlier on. Thus, severe reactors appear to be at increased risk of disabling lung disease if they continue to be exposed.

The risk of byssinosis increases with increasing concentrations of airborne fine dust in the mills. With less than 0.1 mg/cu m fine dust (less than 7 μm), the risk is small. Medical surveillance of textile workers is needed in addition to technical dust control. A functional grading system can assist the early recognition and prevention of disabling lung disease in textile workers.

REFERENCES

1. Arnoldsson H, Bouhuys A, Lindell S-E: Byssinosis. Differential diagnosis from bronchial asthma and chronic bronchitis. Acta Med Scand 173:761–768, 1963
2. Barbero A, Flores R: Dust disease in hemp workers. Arch Environ Health 14: 529–532, 1967
3. Batawi MA El, Din Shash SE: An epidemiological study on aetiological factors in byssinosis. Arch Gewerbepath u Gewerbehyg 19:393–402, 1962
4. Belin L, Bouhuys A, Hoekstra W, Johansson M-B, Lindell S-E, Pool J: Byssinosis in cardroom workers in

Swedish cotton mills. Br J Ind Med 22: 101–108, 1965

5. Berry G, McKerrow CB, Molyneux MKB, Rossiter CE, Tombleson JBL: A study of the acute and chronic changes in ventilatory capacity of workers in Lancashire cotton mills. Br J Ind Med 30:25–36, 1973

6. Bouhuys A: The forced expiratory volume (FEV$_{0.75}$) in healthy males and in textile workers. Am Rev Respir Dis 87:63–68, 1963

7. Bouhuys A: Prevention of Monday dyspnea in byssinosis: a controlled trial with an antihistamine drug. Clin Pharmacol Ther 4:311–314, 1963

8. Bouhuys A, Barbero A, Lindell S-E, Roach SA, Schilling RSF: Byssinosis in hemp workers. Arch Environ Health 14:533–544, 1967

9. Bouhuys A, Barbero A, Schilling RSF, van de Woestijne KP: Chronic respiratory disease in hemp workers. Am J Med 46:526–537, 1969

10. Bouhuys A, Douglas JS, Guyatt AR: Pharmacological modification of histamine-mediated airway responses. J Clin Invest 50:9a, 1971

11. Bouhuys A, van Duyn J, van Lennep HJ: Byssinosis in flax workers. Arch Environ Health 3:499–509, 1961

12. Bouhuys A, Gilson JC, Schilling RSF: Byssinosis in the textile industry; research, prevention and control. Arch Environ Health 21:475–478, 1970

13. Bouhuys A, Hartogensis F, Korfage HJH: Byssinosis prevalence and flax processing. Br J Ind Med 20:320–323, 1963

14. Bouhuys A, Heaphy LJ Jr, Schilling RSF, Welborn JW: Byssinosis in the United States. N Engl J Med 277:170–175, 1967

15. Bouhuys A, Hunt VR, Kim BM, Zapletal A: Maximum expiratory flow rates in induced bronchoconstriction in man. J Clin Invest 48:1159–1168, 1969

16. Bouhuys A, Jönsson R, Lichtneckert S, Lindell S-E, Lundgren C, Lundin G, Ringquist TR: Effects of histamine on pulmonary ventilation in man. Clin Sci 19:79–94, 1960

17. Bouhuys A, Lindell S-E: Release of histamine by cotton dust extracts from human lung tissue in vitro. Experientia 17:211–215, 1961

18. Bouhuys A, Lindell S-E, Lundin G: Experimental studies on byssinosis. Br Med J 1:324–326, 1960

18a. Bouhuys A, Mitchell CA, Schilling RSF, Zuskin E: A physiological study of byssinosis in colonial America. Trans NY Acad Sci 35:537–546, 1973

19. Bouhuys A, Nicholls PJ: The effect of cotton dust on respiratory mechanics in man and in guinea pigs, in Davies CN (ed): Inhaled Particles and Vapours II. London, Pergamon, 1966, pp 75–84

20. Bouhuys A, van de Woestijne KP: Respiratory mechanics and dust exposure in byssinosis. J Clin Invest 49:106–118, 1970

21. Bouhuys A, Wolfson RL, Horner DW, Brain JD, Zuskin E: Byssinosis in cotton textile workers. Respiratory survey of a mill with rapid labor turnover. Ann Intern Med 71:257–269, 1969

21a. Braun DC, Jurgiel JA, Kaschak MC, Babyak MA: Prevalence of respiratory signs and symptoms among U.S. cotton textile workers. J Occup Med 15:414–419, 1973

22. Chu D, Chou TH, Kovacs BA: Isolation of an antihistaminic substance from oak galls. Fed Proc 29:419, 1970

23. Douglas JS, Zuckerman A, Ridgway P, Bouhuys A: Histamine release and bronchoconstriction due to textile dusts and their components. Alicante, Spain, 2nd International Conference on Respiratory Diseases in Textile Workers, 1968, pp 148–155 *

24. DuBois AB, Dautrebande L: Acute effects of breathing inert dust particles and of carbachol aerosol on the mechanical characteristics of the lungs in man. Changes in response after inhaling sympathomimetic aerosols. J Clin Invest 37:1746–1755, 1958

25. Edwards JH, Jones BM: Pseudoimmune precipitation by the isolated byssinosis "antigen". J Immunol 110:498–501, 1973

26. Edwards J, McCarthy P, McDermott M, Nicholls PJ, Skidmore JW: The acute physiological, pharmacological and immunological effects of inhaled cotton dust in normal subjects. J Physiol (Lond) 208:63P–64P, 1970

27. Granerus G, Magnusson R: A method for semiquantitative determination of 1-methyl-4-imidazoleacetic acid in human urine. Scand J Clin Lab Invest 17:483–490, 1965

27a. Guyatt AR, Douglas JS, Zuskin E, Bouhuys A: Lung static recoil and airway obstruction in hemp workers with byssinosis. Am Rev Respir Dis 108: 1111–1115, 1973

28. Hitchcock M, Piscitelli DM, Bouhuys A: Histamine release from human lung by a component of cotton bracts and by compound 48/80. Arch Environ Health 26:177–182, 1973

29. Khogali M: A population study in cotton ginnery workers in the Sudan. Br J Ind Med 26:308–313, 1969

30. Merchant JA, Kilburn KH, Lumsden J, Hamilton J: Preprocessing of cotton to prevent byssinosis assessed in a model cardroom. Am Rev Respir Dis 103: 901–902, 1971

31. Klein FK, Rapoport H, Elliott HW: Cannabis alkaloids. Nature 232:258–259, 1971

32. Lammers B, Schilling RSF, Walford J: A study of byssinosis, chronic respiratory symptoms, and ventilatory capacity in English and Dutch cotton workers, with special reference to atmospheric pollution. Br J Ind Med 21:124–134, 1964

33. Lopez-Merino V, Llopis Lombart R, Flores Marco R, Barbero Carnicero A, Gomez Guillen F, Bouhuys A: Arterial blood gas tensions and lung function during acute responses to hemp dust. Am Rev Respir Dis 107:809–815, 1973

34. Mareska J, Heyman J: Enquête sur le travail et la condition physique et morale des ouvriers employés dans les manufactures de coton, à Gand. Ann Soc Med de Gand 16, part 2:5–245, 1845

35. McCulloch MW, Proctor C, Rand MJ: Evidence for an adrenergic homeostatic bronchodilator reflex mechanism. Eur J Pharmacol 2:214–223, 1967

36. McDermott M, Skidmore JW, Edwards J: The acute physiological, immunological and pharmacological effects of inhaled cotton dust in normal subjects. Alicante, Spain, 2nd International Conference on Respiratory Diseases in Textile Workers, 1968, pp 133–136 *

37. McKerrow CB, McDermott M, Gilson JC, Schilling RSF: Respiratory function during the day in cotton workers: a study in byssinosis. Br J Ind Med 15:75–83, 1958

38. McKerrow CB, Molyneux MKB: The influence of previous dust exposure on the acute respiratory effects of cotton dust inhalation. Alicante, Spain, 2nd International Conference on Respiratory Diseases in Textile Workers, 1968, pp 95–101 *

39. Mekky S, Roach SA, Schilling RSF: Byssinosis among winders in the cotton industry. Br J Ind Med 24:123–132, 1967

40. Mills JE, Sellick H, Widdicombe JG: Activity of lung irritant receptors in pulmonary microembolism, anaphylaxis and drug-induced bronchoconstrictions. J Physiol 203:337–357, 1969

41. Morgagni JB: The Seats and Causes of Diseases Investigated by Anatomy, vol 1, translated by B Alexander. New York, Hafner, 1960

42. Morrow PE: Dynamics of dust removal from the lower airways: Measurements and interpretations based upon radioactive aerosols, in Bouhuys A (ed): Airway Dynamics; Physiology and Pharmacology. Springfield, Charles C Thomas, 1970, pp 299–312

43. Nicholls PJ, Nicholls GR, Bouhuys A: Histamine release by compound 48/80 and textile dusts from lung tissue in vitro, in Davies CN (ed): Inhaled Particles and Vapours, II. London, Pergamon, 1966, pp 69–74

44. Obata Y, Ishikawa Y, Kitazawa R: Studies on the components of the hemp plant (Cannabis sativa L.). II. Isolation and identification of piperidine and several amino acids in the hemp plant. Bull Agr Chem Soc Japan 24:670–672, 1960

45. Popa V, Gavrilescu N, Preda N, Teculescu D, Plecias M, Cirstea M: An investigation of allergy in byssinosis: sensitization to cotton, hemp, flax, and jute antigens. Br J Ind Med 26:101–108, 1969

46. Pottle FA (ed): Boswell in Holland, 1763–1764. New York, McGraw-Hill Paperbacks, McGraw-Hill Book Company, 1956, p 60

47. Ramazzini B: De Morbis Artificum Diatriba, Wright WC (ed). Chicago, University of Chicago Press, 1940

48. Roach SA, Schilling RSF: A clinical and environmental study in byssinosis in

the Lancashire cotton industry. Br J Ind Med 17:1–9, 1960

49. Schilling RSF: Byssinosis in cotton and other textile workers. Lancet 2:261–265, 319–325, 1956

50. Schilling RSF, Bouhuys A, Gilson JC: A report on a conference on byssinosis. Tokyo, XVI International Congress on Occupational Health, September 22–27, 1969, Proc, pp 173–178 †

51. Schilling RSF, Vigliani EC, Lammers B, Valic F, Gilson JC: A report on a Conference on Byssinosis. Madrid, XIV International Congress of Occupational Health, Excerpta Medica International Congress Series No. 62, 2:137–145, 1963

52. Schrag PE, Gullett AD: Byssinosis in cotton textile mills. Am Rev Respir Dis 101:497–503, 1970

53. Simonsson BG, Jacobs FM, Nadel JA: Role of autonomic nervous system and the cough reflex in the increased responsiveness of airways in patients with obstructive airway disease. J Clin Invest 46:1812–1818, 1967

54. Somlyo AP, Somlyo AV: Biophysics of smooth muscle excitation and contraction, in Bouhuys A (ed): Airway Dynamics; Physiology and Pharmacology. Springfield, Charles C Thomas, 1970, pp 209–228

55. Taylor G, Massoud AAE, Lucas F: Studies on the aetiology of byssinosis. Br J Ind Med 28:143–151, 1971

56. Tiller JR, Schilling RSF: Respiratory function during the day in rayon workers —a study in byssinosis. Trans Soc Occup Med 7:161–162, 1957

57. Tuma J, Parker L, Braun DC: The proteolytic enzymes and the prevalence of signs and symptoms in U.S. cotton textile mills. J Occup Med 15:409–413, 1973

58. Valić F, Zuskin E: Effects of different vegetable dust exposures. Brit J Ind Med 29:293–297, 1972

59. Wood CH, Roach SA: Dust in cardrooms; a continuing problem in the cotton spinning industry. Br J Ind Med 21:180–186, 1964

60. Zuskin E, Wolfson RL, Harpel G, Welborn JW, Bouhuys A: Byssinosis in carding and spinning workers. Arch Environ Health 19:666–673, 1969

† Available from: Japan Industrial Safety Association, 35–4, Shiba 5-chome, Minato-ku, Tokyo, 108 Japan.

Chapter 18

Bronchial Asthma

Asthma, which affects some 8.6 million persons in the United States, is one of the most common lung diseases. In addition to claiming at least 4000 lives per year in this country, it is a leading cause of limited activity in persons under 45 years of age.[48]

The main symptoms of asthma—wheezing and shortness of breath—are caused by airway narrowing, which in turn results from airway smooth muscle contraction, secretion of mucus, and thickening of the airway mucosa. The symptoms may occur during brief but often severe episodes (asthma attacks). Between attacks, the patient may have no symptoms. Yet, in symptom-free asthma the underlying disease state that renders the patient susceptible to attacks persists. Other patients with asthma have continuous, but less severe symptoms, often intensified during episodic attacks. Prolonged and severe attacks (status asthmaticus) are a life-threatening condition. Thus, in most patients, asthma is mild and intermittent, in some it leads to frequent and severe illness, and in a few to death.

Present concepts of the pathogenesis of asthma are summarized in Figure 18-1 and its legend. The diagram focuses on airway smooth muscle contraction as the principal cause of airway narrowing. Mucus production (Chap. 2, p. 35) and changes in the airway mucosa undoubtedly contribute to airway narrowing and may be caused, in part, by mechanisms similar to those outlined for smooth muscle contraction in Figure 18-1. This diagram is meant to provide a framework for the more detailed discussions in subsequent sections of this chapter. No attempt has been made to include all factors known or suspected to play a role in asthma.

Early views on the pathogenesis of asthma (asthma nervosum) centered around the concept of an imbalance between vagal and sympathetic (adrenergic) influences on the bronchial tree.[61, 64, 136, 165] After the discovery of anaphylaxis by Portier and Richet (1902), the concept of asthma as a disease characterized by an abnormal sensitivity (allergy) to environmental agents, inhaled or ingested, gained wide acceptance. Today there is no doubt that allergy is an important factor in patients whose asthma attacks are elicited by exposure to antigenic substances,

PATHOGENESIS of ASTHMA

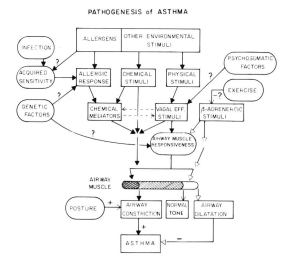

Fig. 18-1. Summary of pathogenetic factors in asthma, with airway muscle contraction, leading to airway constriction, as the end result of the action of environmental stimuli. An abnormal degree of airway muscle contraction occurs when the sum of all contractile stimuli (*black arrowheads*) is increased beyond the level that maintains the normal airway muscle tone, and when this increase is not offset by an appropriate increase in airway dilator stimuli (*white arrowheads*). The contractile stimuli include those exerted by chemical mediators, by vagal efferent stimuli, or by a direct effect of chemical stimuli on the muscle. In turn, these stimuli are released by an allergic response to environmental allergens, by chemically induced release of mediators, or by physical stimuli that increase vagal efferent stimuli via reflex actions. Dilator stimuli result from the relaxant action of β-adrenergic stimuli (circulating catecholamines; neurotransmitters; drugs) on airway muscle; other drug actions omitted from diagram.

Factors that modify airway responses are indicated by ovals. Sensitivity to environmental agents may be acquired through prolonged exposure and perhaps from infections. Genetic factors may help determine the allergic response as well as the responsiveness of airway muscle to constrictor stimuli. Increased airway muscle responsiveness amplifies the effect of contractile stimuli on airway muscle and is promoted by vagal and inhibited by β-adrenergic stimuli. The effects of psychosomatic factors, exercise, and posture are discussed in the text (p. 474).

such as pollens or animal hair (allergens). This type of asthma is often called "extrinsic asthma" and is common among young and otherwise healthy people. In many patients with asthma, however, an association of symptoms with allergen exposure cannot be demonstrated. This group of patients includes older persons with continuous symptoms, often refractory to treatment. For lack of demonstrable extrinsic factors, such patients are often classified as having "intrinsic asthma". However, the term intrinsic asthma is merely an expression of ignorance and should be abandoned. Instead, an attempt should be made, in each case, to determine which pathogenetic factors, including allergy as well as responses to other inhaled agents and physical stimuli, may be important.

Within the last 20 years it has become increasingly clear that the airways of most patients with asthma are abnormally sensitive to a large variety of airway-constrictor stimuli, including chemical substances and physical stimuli as well as allergens. This airway hyperresponsiveness may well be a cardinal feature of asthma. What distinguishes the patient with asthma induced by grass pollen from the patient who responds to the same pollen with hay fever (allergic rhinitis) is probably that the former has hyperresponsive lower airways and the latter has not. Airway hyperresponsiveness may also be a principal cause of asthma in patients without demonstrable allergies; their airways constrict to stimuli (gases, fumes, dusts, cold, exercise) which do not affect others.

Lastly, chemical stimuli may induce airway constriction indistinguishable from that which occurs in allergic asthma in persons who never experience asthma except during these exposures. In these instances, often associated with occupational exposures (e.g., textile dusts, Chap. 17; hairsprays, p. 447), the response is not limited to those with hyperresponsive airways and occurs in most or all persons at risk. Persons with hyperresponsive airways usually avoid these occupations, since they respond more severely to exposure than others.

Thus, the pathogenesis of the asthmatic disease state (i.e., the susceptibility to attacks) as well as of the individual asthmatic attack appears to vary among individuals and may also vary in the same individual at different times. Hence, although classical asthma is easily diagnosed and difficult to confuse with other conditions that cause shortness of breath, it is not surprising that a distinguished panel of experts recently concluded that "asthma could not be defined on the information at present available." [161] Figure 18-1 suggests that any definition should focus on the event common to all forms of bronchial asthma—airway constriction. For instance, asthma is a disease with ". . . widespread narrowing of the bronchial airways, which changes its severity over short periods of time either spontaneously or under treatment and is not due to cardiovascular disease." [33] This definition encompasses all degrees of asthma and does not prejudge its pathogenesis. It may be interpreted to include airway constriction induced by chemical stimuli (e.g., by histamine, cigarette smoke, or hairsprays) in healthy persons who do not have hyperresponsive airways and have never had symptoms of airway obstruction before. Inclusion of this form of asthma in the definition is contrary to current clinical usage, which classifies the effects of these exposures according to the causal agent (e.g., byssinosis). Hence, it is tempting to include airway hyperresponsiveness as a prerequisite for the diagnosis of asthma, but this leads to a circular argument. Normal and increased airway responsiveness are probably part of a continuum of individual sensitivities (p. 445); hyperresponsiveness is the degree of sensitivity that promotes asthma.

For purposes of this chapter, asthma is the complex of symptoms and lung-function changes that results from one or more chains of events as shown in Figure 18-1. The first sections describe the disease, including its epidemiology, pathology, and the lung-function changes it induces. Subsequent sections deal with the mechanisms of pathogenesis: the allergic response, the release of mediators, and the role of the autonomic nervous system, with separate sections on airway smooth muscle responses, interaction between different (chemical and nervous) stimuli, and airway hyperresponsiveness. The final section deals with asthma therapy.

Figure 18-1 explains why bronchodilator drugs are the most common form of therapy in bronchial asthma. When effective, they abolish or decrease airway constriction regardless of its etiology. A more specific treatment directed at the main causal factor is available only in patients with demonstrable allergies (immunotherapy, p. 475) and is often not successful. Development of more effective immunotherapy and of other specific treatment modes aimed at other pathogenetic factors will require more detailed knowledge of each step in the various pathogenetic mechanisms. To utilize such therapies effectively, we must also know more about the relative prevalence of the different mechanisms in the total population of patients with asthma. Hence, research on basic mechanisms in asthma should be pursued in conjunction with epidemiological studies on the prevalence and severity of asthma and on the prevalence of different etiological factors. Such research may succeed in decreasing the morbidity and mortality of this disease. Since asthma is widespread among all age groups, causing considerable distress and economic loss, this research deserves significant effort.

EPIDEMIOLOGY

Most studies on human asthma concern patients seen in hospitals or clinics, a selected group of persons with frequent symptoms or severe illness. This group is probably only the tip of the iceberg. A better perspective on the prevalence of asthma, including its less disabling forms, and of the various etiological factors associated with it, can be obtained from studies in population groups outside hospitals, as in communities or industry (Chap. 13).

Prevalence in Community Populations

In Tecumseh, Michigan, 4.0 percent of men and 4.1 percent of females (all ages) had asthma, diagnosed from history and physical examination.[25] Among young people (6–24 years) the prevalence was higher among men than among women. However, when persons with uncertain diagnoses of asthma were included, the overall prevalence increased to about 10 percent. Obviously, a better definition of asthma prevalence requires more precise, less subjective criteria than a physician's diagnosis. Since there is no agreement on the definition of asthma (p. 443), it is first necessary to describe the prevalence of specific symptoms and etiological factors related to asthma, of lung function changes reversed with bronchodilator drugs, and of airway responses to chemical mediators. This requires use of a standard questionnaire (pp. 307–313) in unselected populations, as well as physiological and pharmacological tests in subgroups of these populations. Table 18-1 contains data from a survey of a rural community (see also Chap. 13, pp. 302, 307), which show that infrequent wheezing occurs among about one-third of all men and women who smoke. Among nonsmokers, about 1 in 7 says he has had wheezing or chest tightness at some time. However, a history of asthma-like symptoms is much more common than a history of asthma. Thus, while many people appear to have some symptoms of asthma, these occur too infrequently or are not severe enough to lead to a clinical diagnosis of asthma.

Clearly, many additional data are required before one can estimate the

Table 18-1
Prevalence of Wheezing and of Asthma in Rural Residents (Lebanon, Connecticut)

| | | Age | | | | | | Total, Ages 15–64 | |
| | | 15–24 | | 25–44 | | 45–64 | | | |
	7–14 *	NS	S	NS	S	NS	S	NS	S
	Males								
n	234	68	46	48	96	38	40	154	182
Wheezing:									
ever (%)	16	12	30 †	15	38 ‡	16	30	14	34 ‡
frequent (%)	5	7	13	4	23 ‡	5	22	6	20 ‡
Asthma (%)	9	7	11	8	2	5	0	7	4
	Females								
n	221	74	22	66	55	41	26	181	103
Wheezing:									
ever (%)	11	8	23	12	33 †	27	38	14	32 ‡
frequent (%)	3	4	18	0	15 ‡	15	15	5	16 ‡
Asthma (%)	2	0	5	2	9	0	0	<1	6 ‡

* Nonsmokers only in this age group; 5 additional subjects smoked cigarettes.
† p < 0.05.
‡ p < 0.01 (χ^2 test), for differences between NS and S.
n=number of subjects in each column. Wheezing: ever=% positive responses to question #30, page 308. Wheezing: frequent=% positive responses to question #34, 1–3, p. 309. Asthma=% positive responses to question #70, page 310.
NS=nonsmokers; S=current cigarette smokers. Ex-, cigar-, or pipe smokers not included in analysis.

prevalence of asthma and assess the relative importance of various etiological factors that cause airway obstruction. Smoking is probably an important cause of wheezing (Table 18-1) and leads to airway obstruction (Chap. 14, p. 321). In populations of textile workers, wheezing and chest tightness are associated with byssinosis (Chap. 17). Depending on one's preferred definition (p. 443), smokers and textile workers may or may not have asthma. Thus, detailed descriptive studies are required before we can improve our definitions of asthma and other disease processes associated with airway obstruction.

Such descriptive data may also reveal whether persons with asthma form a distinct group with characteristics not found in others (bimodal distribution), or whether asthmatic persons are the sensitive individuals among a general population in which airway responsiveness is continuously distributed. In guinea pigs, airway sensitivity to histamine is log-normally distributed (Fig. 18-2). Similar distributions of, for example, histamine releasability from mast cells and of airway responsiveness to mediators might occur in humans. If so, individuals who are prone to mediator release and whose airways respond to small amounts of mediators might be likely to develop asthma. Less responsive individuals might develop wheezing only after strong stimuli, while persons with unresponsive mast cells or airways might not develop asthma even after strong stimuli.

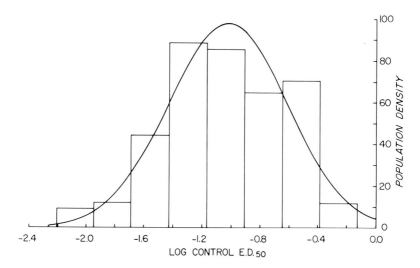

Fig. 18-2. Distribution of ED50 values to histamine aerosols in female albino guinea pigs. Doses of aerosolized histamine which produced a 50% decrease in dynamic lung compliance from baseline values (ED50) were determined from dose-response curves. These data were accumulated into groups and a distribution pattern was constructed by a digital computer. The ordinate is population density (percent population per −0.26 log interval of ED50). A gaussian density function derived from the mean (−1.0354) and variance (0.168) of the log ED50 values is also plotted. The area under the curve is equal to the area under the blocks. The predicted values were not significantly different from the observed values when tested with the χ^2 test. From reference 52.

Prevalence in Occupational Groups

Many substances used or produced in industry cause asthma (Chap. 15). The allergen can often be defined and eliminated, usually by a change of jobs. Also, the exposure is often intensive and frequent, and many exposed persons may be affected. For instance, among 20 bakers, 11 (55 percent) were sensitive to flour in an inhalation provocation test (p. 454).[207] However, since most reports of occupational asthma concern persons who sought medical help, the true prevalence may be higher. A high prevalence of occupational asthma in a group at risk is usually ascribed to sensitization. However, industrial agents may cause asthma on first exposure (e.g., hairspray, see below), suggesting a direct toxic effect. If there is a continuous distribution of airway responsiveness in the general population, industrial exposures could lead to asthma in persons who are not affected by lesser exposures in the home or the community.

A reaginic antibody (p. 453) to castor-bean allergen occurred in the serum of allergic workers in a castor oil factory; the presence of this antibody correlated with their clinical state.[41] Hypersensitivity to nickel salts as a cause of asthma has been demonstrated by provocation tests;[131] asthma caused by platinum salts has been discussed in Chapter 15 (p. 369). Thus, some small-molecular substances in industry may cause asthma via an allergic response (acquired sensitivity), but other chemicals produce similar symptoms, immediately or with a delay, by direct toxic actions on the airways.[162]

Delayed hypersensitivity may play a role in some delayed asthmatic responses to industrial chemicals.[162] Hairspray preparations, which cause acute airway constriction in healthy persons and are a common cause of asthma-like symptoms among beauticians,[211, 214] are examples of agents with direct toxic effects. Twenty seconds' exposure to a spray, directed at the hair, causes decreased flow rates on PEFV curves (Chap. 9), an effect inhibited by atropine (Fig. 18-3). These preparations may act through nonantigenic histamine release in unsensitized human lung tissue,[214] without need for previous sensitization. Soldering flux can induce asthma; the etiological agent is probably aminoethylethanolamine.[186] Other examples of occupational exposures causing asthma occur in grain handlers, laboratory workers (guinea pig hair), printers (gum acacia) and chemical workers (Table 15-2, pp. 353). Few immunological and physiological data are available on most of these conditions, and their prevalence is insufficiently known.

CLINICAL SYNDROME

An attack of bronchial asthma often begins rapidly, with gradually intensifying wheezing and difficult breathing. During a severe attack, the patient is markedly short of breath and breathing is labored. He sits upright and fixes the shoulder girdle with his arms, so that he can use the accessory muscles of inspiration more effectively. There is often some dry cough; during the attack sputum production is usually minimal. An attack may last minutes, hours, or days. When wheezing and dyspnea lessen, there is often expectoration of tenacious white sputum, sometimes in the shape of bronchial casts. Unless infection supervenes, fever does not accompany the attack of asthma. When a patient is examined during an attack, his chest is hyperinflated and he appears to breathe near maximum inspiratory

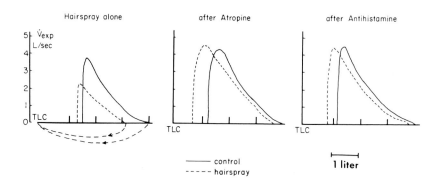

Fig. 18-3. Partial expiratory flow-volume (PEFV) curves in a healthy subject before and immediately after hairspray exposure on three different days: (1) after hairspray alone, (2) with prior administration of atropine (0.5 mg s.c.), and (3) with prior administration of an antihistamine drug (chlorpheniramine maleate, 8 mg). Solid line indicates curve prior to exposure; dashed line, after hairspray exposure. Lung volume (*abscissa*) in liters; all curves superimposed at point of maximum inspiration (TLC), as indicated by dashed inspiratory curves on left-hand graph. Expiratory flow rate (*ordinate*) is in liters per second. Modified from Zuskin et al.[214]

lung volume. On auscultation or even at a distance, one hears inspiratory and expiratory wheezing, musical sounds of varying pitch and loudness.[70] Expiration appears to be prolonged, but this may in part be an acoustic illusion since, normally, breath sounds are almost inaudible near the end of expiration.[22] The patient with a severe attack is often apprehensive and restless. Cyanosis may occur during severe, long-lasting attacks.

In diagnosing asthma, difficulties arise frequently in older patients, in whom chronic bronchitis and emphysema may coexist with partially reversible airway obstruction similar to that found in asthma.[12] The uncomplicated asthma most common among younger people usually poses few problems of differential diagnosis.

Deaths from asthma may have increased in recent years.[182] In a study of 12 patients admitted to a hospital with acute attacks of asthma, all of whom had a normal $FEV_{1.0}$ at some time during the prior 12 months, 3 died of asthma not long after hospital release.[199] At autopsy, the lungs of asthma victims do not collapse when the chest is opened; they remain hyperinflated because the airways are obstructed. They are filled with mucous plugs and the bronchial walls are thickened. Airway smooth muscle cells are increased in size and number.[97] Mucous plugs, which include epithelial and eosinophilic cells, are found from the segmental bronchi down to the terminal bronchioles.[56] The mucosal basement membrane is thickened,[31] the mucous glands are enlarged, and there is edema and cellular infiltration (including mast cells) of the submucosa. In contrast to these extensive changes in the airways, the structure of the lung parenchyma is normal; there may be areas of hyperinflation or atelectasis, but there is usually no parenchymal destruction as in emphysema. The pathology of asthma suggests potential reversibility of most abnormalities except perhaps smooth muscle hyperplasia, so that timely and adequate clinical management should be able to prevent deaths from acute asthma.

LUNG FUNCTION

Breathlessness, shortness of breath, and impeded breathing are subjective sensations that cannot be quantitated. At best, they can be graded according to answers to standard questions (pp. 308–310). In asthma, these sensations are associated with lung-function changes. Although it is difficult to relate descriptions of subjective sensations to results of objective measurements, there is usually a correlation between gross changes in lung function and gross changes in dyspnea and other symptoms (Figs. 18-4, 18-5). In the clinical assessment as well as in experimental studies of asthma, lung-function tests are of value in (1) assessing the degree of airway obstruction (Chap. 9, pp. 197–202) and impairment of gas exchange, (2) measuring airway responses to allergens and other etiological agents, (3) quantitating airway hyperresponsiveness (p. 470), (4) determining the acute effects of bronchodilator treatment, and (5) evaluating the treatment and course of the disease over the longer term. In these applications, functional changes reflect merely the degree of airway obstruction and do not reveal its causes. Rapid reversibility of functional changes implies relaxation of bronchial muscle tone.

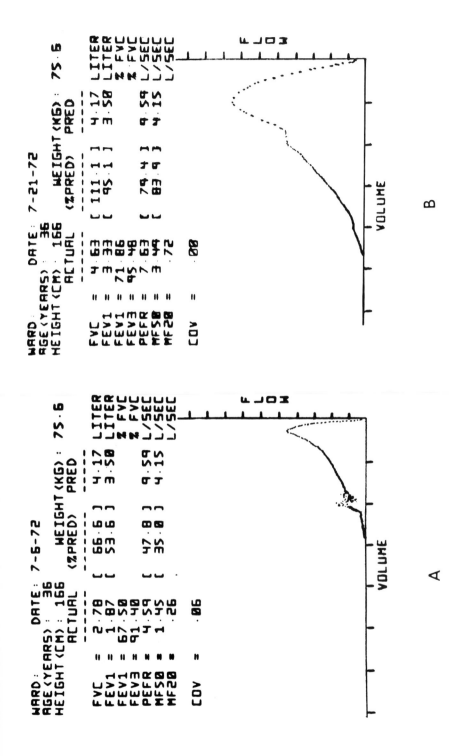

Fig. 18-4. Pulmonary function test computer readout of a 36-year-old man with bronchial asthma (*A*) before and (*B*) after therapy with bronchodilator and corticosteroid drugs, which led to normalization of test results. On 7/6/72 (*A*) the patient had severe dyspnea and wheezing; on 7/21/72 (*B*) he was symptom-free. Each report contains numerical data and MEFV curve based on average expiratory flow rates during the two maximally forced expirations with the highest FEV$_{1.0}$, out of a series of 5 blows. PEFR = PEF; MF50 and MF25 = MEF50% and MEF25%; other abbreviations as in Table 9-1. See Chapter 9, p. 185 for description of test system.

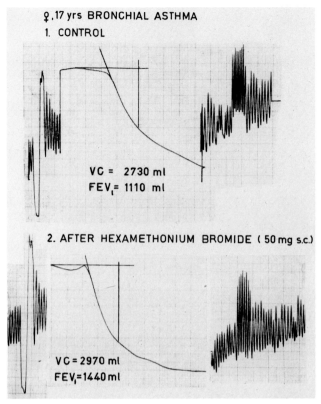

Fig. 18-5. Spirometry tracings of a 17-year-old girl with bronchial asthma before and after hexamethonium bromide administration. Slow vital capacity is recorded on the left of the tracing, forced vital capacity and $FEV_{1.0}$ in the center, and maximal breathing capacity (MBC) maneuver on the right. Note elevated FRC during MBC maneuver prior to administration of hexamethonium. The drug caused marked symptomatic improvement (see also p. 465).

Airway Obstruction

This leads to decreased maximum expiratory flow rates (Chap. 9, p. 197), increased airway resistance (Chap. 8, p. 163), and alterations in static lung volumes (Chap. 7, p. 138). In severe asthma, all indices of expiratory flow limitation ($FEV_{1.0}$, PEF, MEF50%, MEF25%, MMFR; Table 9-1, p. 189) are markedly reduced (Fig. 18-4A). Airway resistance may be very high, and vital capacity is decreased, while residual volume and FRC are increased. During hyperventilation, FRC increases further, to a volume at which higher expiratory flow rates can be achieved (Fig. 18-5A). After effective treatment, all changes return toward normal values (Fig. 18-4B; Fig. 18-5B).

In symptom-free patients, slight functional abnormalities, including reduction of MEF50% and MEF25% (Fig. 18-6),[210] variable increases of airway resistance,[86] and maldistribution of inspired gas [135, 152] (Chap. 4) often persist. Maximum flow rates at low lung volumes (MEF50%, MEF25%) often indicate airway obstruction when other tests are normal.[148, 210]

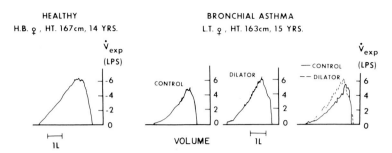

Fig. 18-6. Example of MEFV curves in a patient with bronchial asthma compared with the curve of a healthy child of the same sex and similar height and age. The patient was free of symptoms at the time of study; yet, the shape of the MEFV curve differs from that in the healthy child (see Chap. 1, p. 16). Curves on right side of illustration show improvement of maximum expiratory flow rates on MEFV curve after inhalation of isoproterenol. Modified from reference 210.

Site of Airway Obstruction

Since in severe asthma, airway resistance (mainly reflecting large-airway caliber, p. 161) is increased and maximum expiratory flows (reflecting small-airway caliber, p. 179) are decreased, both large and small airways appear to be narrowed. Although small-airway obstruction probably predominates, the site of airway obstruction may vary.[50] When symptom-free patients are given small doses of histamine aerosol, some respond with decreased flow rates while resistance does not change; in others, resistance increases without changes in flows.[184] Similar dual responses (flow rate and conductance responses) have been observed with methacholine aerosols[30] and with hemp dust exposure (Chap. 17, p. 427). Local variations in smooth muscle responses, or in innervation, might explain these different responses. Animal smooth muscle from large and small airways may respond differently to constrictor agents,[181] but this has not been studied in human airway muscle.

Total Lung Capacity

In adult patients, TLC (plethysmographic method, Chap. 9, p. 185) is about 30 percent larger than predicted.[139] Gas dilution methods may give lower values because of air trapping in poorly ventilated lung spaces. This may occur even in symptom-free patients whose FVC and $FEV_{1.0}$ are normal at the time of study.[210] The increase of TLC is very likely due to the decrease of lung elastic recoil in asthma (see Chap. 7, p. 140). In acute attacks of asthma provoked with allergens, TLC does not increase,[148] and return of the decreased elastic recoil to normal has been observed only over periods of days or weeks (p. 140). Hence, the changes of TLC and of elastic recoil in asthma appear to be relatively slow phenomena. However, a recent study reported significant acute increases in TLC during severe histamine-induced airway constriction in some patients with asthma, suggesting that in some asthmatics, lung recoil may decrease acutely during an attack.[185]

Inspired Gas Distribution

Inspired gas is often distributed unevenly in asthma, even when symptoms are absent.[14, 114, 135, 152] The time constants of different lung zones (p. 63) appear to vary markedly,[156, 193] leading to uneven distribution of inspired O_2 (single- or multiple-breath N_2 washout methods, Chap. 4) and impaired regional distribution of inspired xenon.[84] The multiple-breath N_2 washout method is useful for objective assessment of effects of allergens and constrictor drugs [23, 37] (Figs. 4-10, p. 72, 17-1, p. 420). Results of the single-breath N_2 test are more variable, and do not always reflect improvement after bronchodilator treatment.[73, 98, 193] Inhaled bronchodilator drugs may reach primarily well-ventilated lung zones, sometimes accentuating rather than decreasing ventilation differences between poorly and well-ventilated areas.[193] This might account, in part, for the increased arterial hypoxemia after isoproterenol administration (see below).

Gas Exchange

Arterial hypoxemia is common in bronchial asthma. Since the diffusing capacity (single-breath CO method, Chap. 6) is usually normal,[159] nonuniform ventilation-perfusion relations are the main cause of hypoxemia. During asthma attacks, all indices of unequal $\dot{V}_A/\dot{Q}$ ratios (physiological dead space, A-a D_{O_2}, venous admixture; Chap. 5) are abnormal.[199] The ventilation-perfusion disturbance is caused largely by maldistribution of inspired gas (see above). Constriction of lung blood vessels may, in part, compensate for lack of ventilation in lung zones with severely obstructed airways,[89] but the presence of hypoxemia shows that this compensation is usually incomplete.[154, 166]

Arterial hypoxemia may occur even when airway obstruction appears slight, and it may increase after treatment with bronchodilator drugs even though these decrease obstruction.[115] Since the decrease in Pa_{O_2} is often small and relief of obstruction decreases the work of breathing, the net effect of dilator drugs is usually beneficial.[73] The probable causes of the drop in arterial P_{O_2} after administering dilator drugs include increased uneven gas distribution due to maldistribution of the inhaled aerosol (see above), increased dead space due to increased airway caliber, and increased blood flow through poorly ventilated lung zones.[73, 139] Orciprenaline (p. 477), which has less effect on lung blood vessels than isoproterenol, does not decrease arterial P_{O_2}; hence the effect on lung blood flow may be a major factor.[139]

Arterial P_{CO_2} in asthma is usually either normal or decreased because of hyperventilation. In severe asthma, an increased Pa_{CO_2} indicates ventilatory failure and the need for intensive treatment (p. 475).

IMMUNOLOGY

Allergy

The principal etiological concept of extrinsic asthma is that of the allergic response. Persons with extrinsic asthma are often abnormally sensitive to antigenic material, which may be inhaled or ingested with food. This sensitivity is referred to as allergy, and the antigens involved are called allergens. The constitutional tendency to respond to allergens with formation of antibodies and clinical symptoms is called atopy, an imprecisely defined term.

Immediate Hypersensitivity

The principal immunological response in allergic asthma is called the type I response or immediate hypersensitivity.[75] The role of other responses, in particular delayed (type IV) hypersensitivity, in asthma is not clearly established.[198] Although some allergens elicit a response several hours after exposure, in patients with asthma, it is not certain that the delay is always in the immunological reactions. It may also result from delayed transport of allergens to target cells in the airways.[206] Or, while the immunological response might occur soon after exposure, triggering the attack might require one of the asthma-promoting factors listed in Figure 18-1— for instance, exercise or a change in posture. Consequently, allergen exposure might occur during the day, while the asthma attack occurs later, at night, when the patient lies in bed. One difficulty in linking the immunological response to the appearance of symptoms is that many nonimmunological processes intervene in the response of the airways, either promoting or inhibiting the consequences of the immunological response.

Reagin

The serum of patients with allergic asthma often contains antibodies against the specific allergens that induce asthma in the patient. The presence of these antibodies was first shown with biological methods. For instance, serum of a patient sensitive to rye pollen, when injected into the skin of a healthy person, sensitizes the skin against rye pollen. When a rye pollen extract is injected into the serum injection site, a wheal and flare response results, while other skin sites do not respond (Prausnitz-Küstner test). This test demonstrates that the serum contains a specific factor, called a reaginic antibody or reagin, which sensitizes healthy tissue. More recently, it was shown that this antibody is an immunoglobulin of the IgE class, a heat-labile protein. Procedures that remove or inactivate serum IgE also abolish the capacity of the serum to sensitize healthy skin.[126] In vitro procedures to demonstrate reagins in serum have been developed in recent years (radioallergosorbent method;[1] passive sensitization of lung tissue in vitro[9]).

IgE in Serum

The serum of patients with asthma often contains reagins in quantities sufficient to raise the serum IgE immunoglobulin level.[198] However, there is considerable overlap between the values for total IgE in the serum of healthy persons and those in the serum of patients with asthma.[15, 104, 105] Some patients with asthma have low serum IgE levels, while high IgE levels occur in nonallergic persons with parasitic infections. Not all serum IgE is reagin, and since reagin has to be bound to cells in order to elicit a response, the amount of cell-bound reagin is more relevant than the amount of IgE circulating in serum. For instance, serum IgE may be normal in asthma while leukocyte-bound reagin can be demonstrated.[11]

Cell-bound Reagin

Reagin binds firmly to the surface of mast and basophil cells.[100] Tissue mast cells are probably the main site of reagin binding, which renders them sensitive to subsequent allergen exposure. Cell-bound reagin reacts with its specific allergen on the surface of these target cells and leads to the release of chemical substances (mediators) from these cells. These mediators (p. 455) contract airway smooth muscle, stimulate mucous glands, and cause edema of the airway mucosa.

The presence of cell-bound reagin in airway tissue of an asthmatic patient has been demonstrated by in vitro challenge of the isolated bronchial muscle with the specific allergen.[171] When challenged with the allergen in an organ bath, this tissue releases histamine and the muscle contracts. Bronchial muscle of nonasthmatic persons does not respond to allergen but does contract with histamine.

Cell-bound reagin can also be demonstrated in leukocytes of allergic patients. When leukocytes are incubated with a specific allergen, histamine release occurs, probably due to allergen-reagin binding on the basophil cells.[123] However, since basophils are only about 1 percent of the total number of leukocytes, it is perhaps not surprising that the results of this test are not consistently related to symptoms of allergy.[132]

Nature of Allergens

Pollens, house dust, animal hair, molds, and mites are common allergens. The chemical nature of the allergens in these complex organic materials is unknown. Chemical analysis of house dust has revealed the presence of glycoproteins that attain antigenic properties by a decomposition process.[17] Such molecules can probably derive from a variety of animal or vegetable matter in house dust. How allergens from large particles, such as pollens, which do not penetrate the bronchial tree, reach the airways is not certain.[206]

Provocation Tests

In clinical practice, skin and inhalation tests are commonly used to detect allergies against suspected allergens.

Skin tests. Prick or scratch tests with allergens suggest allergy when a person's skin develops a wheal and flare response. However, these tests may be positive in persons who do not develop asthma on inhalation of the same allergens, and also in persons without any allergic disease.[95] At best, skin tests can suggest which allergens a patient might be sensitive to.

Inhalation tests. These can confirm airway responses to inhaled allergens and may be positive even when skin tests are negative.[36] The tests indicate direct toxic (e.g., to hairspray, Fig. 18-3) as well as allergic responses.

In the laboratory, standard inhalation procedures with aerosolized allergen extracts should be used so that the degree of response to allergens can be compared with that to inert materials in a controlled experiment. Objective and sensitive lung-function tests should be used to test the response (see below) and adequate baseline data should be obtained so that spontaneous variations in airway caliber can be taken into account. Test measurements should be made repeatedly, as long as 6 or more hours after exposure, so that delayed as well as immediate responses can be detected. The tests should be done only in persons whose baseline lung function is sufficient to tolerate a temporary reduction without developing ventilatory insufficiency. Preferably, control function data should be close to normal. In any case, persons with a $FEV_{1.0}$ less than 1.5–2.0 liters, depending on sex and height, should not be given inhalation tests or any other drug that may decrease lung function (e.g., propranolol).

Inhalation of concentrated allergen extracts can lead to severe, even fatal, asthma. Hence, inhalation tests should always be started with minimal amounts of allergen. The use of sensitive function tests to assess the response provides a further margin of safety. In many instances it is preferable to arrange for a provocation test in the environment where the patient experiences asthma, at home or at work. One then has some prior knowledge of timing and degree of response from the patient's history.

Nitrogen washout tests [37] (Chap. 4), airway resistance measurements [207] (Chap. 8), and MEFV or PEFV curves (Chap. 9) are sensitive tests that often detect responses to inhaled agents at dose levels which cause minimal or no symptoms. The $FEV_{1.0}$ is not sensitive enough and detects only severe responses (Fig. 9-15). Hence, to define a response by the criterion of a 10 or 20 percent drop, or more, in $FEV_{1.0}$ implies that only severe and potentially dangerous responses are detected.

Animal Models of Allergic Asthma

In dogs, allergies to nematodes (*Ascaris, Toxocara*) and to grass pollens have similarities to human asthma.[77, 155] The classical animal model of allergic asthma is the guinea pig sensitized with antigen (e.g., egg albumen). Several weeks after sensitization, minute amounts of inhaled or injected antigen cause severe, often fatal, dyspnea and airway constriction [170] and accumulations of mononuclear and eosinophil cells around the bronchi.[58] Functionally, this response resembles severe human asthma. It differs from asthma on several points: (1) the antibody is part of another immunoglobulin fraction (IgG); (2) it can be evoked by soluble antigen-antibody complexes [26] and therefore cell-binding of antibody is not crucial; and (3) the chemical mediators may differ, with histamine being quantitatively more important in the guinea pig than in man.[24, 76] There are indications that the mixture of mediators (histamine, SRS-A) released from sensitized guinea pig lung varies with the strain of animals.

RELEASE OF CHEMICAL MEDIATORS

Antigenic Mediator Release

When allergen and reagin combine on the surface of mast or basophil cells, a selective mediator-release process occurs. Proteins and intracellular enzymes are not released,[107] showing that the cells remain intact. The release process, which requires energy, resembles glandular secretion: discrete granules are exuded from cells, in a process that requires Ca^{++} ions.[69] Next, the granules release their contents via an ion-exchange process.[194]

Mediator release proceeds in distinct steps, each of which can be influenced by chemical agents (Ca^{++}, phenol, salicylates).[170] In addition, the concentration of 3',5' cyclic adenosine monophosphate (3',5' cyclic AMP), a substance that regulates metabolic processes in cells, may influence histamine release.[110] Drugs that increase the 3',5' cyclic AMP level (isoproterenol, theophylline) inhibit release of histamine from sensitized human lung or leukocytes.[8, 10, 121] An analog of 3',5' cyclic AMP (dibutyryl cyclic AMP) inhibits anaphylactic histamine release from the guinea pig uterus.[116] The inhibitory effect of isoproterenol on histamine release from lung or leukocytes is prevented by propranolol, suggesting that the histamine-releasing cells have β-receptor-like drug-binding sites (p. 461). However, comparisons between 3',5' cyclic AMP levels and histamine release have been made only in lung tissue [110] and leukocyte suspensions,[121] both of which contain different types of cells. Thus, it is not certain that changes in 3',5' cyclic AMP levels and changes in histamine release occur in the same cells. For instance, theophylline, which inhibits histamine release, presumably from mast cells, increases the 3',5' cyclic AMP content of airway smooth muscle.[144]

Furthermore, the results of experiments with pure mast cell suspensions differ from those with lung tissue or leukocytes. In mast cells, β-receptor agonists (isoproterenol) as well as β-receptor antagonists (propranolol) inhibit histamine release, and so do α-receptor agonists.[106] Thus, the actions of adrenergic drugs as a group do not support the hypothesis of β-receptor activity in mast cells.

Nonantigenic Histamine Release

Low doses of chemical substances, including compound 48/80, stilbamidine, d-tubocurarine, and morphine,[62] cause selective histamine release from unsensitized mast cells, without intervention of an antigen-antibody reaction. Yet other chemicals, e.g., octylamine, damage mast cells and release mediators as well as other cell contents. Examples of nonantigenic histamine releasers which cause asthma or asthma-like symptoms are described on p. 446. Nonantigenic histamine release may account for asthmatic symptoms as side-effects of drugs.

Nature of Chemical Mediators

Although histamine release has been studied most extensively, a sensitized guinea pig lung also releases other substances that affect airways when challenged with antigen. These include the slow-reacting substance of anaphylaxis (SRS-A), substances of the bradykinin-kallikrein group, prostaglandins (p. 457), and rabbit aorta-contracting substance.[24, 38, 201] Among these, histamine, SRS-A, and prostaglandin $F_{2\alpha}$ contract human airway muscle.[39] SRS-A causes prolonged contraction and may account for persistent airway constriction in asthma. However, the relative roles of histamine, SRS-A, and $PGF_{2\alpha}$ in human asthma are unknown. Histamine and bradykinin may cause mucus secretion and mucosal edema.[24] Bradykinin may be released in human asthma; the kinin content of blood serum is increased in some patients during severe attacks.[2]

Recently, the possible role of prostaglandins as mediators in asthma has aroused much interest. This group of substances, derived from fatty acids, occurs in many body tissues. Lung tissue contains one prostaglandin ($PGF_{2\alpha}$) that contracts and one (PGE_2) that relaxes human bronchial muscle.[188] Another prostaglandin (PGE_1) also relaxes human airway muscle.[117, 173] The site of formation of PGE_2 and $PGF_{2\alpha}$, possibly from arachidonic acid, is not known.[7]

Prostaglandins are released from isolated guinea pig lung in anaphylaxis and after injection of histamine or acetylcholine in the lung blood vessels.[13, 157] This release is due to fresh synthesis of prostaglandins,[158] and occurs not only in the whole lung but also in the isolated trachea of the guinea pig.[150] When the trachea is contracted with histamine or acetylcholine, the effluent of the trachea contracts a rat stomach strip, a preparation uniquely sensitive to prostaglandins (Fig. 18-7). Chromatographic analysis of the effluent has shown the presence of PGE_2 and $PGF_{2\alpha}$.[150] The release appears to depend on the mechanical effect of contraction rather than on specific drug action.[149, 150] Mechanical stimulation of the lungs by squeezing, too, releases prostaglandins.[158] Although the exact site of prostaglandin release is unknown, it probably occurs in the tracheal mucosa, since mechanical stimulation of the mucosa with a glass rod released prostaglandins in the tracheal effluent, while similar stimulation of the outside of the trachea did not.[149]

The severity of allergic responses depends in part on the availability of mediators for release. After repeated antigen challenges in sensitized guinea pigs, the response decreases, presumably because mediator stores are exhausted, although depletion of antibody may also be involved. The amounts of histamine available for release increase with age in rats [145] and vary among different strains of guinea pigs.[187] In this way, age and genetic make-up may affect the severity of allergic responses.

AIRWAY SMOOTH MUSCLE RESPONSES

Contraction of airway smooth muscle (Chap. 2, p. 33) can decrease airway caliber, particularly in airways not supported by cartilage, and it may stabilize large airways during forced expirations (Chap. 8, p. 156). In healthy persons, the role of airway smooth muscle tone is probably of marginal significance (e.g., in regulating gas distribution; Chap. 4, p. 74). Its relaxation causes subtle changes but no gross impairment of lung function. Airway muscle might be a phylogenetic remainder of an important functional tissue in lower animals. For instance, in the lung fish, smooth muscle helps to expel air against the water pressure.[103]

Nervous and humoral stimuli impinge on airway smooth muscle from nerve terminals, the airway lumen, bloodstream, mast cells (during the antigenic or non-antigenic release process), and possibly from other tissue elements (Fig. 18-8). These stimuli are all potential variables and hence results of in vivo experiments on airway muscle tone are often difficult to interpret. Some variables can be studied in isolated smooth muscle preparations (Fig. 18-7, Fig. 18-20), nerve-muscle preparations (Fig. 18-13), and in isolated tracheal segments in vivo (Fig. 1-7, p. 12). Among in vivo techniques with intact animals, breath-by-breath recordings of dynamic lung compliance (Chap. 7, p. 130) and pulmonary resistance (Chap. 8, p. 160) can reveal rapid changes in airway caliber induced by drugs (Fig. 18-9) or in anaphylaxis.[161]

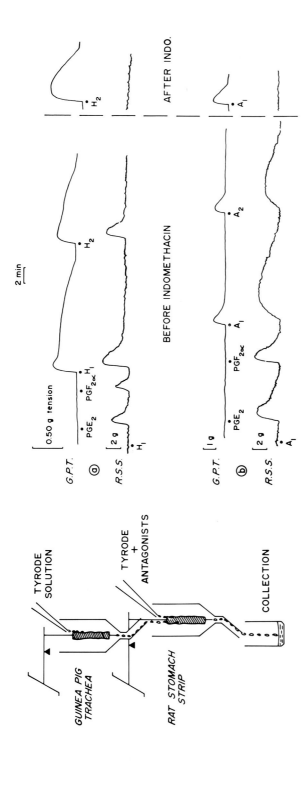

Fig. 18-7. *Left panel*—diagram of the superfused tissue technique. Tyrode solution, after superfusing the guinea pig trachea, drips onto the rat stomach strip, treated with combined antagonists to prevent effects of constrictor agents other than prostaglandins. *Right panel*—release of prostaglandin-like material by the guinea pig trachea (GPT) in 2 different preparations, when contracted with (*a*) histamine and (*b*) acetylcholine. In both cases the rat stomach strip (RSS) is insensitive to direct application of histamine ($H_1 = 100$ μg) or acetylcholine ($A_1 = 10$ ng), but sensitive to prostaglandin E_2 ($PGE_2 = 10$ μg) and prostaglandin $F_{2\alpha}$ ($PGF_{2\alpha} = 10$ ng). When the trachea is contracted with various doses of histamine ($H_1 = 100$ μg, $H_2 = 50$ μg) or acetylcholine ($A_1 = 10$ μg, $A_2 = 5$ μg), the RSS contracts, in a dose-related manner, indicating the release of a prostaglandin-like substance. After indomethacin treatment of the trachea (3 μg/ml/20 min), the tracheal contractions produced by histamine or acetylcholine are increased but the RSS does not contract, indicating that the release of prostaglandin-like substance is abolished. From reference 150.

458

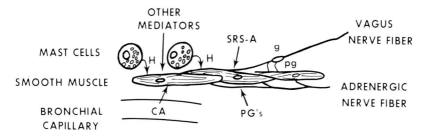

Fig. 18-8. Scheme showing the major stimuli (and some of their sources) that act on airway smooth muscle. H represents histamine; CA, circulating adrenergic agents; g, a parasympathetic ganglion; pg, postganglionic nerve fibers; PG's, prostaglandins; SRS–A, slow-reacting substance of anaphylaxis.

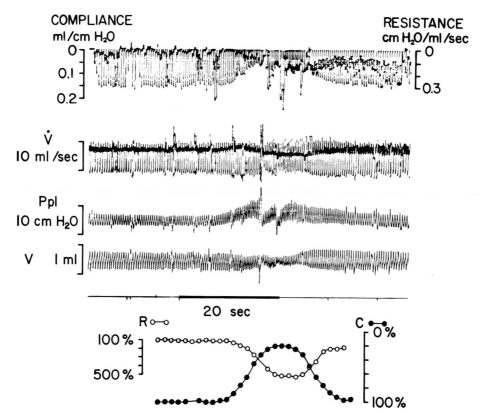

Fig. 18-9. Effect of intravenous histamine (61.6 ng/sec) in a spontaneously breathing, unanesthetized guinea pig. The five panels shown are tidal volume (V), pleural pressure (Ppl), flow (V̇), and computer output showing changes in dynamic lung compliance (C) and airway resistance (R). The lowest panel is a schematic representation of the changes observed in the computer output. Note the decrease in tidal volume, flow rate, and compliance (C), and the increase in resistance (R) after the drug. Responses are evaluated by determining the average dynamic lung compliance (20 breaths) immediately before histamine and the average dynamic lung compliance at the maximum point of response (5 breaths). Values are expressed as percentage of control value, e.g., in Figure 18-11. With aerosols, the average of 20 breaths at the point of maximum response was used since the response lasted longer. From reference 53.

Mechanism of Contraction

The contractile force of smooth muscle is generated by movements of actin and myosin molecules in myofilaments, similar to what happens in striated muscle.[27] The contractile energy is derived from oxidative processes in mitochondria, via synthesis of adenosine triphosphate (ATP) (Fig. 18-10). Calcium ions are crucial in initiating contraction and relaxation. An increased concentration of free Ca^{++} ions in the cell triggers contraction. This increase can result from diffusion of Ca^{++} into the cells from outside or by release from depots within the cell, or both. Many smooth muscle cells contain depots of calcium bound to membranous structures, including the sarcoplasmic reticulum. On relaxation, Ca^{++} is again bound in the depots and diffuses out of the cell cytoplasm (Fig. 18-10).

From outside the cell, contraction can be initiated by electrical stimuli or by drugs.[99] Electrical stimuli depolarize the membrane and cause ion fluxes (Na^+, K^+, and Ca^{++}) which lead to contraction. Drugs attach to binding sites of the cell surface (receptors). Receptor activation by drugs may cause contraction by

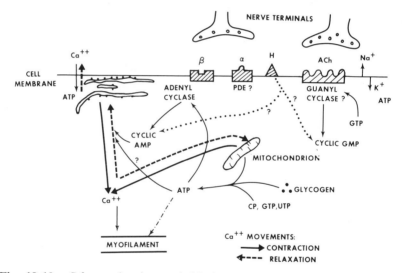

Fig. 18-10. Scheme showing probable interacting mechanisms that influence the contractile state of the myofilaments in airway smooth muscle. The receptor sites are for beta (β) and alpha (α) adrenergic agents, histamine (H), and acetylcholine (ACh). Stimulation of these sites results in fluctuations in intracellular cyclic AMP and possibly in cyclic GMP, and in the level of free ionic calcium (Ca^{++}) in the cell protoplasm. The system is dependent on high-energy phosphate (adenosine triphosphate, ATP), generated in the mitochondria. Ion fluxes (Na^+, K^+, Ca^{++}) incident to depolarization are also shown. PDE = phosphodiesterase; CP = creatinine phosphate; GTP = guanosine triphosphate; UTP = uracil triphosphate. *Heavy drawn arrows,* Ca^{++} movements associated with contraction; *heavy dashed arrows,* those associated with relaxation. β-receptor stimulation activates adenylcyclase, thus increasing intracellular cyclic AMP. This promotes sequestration of Ca^{++} ions in intracellular storage sites. Ca^{++} removal from the cell causes an additional decrease in free intracellular Ca^{++} ions, which leads to myofilament relaxation. The scheme is based on discussions at an informal meeting of smooth muscle physiologists at Yale University, Dec. 3, 1972, and includes contributions from Douglas JS, Fleisch J, Hardman J, Lewis AJ, and Somlyo AV.

depolarization, by causing ion fluxes through an already depolarized membrane, by affecting Ca^{++} movements within the cell, or by combinations of these mechanisms. Thus, drugs cause contraction and relaxation via intermediary processes that link receptors with the metabolic events that act on the myofilaments.

Drug Receptors [60]

These receptors mediate the effects of naturally occurring substances and of drugs that closely resemble them. Receptors can bind only substances that match their own structure, as a key in a lock (receptor specificity, symbolized by different receptor shapes in Fig. 18-10). None of the smooth muscle receptors has been identified chemically; their structures probably differ considerably.[113] The most important receptors in airway smooth muscle are the adrenergic receptors (α and β), the cholinergic receptor (ACh-receptor), and the histamine (H_1) receptor.

Adrenergic receptors mediate effects of catecholamines (norepinephrine, epinephrine) released from adrenergic nerve terminals and from the adrenal medulla (circulating catecholamines). Catecholamine-like drugs (e.g., isoproterenol) also activate these receptors. A-receptors are most sensitive to norepinephrine and least to isoproterenol; β-receptors are most sensitive to isoproterenol and least to norepinephrine. In airway smooth muscle, β-receptors predominate, while α-receptor activity is minimal;[81] β-receptor activity may decrease with age.[3]

How receptor activation leads to muscle contraction or relaxation is far from clear. The β-receptor is linked with the enzyme adenylcyclase, which forms 3',5' cyclic AMP from ATP.[60] B-receptor activation stimulates adenylcyclase and relaxes smooth muscle.[29] In intestinal smooth muscle, β-stimulation raises the 3',5' cyclic AMP level in the cells before the muscle relaxes.[5] The increased cyclic AMP level may promote Ca^{++} binding (Fig. 18-10), initiating relaxation.[6] In guinea pig trachea, too, relaxation is associated with an increased cyclic AMP content,[114] and most cyclic monophosphates relax this muscle.[74, 143, 189] Human bronchial muscle is relaxed by an analog of cyclic AMP (dibutyryl cyclic AMP), which penetrates better into cells than cyclic AMP itself. The action of this analog is not blocked by propranolol, suggesting that it occurs at a site beyond the receptor, in the cell.[113] Thus, much evidence suggests a role for cyclic AMP in the processes mediated by β-receptors, but it is unlikely that its metabolism alone can explain synergistic effects of drugs (see Interaction, p. 465) on airway smooth muscle.[168]

The cholinergic receptor mediates the effect of acetylcholine released from vagal nerve terminals, and that of synthetic choline esters (methacholine and carbamylcholine, or carbachol). The action of acetylcholine is short-lived because it is rapidly destroyed by the enzyme cholinesterase. The action of acetylcholine can be prolonged with physostigmine, a drug that inhibits cholinesterase. The synthetic esters have a prolonged action since they are less rapidly broken down by cholinesterase. Cholinergic stimuli may increase free Ca^{++} levels in the cell; their action may involve a nucleotide similar to cyclic AMP, 3',5' cyclic guanosine monophosphate (cyclic GMP)[82] (Fig. 18-10).

The histamine receptor mediates the action of histamine released from tissue stores or administered as a drug. In most airway muscle preparations, histamine contracts (H_1 receptors), but in some it relaxes the muscle, suggesting that another type of histamine receptor is involved.[65] The action of histamine may include a decrease of 3′,5′ cyclic AMP, perhaps by activation of phosphodiesterase.[96] However, in whole-lung tissue, histamine increases cyclic AMP levels.[153]

Other receptors. How other mediators in asthma (e.g., SRS-A, bradykinin) affect smooth muscle and other cells (mucous glands; mucosa) is not known. Also, how prostaglandins act on airway muscle is not clear; they do not release histamine,[4] and their action is independent of vagal and adrenergic stimuli,[169] and that of PGE_1 is unchanged by α- and β-blockade.[117, 173] Inhibition of neuromuscular transmission may account for the actions of PGE_1 and PGE_2.[85]

Receptor Antagonists

The action of drugs that activate receptors (agonists) is abolished by drugs that bind to the receptors but do not activate their action on the cell (antagonists). Some antagonists cause irreversible receptor activation; more commonly, their binding is reversible and these antagonists compete with agonists for binding sites on the cells. In these instances, whether the action of the agonist or antagonist prevails depends on the relative concentrations of both in the neighborhood of the receptors and on their relative affinities to the receptors. Specific antagonists include propranolol (β-receptor blockade[119]) phentolamine (α-receptor blockade), atropine (cholinergic blockade), and mepyramine (antihistamine drug). In small doses, specific antagonists block the action of only one receptor. Thus, their action supports the concept of specific receptors.

Receptor Activation in Health and in Asthma

In healthy persons, β-receptor blockade does not affect airway caliber.[167, 212, 213] Cholinergic blockade with atropine increases airway caliber[203] (Fig. 17-7). Hence, β-receptor activation is probably minimal, while cholinergic stimuli maintain a degree of smooth muscle tone. There is no evidence that H_1 and α-receptors play a role in physiological conditions, but these can nevertheless mediate effects of drugs (exogenous histamine, norepinephrine, histamine-releasing agents) in healthy persons. Apart from such pharmacological interventions, only the cholinergic receptor appears to be consistently active in healthy persons. When cholinergic blockade is induced (with atropine), airway smooth muscle relaxes and other constrictor stimuli then exert less effect, in man (Fig. 17-7) as well as in animals.[111, 140, 141, 205] Although β-receptor blockade has no direct effect on the airways, in some healthy persons it potentiates the effect of constrictor stimuli (e.g., histamine, textile dust, or cigarette smoke;[213] Fig. 17-8, p. 430). In these persons, airway muscle may be continuously exposed to low-level β-adrenergic stimulation, insufficient to affect airway caliber by itself but sufficient to decrease the effect of constrictor stimuli. A similar potentiation of the effects of histamine by propranolol occurs in unsensitized guinea pigs[51, 52] (Fig. 18-11).

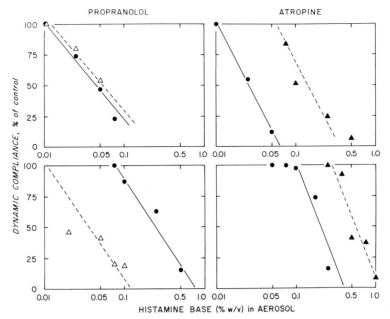

Fig. 18-11. Modification of responses to aerosolized histamine by propranolol and atropine in female albino guinea pigs (one animal per panel). Histamine dose is expressed as concentration of histamine base in nebulized solution. Control responses (●) and responses after propranolol (10 mg/kg intraperitoneally) (△) or atropine (5 mg/kg intraperitoneally) (▲) expressed as percentages of control compliance, on the ordinate. (For method, see Fig. 18-9.) The two upper panels are from animals more sensitive to histamine than those of the two lower panels. Atropine inhibits the histamine response in the sensitive and the insensitive animal (*right-hand panels*). Propranolol potentiates the histamine response in the insensitive (*lower left*) but not in the sensitive (*upper left*) animal. From reference 52.

In patients with asthma, activation of H_1 receptors by histamine released from mast cells (p. 456) is a principal step in the induction of airway constriction. The degree of activation, and hence the severity of the asthma, depends in part on the amounts of histamine that reach the smooth muscle. However, the action of histamine can be potentiated by cholinergic stimuli and inhibited by β-adrenergic stimuli. Although this potentiation or inhibition also occurs in healthy persons (see above), there are quantitative differences between them and patients with asthma. In the latter, propranolol causes airway constriction even without additional exogenous constrictor stimuli.[137] Thus, in asthma, β-receptor stimulation may normally help to oppose the contractile stimuli; when the β-receptors are blocked, the latter prevail and cause airway constriction. In this instance, endogenous cholinergic stimuli may be the main cause of airway constriction, since atropine blocks the propranolol-induced constriction.[80] Since the effect of propranolol is more pronounced in asthmatics than in normal persons, it is likely that in asthma, either the amount of β-adrenergic stimuli is increased, or β-adrenergic receptors are more sensitive to these stimuli. However, one current theory of asthma proposes that β-adrenergic receptors are less rather than more active than normal in this disease.

This theory is discussed in detail on p. 471. The role of α-receptors, if any, in asthma is ill understood, mainly because α-receptor-blocking drugs also have other (e.g., antihistaminic) actions and thus do not provide adequate evidence on α-receptor activity.

Airway caliber in health as well as in asthma is probably determined by the balance between contractile (via H_1 and ACh receptors) and relaxant (via β-receptors) stimuli to airway smooth muscle. In health, cholinergic stimulation appears to maintain the normal smooth muscle tone; in asthma, stimulation of H_1 receptors predominates, with cholinergic and β-adrenergic stimuli acting as potentiating and inhibiting factors, respectively. Stimulation of β-adrenergic receptors with drugs provides powerful symptomatic treatment (p. 476). Small doses of agonists or antagonists, which do not directly contract or relax airway muscle, may potentiate or inhibit the actions of other drugs (interaction; p. 465). Also, the agonist may influence other stimuli: for instance, histamine releases catecholamines from the adrenal medulla, and catecholamines counteract the contractile effect of histamine.[35]

AUTONOMIC NERVOUS SYSTEM OF AIRWAYS

Airway smooth muscle is supplied with vagal and adrenergic motor nerve endings (Fig. 18-8). Afferent vagal nerve fibers, which transmit signals to the central nervous system, are located in the lung parenchyma (inflation and deflation receptors; Chap. 10, p. 211), and in the mucosa of upper airways and the bronchial tree (irritant and cough receptors). Vagal efferent nerve endings are found throughout the bronchial tree; adrenergic nerves have been identified in the trachea (guinea pig) and in the bronchial tree of cats, down to the level of respiratory bronchioles.[45, 147] The afferent receptors have not been identified anatomically; their presence is inferred mainly from physiological experiments.

Role of the Vagus Nerve

Electrical stimulation of the vagus nerve contracts airway smooth muscle [136] (Figs. 1-7, 18-14). Blocking cholinergic stimuli with atropine or through cutting or cooling the vagus nerves inhibits constrictor effects of histamine and allergen challenge.[49, 57, 111, 141, 205, 208] Enhancing cholinergic stimuli with physostigmine potentiates the constrictor effect of histamine.[52] These results show that efferent vagal stimuli promote airway constriction both in animals and in patients challenged with allergens,[208] and in normal persons who respond to histamine or other airway-constrictor agents (Fig. 17-7).

The origin of the vagal stimuli is less clear. They may result from tonic vagal nerve discharge or from reflexly increased vagal activity. Injection of histamine into bronchial arteries of dogs causes constriction of an isolated tracheal segment in the neck,[49] and antigen inhalation into one lung of an allergic dog constricts the other lung.[78] Thus, locally acting histamine or allergen may induce airway constriction elsewhere in the lungs via reflex pathways. However, the afferent nervous pathways of these reflexes have not been identified. Histamine might directly activate irritant receptors, resulting in firing of vagal afferents.[140] However, while histamine acts in 5–10 seconds (Fig. 18-9), the afferent fibers fire only after a latency of 30 seconds–2 minutes.[140, 172] Vagal afferent firing may result from muscle contraction.[18] Thus, increased vagal efferent discharge might result from stimuli arising in contracting airways, and this could prolong and increase the contraction locally and elsewhere in the airways (positive feedback[205]). Consequently, there may be no need to assume that histamine or other mediators act directly on afferent receptors.

Role of the Adrenergic System

Electric stimulation of adrenergic (sympathetic) nerve fibers relaxes airway smooth muscle (Fig. 1-7, p. 12). The evidence that β-stimulation is minimal in healthy persons and demonstrable (by the effect of β-blockade) in asthma, as well as the potentiation of airway constriction by β-blockade, has already been discussed (p. 462). The β-adrenergic stimuli, which normally counteract the action of constrictor agents, are probably provided by circulating catecholamines rather than by adrenergic transmitter release from nerve endings in airways. Guanethidine, which blocks only the latter, potentiates histamine responses less than propranolol, which blocks the action of all β-adrenergic stimuli.[52] Bilateral adrenalectomy potentiates histamine responses in guinea pigs, which supports a role for circulating catecholamines.[28] Since disruption of lung afferents does not potentiate histamine responses,[51] it is unlikely that the potentiation of histamine responses by β-blockade results from a bronchodilator reflex elicited by histamine.[133]

Effects of Autonomic Ganglion Blockade

Hexamethonium, a drug that blocks stimulus transmission in autonomic ganglia, reduces the effect of histamine in patients with asthma[23] (Fig. 18-12) and can induce bronchodilatation in spontaneous asthma[92] (Fig. 18-5). Hexamethonium also reduces the effects of histamine, choline esters, and anaphylaxis in guinea pigs.[51, 52, 90] Since the drug has no effect on airway smooth muscle, its action demonstrates that autonomic nerve pathways contribute to the histamine response in asthma. Presumably, blockade of vagal ganglia by hexamethonium reduces cholinergic stimulation of airways and hence the histamine response, by eliminating interaction between acetylcholine and histamine (see next section).

STIMULUS INTERACTION

The preceding discussion shows that effects of contractile stimuli (histamine) can be enhanced by cholinergic and reduced by β-adrenergic stimuli. In intact guinea pigs, cholinergic blockade inhibits, while β-adrenergic blockade often potentiates, histamine responses[52] (Fig. 18-11). Enhancement of cholinergic stimuli with physostigmine potentiates while β-adrenergic drugs inhibit histamine contractions.[52] Thus, the action of histamine on guinea pig airways appears to depend on the balance between vagal and β-adrenergic stimuli. Variations in this balance may explain why histamine responses vary greatly in individual animals (Fig. 18-2), while in vitro responses of their tracheal muscle to histamine vary much less.[54]

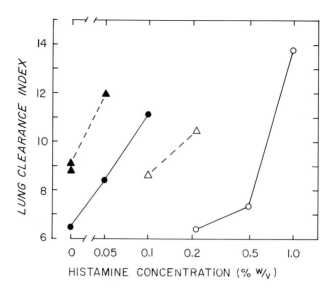

Fig. 18-12. Histamine dose-response curves in two symptom-free patients (△ and ○) with asthma, before (*filled symbols*) and after (*open symbols*) administration of hexamethonium bromide in divided doses, subcutaneously (see reference 23 for details). Before hexamethonium administration, both patients are highly sensitive to histamine; afterward, their sensitivity decreases by a factor 4 to 10. For example, after hexamethonium administration, one patient (○) had a minimal histamine response to 0.5% histamine (5 mg/ml); before hexamethonium administration, he reacted to 0.05% (0.5 mg/ml) with a slightly larger increase of the lung clearance index (see Chap. 4, p. 71, for definition of this index).

Thus, the presence of varying vagal and β-adrenergic stimuli may increase the range of variability of airway responses in vivo.

Atropine inhibits the histamine response of guinea pigs in both histamine-sensitive and insensitive animals, while the potentiating effect of propranolol is most pronounced in histamine-insensitive animals [52] (Fig. 18-11). Thus, among individual guinea pigs, β-adrenergic stimuli appear to vary more than cholinergic stimuli. The wide dispersion of histamine sensitivity in guinea pigs (Fig. 18-2) may largely reflect variations in the amounts of circulating catecholamines (p. 464) or variations in β-receptor sensitivity, or both. Histamine-sensitive guinea pigs have tracheal β-receptors which, in vitro, respond less to isoproterenol than those of histamine-insensitive animals.[54] However, the comparison of in vivo and in vitro responses to histamine suggests that variations in β-adrenergic stimuli reaching the muscle in vivo play a role in addition to variations in β-receptor response.

The effects of atropine, propranolol, and other drugs on histamine responses in vivo [52] (Fig. 18-11) occur with dose levels which by themselves do not affect airway caliber. Thus, cholinergic and β-adrenergic receptors appear to influence histamine responses at subthreshold stimulation levels. The interaction between cholinergic stimuli and histamine can be studied in experiments with an isolated

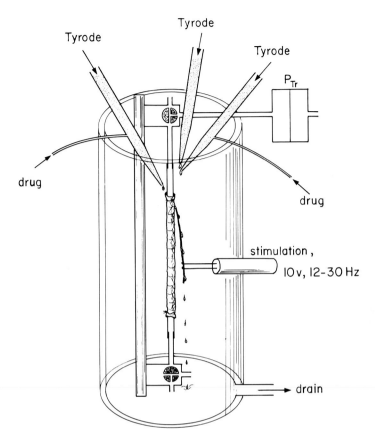

Fig. 18-13. Nerve-muscle preparation of isolated guinea pig trachea, connected at one end to pressure transducer for recording of intratracheal pressure (Ptr). Drugs are added to the superfused warm, oxygenated Tyrode solution. Nerve stimulation parameters are also shown. From reference 88.

guinea pig trachea nerve-muscle preparation (Fig. 18-13). In this preparation, subthreshold doses of histamine enhance the effect of stimulation of the peripheral vagal nerve stump (Fig. 18-14). A similar interaction occurs when subthreshold doses of histamine are combined with methacholine (an acetylcholine analog); the contraction obtained with both drugs is larger than the sum of the contractions induced by each (Fig. 18-15). That this interaction also occurs in man is shown by the results of Fig. 18-16, in which inhalation of an aerosol containing histamine and methacholine produced a larger constrictor effect than inhalation of each drug separately.[142]

The mechanism of interaction between histamine and cholinergic stimuli is not known. It may occur at the level of the receptors or of the intracellular processes that follow receptor activation. Both receptors may act on intracellular events (Ca^{++} transport or $3',5'$ cyclic AMP metabolism, or both), which are crucial in the contraction process, resulting in a larger contractile response than when each receptor is activated separately. Experiments with other smooth muscles (guinea

RESPONSES to NERVE STIMULATION

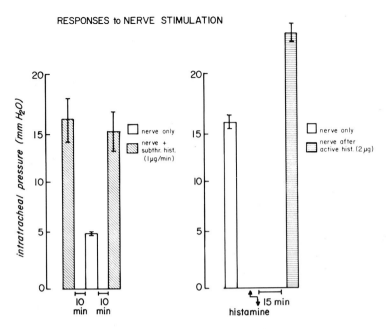

Fig. 18-14. Response of superfused tracheal preparations (Fig. 18-13) to vagus nerve stimulation and histamine. *Left graph:* white bar shows mean value of control vagal stimulation. Hatched bars indicate increased effect of stimulation when an inactive dose of histamine was being superfused. *Right graph:* white bar—control vagal stimulation. After relaxation, the preparation was contracted with histamine (between arrows). After 15 minutes, the trachea had relaxed to baseline pressure. Even so, vagal stimulation had an increased effect at this time (hatched bar, mean of 3 contractions over a period of 30 minutes). Modified from reference 88.

TRACHEAL RESPONSE to METHACHOLINE and SUBTHRESHOLD HISTAMINE

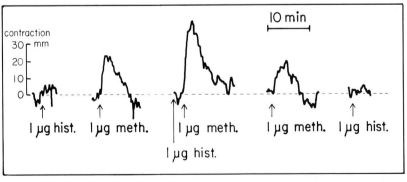

meth.= methacholine   hist.= histamine

Fig. 18-15. Response of the superfused trachea (Fig. 18-13) to an inactive dose of histamine, an active dose of methacholine, and to the same dose of histamine followed 30 seconds later by the same dose of methacholine. A potentiation of approximately 100% is seen. From reference 88.

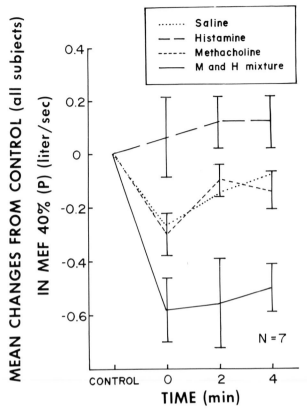

Fig. 18-16. Change in flow rates on PEFV curves (Chap. 9) after inhalation of histamine and methacholine aerosols administered separately and together in 7 healthy subjects (mean ± standard error). For definition of MEF 40% (P), see Table 9-1, p. 189. The decreases seen after the simultaneous administration of these two agents is greater than the algebraic sum of the effects of the drugs administered separately. Data of CA Mitchell et al.[142]

pig vas deferens and seminal vesicle) have shown similar patterns of interaction, for instance, between adrenergic nerve stimuli and histamine.[177, 178]

Recent work has shown that locally released prostaglandins (p. 457) may modulate the action of contractor stimuli on airway smooth muscle. The synthesis, and thus the release, of prostaglandins are inhibited by anti-inflammatory drugs, indomethacin and aspirin.[39, 200] In the guinea pig trachea, these drugs reduce the contractile effect of low histamine doses, while potentiating the effect of large histamine concentrations (Fig. 18-17). Thus, the histamine dose-response curve becomes steeper.[150] If prostaglandins also are released in human airways, it is conceivable that this plays a role in asthma. For instance, increased $PGF_{2\alpha}$ synthesis might enhance the effect of contractile stimuli and might also explain hyperresponsiveness to $PGF_{2\alpha}$ in asthma.[127]

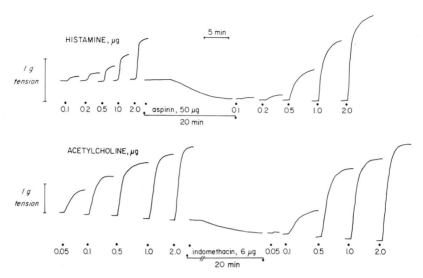

Fig. 18-17. Effects of aspirin (*upper record*) and indomethacin (*lower record*) on histamine (H)- or acetylcholine (ACh)-induced contractions, and on the basal tone of the spirally cut guinea pig trachea. Aspirin and indomethacin decrease the basal tone of the trachea. They reduce the effect of low concentrations of H (0.1 μg) and ACh (0.05 and 0.1 μg) and increase the effect of higher concentrations (0.5–2.0 μg H and ACh). From reference 150.

AIRWAY HYPERRESPONSIVENESS

In patients with asthma, drugs like histamine and choline esters cause airway-constrictor responses in doses far below those required to elicit similar effects in nonasthmatic persons.[23, 30, 43, 195] This hyperresponsiveness exists even in patients who have been symptom-free, or nearly so, for many years.[23, 30] Patients with asthma may also be more sensitive than normal persons to other stimuli, including inhalation of cold air and citric acid aerosol.[176] In addition, asthmatic patients are extremely sensitive to inhalation of $PGF_{2\alpha}$, a prostaglandin that contracts airway muscle (p. 457). Changes in airway resistance revealed that asthmatic patients were about 8000 times more sensitive to $PGF_{2\alpha}$ and only about 10 times more sensitive to histamine than nonasthmatic persons.[127]

Studies on airway hyperresponsiveness have usually concerned patients with asthma who sought medical help. Although their response to constrictor stimuli is usually much more pronounced than that of healthy nonasthmatic subjects, little is known about the responsiveness of persons with infrequent or subclinical asthma. Thus, the hyperresponsiveness of asthmatics might represent the far end of a continuous distribution of sensitivity to constrictor stimuli among the general population as, e.g., the response to histamine in guinea pigs (Fig. 18-2). If this is true, there is no clear differentiation between hyperresponsive and normally responsive persons (see also p. 443).

Clinical Significance

In persons who have no demonstrable allergies, increased response to airway-constrictor stimuli may be the principal cause of asthma. In allergic persons, airway responses to mediators may determine the frequency and severity of asthma. Absence of hyperresponsiveness may explain why healthy persons made allergic with modified allergens did not develop asthma,[126] and why many allergic persons suffer only from hay fever and not from asthma. In guinea pigs, histamine sensitivity correlates with the severity of the anaphylactic response, suggesting that histamine sensitivity may, in part, determine the effect of the antigen challenge.[160]

Assessment of Hyperresponsiveness

Effects of constrictor and dilator drugs depend on the initial airway caliber.[23, 72] Therefore, airway responses in asthma should be studied in a symptom-free period when control function data are normal. Otherwise, spuriously enhanced responses are likely. Posture should also be controlled[20] (Fig. 18-18). Sensitive tests, such as N_2 washout and MEFV or PEFV curves, are more suitable to assess responses than the $FEV_{1.0}$.

Mechanisms of Hyperresponsiveness

Why airways of asthmatic persons are hyperresponsive to stimuli is one of the most important questions concerning the pathogenesis of bronchial asthma. Scattered data in the literature suggest that, in vitro, airway muscle from asthma patients is not more sensitive to histamine than that of nonasthmatics. Hence, it is likely that humoral or nervous factors cause the markedly increased response to histamine in asthma patients in vivo. Several hypotheses have been proposed to account for the in vivo hyperresponsiveness:

1. Anaphylactic sensitization of guinea pigs does not lead to long-term histamine or acetylcholine hyperresponsiveness.[161] Thus, the phenomenon may be independent of immunological processes.

2. Increased formation or decreased breakdown of mediators might lead to high tissue levels of mediators, so that a smaller dose of histamine or acetylcholine could elicit airway constriction. However, available evidence suggests that the metabolism of histamine in asthma is normal.[55, 87]

3. Partial blockade of β-receptors[165, 190] could render airway smooth muscle more sensitive to histamine and other constrictor stimuli. Variations in β-receptor responses occur among guinea pigs,[54, 196] but although some responses to β-adrenergic stimuli (e.g., adenylcyclase activation in leukocytes[124]) may be decreased in asthma, isoproterenol usually causes marked airway dilatation (Figs. 18-19, 18-21). The effect of propranolol in asthma suggests increased rather than decreased β-stimulation (p. 463). Thus, there is at present no evidence that β-receptors in airways are less responsive in asthmatics than in normal persons. In addition, in healthy persons β-blockade does not potentiate constrictor responses sufficiently to explain airway hyperresponsiveness in asthma[209, 213] (Fig. 17-8, p. 430).

4. Increased efferent vagal stimuli, induced either by tonic nerve activity[64] or by reflex,[176] might explain hyperresponsiveness, since vagal stimuli increase hista-

mine responses (p. 464). Sensitization of cough receptors has been postulated as a source of increased afferent vagal stimuli in asthma.[176] After hexamethonium (p. 465), histamine responses of asthmatic patients become similar to those of normals (Table 18-2), and atropine inhibits allergen and histamine responses in asthma.[57, 208] Thus, increased vagal efferent stimuli may largely explain histamine hyperresponsiveness in asthma. The origin of the vagal stimuli has already been discussed (p. 464). Interaction between histamine and vagal stimuli on the smooth muscle cell (p. 465) probably determines the increased response of the airways to histamine, and similar interactions may occur with other constrictor stimuli.

5. Increased vagal tone can explain histamine hyperresponsiveness but not the much greater degree of hypersensitivity to $PGF_{2\alpha}$ in asthma.[127] The latter may be related to increased prostaglandin synthesis in airway tissue (p. 469).

OTHER FACTORS IN PATHOGENESIS OF ASTHMA

Genetic Factors

Asthma often runs in families. However, this may be due to common environmental factors as well as to gene heritage. Among pairs of monozygotic twins, whose genetic make-up is similar, cases of only one twin having asthma are common.[19] Sometimes both twins have allergies but only one has asthma. In these instances, only the asthmatic twin has hyperresponsive airways.[66] Since asthma results from a chain of immunological events and tissue responses, many genes may be involved as determinants of various links in this chain. Thus, geneticists have concluded that the familial occurrence of asthma does not conform to any simple, well-defined pattern of inheritance.[19]

In guinea pigs, strains sensitive to chemical mediators can be developed by inbreeding techniques.[191] The sensitivity of these animals does not result from antigenic sensitization, and it is likely that increased responsiveness to the chemical mediators is the main reason why these animals are more sensitive to anaphylaxis than are animals belonging to mediator-insensitive strains.[161, 191]

Table 18-2
Effect of Hexamethonium Bromide on Histamine Sensitivity

Subjects	Histamine Threshold Dose (mg/ml) *	
	Mean	Range
6 healthy nonasthmatic subjects	7.2	2.5–15.0
6 symptom-free asthmatics with normal control function data	1.4	0.05–5.0
Same 6 asthmatics after hexamethonium (divided doses s.c.)	6.2	2.5–10.0

* Smallest dose that caused significant change of nitrogen washout curve. Methods and procedures—as described in reference 23. (The data are from an additional group of subjects and patients not included in that reference.)

Infection

Many patients with asthma say their asthma began after a cold or airway infection. However, it is not clear how inflammatory and immunological events due to infections lead to asthma after the infection is past. In some unknown way, these events might lead to hyperresponsive airways (see p. 470), but many other hypotheses equally speculative and difficult to test can be made. Allergy to bacterial antigens has not been clearly demonstrated.

Time of Day

Attacks of asthma frequently begin at night, during sleep. In some patients this may be due to allergen exposure (e.g., from bedding materials). Diurnal variations in, for example, adrenocortical secretions, may also be responsible for the timing of the attacks.[183] Others have concluded that nocturnal attacks are not clearly related to the stage of sleep or to circadian changes in adrenal secretions.[109] Posture may be important: healthy persons as well as asthmatics are more sensitive to the effect of inhaled histamine when supine or in a head-down posture than

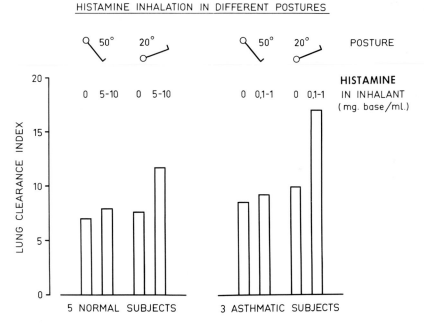

Fig. 18-18.   Average values of the lung clearance index (LCI; Chap. 4, p. 71) in normal and asthmatic subjects in two different positions, with and without inhalation of a histamine aerosol. An increased LCI indicates more uneven gas distribution caused by airway obstruction (p. 74). Inhaled histamine concentrations were 5 or 10 mg base per ml in normal subjects. In the asthmatic patients, either 0.1 (two subjects) or 1 mg per ml (one subject) was administered. In both healthy and asthmatic subjects the increase of LCI was significantly greater when histamine was administered in the head-down position than when given while the subject was upright. From reference 20.

when upright [20] (Fig. 18-18). Thus, the nocturnal attacks may, in part, occur because the airways undergo greater narrowing during recumbency. Since the relation of nocturnal asthma to allergen exposure is usually not evident, it is not clear what constricts the airways. Normal or increased vagal tone may be responsible, with its effect being enhanced by posture, as for histamine.

Exercise

Many patients with asthma have attacks shortly after physical exertion. After exercise on a bicycle or treadmill, most patients with asthma, unlike nonasthmatic persons, have a decreased $FEV_{1.0}$, maximally 5–10 minutes after exercise.[32, 67] Swimming has, for unclear reasons, less effect than bicycling or running. Exercise asthma can be prevented by isoproterenol,[34] disodiumcromoglycate,[163] or epinephrine, but not by atropine, hydrocortisone, or an antihistamine drug.[138] Measurements of MMFR (Table 9-1, p. 189) show decreases after exercise in cigarette smokers.[118] Most healthy subjects do not develop asthma-like function changes after β-blockade with propranolol,[209] but about 15 percent do.[108]

The mechanisms of exercise-asthma are unclear. Hyperventilation without exercise does not consistently decrease the $FEV_{1.0}$ in asthmatics.[34, 202] The asthmatic response decreases after repeated bouts of exercise, suggesting that mediator stores (p. 457) become exhausted.[138] During exercise, the adrenal medulla releases increased amounts of catecholamines into the bloodstream; these counteract the action of constrictor agents on airway muscle. The adrenal medulla of asthmatics may respond less to stress than that of normals.[128] Therefore, postexercise exhaustion of catecholamine stores may remove a muscle-relaxing stimulus and thus lead to airway constriction.

Psychosomatic Factors

Many clinicians are impressed with the associations between personality traits, psychotraumatic events, and asthma attacks. In laboratory experiments, attacks can sometimes be induced by placebo inhalations if the patient is led to believe that the aerosol contains an allergen.[125] There are anatomic substrates for effects of events in the brain on the caliber of airways, via the vagus nerve. In animals, electrical stimulation of the cerebral cortex can lead to airway constriction, as shown by Francois-Franck in 1888.[71] It may also be that increases in vagal nerve impulses normally accompany emotional or other psychological events linked to brain processes, and that these lead to asthma only in persons with hyperresponsive airways (see p. 470). In any case, whether induced by psychosomatic mechanisms or otherwise, treatment of acute asthma requires relief of airway obstruction by medical means.

Aspirin Intolerance

Some patients with asthma develop attacks after ingestion of aspirin. Even among persons without evident aspirin intolerance, a challenge test (640 mg aspirin orally) often causes airway constriction,[134] and indomethacin may do the same.[179] How aspirin and indomethacin cause asthma is unknown. If these drugs act through inhibition of prostaglandin synthesis, their best known action, one might assume that aspirin- or indomethacin-sensitive patients are normally protected against constrictor stimuli by increased synthesis of PGE_2 in the airways.

THERAPY

This section discusses the physiological and pharmacological basis of therapy rather than individual indications for different drugs and procedures. Many patients with asthma can be treated effectively with bronchodilator drugs; others require combinations of bronchodilators and steroids. Prolonged and severe attacks of asthma (status asthmaticus) call for intensive treatment with bronchodilators (aminophylline intravenously), corticosteroids, and oxygen. Widespread mucus plugging of airways is a principal cause of persistent airway obstruction and may cause fatal ventilatory failure. Thus, frequent blood gas monitoring is needed, and airway intubation, assisted ventilation, and bronchial lavage should be considered when the arterial P_{CO_2} rises, as an indication of ventilatory failure.[59, 83, 91]

Avoidance of Allergen Exposure

Persons with known allergies can prevent asthma by avoiding the pertinent allergen. Restrictions of activities (diet, domestic environments, jobs, household pets) are rational if provocation with the allergen causes airway constriction; they should not be prescribed solely on the basis of positive skin tests.

Immunotherapy

Repeated injections with allergen solutions may lessen the response to allergen exposure (desensitization[130]) and, at least in hay fever, this treatment reduces the amount of IgE antibodies.[122] For the treatment of asthma, desensitization is a controversial method. The criteria for clinical improvement are ill defined and few studies have been sufficiently controlled. However, desensitization against grass pollens, ragweed, and house dust may have some merit.[146] Bacterial vaccines are ineffective.

Bronchodilator Drugs

Airway caliber in asthma can be increased by drugs that inhibit the actions of chemical mediators on smooth muscle, by direct antagonism (antihistamine drugs), or by increasing β-adrenergic stimuli (β-stimulants), reducing cholinergic stimuli (anticholinergic drugs), or with phosphodiesterase-inhibiting drugs.

Antihistamine drugs are rarely used alone in asthma. They are relatively ineffective, although no controlled trials appear to have been reported. Their ineffectiveness might be related to insufficient concentrations in the airway tissues[46] or to the constrictor effect of other mediators not antagonized by these drugs (e.g., SRS-A, p. 456).

B-stimulant drugs are highly effective bronchodilators, often reducing symptoms and improving function in minutes. Isoproterenol, which not only relaxes airway muscle but also inhibits histamine release (p. 456), increases airway conductance and maximum expiratory flow rates in asthma (Fig. 18-19). In healthy persons, isoproterenol may render large airways more collapsible, thus reducing maximum flows (Chap. 8, p. 156). Phenylephrine, which constricts mucosal blood vessels, enhances the dilator effect of isoproterenol.[34] Aerosol administration deposits drugs close to their target cells in the airways.[53, 93] Nebulizers producing 2–5 μm diameter particles are preferable; larger particles are deposited in upper airways where they exert no useful action [21] (p. 271). Aerosol administration of isoproterenol by hand nebulizers is just as effective as aerosolization by pressure breathing devices.[34]

Frequent and prolonged use of β-stimulants often leads to decreased effective-

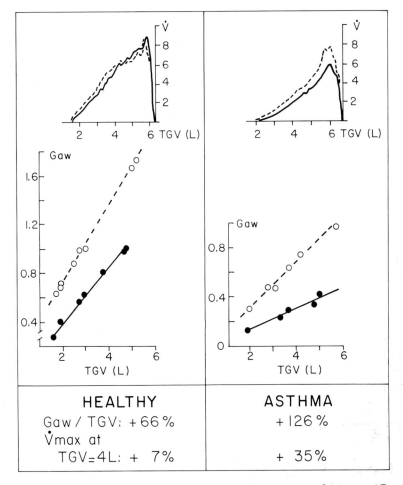

Fig. 18-19. MEFV curves (*top section*) and airway conductance (Gaw) as a function of thoracic gas volume (TGV) (*bottom section*) before (*solid line*) and after (*dashed line*) inhalation of isoproterenol in a healthy and an asthmatic subject. In both, conductance increases; flow rates on MEFV curves increase only in the asthmatic. Modified from Bouhuys A, Prog. Respir. Res. 4: 24–38, 1969.

ness, and overuse of isoproterenol may have contributed to increased asthma mortality in some countries.[182] In guinea pigs, intensive treatment with isoproterenol increases the lethal effect of histamine.[40, 120] In vitro, desensitization against isoproterenol can be produced in rat aortic muscle and in guinea pig and rat trachea [68, 120] (Fig. 18-20). Other drugs which, like isoproterenol, increase 3',5' cyclic AMP levels in cells can also desensitize the trachea against isoproterenol. The mechanism of desensitization is as yet unknown.

The short-lasting action of isoproterenol (5–30 minutes) promotes frequent use and hence the chance of desensitization. Orciprenaline is about as potent but its effect lasts much longer.[94] Orciprenaline, salbutamol, and terbutaline are more selective in their effect on the airways and have less effect on the force and rate of cardiac contraction than isoproterenol.[102, 204] The selectivity of these newer β-stimulants is a practical advantage. Its explanation in terms of two types of β-receptors (β_1-receptors in the heart; β_2-receptors in the airways) may be too simplistic.[16, 79]

Anticholinergic drugs, in particular atropine, have a bronchodilator effect in asthma [42, 197] but also undesirable side-effects (dry mouth, drying of secretions). A phenothiazine compound with antihistamine and anticholinergic properties (Multergan®) often improves lung function in older patients more than isoproterenol.[175, 192]

Phosphodiesterase (PDE)-inhibiting drugs may cause bronchodilatation by increasing the intracellular level of 3',5' cyclic AMP, through inhibition of the enzymes that decompose cyclic AMP. One of these drugs, theophylline (a component of aminophylline), causes marked airway dilatation after intravenous injection.[42] Since there are discrepancies between their enzyme-inhibiting and broncho-

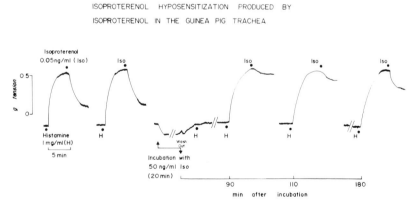

ISOPROTERENOL HYPOSENSITIZATION PRODUCED BY
ISOPROTERENOL IN THE GUINEA PIG TRACHEA

Fig. 18-20. Effect of incubation of guinea pig trachea with isoproterenol (50 ng/ml for 20 minutes) on isoproterenol relaxations (0.05 ng/ml) superimposed on histamine contractions (H; 1 μg/ml). The time course after washout is represented by the horizontal line. Ninety minutes after incubation, isoproterenol causes only minimal relaxation of the histamine-contracted trachea, compared with the two control responses at left. The relaxant response gradually increases again over a 90 minute period. Data of Lewis et al.[120]

dilator properties, it is not certain that the therapeutic effects of PDE-inhibiting drugs depend solely on inhibition of this enzyme system.[47, 174]

Corticosteroid Drugs

Treatment with these drugs (e.g., prednisolone) is often indispensable when bronchodilator drugs cause insufficient improvement. In older patients with airway obstruction, corticosteroids sometimes cause marked and unexpected improvement.[42] The mode of action of corticosteroids on the airways may include reduced mucosal swelling and secretion as a part of the general anti-inflammatory properties of these drugs.

Disodiumcromoglycate (DSCG)

This drug inhibits the release of histamine from mast cells by compound 48/80 in vitro, and appears to stabilize mast cells.[151] It also inhibits the effect of exogenous histamine in patients with asthma,[112] and it often abolishes the effect of allergen challenge in these patients.[63] DSCG is not a bronchodilator drug; side-effects are practically absent. Several clinical trials with DSCG have shown that it is effective in about 30 percent[101] of patients with asthma, but few objective data on its clinical effectiveness are available. Small improvements in $FEV_{1.0}$ and FVC have been reported.[101] Other reports conclude that DSCG allows patients with severe asthma to reduce their doses of corticosteroids.[129]

Ascorbic Acid (Vitamin C)

In healthy persons, 500 mg ascorbic acid inhibits the constrictor effect of histamine. Ascorbic acid also reduces in vitro effects of several airway muscle-contractor agents. The effectiveness of this physiological substance in asthma needs to be investigated.[212]

Prostaglandins

PGE_1 and PGE_2 (by aerosol) induce airway dilatation in asthma.[44] PGE_1 (1–2 $\mu g/ml$) relaxes human bronchial muscle.[173] PGE_2 is about ten times more potent than isoproterenol in reducing $PGF_{2\alpha}$-induced airway constriction in non-asthmatic persons.[180] In cats and guinea pigs, PGE_1 and PGE_2 aerosols are also more potent than isoproterenol aerosols.[117, 169] Intravenously, prostaglandins are much less active since they are inactivated during passage through lung blood vessels.[159, 169] The role of prostaglandins E in the clinical management of asthma is not yet established.

Assessment of Therapy

In patients with asthma, lung-function tests should be used to (1) assess the patient's condition when first seen, (2) assess improvement during therapy, and (3) document lung function when the patient is symptom-free. The latter is important to distinguish reversible airway constriction from other conditions that impair lung function. If function is normal in the absence of symptoms, this may help convince the patient that the condition can be treated and is functionally fully reversible (Fig. 18-4). A comparison of MEFV curves and spirographic data before and after inhalation of a bronchodilator drug can show reversibility of airway obstruction. This comparison is facilitated by superimposition of consecutive MEFV curves before and after treatment (Fig. 18-21).

SUMMARY

Asthma, a common and sometimes disabling or fatal disease, is characterized by reversible airway constriction, leading to wheezing, shortness of breath, and sometimes ventilatory failure. Environmental agents, including allergens, are important etiological factors, but genetic factors, airway infections, and psychosomatic factors may play a role as well. How these factors cause airway constriction is shown diagrammatically in Figure 18-1. Allergens react with mast-cell-bound reagins in airway tissue, leading to release of chemical mediators that contract airway muscle, stimulate mucus secretion, and promote mucosal edema. Chemical agents may act directly on the mast cells, while physical stimuli may constrict airways via a vagal reflex. The effect of these constrictor stimuli is opposed by airway dilator, mainly β-adrenergic, stimuli. In healthy persons, vagal efferent (cholinergic) stimuli maintain the normal airway muscle tone; β-adrenergic stimulation is minimal. When the balance between constrictor and dilator stimuli is disturbed by increasing chemical or vagal constrictor stimuli, or by decreasing β-adrenergic stimulation (by β-blockade), airway muscle tone increases and may induce perceptible airway constriction. In asthmatics, increased constrictor stimuli impinge on airway muscle, shifting the balance in the direction of airway constriction. In addition, the airways of patients with asthma are much more sensitive to constrictor stimuli than those of normals. To a large extent, this hyperresponsiveness may be caused by increased cholinergic stimulation; alteration in prostaglandin metabolism may also play a role. Partial blockade of β-receptors might also account for hyperresponsiveness but has not been demonstrated in airway muscle; other data suggest increased β-receptor activity in asthma. Interpretation of airway responses to constrictor stimuli is complicated by interaction between chemical and nervous stimuli on airway muscle. Local release of prostaglandins provides an additional mechanism for modulation of constrictor responses. Therapy for asthma is usually directed primarily at reversing airway constriction with bronchodilator drugs. Specific therapy directed against one of the several pathogenetic mechanisms is available only in patients with demonstrable allergies. In others, asthma attacks can be prevented by avoiding domestic or occupational exposure to allergens and inhaled constrictor agents.

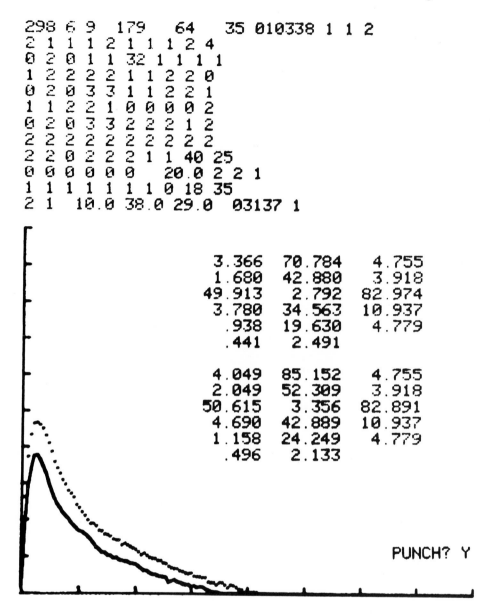

```
298 6 9   179    64    35 010338 1 1 2
2 1 1 1 2 1 1 1 2 4
0 2 0 1 1 32 1 1 1 1
1 2 2 2 2 1 1 2 2 0
0 2 0 3 3 1 1 2 2 1
1 1 2 2 1 0 0 0 0 2
0 2 0 3 3 2 2 2 1 2
2 2 2 2 2 2 2 2 2 2
2 2 0 2 2 2 1 1 40 25
0 0 0 0 0 0    20.0 2 2 1
1 1 1 1 1 1 1 0 18 35
2 1   10.0 38.0 29.0   03137 1
```

```
          3.366  70.784    4.755
          1.680  42.880    3.918
         49.913   2.792   82.974
          3.780  34.563   10.937
           .938  19.630    4.779
           .441   2.491

          4.049  85.152    4.755
          2.049  52.309    3.918
         50.615   3.356   82.891
          4.690  42.889   10.937
          1.158  24.249    4.779
           .496   2.133
```

PUNCH? Y

Fig. 18-21. Data output from computer test system (Chap. 9 p. 185) in a cotton cardroom worker, with MEFV curves before (*drawn line*) and after (*dashed line*) isoproterenol inhalation superimposed. Data in left upper corner are identification and questionnaire (Chap. 13; p. 307) data. Data at right are numerical function values before (*top block*) and after (*lower block*) isoproterenol inhalation. Values in each block (from above down) are FVC, $FEV_{1.0}$, $FEV_{1.0}/FVC$ ratio, PEF, MEF50%, and MEF25%. *Left column:* test data; *right column:* predicted values; *middle column:* test data as a percentage of predicted values.

REFERENCES

1. Aas K: The Biochemical and Immunological Basis of Bronchial Asthma. Springfield, Charles C Thomas, 1972
2. Abe K, Watanabe N, Kumagai N, Mouri T, Seki T, Yoshinaga K: Circulating plasma kinin in patients with bronchial asthma. Experientia 23:626–627, 1967
3. Aberg G, Adler G, Ericsson E: The effect of age on β-adrenoceptor activity in tracheal smooth muscle. Br J Pharmacol 47:181–182, 1973
4. Albro P, Thomas R, Fishbein L: Prostaglandins: Action in mast cells in vitro. Prostaglandins 1:133–144, 1972
5. Andersson R: Role of cyclic AMP and Ca⁺⁺ in the metabolic and relaxing effects of catecholamines in intestinal smooth muscle. Acta Physiol Scand 85:312–322, 1972
6. Andersson R, Nilsson K: Cyclic AMP and calcium in relaxation in intestinal smooth muscle. Nature [New Biol] 238:119–120, 1972
7. Änggård E, Samuelsson B: Biosynthesis of prostaglandins from arachidonic acid in guinea pig lung. J Biol Chem 240:3518–3521, 1965
8. Assem ESK, Pickup PM, Schild HO: The inhibition of allergic reactions by sympathomimetic amines and methylxanthines. Br J Pharmacol 39:212P–213P, 1970
9. Assem ESK, Schild HO: Detection of allergy to penicillin and other antigens by in vitro passive sensitization and histamine release from human and monkey lung. Br Med J 3:272–276, 1968
10. Assem ESK, Schild HO: Inhibition by sympathomimetic amines of histamine release induced by antigen in passively sensitized human lung. Nature 224:1028–1029, 1969
11. Assem ESK, Turner Warwick M, Cole P, Shaw KM: Reversed anaphylactic reaction of leucocytes in intrinsic asthma. Clin Allergy 1:353–361, 1971
12. Astin TW: Reversibility of airways obstruction in chronic bronchitis. Clin Sci 42:725–733, 1972
13. Bakhle YS, Smith TW: Release of spasmogenic substances induced by vasoactive amines from isolated lungs. Br J Pharmacol 46:543P–544P, 1972
14. Beale HD, Fowler WS, Comroe JH Jr: Pulmonary function studies in 20 asthmatic patients in the symptom-free interval. J Allergy 23:1–10, 1952
15. Berg T, Johansson SGO: IgE concentrations in children with atopic diseases. Int Arch Allergy Appl Immunol 36:219–232, 1969
16. Bernecker C, Roetscher I: The beta-blocking effect of practolol in asthmatics. Lancet 2:662, 1970
17. Berrens L: The allergens in house dust. Progress in Allergy. 14:259–339, 1970
18. Bevan JA: Tonically active vagal pulmonary afferent neurones. Life Sci 4:2289–2294, 1965
19. Bias WB: The genetic basis of asthma, in Austen KF, Lichtenstein LM (eds): Asthma: Physiology, Immunopharmacology and Treatment. New York, Academic Press, 1973
20. Bouhuys A: Effect of posture in experimental asthma in man. Am J Med 34:470–476, 1963
21. Bouhuys A: Isoprenaline-inhalatie bij asthma bronchiale. Ned Tijdschr Geneeskd 107:1739–1742, 1963
22. Bouhuys A: The clinical use of pneumotachography. Acta Med Scand 159:91–103, 1957
23. Bouhuys A, Jönsson R, Lichtneckert S, Lindell S-E, Lundgren C, Lundin G, Ringquist TR: Effects of histamine on pulmonary ventilation in man. Clin Sci 19:79–94, 1960
24. Brocklehurst WE: The pharmacology of asthma and possible therapeutic developments, in: Porter R, Birch J (eds): Identification of Asthma. Ciba Foundation, Baltimore, Williams & Wilkins Company, 1971, pp 132–142
25. Broder I, Barlow PP, Horton RJM: The epidemiology of asthma and hay fever in a total community, Tecumseh, Michigan. J Allergy 33:513–523, 1962
26. Broder I, Schild HO: The action of soluble antigen-antibody complexes in perfused guinea-pig lung. Immunology 8:300–318, 1965
27. Bülbring E, Brading AF, Jones AW,

Tomita T: Smooth Muscle. London, Edward Arnold Ltd, 1970

28. Burden DT, Parkes MW, Gardiner DG: Effect of β-adrenoceptive blocking agents on the response to bronchoconstrictor drugs in the guinea pig air overflow preparation. Br J Pharmacol 41: 122–131, 1971

29. Burges RA, Blackburn KJ: Adenyl cyclase and the differentiation of β-adrenoreceptors. Nature [New Biol] 235:249–250, 1972

30. Cade JF, Woolcock AJ, Rebuck AS, Pain MCF: Lung mechanics during provocation of asthma. Clin Sci 40: 381–391, 1971

31. Callerame ML, Condemi JJ, Bohrod MG, Vaughan JH: Immunologic reactions of bronchial tissues in asthma. N Engl J Med 284:459–464, 1971

32. Chan-Yeung MMW, Vyas MN, Grzybowski S: Exercise-induced asthma. Am Rev Respir Dis 104:915–923, 1971

33. CIBA Guest Symposium: Terminology, definitions, and classification of chronic pulmonary emphysema and related conditions. Thorax 14:286–299, 1959

34. Cohen AA, Hale FC: Comparative effects of isoproterenol aerosols on airway resistance in obstructive pulmonary diseases. Am J Med Sci 249:309–315, 1965

35. Colebatch HJH: The humoral regulation of alveolar ducts, in: Bouhuys A (ed), Airway Dynamics: Physiology and Pharmacology. Springfield, Charles C Thomas Publisher, 1970, pp 169–189

36. Colldahl H (ed): Inhalation Tests. Acta Allergol (Kbh) 22 (suppl 8): 7–152, 1967

37. Colldahl H, Lundin G: Ventilatory studies of lungs in asthma. Acta Allergol (Kbh) 5:37–51, 1952

38. Collier HOJ, James GWL: Humoral factors in airway function, with particular reference to anaphylaxis in the guinea pig, in: Bouhuys A (ed), Airway Dynamics: Physiology and Pharmacology. Springfield, Charles C Thomas, 1970, pp 239–252

39. Collier HOJ, Sweatman WJF: Antagonism by fenamates of prostaglandin F$_{2\alpha}$ and of slow reacting substance on human bronchial muscle. Nature 219: 864–865, 1968

40. Conolly ME, Davies DS, Dollery CT, George CF: Resistance to β-adreno-

ceptor stimulants (a possible explanation for the rise in asthma deaths). Br J Pharmacol 43:389–402, 1971

41. Coombs RRA, Hunter A, Jonas WE, Bennich H, Johansson SGO, Panzani R: Detection of IgE (IgND) specific antibody (probably reagin) to castor-bean allergen by the red-cell-linked antigen-antiglobulin reaction. Lancet 1:1115–1118, 1968

42. Crompton GK: A comparison of responses to bronchodilator drugs in chronic bronchitis and chronic asthma. Thorax 23:46–55, 1968

43. Curry JJ: The action of histamine on the respiratory tract in normal and asthmatic subjects. J Clin Invest 25: 785–791, 1946

44. Cuthbert MF: Bronchodilator activity of aerosols of prostaglandins E$_1$ and E$_2$ in asthmatic subjects. Proc R Soc Med 64:15–16, 1971

45. Dahlström A, Fuxe K, Hökfelt T, Norberg K-A: Adrenergic innervation of the bronchial muscle of the cat. Acta Physiol Scand 66:507–508, 1966

46. Dale HH: Antihistamine substances. Br Med J 2:281–283, 1948

47. Davies GE, Rose FL, Somerville AR: New inhibitor of phosphodiesterase with anti-bronchoconstrictor properties. Nature [New Biol] 234:50–51, 1971

48. Davis DJ: NIAID initiatives in allergy research. J Allergy Clin Immunol 49: 323–328, 1972

49. DeKock MA, Nadel JA, Zwi S, Colebatch HJH, Olsen CR: New method for perfusing bronchial arteries: histamine bronchoconstriction and apnea. J Appl Physiol 21:185–194, 1966

50. Despas PJ, Leroux M, Macklem PT: Site of airway obstruction in asthma as determined by measuring maximal expiratory flow breathing air and a helium-oxygen mixture. J Clin Invest 51: 3235–3243, 1972

51. Diamond L: Potentiation of bronchomotor responses by beta adrenergic antagonists. J Pharmacol Exp Ther 181: 434–445, 1972

52. Douglas JS, Dennis MW, Ridgway P, Bouhuys A: Airway constriction in guinea pigs: interaction of histamine and autonomic drugs. J Pharmacol Exp Ther 184:169–179, 1973

53. Douglas JS, Dennis MW, Ridgway P, Bouhuys A: Airway dilatation and con-

striction in spontaneously breathing guinea pigs. J Pharmacol Exp Ther 180:98–109, 1972

54. Douglas JS, Lewis AJ, Orehek J, Bouhuys A: Histamine responses of guinea pig airways *in vivo* and *in vitro*. J Clin Invest 52:24a, 1973

55. Dowell RC, Kerr JW, Park VA: The metabolism of C^{14} histamine in subjects with bronchial asthma. J Allergy 38:290–298, 1966

56. Dunnill MS: The pathology of asthma, in Porter R, Birch J (eds): Identification of Asthma. Ciba Foundation, Baltimore, Williams and Wilkins Company, 1971, pp 35–40

57. Duron B, Humbert J: Effets de l'atropine sur la réponse bronchique aux aérosols d'acétylcholine et d'histamine chez l'asthmatique. Compt Rend Soc Biol (Paris) 164:1086–1091, 1970

58. Eastham WN, Muller HK: Changes in guinea-pig lungs following the inhalation of powdered egg albumen. Pathology 4:235–241, 1972

59. Editorial: Assessment and management of severe asthma. Lancet 1:1055–1056, 1972

60. Ehrenpreis S, Fleisch JH, Mittag TW: Approaches to the molecular nature of pharmacological receptors. Pharmacol Rev 21:131–181, 1969

61. Einthoven W: Ueber die Wirkung der Bronchialmuskeln, nach einer neuen Methode untersucht, und ueber Asthma nervosum. Arch Ges Physiol 51:367–445, 1892

62. Ellis HV III, Johnson AR, Moran NC: Selective release of histamine from rat mast cells by several drugs. J Pharmacol Exp Ther 175:627–631, 1970

63. Engström I, Vejmolova J: The effect of disodium cromoglycate on allergen challenge in children with bronchial asthma. Acta Allergol (Kbh) 25:382–391, 1970

64. Eppinger H, Hess L: Vagotonia. A Clinical Study in Vegetative Neurology, ed 2. New York, Nervous and Mental Disease Publishing Company, 1917

65. Eyre P: Cutaneous vascular permeability factors (histamine, 5-hydroxytryptamine, bradykinin) and passive cutaneous anaphylaxis in sheep. J Pharm Pharmacol 22:104–109, 1970

66. Falliers CJ, de A Cardoso RR, Bane HN, Coffey R, Middleton E Jr: Discor-

dant allergic manifestations in monozygotic twins: genetic identity versus clinical, physiologic, and biochemical differences. J Allergy 47:207–219, 1971

67. Fitch KD, Morton AR: Specificity of exercise in exercise-induced asthma. Br Med J 4:577–581, 1971

68. Fleisch JH, Titus E: The prevention of isoproterenol desensitization and isoproterenol reversal. J Pharmacol Exp Ther 181:425–433, 1972

69. Foreman JC, Mongar JL: The role of the alkaline earth ions in anaphylactic histamine secretion. J Physiol (London) 224:753–769, 1972

70. Forgacs P: Lung sounds. Br J Dis Chest 63:1–12, 1969

71. Francois-Frank CA: Influence des excitations du cerveau sur les principales fonctions organiques. Compt Rend Soc Biol 40:27–43, 1888

72. Gayrard P, Orehek J, Charpin J: Influence de la valeur fonctionnelle de départ sur l'effet bronchodilatateur d'un stimulant bêta-adrénergique dans l'asthme. Respiration 29:247–256, 1972

73. Gazioglu K, Condemi JJ, Hyde RW, Kaltreider NL: Effect of isoproterenol on gas exchange during air and oxygen breathing in patients with asthma. Am J Med 50:185–190, 1971

74. Geddes BA, Patterson NAM, Lefcoe NM: Effects of dibutyryl cyclic AMP and cyclic GMP on isolated guinea pig trachea. Proceedings Canadian Federation of Biological Sciences 15:603a, 1972

75. Gell PGH, Coombs RRA: Clinical Aspects of Immunology. Oxford, Blackwell, 1968

76. Giertz H, Hahn F, Bernauer W: Wirkung von Histamin und Serotonin und Mastzellfunktion in der Lunge; Dargestellt am Beispiel der Meerschweinchenanaphylaxie. Beitr Klin Tuberk 138:297–305, 1968

77. Gold WM, Kessler G-F, Yu DYC, Frick OL: Pulmonary physiologic abnormalities in experimental asthma in dogs. J Appl Physiol 33:496–501, 1972

78. Gold WM, Kessler G-F, Yu DYC: Role of vagus nerves in experimental asthma in allergic dogs. J Appl Physiol 33:719–725, 1972

79. Grana E, Cattarini Mastelli O, Zonta F, Lucchelli A, Santagostino MG: The selectivity of β-adrenergic compounds.

II. Studies on the mimetic compound Salbutamol and the lytic compound practolol. Farmaco (Sci) 27:842–854, 1972

80. Grieco MH, Pierson RN Jr: Mechanism of bronchoconstriction due to beta adrenergic blockade. J Aller Clin Immunol 48:143–152, 1971

81. Guirgis HM, McNeill RS: The nature of the adrenergic receptors in isolated human bronchi. Thorax 24:613–615, 1969

82. Hardman J: Role of cyclic AMP, cyclic GMP and smooth muscle system, in Austen KF, Lichtenstein LM (eds): Asthma: Physiology, Immunopharmacology and Treatment. New York, Academic Press, 1973

83. Harris MC: Are bronchodilator aerosol inhalations responsible for an increase in asthma mortality? Ann Allergy 29: 250–256, 1971

84. Heckscher T, Bass H, Oriol A, Rose B, Anthonisen NR, Bates DV: Regional lung function in patients with bronchial asthma. J Clin Invest 47:1063–1070, 1968

85. Hedqvist P, von Euler US: Prostaglandin controls neuromuscular transmission in guinea-pig vas deferens. Nature [New Biol] 236:113–115, 1972

86. Heim E, Constantine H, Knapp PH, Graham WGB, Globus GG, Vachon L, Nemetz SJ: Airway resistance and emotional state in bronchial asthma. Psychosom Med 29:450–467, 1967

87. Helander E, Lindell S-E, Nilsson K, Westling H: Catabolism of C-14-labelled histamine in patients with allergic diseases. Acta Allergol (Kbh) 17: 86–97, 1962

88. Helgerson RB: Interaction between nervous stimuli and humoral agonists on airway smooth muscle. MD thesis, Yale University, 1971

89. Henderson LL, Tauxe WN, Hyatt RE: Lung scanning of asthmatic patients with 131-I-MAA. South Med J 60:795–804, 1967

90. Herxheimer H: Bronchoconstrictor agents and their antagonists in the intact guinea pig. Arch Int Pharmacodyn 106: 371–380, 1956

91. Herxheimer H: How to prevent death from bronchial asthma. Folia Allergol 18:362–366, 1971

92. Herxheimer H: The influence of hexa-

methonium on the vital capacity in bronchial obstruction. Abstracts of Communications, 19th International Physiological Congress, Montreal, 1953, p 459

93. Herxheimer H: The protective action of antihistaminic and sympathomimetic aerosols in anaphylactic microshock of the guinea-pig. Br J Pharmacol 8:461–465, 1953

94. Holmes TH: A comparative clinical trial of metaproterenol and isoproterenol as bronchodilator aerosols. Clin Pharmacol Ther 9:615–624, 1968

95. Holt LE Jr: A nonallergist looks at allergy. N Engl J Med 276:1449–1454, 1967

96. Honeyman T, Goodman HM: Histamine activates cyclic nucleotide phosphodiesterase. Fed Proc 30:435a, 1971

97. Hossain S: Quantitative measurement of bronchial muscle in men with asthma. Am Rev Respir Dis 107:99–109, 1973

98. Hsieh Y-C, Frayser R, Ross JC: The effect of cold-air inhalation on ventilation in normal subjects and in patients with chronic obstructive pulmonary disease. Am Rev Respir Dis 98:613–622, 1968

99. Hurwitz L, Suria A: The link between agonist action and response in smooth muscle. Annu Rev Pharmacol 11:303–326, 1971

100. Ishizaka K, Ishizaka T: Role of IgE and IgG antibodies in reaginic hypersensitivity in the respiratory tract, in Austen KF, Lichtenstein LM (eds): Asthma: Physiology, Immunopharmacology and Treatment. New York, Academic Press, 1973

101. Irani FA, Jones NL, Gent M, Newhouse MT: Evaluation of disodium cromoglycate in intrinsic and extrinsic asthma. Am Rev Respir Dis 106:179–185, 1972

102. Jack D: Selectively acting β-adrenoreceptor stimulants in asthma, in Austen KF, Lichtenstein LM (eds): Asthma: Physiology, Immunopharmacology and Treatment. New York, Academic Press, 1973

103. Johansen K, Reite OB: Effects of acetylcholine and biogenic amines on pulmonary smooth muscle in the African lungfish, Protopterus Aethiopicus. Acta Physiol Scand 71:248–252, 1967

104. Johansson SGO, Bennich H: Studies on a new class of human immunoglobulins,

in Killander J (ed): Gamma Globulins. Nobel Symposium 3, Stockholm, Almquist & Wiksell, 1967

105. Johansson SGO, Mellbin T, Vahlquist B: Immunoglobulin levels in Ethiopian preschool children with special reference to high concentrations of immunoglobulin E (IgND). Lancet 1:1118–1121, 1968

106. Johnson AR, Moran NC: Inhibition of the release of histamine from rat mast cells: The effect of cold and adrenergic drugs on release of histamine by compound 48/80 and antigen. J Pharmacol Exp Ther 175:632–640, 1970

107. Johnson AR, Moran NC: Selective release of histamine from rat mast cells by compound 48/80 and antigen. Am J Physiol 216:453–459, 1969

108. Jones RS: Significance of effect of beta blockade on ventilatory function in normal and asthmatic subjects. Thorax 27:572–576, 1972

109. Kales A, Beall GN, Bajor GF, Jacobson A, Kales JD: Sleep studies in asthmatic adults: Relationship of attacks to sleep stage and time of night. J Allergy 41:164–173, 1968

110. Kaliner M, Orange RP, Austen KF: Immunological release of histamine and slow reacting substance of anaphylaxis from human lung. J Exp Med 136:556–567, 1972

111. Karczewski W, Widdicombe JG: The role of the vagus nerves in the respiratory and circulatory responses to intravenous histamine and phenyl diguanide in rabbits. J. Physiol (Lond) 201:271–291, 1969

112. Kerr JW, Govindaraj M, Patel KR: Effect of alpha-receptor blocking drugs and disodium cromoglycate on histamine hypersensitivity in bronchial asthma. Br Med J 2:139–141, 1970

113. Kier LB: Receptor mapping using molecular orbital theory, in Danielli JF, Moran JF, Triffle DJ (eds): Fundamental Concepts in Drug-Receptor Interactions. New York, Academic Press, 1970, pp 15–45

114. Kjellman B: Lung function in children with bronchial asthma and recurrent pneumonia. Scand J Respir Dis 50:28–40, 1969

115. Knudson RJ, Constantine HP: An effect of isoproterenol on ventilation-per-fusion in asthmatic versus normal subjects. J Appl Physiol 22:402–406, 1967

116. Okazaki T, Namae E: Enhancement of anaphylaxis of isolated smooth muscle by adenosine phosphates and inhibition of anaphylactic mechanisms by adenosine-3'5'-cyclic monophosphate. Experientia 28:426–427, 1972

117. Large BJ, Leswell PF, Maxwell DR: Bronchodilator activity of an aerosol of prostaglandin E_1 in experimental animals. Nature 224:78–80, 1969

118. Lefcoe NM, Carter RP, Ahmad D: Postexercise bronchoconstriction in normal subjects and asthmatics. Am Rev Respir Dis 104:562–567, 1971

119. Levy B, Wilkenfeld BE: The actions of selective β-receptor antagonists on the guinea pig trachea. Eur J Pharmacol 11:67–74, 1970

120. Lewis AJ, Douglas JS, Bouhuys A: Adrenergic hyposensitization in the guinea pig in vitro and in vivo. Physiologist 15:197a, 1973

121. Lichtenstein LM: The control of IgE mediated histamine release: implications for the study of asthma, in Austen KF, Lichtenstein LM (eds): Asthma: Physiology, Immunopharmacology and Treatment. New York, Academic Press, 1973

122. Lichtenstein LM, Ishizaka K, Norman PS, Sobotka AK, Hill BM: IgE antibody measurements in ragweed hay fever: Relationship to clinical severity and the results of immunotherapy. J Clin Invest 52:472–482, 1973

123. Lichtenstein LM, Norman PS, Winkenwerder WL, Osler AG: In vitro studies of human ragweed allergy: changes in cellular and humoral activity associated with specific desensitization. J Clin Invest 45:1126–1136, 1966

124. Logsdon PJ, Middleton E Jr, Coffey RG: Stimulation of leukocyte adenyl cyclase by hydrocortisone and isoproterenol in asthmatic and nonasthmatic subjects. J Allergy Clin Immunol 50:45–56, 1972

125. Luparello T, Lyons HA, Bleecker ER, McFadden ER Jr: Influences of suggestion on airway reactivity in asthmatic subjects. Psychosom Med 30:819–825, 1968

126. Marsh DG, Lichtenstein LM, Norman PS: Induction of IgE-mediated immediate hypersensitivity to group I rye

grass pollen allergen and allergoids in non-allergic man. Immunology 22: 1013–1028, 1972

127. Mathé AA, Hedqvist P, Holmgren A, Svanborg N: Bronchial hyperreactivity to prostaglandin $F_{2\alpha}$ and histamine in patients with asthma. Br Med J 1:193–196, 1973

128. Mathé AA, Knapp PH: Decreased plasma free fatty acids and urinary epinephrine in bronchial asthma. N Engl J Med 281:234–238, 1969

129. Mathison DA, Condemi JJ, Lovejoy FW Jr, Vaughan JH: Cromolyn treatment of asthma. JAMA 216:1454–1458, 1971

130. McAllen MK, Heaf PJD, McInroy P: Depot grass-pollen injections in asthma. Br Med J 1:22–25, 1967

131. McConnell LH, Fink JN, Schlueter DP, Schmidt MG Jr: Asthma caused by nickel sensitivity. Ann Intern Med 78:888–890, 1973

132. McCourtie DRM, Elder HW, Broder I: Leukocyte histamine release in clinical assessment of subjects with ragweed respiratory allergy. Int Arch Allergy Appl Immunol 44:294–301, 1973

133. McCulloch MW, Proctor C, Rand MJ: Evidence for an adrenergic homeostatic bronchodilator reflex mechanism. Eur J Pharmacol 2:214–223, 1967

134. McDonald JR, Mathison DA, Stevenson DD: Aspirin intolerance in asthma: detection by oral challenge. J Allergy Clin Immunol 50:198–207, 1972

135. McFadden ER Jr, Lyons HA: Airway resistance and uneven ventilation in bronchial asthma. J Appl Physiol 25: 365–370, 1968

136. MacGillavry ThH: L'influence du spasme bronchique sur la respiration. Arch Néerl Sci 12:445–456, 1877

137. McNeill RS: Effect of β-adrenergic-blocking agent, propranolol, on asthmatics. Lancet 2:1101–1102, 1964

138. McNeill RS, Nairn JR, Millar JS, Ingram CG: Exercise-induced asthma. Q J Med 35:55–67, 1966

139. Meisner P, Hugh-Jones P: Pulmonary function in bronchial asthma. Br Med J 1:470–475, 1968

140. Mills JE, Sellick H, Widdicombe JG: Activity of lung irritant receptors in pulmonary microembolism, anaphylaxis and drug-induced bronchoconstrictions. J Physiol (Lond) 203:337–357, 1969

141. Mills JE, Widdicombe JG: Role of the vagus nerves in anaphylaxis and histamine-induced bronchoconstrictions in guinea pigs. Br J Pharmacol 39:724–731, 1970

142. Mitchell CA, Piscitelli D, Bouhuys A: Interaction of humoral agents on airway smooth muscle responses in man. Physiologist 15:219, 1972

143. Moore PF, Iorio LC, McManus JM: Relaxation of the guinea pig tracheal chain preparation by $N^6,2'-0$–dibutyryl $3',5'$-cyclic adenosine monophosphate. J Pharm Pharmacol 20:368–372, 1968

144. Murad F: Cyclic AMP levels in tracheal preparations: effects of epinephrine, (EPI) theophylline and prostaglandin E_1. Clin. Res 21:73, 1973

145. Muus P, Lewis AJ, Douglas JS, Bouhuys A: Contenu en histamine du poumon du rat et sa libération par le 48–80: variations en fonction de l'âge et du sexe. J Physiol (Paris) 65:459A–460A, 1972

146. Norman PS: A review of immunotherapy in asthma, in Austen KF, Lichtenstein LM (eds): Asthma: Physiology, Immunopharmacology and Treatment. New York, Academic Press, 1973

147. O'Donnell SR, Saar N: Histochemical localization of adrenergic nerves in the guinea-pig trachea. Br J Pharmacol 47: 707–710, 1973

148. Olive JT Jr, Hyatt RE: Maximal expiratory flow and total respiratory resistance during induced bronchoconstriction in asthmatic subjects. Am Rev Respir Dis 106:366–376, 1972

149. Orehek J, Douglas JS, Bouhuys A: The effect of anti-inflammatory drugs upon responses of the guinea pig trachea in vitro to contractile agonists. (In preparation)

150. Orehek J, Douglas JS, Lewis AJ, Bouhuys A: Prostaglandin regulation of airway smooth muscle tone. Nature [New Biol] 245:84–85, 1973

151. Orr TSC, Hall DE, Gwilliam JM, Cox JSG: The effect of disodium cromoglycate on the release of histamine and degranulation of rat mast cells induced by compound 48/80. Life Sci I, 10: 805–812, 1971

152. Orzalesi MM, Cook CD, Hart MC: Pulmonary function in symptom-free asthmatic patients. Acta Paediatr Scand 53:401–407, 1964

153. Palmer GC: Characteristics of the hormonal induced cyclic adenosine 3',5'-monophosphate response in the rat and guinea pig lung *in vitro*. Biochim Biophys Acta 252:561–566, 1971

154. Palmer KNV, Diament ML: Spirometry and blood-gas tensions in bronchial asthma and chronic bronchitis. Lancet 2:383–384, 1967

155. Patterson R, Roberts M, Pruzansky JJ: Comparisons of reaginic antibodies from three species. J Immunol 102:466–475, 1969

156. Petit J-M: Physiopathologie de la Dyspnée Chez l'Asthmatique. Brussels, Arscia, 1966

157. Piper PJ, Vane JR: Release of additional factors in anaphylaxis and its antagonism by anti-inflammatory drugs. Nature [Lond] 223:29–35, 1969

158. Piper P, Vane J: The release of prostaglandins from lung and other tissues. Ann NY Acad Sci 180:363–385, 1971

159. Piper PJ, Vane JR, Wyllie JH: Inactivation of prostaglandins by the lungs. Nature 225:600–604, 1970

160. Popa V, Douglas JS, Bouhuys A: Airway responses to histamine, acetylcholine, and antigen in sensitized guinea pigs. J Lab Clin Med (In press)

161. Popa V, Douglas JS, Bouhuys A: Airway responses to histamine, acetylcholine, and propranolol in anaphylactic hypersensitivity in guinea pigs. J Allergy Clin Immunol 51:344–356, 1973

162. Popa V, Teculescu D, Stănescu D: Bronchial asthma and asthmatic bronchitis determined by simple chemicals. Dis Chest 56:395–404, 1969

163. Poppius H, Muittari A, Kreus K-E, Korhonen O, Viljanen A: Exercise asthma and disodium cromoglycate. Br Med J 4:337–339, 1970

164. Porter R, Birch J (eds): Identification of Asthma. Ciba Foundation. Baltimore, Williams & Wilkins Company, 1971

165. Reed CE: The role of the autonomic nervous system in the pathogenesis of bronchial asthma. Is the abnormal bronchial sensitivity due to beta adrenergic blockade? Excerpta Med Int Congr Series 162:402–415, 1968

166. Rees HA, Millar JS, Donald KW: A study of the clinical course and arterial blood gas tensions of patients in status asthmaticus. Q J Med 37:541–561, 1968

167. Richardson PS, Sterling GM: Effects of β-adrenergic receptor blockade on airway conductance and lung volume in normal and asthmatic subjects. Br Med J 3:143–145, 1969

168. Robison GA, Butcher RW, Sutherland EW: On the relation of hormone receptors to adenyl cyclase in Danielli JF, Moran JF, Triggle DJ (eds): Fundamental Concepts in Drug-receptor Interactions. New York, Academic Press, 1970, pp 59–91

169. Rosenthale ME, Dervinis A, Kassarich J: Bronchodilator activity of the prostaglandins E_1 and E_2. J Pharmacol Exp Ther 178:541–548, 1971

170. Schild HO: Biochemical and immunological mechanisms of allergic disease, in: Bouhuys A (ed), Airway Dynamics: Physiology and Pharmacology. Charles C Thomas, Springfield, 1970, pp 229–238

171. Schild HO, Hawkins DF, Mongar JL, Herxheimer H: Reactions of isolated human asthmatic lung and bronchial tissue to a specific antigen; histamine release and muscular contraction. Lancet 2: 376–382, 1951

172. Sellick H, Widdicombe JG: Stimulation of lung irritant receptors by cigarette smoke, carbon dust, and histamine aerosol. J Appl Physiol 31:15–19, 1971

173. Sheard P: The effect of prostaglandin E_1 on isolated bronchial muscle from man. J Pharm Pharmacol 20:232–233, 1968

174. Sheppard H: Phosphodiesterase inhibitors and analogues of cyclic AMP as potential agents for the treatment of asthma, in Austen KF, Lichtenstein LM (eds): Asthma: Physiology, Immunopharmacology and Treatment. New York. Academic Press, 1973

175. Simonsson BG: Effect of multergan on ventilatory capacities in patients with generalized airways obstruction. Acta Allergol (Kbh) 19:305–310, 1964

176. Simonsson BG, Jacobs FM, Nadel JA: Role of autonomic nervous system and the cough reflex in the increased responsiveness of airways in patients with obstructive airway disease. J Clin Invest 46:1812–1818, 1967

177. Sjöstrand NO, Swedin G: Potentiation by smooth muscle stimulants of the hy-

pogastric nerve—Vas deferens preparation from normal and castrated guinea pigs. Acta Physiol Scand 74:472–479, 1968

178. Sjöstrand NO, Swedin G: Potentiation by various smooth muscle stimulants of an isolated sympathetic nerve-seminal vesicle preparation from the guinea pig. Acta Physiol Scand 80:172–177, 1970

179. Smith AP: Response of aspirin-allergic patients to challenge by some analgesics in common use. Br Med J 2:494–496, 1971

180. Smith AP, Cuthbert MF: Antagonistic action of aerosols or prostaglandins $F_{2\alpha}$ and E_2 on bronchial muscle tone in man. Br Med J 3:212–213, 1972

181. Somlyo AP, Somlyo AV: Biophysics of smooth muscle excitation and contraction, in Bouhuys A (ed): Airway Dynamics Physiology and Pharmacology. Springfield, Charles C Thomas, 1970, pp 209–228

182. Speizer FE, Doll R, Heaf P: Observations on recent increase in mortality from asthma. Br Med J 1:335–339, 1968

183. Sperber PA: The allergist and the biological time clock. Ann Allergy 30: 642–644, 1972

184. Stănescu DC, Brasseur LA: Maximal expiratory flow rates and airway resistance following histamine aerosols in asthmatics. Scand J Respir Dis (In press.)

185. Stănescu DC, Frans A, Brasseur L: Acute increase of total lung capacity in asthma following histamine aerosols. Bull Physiopathol Respir (Nancy) 9: 523–530, 1973

186. Sterling GM: Asthma due to aluminum soldering flux. Thorax 22:533–537, 1967

187. Stone SH, Liacopoulos P, Liacopoulos-Briot M, Neveu T, Halpern BN: Histamine: Differences in amount available for release in lungs of guinea pigs susceptible and resistant to acute anaphylaxis. Science 146:1061–1062, 1964

188. Sweatman WJF, Collier HOJ: Effects of prostaglandins on human bronchial muscle. Nature 217:69, 1968

189. Szaduykis-Szadurski L, Weimann G, Berti F: Pharmacological effects of cyclic nucleotides and their derivatives on tracheal smooth muscle. Pharmacol Res Comm 4:63–69, 1972

190. Szentivanyi A: The beta-adrenergic theory of the atopic abnormality in bronchial asthma. J Allergy 42:203–232, 1968

191. Takino Y, Sugahara K, Horino I: Two lines of guinea pigs sensitive and nonsensitive to chemical mediators and anaphylaxis. J Allergy 47:247–261, 1971

192. Tammeling GJ, Sluiter HJ, Hilvering C, Berg WC: Transpulmonary pressure at full inspiration and dynamics of the airways in patients with obstructive lung disease. Am Rev Respir Dis 103:38–48, 1971

193. Teculescu D, Popescu I Gr: Pulmonary function studies in bronchial asthma during the free interval. IV. Distribution of inspired gas. Rev Roum Med Intern 8:37–52, 1971

194. Thon IL, Uvnás B: Degranulation and histamine release. Two consecutive steps in the response of rat mast cells to compound 48/80. Acta Physiol Scand 71:303–315, 1967

195. Tiffeneau R: Examen Pulmonaire de l'Asthmatique. Paris, Masson & Cie, 1957

196. Townley RG, Trapani IL, Szentivanyi A: Sensitization to anaphylaxis and to some of its pharmacological mediators by blockade of the beta adrenergic receptors. J Allergy 39:177–197, 1967

197. Trechsel K, Bachofen H, Scherrer M: Die bronchodilatatorische Wirkung der Asthmazigarette. Schweiz Med Wochenschr 103:415–418, 1973

198. Turner Warwick M: Provoking factors in asthma. Br J Dis Chest 65:1–20, 1971

199. Valabhji P: Gas exchange in the acute and asymptomatic phases of asthma breathing air and oxygen. Clin Sci 34: 431–440, 1968

200. Vane JR: Inhibition of prostaglandin synthesis as a mechanism of action for aspirin-like drugs. Nature [New Biol] 231:232–235, 1971

201. Vane JR: Mediators of the anaphylactic reaction, in Porter R, Birch J (eds): Identification of Asthma. Ciba Foundation, Baltimore, Williams & Wilkins Company, 1971, pp 121–131

202. Vassallo CL, Gee JBL, Domm BM: Exercise-induced asthma: observations regarding hypocapnia and acidosis. Am Rev Respir Dis 105:42–49, 1972

203. Vincent NJ, Knudson R, Leith DE, Macklem PT, Mead J: Factors influencing pulmonary resistance. J Appl Physiol 29:236–243, 1970

204. Warrell DA, Robertson DG, Newton-Howes J, Conolly ME, Paterson JW, Beilin LJ, Dollery CT: Comparison of cardiorespiratory effects of isoprenaline and salbutamol in patients with bronchial asthma. Br Med J 1:65–70, 1970

205. Widdicombe JG, Sterling GM: The autonomic nervous system and breathing. Arch Intern Med 126:311–329, 1970

206. Wilson AF, Novey HS, Berke RA, Surprenant EL: Deposition of inhaled pollen and pollen extract in human airways. N Engl J Med 288:1056–1058, 1973

207. Woitowitz H-J, Woitowitz RH, Schäcke G: Arbeitsmedizinische Aspekte des allergischen Asthma bronchiale durch Mehlberufe. Dtsch Med Wochenschr 96:276–280, 1971

208. Yu DYC, Galant SP, Gold WM: Inhibition of antigen-induced bronchoconstriction by atropine in asthmatic patients. J Appl Physiol 32:823–828, 1972

209. Zaid G, Beall GN: Bronchial response to beta-adrenergic blockade. N Engl J Med 275:580–584, 1966

210. Zapletal A, Motoyama EK, Gibson LE, Bouhuys A: Pulmonary mechanics in asthma and cystic fibrosis. Pediatrics 48:64–72, 1971

211. Zuskin E: Exposures to inhalants in the home. Presented at the Symposium on Environmental Health in the Americas, Mexico City, July 3–4, 1973

212. Zuskin E, Lewis AJ, Bouhuys A: Inhibition of histamine-induced airway constriction by ascorbic acid. J Allergy Clin Immunol 51:218–226, 1973

213. Zuskin E, Mitchell CA, Bouhuys A: Interaction between effects of beta blockade and cigarette smoke on airways. J Appl Physiol (In press)

214. Zuskin E, Bouhuys A: Acute airway responses to hairspray preparations. N Engl J Med (In press)

Index

       b
       c
   6   d
   7   e
   8   f
   9   g
   0   h
   1   i
 8 2 j

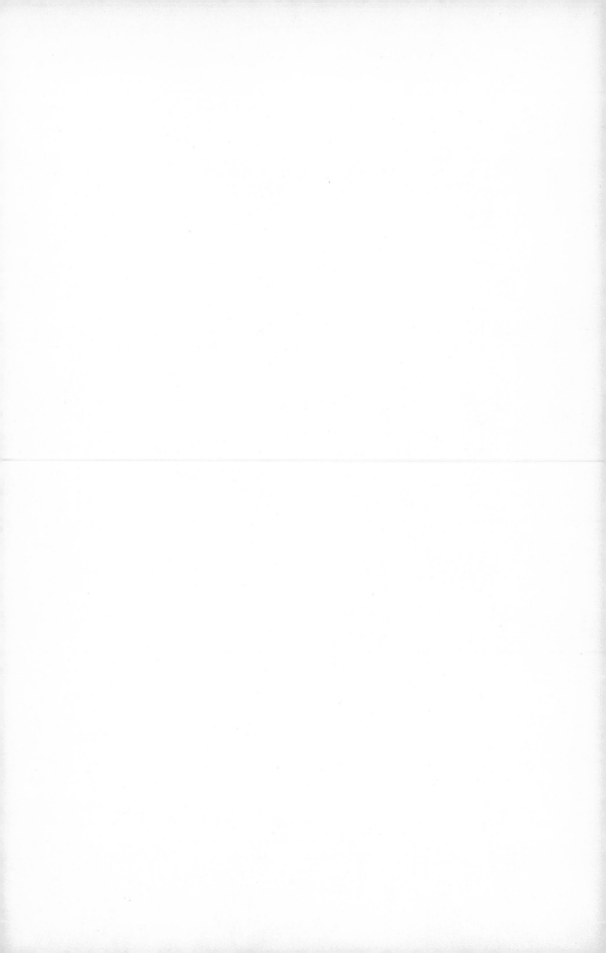